New Horizons in Predictive Drug Metabolism and Pharmacokinetics

RSC Drug Discovery Series

Editor-in-Chief
Professor David Thurston, *King's College, London, UK*

Series Editors:
Professor David Rotella, *Montclair State University, USA*
Professor Ana Martinez, *Centro de Investigaciones Biologicas-CSIC, Madrid, Spain*
Dr David Fox, *Vulpine Science and Learning, UK*

Advisor to the Board:
Professor Robin Ganellin, *University College London, UK*

Titles in the Series:
 1: Metabolism, Pharmacokinetics and Toxicity of Functional Groups
 2: Emerging Drugs and Targets for Alzheimer's Disease; Volume 1
 3: Emerging Drugs and Targets for Alzheimer's Disease; Volume 2
 4: Accounts in Drug Discovery
 5: New Frontiers in Chemical Biology
 6: Animal Models for Neurodegenerative Disease
 7: Neurodegeneration
 8: G Protein-Coupled Receptors
 9: Pharmaceutical Process Development
10: Extracellular and Intracellular Signaling
11: New Synthetic Technologies in Medicinal Chemistry
12: New Horizons in Predictive Toxicology
13: Drug Design Strategies: Quantitative Approaches
14: Neglected Diseases and Drug Discovery
15: Biomedical Imaging
16: Pharmaceutical Salts and Cocrystals
17: Polyamine Drug Discovery
18: Proteinases as Drug Targets
19: Kinase Drug Discovery
20: Drug Design Strategies: Computational Techniques and Applications
21: Designing Multi-Target Drugs
22: Nanostructured Biomaterials for Overcoming Biological Barriers
23: Physico-Chemical and Computational Approaches to Drug Discovery
24: Biomarkers for Traumatic Brain Injury
25: Drug Discovery from Natural Products
26: Anti-Inflammatory Drug Discovery
27: New Therapeutic Strategies for Type 2 Diabetes: Small Molecules
28: Drug Discovery for Psychiatric Disorders
29: Organic Chemistry of Drug Degradation
30: Computational Approaches to Nuclear Receptors

How to obtain future titles on publication:
A standing order plan is available for this series. A standing order will bring delivery of each new volume immediately on publication.

For further information please contact:
Book Sales Department, Royal Society of Chemistry, Thomas Graham House, Science Park, Milton Road, Cambridge, CB4 0WF, UK
Telephone: +44 (0)1223 420066, Fax: +44 (0)1223 420247,
Email: booksales@rsc.org
Visit our website at www.rsc.org/books

New Horizons in Predictive Drug Metabolism and Pharmacokinetics

Edited by

Alan G. E. Wilson
Lexicon Pharmaceuticals, Texas, USA
Email: awilson@lexpharma.com

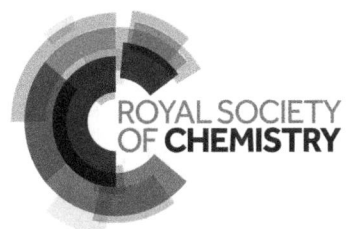

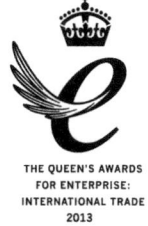

RSC Drug Discovery Series No. 49

Print ISBN: 978-1-84973-828-6
PDF eISBN: 978-1-78262-237-6
ISSN: 2041-3203

A catalogue record for this book is available from the British Library

Published by The Royal Society of Chemistry,
Thomas Graham House, Science Park, Milton Road,
Cambridge CB4 0WF, UK

Registered Charity Number 207890

For further information see our web site at www.rsc.org

Printed in the United Kingdom by CPI Group (UK) Ltd, Croydon, CR0 4YY, UK

Foreword

It is a measure of the maturity of a branch of science as to how successfully it is able to predict the phenomena with which it deals. The development of a science proceeds in a series of steps; firstly, the observation and description of phenomena, then the development of an understanding of the origin of these phenomena and finally the emergence of a theoretical basis for the phenomena, which in turn provides a basis for *a priori* prediction. Experience across a wide range of sciences shows that this growth in the extent and depth of knowledge relies upon the interaction of experimental and theoretical approaches. The development of drug metabolism and pharmacokinetics, which depends upon progress in a group of chemical and biological sciences, illustrates this sequence very well.

The first experiments to elucidate the fate of foreign compounds in living organisms in the nineteenth century led to the description of the vast majority of the metabolic pathways for foreign compounds along with the recognition of the routes for their elimination. Although it was assumed that these pathways were mediated by enzymes, the basis for this did not emerge until the 1950s. Later, from the 1970s onwards, it became clear that these enzymes are not single entities but exist in families of closely related proteins. From the 1990s, the very rapid growth of knowledge in molecular genetics facilitated huge developments, providing a mechanistic basis to understand the myriad of genetic and environmental factors that had been observed to influence the disposition of foreign compounds.

Efforts to describe the physiological disposition of xenobiotics lagged somewhat behind. In the 1950s, it was shown that passage across membranes, the basis of absorption, distribution and excretion, was principally a passive process, in which unionized molecules passed through lipid-rich membranes, while ionized molecules did not. These models were refined by the inclusion of other physicochemical properties of drugs, notably lipid

RSC Drug Discovery Series No. 49
New Horizons in Predictive Drug Metabolism and Pharmacokinetics
Edited by Alan G. E. Wilson
© The Royal Society of Chemistry 2016
Published by the Royal Society of Chemistry, www.rsc.org

solubility, as well as both intra- and extracellular protein binding. However, it was evident that this framework did not describe the behaviour of all molecules and a fuller understanding emerged from the discovery of families of membrane transporter systems responsible for the import and export of xenobiotics from cells.

The mathematical modelling of drug disposition has a long history. The first attempts to describe blood levels of drugs led to compartmental models providing important insights into drug disposition. However, these models had no anatomical basis and could not be easily related to the chemical and biological aspects of drug metabolism mentioned above. The application of engineering principles refined these models, giving them more biological relevance in the form of pharmacokinetic–pharmacodynamic models linking drug disposition to drug effect.

Alongside progress in our ability to describe and understand biological systems, we have seen comparable advances in chemistry, particularly in computational chemistry. These allow the visualisation of the molecular structure and relevant physicochemical properties of both small molecule substrates, and the enzyme and transporter macromolecules with which they have key interactions. Insights into the molecular mechanisms of the function of these enzymes and transporters provide further foundations for predictive drug metabolism and disposition.

It is relatively rare to find that the fate of a drug in the body is dominated by a single mechanism; in general, the problem is describing the complex and subtle interactions between a very large number of processes, some passive, and many mediated by enzymes and transporters. The ability to handle very large datasets and the emergence of new paradigms in systems biology has transformed our ability to describe and predict biological systems, integrating reductionist and holistic approaches. The goal of achieving the *a priori* prediction of the metabolism and pharmacokinetics of a new drug thus becomes a feasible ambition.

This timely volume represents an authoritative summary of recent progress in relevant fields and the opportunities that exist for further developments from an international group of experts in predictive drug metabolism and pharmacokinetics, many of whom have made major contributions to the subject. I commend the initiative of the editor and publisher in bringing this volume together as well as the efforts of the contributors in producing a book that will be a point of reference for many scientists in academia, and the pharmaceutical and other industries where an understanding of the fate of drugs and xenobiotics is critical, as well as for regulators charged with making key decisions on the use of such compounds. This is a very rich volume that will provide the specialist and general reader alike with an immense amount of interest.

John Caldwell,
Emeritus Professor
University of Liverpool, United Kingdom

Preface

Since the pioneering work and treatise by authors such as Tecwyn Williams, Dennis Parke, Bernard Brodie Milo Gibaldi, and other global leaders, a plethora of reviews and books have been published on absorption, distribution, metabolism, elimination and pharmacokinetics (ADME/PK). It may, therefore, seem foolhardy to think that a book on predictive ADME and PK could add substantially to the literature and assist in the shifting focus we are seeing in the pharmaceutical, chemical and life science industries towards predictive approaches. However, it is a testimony to a field that had its origins in the 19th century that it continues to evolve in sophistication, understanding and in its multi-disciplinary impact, and continues to be a critical component in the efficacy and safety of drugs, chemicals, and biologics. For those of us who have had the pleasure of working in this field, it has been a most rewarding experience and journey, since we have seen the continuing awareness and impact that our science has made to the safety and efficacy of new chemical entities. Perhaps there is no better example of this than the impact the introduction of high-throughput ADME screening has made in reducing ADME/PK related attrition in the pharmaceutical and biotechnology industries. However, despite this, a significant challenge still exists to improve the success rates of our discovery and development processes to allow patients faster access to safe and effective drugs. The high rate of attrition of promising drug candidates continues to be a major issue in meeting the medical needs of our patients and the future success of the pharmaceutical industry.

The current focus and urgency in the pharmaceutical industry is to shorten the time lines for all aspects of drug discovery and to improve the ability to filter out early potential ADME/PK, safety, and efficacy issues. We are therefore seeing increasing interest and focus on predictive approaches. These predictive approaches are completed in the early drug discovery phase and will

RSC Drug Discovery Series No. 49
New Horizons in Predictive Drug Metabolism and Pharmacokinetics
Edited by Alan G. E. Wilson
© The Royal Society of Chemistry 2016
Published by the Royal Society of Chemistry, www.rsc.org

gain increasing importance in the coming years in allowing early identification of potential ADME/PK issues.

This book presents a comprehensive treatise by leading experts on the current issues and challenges facing drug metabolism and PK (ADME/PK), and the role of predictive models in drug discovery and development in improving the success rate and safety assessment of pharmaceuticals. The hope of this book is that it will assist in the continuing paradigm shift of the incorporation of ADME/PK prediction and assessment into the drug discovery and development process, and in the overall paradigm of exposure assessment. The authors not only discuss the current state of the art methodologies, but perhaps more importantly focus on the future needs in ADME/PK that are likely to improve our prediction and optimization of ADME/PK, efficacy and human safety. The authors of the various chapters represent leading experts and investigators in the respective areas.

As mentioned previously, many books have been published over the past century in the field of drug metabolism and PK, these not only add to our continuing understanding of the complexity of the field within which we are privileged to work, but also add to the impact that our field has on improving human health and the environment in which we live. Any book of this nature is only as good as the expertise and vision of the contributing authors and I am deeply indebted to all of the experts who have contributed to making this book such a rewarding experience and a valuable addition to the field of ADME/PK.

Alan G. E. Wilson
Texas, USA

Acknowledgements

I personally want to thank all of the authors for providing their time and expertise in the completion of this book, and the Royal Society of Chemistry for giving me the opportunity to compile and edit this book on *New Horizons in Predictive Drug Metabolism and Pharmacokinetics* in the RSC Drug Discovery Series. A special thanks goes to Ayako Shinomiya Takei, who assisted me in the review and editing of the chapters. And finally, to the reader, I hope you will find this book of value to you in your quest for understanding the absorption, distribution, metabolism, elimination and pharmacokinetics of chemical entities, and as enjoyable to read as it was to compile.

This book is dedicated to my daughter Julia, my grandson Iain, and to the memory of my beloved Mary.

RSC Drug Discovery Series No. 49
New Horizons in Predictive Drug Metabolism and Pharmacokinetics
Edited by Alan G. E. Wilson
© The Royal Society of Chemistry 2016
Published by the Royal Society of Chemistry, www.rsc.org

Contents

RSC Drug Discovery Series No. 49
New Horizons in Predictive Drug Metabolism and Pharmacokinetics
Edited by Alan G. E. Wilson
© The Royal Society of Chemistry 2016
Published by the Royal Society of Chemistry, www.rsc.org

CHAPTER 1

How Physicochemical Properties of Drugs Affect Their Metabolism and Clearance

MARIA KARLGREN[a] AND CHRISTEL A. S. BERGSTRÖM[*a]

[a]Department of Pharmacy, Uppsala University, Biomedical Centre P.O. Box 580, Husargatan 3, SE-75123 Uppsala, Sweden
*E-mail: Christel.Bergstrom@farmaci.uu.se

1.1 Introduction

The physicochemical properties of compounds have been used for more than a century to predict or estimate pharmacokinetic processes. The most well known property is lipophilicity, often defined as the partition coefficient between octanol and water. This property is related to passive diffusion across cell membranes, solubility, interaction with receptors, metabolism and toxicity. To activate proteins, *e.g.* receptors and enzymes, the compound needs to bind to a binding pocket. Besides lipophilicity, physicochemical properties of importance for binding include molecular size, hydrogen bond acceptors/donors and charge. This chapter discusses the physicochemical properties of importance for drug metabolism. The primary organ for drug metabolism is the liver and to reach the liver the compound must cross cellular barriers. Absorption from the gastrointestinal tract (GIT) is therefore of critical importance for orally administered drugs, before distribution into and out of the liver can occur. We introduce the GIT in this chapter, and all

RSC Drug Discovery Series No. 49
New Horizons in Predictive Drug Metabolism and Pharmacokinetics
Edited by Alan G. E. Wilson
© The Royal Society of Chemistry 2016
Published by the Royal Society of Chemistry, www.rsc.org

of these processes are discussed in detail in other chapters. Thereafter we describe the enzymes responsible for drug metabolism in different tissues; the biology of these enzymes is further discussed in later chapters. Finally, the role of the enzymes and that of transporters in drug clearance is presented together with an analysis of the structural features of molecules of importance for binding to enzymes and transporters.

1.2 Intestinal Absorption, Liver Disposition and Enzyme Expression

Only free molecules can pass through cell barriers and, hence, only the unbound fraction of drugs can pass over the intestinal epithelium. Solubility governs the concentration reached in the intestinal fluid and is therefore a major driving force for the absorption. Hydrophilic and small molecules may be absorbed by diffusing through the paracellular route. This transport route has limited capacity as its total surface area is much smaller than that of the transcellular (membrane related) pathway. Furthermore, the tight junction reduces the pore size. In the small intestine compounds greater than 4 Å have limited permeability through this pathway whereas those greater than 15 Å are excluded from permeation.[1] To cross the cell membrane compounds have several options. The two most common pathways are passive diffusion through the lipoidal membrane or active transport mediated by transport proteins. The impact of these pathways is heavily debated. Kell and coworkers have challenged the theory that the majority of drugs use lipoidal passive diffusion to pass through cells.[2-4] Their hypothesis is that most of the transport across cells involves active processes and transport proteins. This debate has spurred research to determine to what extent the two pathways are involved in drug distribution.[5,6]

Once the compound has traversed the luminal membrane, it may either diffuse through the cytosol and cross the serosal membrane, or interact with enzymes, intracellular organelles (lysosomes, endoplasmic reticulum) or the cell nuclei. It has been proposed that there is a substrate overlap between cytochrome P450 3A4 (CYP3A4) and the efflux protein P-glycoprotein [P-gp; also known as multidrug resistance protein 1 (MDR1)]. Hence, these two different pathways may have synergistic effects in the clearance and detoxification of certain compounds.

When the compound has crossed the intestinal epithelium it reaches the portal vein from where the systemic circulation transports it to the main metabolic organ in the body—the liver. The compound can then reach the cytosol by either passive or active transport mechanisms across the basolateral membrane facing the bloodstream. The capacity of the liver as a detoxification organ is remarkable. Even compounds with high protein binding can be extracted to a large extent by the liver. This can be exemplified by atorvastatin, the cholesterol-lowering compound marketed as LIPITOR®. A high fraction of atorvastatin is absorbed from the intestine but is also highly bound (98%) to proteins in the blood. Therefore, only 2% is available in an unbound free form that can permeate the cell membrane. In spite of this, the absolute bioavailability after oral administration is only 14%. This low number is a result of the cooperation between active influx transporters [mainly organic anion-transporting polypeptides (OATP) 1B1 and 1B3] in the basolateral membrane and CYP3A4 in the cytosol. In addition to these processes, atorvastatin is thereafter cleared from the hepatocytes through canalicular efflux by P-gp. The drug transporters and metabolic enzymes in the gut and liver that are crucial for the first-pass effect are shown in Figure 1.1. The metabolic capacity of the gut and liver are discussed in more detail below.

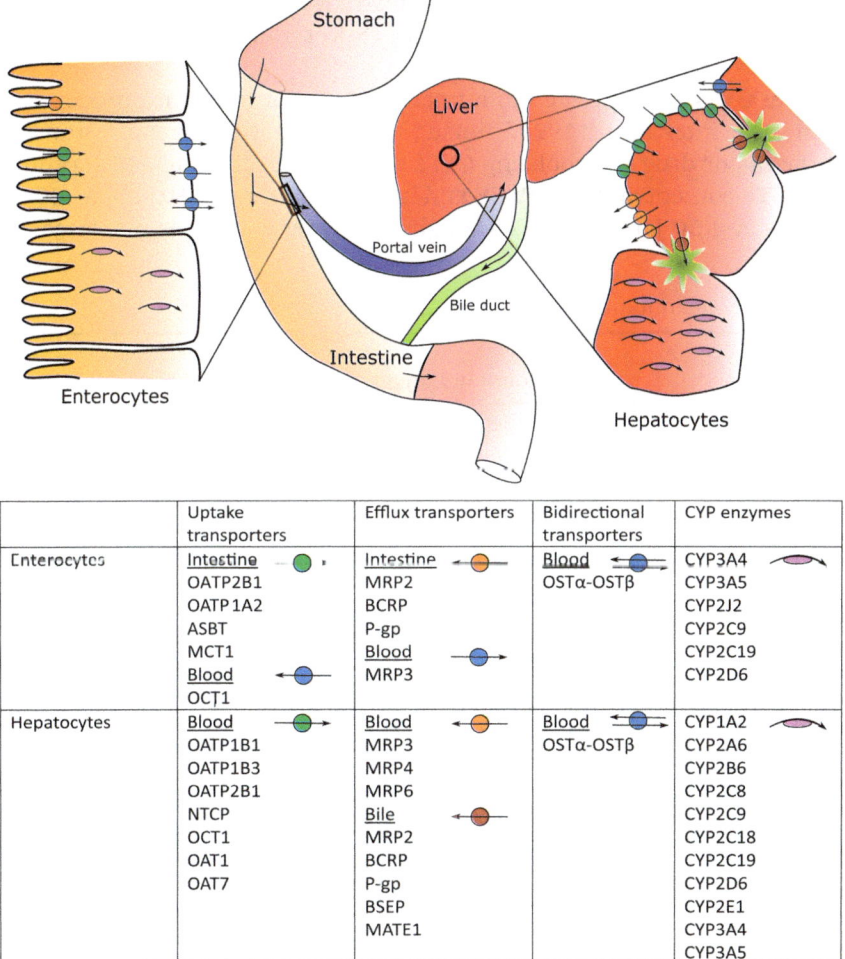

	Uptake transporters	Efflux transporters	Bidirectional transporters	CYP enzymes
Enterocytes	Intestine OATP2B1 OATP1A2 ASBT MCT1 Blood OCT1	Intestine MRP2 BCRP P-gp Blood MRP3	Blood OSTα-OSTβ	CYP3A4 CYP3A5 CYP2J2 CYP2C9 CYP2C19 CYP2D6
Hepatocytes	Blood OATP1B1 OATP1B3 OATP2B1 NTCP OCT1 OAT1 OAT7	Blood MRP3 MRP4 MRP6 Bile MRP2 BCRP P-gp BSEP MATE1	Blood OSTα-OSTβ	CYP1A2 CYP2A6 CYP2B6 CYP2C8 CYP2C9 CYP2C18 CYP2C19 CYP2D6 CYP2E1 CYP3A4 CYP3A5

Figure 1.1　Overview of transporters and CYP enzymes of importance for drug absorption, liver distribution and hepatic elimination.

1.3　Metabolic Capacity of the Intestine and Liver

The intestine is the most important extrahepatic site of drug metabolism and its involvement in the first-pass metabolism of orally administered drugs makes it a major determinant of drug bioavailability. The most abundant CYP in the small intestine is CYP3A, constituting 50–82% of the intestinal CYP content.[7-10] However, compared with the liver, the total mass of CYP3A in the small intestine corresponds to only about 1% of the hepatic CYP3A levels.[9,11] Other CYPs expressed in the small intestine, as determined using immunoblotting or liquid chromatography-tandem mass spectrometry (LC-MS/MS)-based protein quantification, are CYP2C9, CYP2C19, CYP2D6 and CYP2J2 (Table 1.1).[7,8] Their expression levels vary in the different regions of the intestine. CYP3A, CYP2C and CYP2D6 show highest expression in the proximal intestinal region and decreasing levels in the distal regions.[9,12] For CYP2J2, the expression is constant throughout the GIT.[13]

More CYPs are expressed in human liver and at higher expression levels than in the intestine. In 1994 Shimada *et al.* determined the expression levels of the major drug metabolizing CYPs in human liver using P450-spectra of total CYP content and SDS-PAGE and immunoblotting in 60 people (30 Caucasians and 30 Japanese).[15] Although the expression levels displayed both

Table 1.1　Quantitative expression of CYPs in human intestine.

CYP isoform	Amount in human intestinal microsomes			
Total CYP	61 (Immunoquantified)	No data	No data	No data
CYP2C9	11 ± 0.5	15% of total CYP	2.96	4.27 ± 0.97	0.32 ± 0.18
CYP2C19	2.1 ± 0.1	2.9% of total CYP		2.79 ± 1.32	1.43 ± 0.25
CYP2D6	0.7 ± 0.01	1% of total CYP	2.25	<LLOQ[a]	<LLOQ[a]
CYP2J2	1.0 ± 0.1	1.4% of total CYP	2.92		
CYP3A4	58 ± 1.0	80% of total CYP	26.3	18.7 ± 6.26	1.85 ± 0.36
CYP3A5	16 ± 0.3		1.44	<LLOQ[a]	<LLOQ[a]
Unit	pmol mg^{-1} protein		fmol µg^{-1} protein	pmol mg^{-1} protein	pmol mg^{-1} protein
References	8		14	7	7
Number of samples	Pooled microsomes from 31 donors (11 for CYP3A5)		Pooled microsomes from 8 donors	Pooled microsomes from 8 donors	Self-prepared microsomes from 3 donors
Method of detection	Western blot		LC-MS/MS	LC-MS/MS	LC-MS/MS

[a]LLOQ: lower limit of quantification.

interindividual and interethnic variations, the average expressions levels in comparison with total CYP content were: CYP3A (28.8%) > CYP2C (18.2%) > CYP1A2 (12.7%) > CYP2E1 (6.6%) > CYP2A6 (4.0%) > CYP2D6 (1.5%) > CYP2B6 (0.2%). Since then the methodological development of more sophisticated methods, *e.g.* different types of LC-MS/MS-based proteomics, has allowed quantification of CYPs.[7,14,16,17] Although the quality of the LC-MS/MS analyses may vary due to the level of method validation *etc.*, the results are consistent with those obtained by Shimada *et al.* that identified the CYP3A and CYP2C families as the most abundant hepatic CYPs (Table 1.2). All tissues have enzymatic activity to some extent; however, the gut and the liver are the two most important metabolic tissues. An overview of the metabolic profile of different tissues is provided in Table 1.3. It should be noted that not only the type of enzymes differs between tissues; the expression levels of these enzymes differ as well.

Although the abundance of CYPs is of major interest it does not provide the full picture of the importance of the specific CYP enzymes for drug metabolism. One striking example showing discrepancy between expression levels and importance is the CYP2D6 enzyme. This enzyme is only expressed in low levels in human liver (1.5–2% of the total CYP content). However, it is one of the major drug-metabolizing enzymes and metabolizes up to 25% of clinically used drugs.[31–34] Another example is CYP1A2. It constitutes approximately 18% of the human hepatic CYP content,[15] but its relative importance in drug metabolism is only 3–9% (Table 1.4).[32–34]

1.4   Pharmacogenomics

In addition to interindividual variation in expression levels, many drug-metabolizing enzymes, and especially some of the CYPs, are highly polymorphic. Approximately 40% of CYP-dependent phase I metabolism is performed by polymorphic CYPs, including CYP2D6, CYP2C9, CYP2C19 and CYP2B6.[36] For CYP2D6 more than 100 different alleles and suballeles have been identified. These include alleles where the entire *CYP2D6* gene is deleted, alleles with duplicated or multiduplicated *CYP2D6* genes, and alleles containing single-nucleotide polymorphisms (SNPs).[36] Such gene variants may of course have a major impact on the pharmacokinetics and may result in adverse effects of drugs that are CYP2D6 substrates (*cf.*[37,38]). A classic example of this is the prodrug codeine, which is activated by CYP2D6 into the active drug morphine. For people who are poor CYP2D6 metabolizers, *i.e.* their *CYP2D6* genes are deleted or contain mutations leading to non-functional enzymes, codeine does not give the desired analgesic effect.[39] On the contrary, for individuals with alleles with duplicated or multiduplicated *CYP2D6* genes, *i.e.* ultra-rapid metabolizers, codeine is activated rapidly, which can lead to codeine toxicity and central nervous system depression.[40] There are also a few cases of infant mortality where ultra-rapid metabolizer mothers treated with codeine transferred fatally high morphine concentrations to their breastfed infants.[41–43]

Table 1.2 Quantitative expression of CYPs in human liver.

CYP isoform	Amount in human liver					
Total CYP determined spectrally	0.344 ± 0.167	411	255 ± 17	534	No data	No data
CYP1A2	0.042 ± 0.023	17.7 ± 0.6		45	12.8 ± 0.17	19.0
CYP2A6	0.014 ± 0.013	49.2 ± 1.7		68		61.1
CYP2B6	0.001 ± 0.002	6.86 ± 0.44		39	9.59 ± 0.38	29.3
CYP2D6	0.005 ± 0.004	11.5 ± 0.3		10	9.34 ± 0.15	38.6
CYP2C	0.060 ± 0.027					
CYP2C8		29.3 ± 0.6	11.5 ± 2.9	64	26.9 ± 0.54	55.8
CYP2C9		80.2 ± 1.4	88.5 ± 8.7	96	37.3 ± 2.50	93.0
CYP2C18						2.82
CYP2C19		3.64 ± 0.22	17.8 ± 3.3	19	2.18 ± 0.18	15.6
CYP2E1	0.022 ± 0.012	51.3 ± 0.9		49	65.3 ± 1.52	103
CYP2J2	0.096 ± 0.100					4.95
CYP3A (3A4/3A5)						
CYP3A4		64.0 ± 1.9		108	32.6 ± 0.38	109
CYP3A5		3.54 ± 0.28		1	1.96 ± 0.05	7.24
CYP3A7						11.4
CYP4A11						16.5
CYP51A1						4.89
Unit	nmol mg⁻¹ protein	pmol mg⁻¹ protein	pmol mg⁻¹ protein	pmol mg⁻¹ protein	pmol mg⁻¹ protein	fmol µg⁻¹ protein
References	15	16	18	19	7	14
Number of liver specimens	60	10	17	No data	25	50
Method of detection	Immunochemical	LC-MS/MS	Immunochemical	Immunochemical	LC-MS/MS	LC-MS/MS

Table 1.3   Overview of CYPs (family 1–3) expressed in hepatic and extrahepatic tissues.

CYP isoform	Gastrointestinal tract	Liver	Brain[b]	Kidney	Heart	Skin[e]	Respiratory tract[e]
CYP1A1			X	X	X		X
CYP1A2		X	X		X[d]		X
CYP1B1			X	X	X	X	X
CYP2A6		X				X	X
CYP2A13							X
CYP2B6		X	X	X	X[d]	X	X
CYP2C8		X		X[c]	X		X
CYP2C9	X	X		X[c]	X	X	
CYP2C18		X				X	X
CYP2C19	X	X	X			X	
CYP2D6	X	X	X		X	X	X
CYP2E1		X	X		X[d]	X	X
CYP2F1							X
CYP2J2	X			X[c]	X	X	X
CYP2S1						X	X
CYP2R1						X	
CYP2U1			X			X	
CYP2W1						X	
CYP3A						X	
CYP3A4	X	X	X	X[c]	X		X
CYP3A5	X	X	X	X			X
CYP3A7[a]		X					
CYP3A43			X				
References	7,8,14	7,14–16,18–20	21–25	26	27	28 and 29	30

[a]Major CYP3A enzyme expressed in fetal liver.
[b]Expression levels vary greatly between different brain regions and cell types.
[c]Data regarding human kidney expression are conflicting.
[d]Not seen in healthy human heart.
[e]mRNA and/or protein expression.

For other CYPs, *e.g.* CYP2C9, CYP2C19 and CYP2B6, many variant alleles and suballeles have been described, some of which have significant clinical impact. The most well known clinical CYP2C examples are the *CYP2C9* polymorphisms involved in warfarin metabolism[44,45] and *CYP2C19* polymorphisms associated with clopidogrel activation.[46,47] Both of these were highlighted in 2011 as important pharmacogenomics biomarkers.[37] The warfarin (COUMADIN®) and the clopidogrel (PLAVIX®) Food and Drug Administration (FDA) drug labels have been updated to contain recommendations for initial doses based on *e.g.* *CYP2C9* genotype[48] and a warning about diminished effectiveness in CYP2C19 poor metabolizers,[49] respectively. A complete and updated overview of CYP and CYP oxidoreductase (POR) polymorphisms can be found on the home page of The Human Cytochrome P450 (CYP) Allele Nomenclature Committee (http://www.cypalleles.ki.se).

Table 1.4 Relative contribution of the CYP isoforms to hepatic drug metabolism.

CYP isoform	Relative contribution to hepatic drug metabolism (%)			
CYP3A (3A4/3A5)	51	46	53	30.2
CYP2D6	24	12	25	20
CYP2C	19	—	18	—
CYP2C8	—	—	—	4.7
CYP2C9	—	16	—	12.8
CYP2C19	—	12	—	6.8
CYP1A	—	9	—	—
CYP1A2	5	—	3	8.9
CYP2E1	1	2	—	3
CYP2A6	—	—	—	3.4
CYP2B6	—	2	—	7.2
CYP2J2	—	—	—	3
References	33	32	34	35
Number of drugs studied	All prescribed drugs	200 drugs (of which ~100 cleared by CYP-mediated metabolism)	315 drugs (of which 175 cleared by CYP-mediated metabolism)	248 drugs cleared by CYP-mediated metabolism

1.5 Molecular Features of Importance for Transporter Interactions: Substrates *Versus* Inhibitors

Many substrates and inhibitors have been identified for transporters that are of importance for drug distribution into and out of cells. For a selection of these, see Table 1.5. While a substrate of the transporter can also be an inhibitor of the transport protein and block transport of other compounds, compounds that have been identified as inhibitors may not be transported. The latter is related to the inactivation of the transport protein by binding to sites other than the one crucial for mediating transport. Interaction with the transport-mediating site allows the drug compound (or its metabolite) to traverse the lipophilic membrane. Hence, the molecular requirements of the different transporters have been studied to better understand what physicochemical properties of a compound will result in them being actively transported by a particular transport protein. While metabolism is a chemical reaction that turns a substrate into a product that is chemically different, the substrates of transport proteins remain the same; no chemical reaction occurs. However, the terminology of transporters and experimental procedures to study transport have been inspired by those in the metabolism field. So, for example, the Michaelis–Menten equation is often used to describe the efficiency of transporters to flux compounds across the membrane.

The structural requirements for transport by influx and efflux transport proteins have been heavily studied. The majority of studies have been

Table 1.5 Transporters of clinical relevance for drug clearance, expressed in the gut and liver.[a]

Transporters	Gut	Liver	Selected substrates	Selected inhibitors
Influx				
ASBT (SLC10A2)	X		Bile salts	Cyclosporin A
MCT1 (SLC16A1)	X		Nateglinide	Nateglinide
NTCP (SLC10A1)		X	Bile salts	Bumetanide, chlorpropamide, cyclosporin A, furosemide, ketoconazole, progesterone
OAT2 (SLC22A7)		X	Methotrexate, tetracycline, theophylline	Cefamandole, cefoperazone, cefotaxime, cephaloridine, cephalothin, cilastatin, clarithromycin, erythromycin, ganciclovir, minocycline, oxytetracycline, pravastatin, probenecid
OATP1A2 (SLCO1A2)	X		Enalapril, fexofenadine, pravastatin, rifampicin	Dexamethasone, erythromycin, ketoconazole, lovastatin, naloxone, nelfinavir, quinidine, rifampicin, ritonavir, saquinavir, verapamil
OATP1B1 (SLCO1B1)		X	Atorvastatin, benzylpenicillin, cerivastatin, irinotecan, methotrexate, pitavastatin, pravastatin, rifampicin, simvastatin	Cyclosporin A, indinavir, lovastatin, nelfinavir, pioglitazone, pravastatin, quinidine, rapamycin, ritonavir, rosiglitazone, saquinavir, troglitazone
OATP1B3 (SLCO1B3)		X	Digoxin, methotrexate, pioglitazone, pitavastatin, rifampicin	Rifampicin
OATP2B1 (SLCO2B1)	X	X	Benzylpenicillin, glibenclamide, ibuprofen, fexofenadine, pravastatin, rifampicin, tolbutamide	Tangeretin, rifamycin
OCT1 (SLC22A1)	X	X	Acyclovir, cimetidine, cisplatin, ganciclovir	Amiloride, chlorpromazine, clonidine, desipramine, disopyramide, metformin, midazolam, prazosin, progesterone, quinidine, ranitidine, verapamil
OCT3 (SLC22A3)	X		Carboplatin, cimetidine, cisplatin	Clonidine, desipramine, imipramine, prazosin, progesterone
OCTN2 (SLC22A5)	X		Cimetidine, valproic acid	Aldosterone, amphetamine, ampicillin, cefadroxil, cefdinir, cefepime, cefixime, cefluprenam, cefoselis, cefsulodin, ceftazidime, cephalexin, cephalothin, clonidine, cyclacillin, desipramine, furosemide, lomefloxacin, norfloxacin, benzylpenicillin, probenecid, verapamil
PEPT1 (SLC15A1)	X		Benzylpenicillin, cefadroxil, cefixime, ceftibuten, enalapril, faropenem, lisinopril, temocapril, valacyclovir	Amoxicillin, ampicillin, captopril, cefadroxil, cefluprenam, cefotaxime, cefpirome, cefsulodin, ceftazidime, ceftriaxone, cefuroxime, cephadroxil, cephalexin, cephaloridine, cloxacillin, cyclacillin, dicloxacillin, glycylsarcosine, L-dopa, metampicillin, moxalactam

(continued)

Table 1.5 (*continued*)

Transporters	Gut	Liver	Selected substrates	Selected inhibitors
Efflux				
BCRP (ABCG2)	X	X	Cerivastatin, daunorubicin, glibenclamide, lamivudine, methotrexate, mitoxantrone, prazosin, pravastatin, tamoxifen, topotecan	Cyclosporin A, doxorubicin, nelfinavir, novobiocin, omeprazole, pantoprazole, ritonavir, saquinavir, silybin, silymarin, verapamil
BSEP (ABCB11)		X	Daunorubicin, doxorubicin, vincristine	Chlorpromazine, cimetidine, clofazimine, cyclosporin A, glibenclamide, ketoconazole, paclitaxel, progesterone, quinidine, reserpine, tamoxifen, troglitazone, valinomycin, verapamil, vinblastine
P-gp, MDR1 (ABCB1)	X	X	Acetaminophen, acetylsalicylic acid, albendazole, aldosterone, atenolol, carbamazepine, chlorpromazine, ciprofloxacin, clozapine, cyclosporin A, daunorubicin, diazepam, digoxin, dipyridamole, docetaxel, emetine, fluconazole, flumazenil, fluoxetine, haloperidol, hydrocortisone, ibuprofen, imatinib, ivermectin, ketamine, loperamide, losartan, naloxone, neostigmine, nitrazepam, olanzapine, paclitaxel, quinidine, risperidone, scopolamine, sumatriptan, valinomycin, verapamil, vinblastine	Amiodarone, amitriptyline, astemizole, atorvastatin, bromocriptine, buspirone, candesartan, captopril, cimetidine, clarithromycin, clofazimine, clotrimazole, desipramine, desloratadine, dexamethasone, diclofenac, erythromycin, felodipine, fentanyl, glibenclamide, indinavir, itraconazole, ketoconazole, lidocaine, lopinavir, loratadine, lovastatin, methadone, metoprolol, miconazole, morphine, nelfinavir, nicardipine, nifedipine, norverapamil, omeprazole, pantoprazole, ranitidine, reserpine, ritonavir, saquinavir, simvastatin, sirolimus, spironolactone, tamoxifen, terfenadine, verapamil, vincristine
MRP2 (ABCC2)	X	X	Cerivastatin, etoposide, indinavir, methotrexate, pravastatin, ritonavir, saquinavir, vinblastine, vincristine	Benzbromarone, cyclosporin A, furosemide, lovastatin acid, probenecid, quinidine, reserpine, sulfinpyrazone, verapamil
MRP3 (ABCC3)	X	X	Etoposide, glibenclamide, glutathione, methotrexate	Benzbromarone, doxorubicin, indomethacin, probenecid, verapamil, vincristine
MRP4 (ABCC4)		X	Adefovir, methotrexate	Benzbromarone, celecoxib, diclofenac, dipyridamole, ibuprofen, indomethacin, indoprofen, ketoprofen, probenecid, rofecoxib, sildenafil, verapamil
MRP6 (ABCC6)		X	Cisplatin, daunorubicin, doxorubicin, etoposide, teniposide	Benzbromarone, indomethacin, probenecid, sulfinpyrazone

[a]Data on clinically relevant transporters were taken from ref. 70–73. Representative examples of substrates and inhibitors for each of the transport proteins were extracted from the database established by Prof. Sugiyama (http://togodb.dbcls.jp/tpsearch/). Substrates also being identified as inhibitors are not listed. Note that inhibitors listed may be substrates but to date only data on inhibition are available in the open literature.

directed towards investigation of transport protein inhibition. The reason for this is mainly methodological issues associated with substrate assays. While analyses of molecular features of substrates require determination of the intracellular concentration of a large number of compounds, inhibition assays rely on screening a large number of compounds for their inhibition of the transport of one substrate. Hence, analytical demands for the latter are reduced and a higher throughput mode is possible. The most important transport proteins for clearance are discussed below.

1.5.1 Efflux Proteins

1.5.1.1 P-gp Substrate Recognition Pattern

One of the most studied transport proteins is the efflux protein P-gp since it is important for drug distribution to several tissues, including the gut and liver. Drug–drug interactions (DDIs) have also been identified that are mediated by P-gp. Among the most well known are those that occur between digoxin and the P-gp inhibitors amiodarone, cyclosporin A, quinine and verapamil.[50] Seelig and coworkers were pioneers in the study of the recognition pattern of P-gp (*cf.*[51,52]). Based on studies of ~100 compounds, they suggested that a special spatial separation of electron donor groups is required for compounds to be transported by P-gp. Their work was followed by a number of structure–activity relationship (SAR) studies in which P-gp substrates are predicted on the basis of chemical information calculated from the molecular structure. The SAR models are typically classification models used to distinguish compounds that are substrates from those that are not transported by the P-gp. One classification model used the sum of atomic electrotopological states (MolES), a descriptor of molecular bulkiness, to predict substrates.[53] Compounds with a MolES >110 are regarded as substrates for P-gp whereas a MolES <49 indicates non-substrates. For compounds with a value between 49 and 110 other descriptors are needed to identify whether they would be substrates.[53] A similar study using a classification approach established the rule of four.[54] This rule states the following: compounds with (N + O) $\geq$ 8, molecular weight > 400 and acid pK_a > 4 are likely to be P-gp substrates. Compounds with (N + O) $\leq$ 4, molecular weight < 400 and base pK_a < 8 are likely to be non-substrates. Both of these SAR studies identified that P-gp transports larger molecules. Furthermore, it seems that compounds with many hydrogen bonds, and to some extent negative charges, are transportable by P-gp. The non-substrates have fewer hydrogen bond acceptors and are neutral, or at least not highly positively charged. The importance of N and O demonstrated by this study confirms the work by Seelig and colleagues. Finally, P-gp substrates are amphipathic and lipophilic.[55] It has been suggested that the substrate binding pocket sits inside the cellular membrane and needs to be accessed by distribution into the lipid bilayer.[56–58] Based on this, the lipophilic and amphiphilic nature of the substrates is to be expected.

1.5.1.2   Inhibition of P-gp, BCRP, MRPs, BSEP: Specificity and Overlap

While it is important to understand molecular features that result in substances being substrates to efflux proteins, it is also of interest to look at which molecular features lead to inhibition of transport. Inhibition may result in severe DDIs. Inhibitors may be competitive (they bind to the same binding site as the substrate) or non-competitive (they bind to another site on the transport protein and thereby block the transport). Therefore, a substrate may inhibit the transport of another substrate, and an inhibitor is not necessarily transported by the protein. Artursson and colleagues have explored large compound series to identity inhibitors of the transport proteins most important for drug disposition. They identified specific molecular requirements of the different transporters and the extent to which the molecular requirements for inhibition of these transporters overlap. For example, the ABC transporters P-gp, breast cancer resistance protein (BCRP), multidrug resistance-associated protein 2 (MRP2) and bile salt export pump (BSEP), all of which are expressed in the canalicular membrane of the hepatocyte, have a significant overlap of inhibitors, *i.e.* the same compound may block several of these transporters at the same time. The impact on drug clearance, for instance from hepatocytes to bile, may therefore be greatly affected. Such inhibition may also result in reduced enterohepatic recycling of endogenous substances such as bile acids and bilirubin, which can result in, among others, fatal cholestasis.[59] In a study of 122 compounds, all tested for their inhibition of P-gp, BCRP and MRP2, molecular features of specific inhibitors (interacting with only one of the transporters) and of those that interacted with all three transporters were identified.[60] The inhibitors of P-gp were lipophilic, non-polar and had higher structure connectivity. BCRP inhibitors were also more lipophilic than non-inhibitors and the number of aromatic rings correlated positively with inhibition. Inhibitors of MRP2 had similar properties; lipophilicity and unsaturated bonds (double bonds) positively correlated with inhibition, as did shape. Thus, inhibitors of P-gp, BCRP and MRP2 are all lipophilic and aromatic, but to different degrees. The specific inhibitors of P-gp are less aromatic than those of MRP2 and BCRP, and the BCRP inhibitors generally have more aromatic nitrogens than the P-gp inhibitors. P-gp inhibitors are the most lipophilic ($\log D_{pH7.4}$ of 2.3) followed by BCRP ($\log D_{pH7.4}$ of 1.9) and MRP2 ($\log D_{pH7.4}$ of 1.2). By contrast, multi-specific inhibitors, *i.e.* compounds that inhibit all three proteins, are 100- to 1000-fold more lipophilic ($\log D_{pH7.4}$ of 4.5).[60]

Another study investigated 250 compounds for their inhibition of BSEP. Of the 86 inhibitors identified, 58% were neutral at physiological pH, 36% were negatively charged and only 6% were positively charged. By contrast, BSEP substrates are typically monovalent, negatively charged bile acids. BSEP inhibition is also favored by lipophilicity, hydrophobicity and number of halogens. Reciprocally, hydrophilicity and hydrogen bond acceptors negatively correlate with inhibition.[61]

1.5.2   Uptake Transporters

1.5.2.1   *Inhibition of OATP1B1, OATP1B3, OATP2B1: Specificity and Overlap*

There are a number of studies on the inhibition of OATP uptake transporters, particularly OATP1B1 (which is the most important hepatic OATP). Two studies by Karlgren *et al.* investigated the inhibition of OATP1B1 by 146 compounds and the inhibition of OATP1B1, OATP1B3 and OATP2B1 by 225 compounds.[62,63] In both studies, a significantly larger proportion of the inhibitors were negatively charged compounds compared with the non-inhibitors. This is not surprising given that OATPs are known to primarily transport anionic drugs. Furthermore, these studies showed that compared with the non-inhibitors, the OATP inhibitors had a significantly higher lipophilicity (mean NNLogP of 3.6–4.0 *vs.* 2.3–2.7), larger molecular weight (mean weight of 481–514 *vs.* 325–336 g mol^{-1}) and a larger polar surface area (PSA; mean PSA of 115–142 *vs.* 66–74 Å^2).[62,63] OATP1B1 inhibitors also displayed a lower mean square distance index (MSD), a topological distance descriptor normalized for size.[63] Inhibitors of OATP1B3—but not of OATP1B1 and OATP2B1—had more hydrogen bond donors than the non-inhibitors, whereas the OATP2B1 inhibitors were less dependent on polarity than those of OATP1B1 and OATP1B3.[62] These findings were confirmed by an *in vitro* study of 2000 compounds on OATP1B1 and OATP1B3.[64] It was also found that a low number of aromatic bonds (<7) correlated positively with OATP1B1 inhibition but negatively with OATP1B3 inhibition, whereas a log *D* value of >7.5 and 3–4 hydrogen bond donors correlated positively with OATP1B3 inhibition. Interestingly, due to the high number of compounds investigated, they could also identify substructures that favored inhibition of a specific transporter or favored inhibition of both OATP1B transporters.

The three OATP transporters share many inhibitors. Two examples are atazanavir and ritonavir, which are considered general OATP inhibitors.[62] In one study of 91 identified inhibitors, 42 were common for OATP1B1 and OATP1B3. Of these 42 inhibitors, 16 did not inhibit OATP2B1. By contrast, only 9 of the inhibitors were identified as inhibitors of OATP1B1 and OATP2B1 but not OATP1B3. Only one compound, nefazodone, interacted with both OATP1B3 and OATP2B1 but did not inhibit OATP1B1.

Many of the compounds identified as inhibitors of the OATP transporters are also inhibitors or substrates of other transporters or metabolizing enzymes. For example, the FDA and/or the European Medicines Agency (EMA) list that 67 of the 225 compounds included in the studies above are substrates, inhibitors or inducers of CYP enzymes. Of these 67 compounds, 21 compounds were also identified as inhibitors of one or more OATP transporters.[62] The largest overlap was for OATPs and CYP2C8, followed by OATPs and CYP3A4. Previously it was suggested that there was a substrate overlap between OATP1B1 and the efflux transporter MRP2.[65] However, an investigation of common inhibitors of OATP1B1 and MRP2 found no such corresponding overlap of inhibitors.[63]

1.5.2.2   Inhibition of OCT1

Organic cation transporter 1 (OCT1) is the major cationic uptake transporter in the liver. An investigation of 191 compounds identified 62 as inhibitors of OCT1.[66] These inhibitors tended to be positively charged (66%) or neutral (32%) at physiological pH. They were more lipophilic (mean ClogP of 3.50 vs. 1.43), had a lower PSA (mean PSA of 42.9 vs. 95.5), and a lower number of both hydrogen bond donors (1.07 vs. 2.66) and acceptors (3.38 vs. 5.09) than the non-inhibitors.[66] These results agree with a previous study of OCT1 inhibition that used a more homogeneous dataset ($n = 30$).[67] The results also support previous observations that a positive charge is important for interactions with the OCT1 transporter.[68,69]

1.6   Molecular Features of Importance for Enzyme Interactions: Substrates *Versus* Inhibitors

Table 1.6 presents a representative sample of the many substrates and inhibitors of the enzymes responsible for drug metabolism. The liver is the organ with the highest metabolic capacity (Table 1.4). The enzymes of highest importance for drug metabolism in this tissue are CYP3A4, CYP2C9, CYP2C19 and CYP2D6. Below we discuss the molecular features of the substrates and inhibitors of these four enzymes. We focus on CYP3A4 as this enzyme is of the greatest importance for drug metabolism and therefore the most studied.

1.6.1   CYP3A4

The binding pocket of CYP3A4 is quite large. Pharmacophore modeling has been used to reveal the molecular requirements of compounds that bind and activate the enzyme.[74] Information extracted from 38 compounds and the software Catalyst showed that the large binding pocket required interaction with a hydrophobic fragment and hydrogen bond interactions through a hydrogen bond donor and a hydrogen bond acceptor. These different features require a particular spatial distribution in the molecule to interact with the binding pocket. The pharmacophore was later regenerated in a study by Norinder, who also identified another pharmacophore with similar accuracy.[75] Norinder included more hydrophobic interaction points (three hydrophobic fragments) and only one hydrogen bond acceptor to achieve the same quality of pharmacophore as the previous one. This shows the complexity in identifying the molecular features that characterize substrates. A more complex approach, also using pharmacophore modeling, identifies structures vulnerable to metabolism and the reactive site. This methodology calculates the fingerprint of both the enzyme and the substrate. The calculations are

Table 1.6 Substrates and inhibitors of CYP enzymes of importance for drug clearance in the gut and liver.[a]

CYP isoform	Substrates	Inhibitors
CYP1A2	Amitriptyline, caffeine, clomipramine, clozapine, cyclobenzaprine, duloxetine, estradiol, fluvoxamine, haloperidol, mexiletine, nabumetone, naproxen, olanzapine, ondansetron, phenacetin, propranolol, riluzole, ropivacaine, tacrine, theophylline, tizanidine, triamterene, verapamil, (R)-warfarin, zileuton, zolmitriptan	Amiodarone, ciprofloxacin, cimetidine, efavirenz, fluoroquinolones, furafylline, interferon, methoxsalen, mibefradil, ticlopidine
CYP2B6	Artemisinin, bupropion, cyclophosphamide, efavirenz, ifosfamide, ketamine, meperidine, methadone, nevirapine, propafol, selegiline, sorafenib	Clopidogrel, thiotepa, ticlopidine, voriconazole
CYP2C8	Amodiaquine, cerivastatin, paclitaxel, repaglinide, sorafenib, torsemide	Gemfibrozil, glitazones, montelukast, quercetin, trimethoprim
CYP2C9	Amitriptyline, celecoxib, diclofenac, fluoxetine, fluvastatin, glimepiride, glipizide, glyburide, ibuprofen, irbesartan, lornoxicam, losartan, meloxicam, S-naproxen, nateglinide, phenytoin-4-OH2, piroxicam, rosiglitazone, suprofen, tamoxifen, tolbutamide, torsemide, valproic acid, S-warfarin, zakirlukast	Amiodarone, efavirenz, fenofibrate, fluconazole, fluvoxamine, isoniazid, lovastatin, metronidazole, paroxetine, phenylbutazone, probenicid, sertraline, sulfamethoxazole, sulfaphenazole, teniposide, voriconazole
CYP2C19	Amitriptyline, carisoprodol, citalopram, chloramphenicol, clomipramine, clopidogrel, cyclophosphamide, diazepam, esomeprazole, hexobarbital, indomethacin, labetalol, lansoprazole, S-mephenytoin, R-mephobarbital, moclobemide, nelfinavir, nilutamide, omeprazole, pantoprazole, phenobarbitone, primidone, progesterone, proguanil, propranolol, teniposide, R-warfarin, voriconazole	Cimetidine, esomeprazole, felbamate, fluoxetine, fluvoxamine, isoniazid, ketoconazole, modafinil, oxcarbazepine, probenecid, ticlopidine, topiramate
CYP2D6	Alprenolol, amphetamine, amitriptyline, aripiprazole, atomoxetine, bufuralol, carvedilol, chlorpheniramine, chlorpromazine, clonidine, codeine, clomipramine, debrisoquine, desipramine, dexfenfluramine, dextromethorphan, donepezil, duloxetine, flecainide, fluvoxamine, fluoxetine, haloperidol, imipramine, lidocaine, metoclopramide, S-metoprolol, methoxyamphetamine, mexiletine, minaprine, nebivolol, nortriptyline, ondansetron, oxycodone, paroxetine, perhexiline, perphenazine, phenacetin, phenformin, promethazine, propafenone, propranolol, risperidone, sparteine, tamoxifen, thioridazine, timolol, tramadol, venlafaxine, zuclopenthixol	Amiodarone, bupropion, cinacalcet, cimetidine, celecoxib, citalopram, clemastine, cocaine, diphenhydramine, doxepin, doxorubicin, escitalopram, halofantrine, hydroxyzine, levomepromazine, methadone, metoclopramide, mibefradil, midodrine, moclobemide, quinidine, ranitidine, ritonavir, sertraline, terbinafine, ticlopidine, tripelennamine

(continued)

Table 1.6 *(continued)*

CYP isoform	Substrates	Inhibitors
CYP2E1	Acetaminophen, aniline, benzene, chlorzoxazone, enflurane, ethanol, N,N-dimethylformamide, halothane, isoflurane, methoxyflurane, sevoflurane, theophylline	Diethyl-dithiocarbamate, disulfiram
CYP3A4/3A5/3A7	Alfentanil, alprazolam, amlodipine, aprepitant, aripiprazole, astemizole, atorvastatin, boceprevir, buspirone, carbamazepine, cafergot, caffeine → TMU, cerivastatin, clarithromycin, chlorpheniramine, cilostazol, cisapride, cocaine, codeine-N-demethylation, cyclosporine, dapsone, dexamethasone, dextromethorphan, diazepam, diltiazem, docetaxel, domperidone, eplerenone, erythromycin, estradiol, felodipine, fentanyl, finasteride, gleevec, haloperidol, hydrocortisone, indinavir, irinotecan, lercanidipine, lidocaine, lovastatin, methadone, midazolam, nateglinide, nelfinavir, nevirapine, nifedipine, nisoldipine, nitrendipine, ondansetron, pimozide, progesterone, propranolol, quetiapine, quinidine, quinine, risperidone, ritonavir, romidepsin, salmeterol, saquinavir, sildenafil, simvastatin, sirolimus, sorafenib, tacrolimus, tamoxifen, taxol, telaprevir, telithromycin, terfenadine, testosterone, torisel, trazodone, triazolam, vemurafenib, verapamil, vincristine, zaleplon, ziprasidone, zolpidem	Amiodarone, chloramphenicol, cimetidine, ciprofloxacin, delavirdine, diethyl-dithiocarbamate, fluconazole, fluvoxamine, gestodene, imatinib, itraconazole, ketoconazole, nefazodone, mibefradil, mifepristone, norfloxacin, norfluoxetine, suboxone, voriconazole

[a]Data on CYP substrates and inhibitors were taken from the cytochrome P450 drug interaction table established by Prof. Flockhart. Flockhart DA. Drug Interactions: Cytochrome P450 Drug Interaction Table. Indiana University School of Medicine (2007). http://medicine.iupui.edu/clinpharm/ddis/clinical-table/, accessed 2014-12-09. http://togodb.dbcls.jp/tpsearch/.

based on GRID methodology, *i.e.* the enzyme fingerprints are calculated by the GRID flexible molecular interaction fields and the substrate fingerprints are obtained through GRID probe pharmacophore recognition. The latter calculates hydrophobicity, hydrogen bond donors and acceptors, and charge to obtain a fingerprint of each atom in the molecule. These descriptors are then assessed for their capacity to interact with the reactive heme atom of the enzyme. This is performed through assessment of how accessible they are for interactions with the heme. This fingerprint method has resulted in the software MetaSite for prediction of vulnerable sites for CYP metabolism of CYP3A4, CYP2C9 and CYP2D6 (see Section 1.7.1).[76–78]

Another method to predict the site of metabolism (SOM) in a drug molecule was developed at the University of Copenhagen. Their approach uses quantum chemical calculations with the density functional method B3LYP to estimate the activation energy required for different atoms to become the SOM. The group has also tested less time-consuming calculations by making use of the semi-empirical AM1 method.[79] Using the two methods together, the following descriptors were calculated for the substrate and the radical obtained after dehydration: the Mulliken charges on the carbon and hydrogen atoms involved in the reaction; the spin of the carbon atom in the radical; the energies of the highest occupied molecular orbital (HOMO) and lowest unoccupied molecular orbital (LUMO); and the energy difference between these two orbitals. The coefficients for the hydrogen 1s and carbon 2p atomic orbitals in the HOMO and LUMO were also calculated. Their analyses of computational models of different complexity revealed that simpler and less computationally demanding methods could be used to identify SOM. This spurred many articles (*cf.*[80–82]) as well as the development of the software SMARTCyp, further discussed in Section 1.7.2.

Inhibitors of CYP3A4 have been studied extensively. Datasets in earlier studies often had fewer than 30 compounds and, based on these, typically linear SAR models were developed. These studies identified lipophilicity as an important descriptor for achieving inhibition.[75,83,84] Later studies used datasets with several hundreds of compounds. The aim of these was to find molecular motifs of importance for CYP3A4 inhibition or to develop global computational models for predicting the risk that a new compound might be a CYP3A4 inhibitor. AstraZeneca studied 463 compounds for their CYP3A4 inhibition and the response data were analyzed by either partial least squares or regression tree methodology.[85] The modeling used molecular descriptors based on atoms and fragments as input. The greater the aromaticity and lipophilicity, the more potently the compound inhibited CYP3A4. Furthermore, neutral compounds and bases inhibited CYP3A4 whereas negatively charged compounds bound to other isozymes. Another study of 741 compounds developed a classification model to distinguish inhibitors from non-inhibitors. The model was then validated with a test set of 186 compounds. The recognition rate of the model was relatively high and 73% of the compounds were correctly identified as either inhibitors or non-inhibitors. The final model was based on constitutional, electrostatic and geometric descriptors. Examples of these are molecular weight, flexibility (number of flexible bonds, rigid bonds and rings), charge, lipophilicity and van der Waals surface area. This model identified that inhibitors are larger than non-inhibitors and extracted a cut-off value of 354 g mol^{-1}. Inhibitors are also more hydrophobic and have fewer chargeable groups, the latter being <5% of the molecular composition for inhibitors. Another molecular property that discriminates inhibitors from non-inhibitors is the number of nitrogens; a compound with more than two nitrogens does not inhibit CYP3A4.[86] A study of 1756 compounds on the inhibition of CYP3A4 concluded that the models for prediction of CYP3A4 inhibition must be based on algorithms that can handle the complexity of enzymatic inhibition and the resulting non-linear data.[87]

1.6.2   CYP2C9, CYP2C19 and CYP2D6

Computational analyses of pharmacophore modeling, protein conformation analyses and multivariate data analyses have identified that substrates to CYP2C9 are hydrophobic (up to two functions), and include at least one hydrogen bond donor and one hydrogen bond acceptor.[88–91] Substrates of CYP2C9 are favored by being negatively charged but metabolism by CYP2C19 enzyme is not. Substrates of CYP2D6 often contain overlapping hydrophobic features, a hydrogen bond donor function well separated from the hydrophobic features and negative molecular electrostatic potential.[92,93] The hydrophobic domain near the oxidation site interacts with a large, flat and lipophilic region of the CYP2D6 that contains residues Leu121, Leu213, Ala305, Val370 and Thr309. The hydrogen bond donor group can have two different spatial locations from the hydrophobic region. Substrates with the nitrogen atom positioned 10 Å from the oxidation center interact with CYP2D6 through hydrogen bonds between the nitrogen and Glu216 and Gln117. Other substrates have the nitrogen atom positioned 5 or 7 Å away from the oxidation center and the nitrogen interacts only with the Asp301 residue of CYP2D6.[93]

Gleeson and colleagues studied a dataset of 457 compounds to predict CYP2C9 inhibitors.[85] Molecular features that correlated with CYP2C9 inhibition were lipophilicity, aromaticity and non-ionizability. The enzyme was also found to be inhibited by negatively charged compounds, a finding also confirmed by Manga et al.[94] Pharmacophore models based on three different datasets (n = 9, 29 and 13, respectively) each generated a different pharmacophores that inhibited CYP2C9. The pharmacophores differed from each other spatially and in other important molecular features.[95] All three pharmacophore models included one hydrophobic pocket and one hydrogen bond acceptor but they differed in number of hydrophobic pockets (1–2), hydrogen bond acceptors (1–2) and whether they had hydrogen bond donors. There is a large overlap in the physicochemical properties of inhibitors of CYP2C9 and CYP2C19. For example, Gleeson et al., who used a dataset of 369 compounds, found that CYP2C19 is also inhibited by lipophilic and aromatic compounds.[85] However, CYP2C19 has a preference for neutral compounds.

The overlap between these two enzymes is understandable as they share 95.7% homology—only 43 of their 490 amino acids differ from each other.[96] Studies of CYP2C19 have also revealed that stronger inhibitors are more lipophilic at the N-3 position. The binding affinity of the inhibitors also increases with the degree of steric bulk. This is a result of the general entropic effect associated with solvation where the increased order of the bulk water for larger compounds favors binding of such molecules to the enzyme.

In contrast to the CYP3A4, CYP2C9 and CYP2C19 inhibitors, the role of lipophilicity for inhibition of CYP2D6 is less clear. Using a dataset of 170 compounds, Gleeson *et al.* identified that inhibitors of this enzyme are aromatic structures with weak basic functions, but not lipophilic *per se.*[85] Groot *et al.* reviewed different models for the prediction of CYP2D6 inhibitors (and substrates).[92] Based on 3500 compounds, they extracted the following rules for inhibitors: (i) inhibitors are weak bases (92% of the compounds with CYP2D6 IC_{50} < 1 mM were weak bases); and (ii) decreasing polarity, as measured by the total PSA (TPSA), increases CYP2D6 inhibition (*e.g.* 73% of the weak bases had CYP2D6 IC_{50} < 10 mM when the TPSA was <50 Å^2). In comparison, this number was 37% when TPSA was >100 Å^2. In contrast to the study by Gleeson *et al.* Groot and coworkers found that lipophilicity was positively related to inhibition. The majority (73%) of the weak bases with a calculated $\log P$ of 3–5 had CYP2D6 IC_{50} < 10 mM, whereas this number was 45% for the weak bases with a $\log P$ of 1–3.

1.7   Software

A number of different methods and software are available for the prediction of metabolism. These enable predictions of metabolic sites, metabolic reactions and products, mechanisms, and enzyme dynamics. More traditional structure–activity approaches are also used and models have been developed to predict CYP inducers and inhibitors. An extensive list of software can be found in the article published by Kirchmair and coworkers.[97] Three commonly used pieces of software that make use of a combination of different *in silico* approaches are MetaSite, SMARTCyp and StarDrop. These are briefly described below.

1.7.1   MetaSite

MetaSite (Molecular Discovery, Italy) predicts phase I metabolism mediated by CYP enzymes and flavin-containing monooxygenases. It predicts the binding between substrates and enzymes (a thermodynamic factor) and the chemical transformation (a kinetic factor). The predictions are obtained by a combination of molecular interaction fields that analyze ligand and enzyme properties, together with quantum mechanics and knowledge-based components that relate to the kinetics of metabolism (*i.e.* the reactivity). The software enables identification of molecular sites vulnerable to metabolism so that medicinal chemists can redesign structures that are rapidly cleared through metabolism. To further improve predictions of metabolism patterns and reactivity, Molecular Discovery has formed a human CYP consortium with some pharmaceutical companies. The overarching goal of this consortium is to produce high-quality experimental data to improve predictions for metabolic rate, site and reaction pathways, and the likelihood of a compound being a substrate/inhibitor for a specific enzyme. Information about the program can be found on the MetaSite webpage (http://www.moldiscovery.com/software/metasite).

1.7.2   SMARTCyp and StarDrop

The software SMARTCyp originates from the University of Copenhagen. It includes a fragment-based database for which the density functional theory activation energy has been calculated. This database is then used to match structural fragments of drug molecules to estimate CYP3A4-, CYP2D6- and CYP2C9-mediated transformation. Data from 211 transitions were used to develop the fragment-based energy rules. To rank the SOM in the molecules, an accessibility descriptor is used.

Figure 1.2 shows clopidogrel, an antithrombosis drug discussed in the pharmacogenomics Section (1.4). SMARTCyp provides probability estimations of a particular atom being the site of enzymatic activation. For clopidogrel, which is composed of 18 heteroatoms, the atoms are numbered 1 to 18. The estimation is based on three factors related to the molecular structure: activation energy, accessibility and solvent-accessible surface area. The

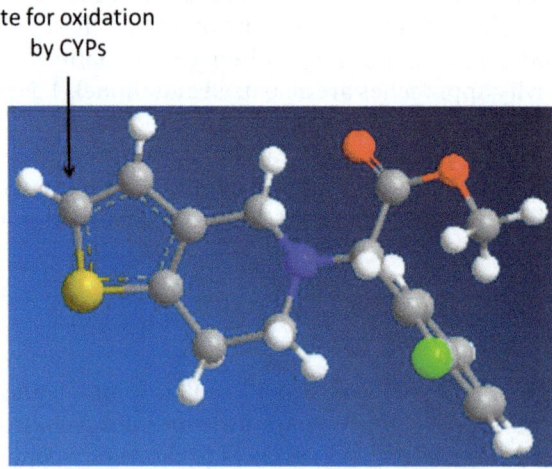

Figure 1.2   Clopidogrel's main site for enzymatic degradation. SMARTCyp predicts the probability of this atom being the site of metabolism to be among the top 33% (with CYP2D6 the highest probability; and for CYP2C9 and CYP3A4 ranked as atoms 5 and 6, respectively, out of 18). Predictions are based on the methodology described by Rydberg and coworkers.[80]

activation energy is the approximate energy required for the reaction of the catalytic site of the enzyme (*i.e.* CYP3A4, CYP2C9 or CYP2D6) to occur at this atom. Accessibility is a measure of the distance of the particular atom from the center of the molecule and always has a number between 0.5 (atom is positioned in the center) and 1.0 (atom is positioned at the far end of the molecule). The solvent-accessible surface area is the total surface area of that particular atom exposed to *e.g.* water and thereby accessible for interaction with the enzyme. This surface area is predicted from 2D molecular topology descriptors. CYP3A4 and CYP3A5 are the most important enzymes for hepatic metabolism of clopidrogel.[98] Clopidogrel is a prodrug and requires enzymatic activation *in vivo*, the atom of importance for this is the carbon next to the sulfur in the thiophene group (Figure 1.2).[99] It should be noted that *in vivo* about 85% of clopidogrel is inactivated by hydrolysis of the ester group, *i.e.* this ester is necessary to obtain active inhibition of platelet aggregation. This type of reaction is not predictable by the SMARTCyp software.

Similar to SMARTCyp, the software Stardrop (Optibrium, UK) predicts reaction sites. It makes use of quantum mechanics calculations to predict metabolic sites and their vulnerability to different CYPs. This software has also been suggested as a useful tool in the redesign of enzymatically liable molecules. The accuracies of the predictions of SMARTCyp and StarDrop are similar.[80]

1.8   Conclusion

This chapter has reviewed the physicochemical properties of compounds that determine their interaction with transport proteins and the enzymes involved in drug clearance. Lipophilicity is an important physicochemical property resulting in interaction and, in particular, inhibition of both transport proteins and enzymes. Other specific features of the substrates and inhibitors are summarized below.

- Substrates to OATP1B1, OATP2B1 and OATP1B3 are negatively charged. Inhibitors of these transport proteins are lipophilic (~log P 4), large (~500 g mol^{-1}) and polar ~120 Å^2, although OATP2B1 inhibitors are less dependent on polarity than those of OATP1B1 and OATP1B3. Inhibitors of OATP1B3 have a larger number of hydrogen bond donors (3–4). A low number of aromatic bonds (<7) increases the risk of OATP1B1 inhibition, but reduces the risk of OATP1B3 inhibition.
- Substrates to OCT1 are cationic and, hence, many of the inhibitors also carry a positive charge. Furthermore, inhibitors are lipophilic (log P of 3.50) and less polar (PSA of 43), with a lower number of hydrogen bond donors (1) and acceptors (~3) than the non-inhibitors.
- P-gp substrates require specific hydrogen bond interactions and compounds with (N + O) ≥ 8, molecular weight > 400 g mol^{-1} and acid pK_a > 4 are likely to be P-gp substrates. Inhibitors of P-gp and other efflux proteins (BCRP and MRP2) are lipophilic and aromatic. P-gp is

the most lipophilic ($\log D_{pH7.4}$ of 2.3) followed by BCRP ($\log D_{pH7.4}$ 1.9) and MRP2 ($\log D_{pH7.4}$ of 1.2). Multi-specific inhibitors are 100- to 1000-fold more lipophilic ($\log D_{pH7.4}$ of 4.5). Specific inhibitors of P-gp are less aromatic than those of MRP2 and BCRP. In addition, BCRP inhibitors have a greater number of aromatic nitrogens than P-gp inhibitors.

- Studies of CYP substrates have identified the importance of an acidic function, hydrogen bond donors and hydrogen bond acceptors for CYP2C9, a weak basic function (*i.e.* cationic charge), and aromatic ring features for CYP2D6 and hydrophobic features for CYP3A4.
- Inhibition of CYP2C9, CYP2C19, CYP2D6 and CYP3A4 is highly related to the lipophilicity and aromaticity of the drug—inhibition increases with lipophilicity for all four enzymes. Inhibitors of CYP2C9 and CYP2C19 have common features; however, CYP2C9 prefers negatively charged compounds whereas CYP2C19 is inhibited by neutral compounds. Inhibition of CYP3A4, which is the most studied enzyme, is favored by aromatic structures, larger molecules (molecular weight > 354 g mol^{-1}) and compounds with a low number of nitrogens (<2).

The literature on substrates and inhibitors of the transporters and CYP enzymes suggests that different computational approaches are required to arrive at reliable and robust predictions of interactions. Increasing the prediction accuracy of SOM and the development of quantitative models, for the prediction of *e.g.* IC$_{50}$ values, will require elucidation of the pathway (competitive/non-competitive inhibition and binding site of the enzyme for substrates) based on large, high-quality datasets. In addition, the interplay between transporters and enzymes needs further attention to understand how drug-like compounds access the intracellular enzymes.

Acknowledgements

We are grateful to Ms Andrea Treyer for producing Figure 1.1 and Ms Paulina Jakubiak for help compiling the tables.

References

1. J. L. Madara and K. Dharmsathaphorn, *J. Cell Biol.*, 1985, **101**, 2124.
2. P. D. Dobson and D. B. Kell, *Nat. Rev. Drug Discovery*, 2008, 7, 205.
3. D. B. Kell, *Trends Pharmacol. Sci.*, 2015, **36**, 15.
4. D. B. Kell, P. D. Dobson and S. G. Oliver, *Drug Discovery Today*, 2011, **16**, 704.
5. L. Di, P. Artursson, A. Avdeef, G. F. Ecker, B. Faller, H. Fischer, J. B. Houston, M. Kansy, E. H. Kerns, S. D. Kramer, H. Lennernas and K. Sugano, *Drug Discovery Today*, 2012, **17**, 905.
6. D. Smith, P. Artursson, A. Avdeef, L. Di, G. F. Ecker, B. Faller, J. B. Houston, M. Kansy, E. H. Kerns, S. D. Kramer, H. Lennernas, H. van de Waterbeemd, K. Sugano and B. Testa, *Mol. Pharmaceutics*, 2014, **11**, 1727.

7. C. Groer, D. Busch, M. Patrzyk, K. Beyer, A. Busemann, C. D. Heidecke, M. Drozdzik, W. Siegmund and S. Oswald, *J. Pharm. Biomed. Anal.*, 2014, **100**, 393–401.
8. M. F. Paine, H. L. Hart, S. S. Ludington, R. L. Haining, A. E. Rettie and D. C. Zeldin, *Drug Metab. Dispos.*, 2006, **34**, 880.
9. M. F. Paine, M. Khalighi, J. M. Fisher, D. D. Shen, K. L. Kunze, C. L. Marsh, J. D. Perkins and K. E. Thummel, *J. Pharmacol. Exp. Ther.*, 1997, **283**, 1552.
10. P. B. Watkins, S. A. Wrighton, E. G. Schuetz, D. T. Molowa and P. S. Guzelian, *J. Clin. Invest.*, 1987, **80**, 1029.
11. J. Yang, G. T. Tucker and A. Rostami-Hodjegan, *Clin. Pharmacol. Ther.*, 2004, **76**, 391.
12. I. de Waziers, P. H. Cugnenc, C. S. Yang, J. P. Leroux and P. H. Beaune, *J. Pharmacol. Exp. Ther.*, 1990, **253**, 387.
13. D. C. Zeldin, J. Foley, S. M. Goldsworthy, M. E. Cook, J. E. Boyle, J. Ma, C. R. Moomaw, K. B. Tomer, C. Steenbergen and S. Wu, *Mol. Pharmacol.*, 1997, **51**, 931.
14. K. Nakamura, M. Hirayama, S. Ito and S. Ohtsuki, *Poster presented at the 19th ISSX conference in San Francisco*, 2014.
15. T. Shimada, H. Yamazaki, M. Mimura, Y. Inui and F. P. Guengerich, *Pharmacol. Exp. Ther.*, 1994, **270**, 414.
16. H. Kawakami, S. Ohtsuki, J. Kamiie, T. Suzuki, T. Abe and T. Terasaki, *J. Pharm. Sci.*, 2011, **100**, 341.
17. A. Vildhede, J. R. Wisniewski, A. Noren, M. Karlgren and P. Artursson, *J. Proteome Res.*, 2015, **14**, 3305.
18. J. M. Lasker, M. R. Wester, E. Aramsombatdee and J. L. Raucy, *Arch. Biochem. Biophys.*, 1998, **353**, 16.
19. M. Ingelman-Sundberg, *Naunyn-Schmiedeberg's Arch. Pharmacol.*, 2004, **369**, 89.
20. S. C. Sim, R. J. Edwards, A. R. Boobis and M. Ingelman-Sundberg, *Pharmacogenet. Genomics*, 2005, **15**, 625.
21. E. Hedlund, J. A. Gustafsson and M. Warner, *Curr. Drug Metab.*, 2001, **2**, 245.
22. M. Karlgren, M. Backlund, I. Johansson, M. Oscarson and M. Ingelman-Sundberg, *Biochem. Biophys. Res. Commun.*, 2004, **315**, 679.
23. S. Miksys and R. F. Tyndale, *J. Psychiatry Neurosci.*, 2013, **38**, 152–163.
24. S. L. Miksys and R. F. Tyndale, *J. Psychiatry Neurosci.*, 2002, **27**, 406.
25. V. Ravindranath and H. W. Strobel, *Expert Opin. Drug Metab. Toxicol.*, 2013, **9**, 551.
26. K. M. Knights, A. Rowland and J. O. Miners, *Br. J. Clin. Pharmacol.*, 2013, **76**, 587.
27. K. R. Chaudhary, S. N. Batchu and J. M. Seubert, *IUBMB Life*, 2009, **61**, 954.
28. N. Ahmad and H. Mukhtar, *J. Invest. Dermatol.*, 2004, **123**, 417.
29. L. Du, S. M. Hoffman and D. S. Keeney, *Toxicol. Appl. Pharmacol.*, 2004, **195**, 278.
30. X. Ding and L. S. Kaminsky, *Annu. Rev. Pharmacol. Toxicol.*, 2003, **43**, 149.

31. W. E. Evans and M. V. Relling, *Science*, 1999, **286**, 487.
32. L. C. Wienkers and T. G. Heath, *Nat. Rev. Drug Discovery*, 2005, **4**, 825.
33. C. R. Wolf and G. Smith, *Br. Med. Bull.*, 1999, **55**, 366.
34. R. J. Bertz and G. R. Granneman, *Clin. Pharmacokinet.*, 1997, **32**, 210.
35. U. M. Zanger and M. Schwab, *Pharmacol. Ther.*, 2013, **138**, 103–141.
36. M. Ingelman-Sundberg, M. Oscarson and R. A. McLellan, *Trends Pharmacol. Sci.*, 1999, **20**, 342–349.
37. S. C. Sim and M. Ingelman-Sundberg, *Trends Pharmacol. Sci.*, 2011, **32**, 72.
38. S. C. Sim, M. Kacevska and M. Ingelman-Sundberg, *Pharmacogenomics J.*, 2013, **13**, 1.
39. M. Eichelbaum and B. Evert, *Clin. Exp. Pharmacol. Physiol.*, 1996, **23**, 983.
40. P. Dalen, C. Frengell, M. L. Dahl and F. Sjoqvist, *Ther. Drug Monit.*, 1997, **19**, 543.
41. G. Koren, J. Cairns, D. Chitayat, A. Gaedigk and S. J. Leeder, *Lancet*, 2006, **368**, 704.
42. P. Madadi, G. Koren, J. Cairns, D. Chitayat, A. Gaedigk, J. S. Leeder, R. Teitelbaum, T. Karaskov and K. Aleksa, *Can. Fam. Physician*, 2007, **53**, 33.
43. P. Madadi, C. J. Ross, M. R. Hayden, B. C. Carleton, A. Gaedigk, J. S. Leeder and G. Koren, *Clin. Pharmacol. Ther.*, 2009, **85**, 31.
44. H. Furuya, P. Fernandez-Salguero, W. Gregory, H. Taber, A. Steward, F. J. Gonzalez and J. R. Idle, *Pharmacogenetics*, 1995, **5**, 389.
45. A. K. Daly, *Arch. Toxicol.*, 2013, **87**, 407.
46. J. L. Mega, T. Simon, J. P. Collet, J. L. Anderson, E. M. Antman, K. Bliden, C. P. Cannon, N. Danchin, B. Giusti, P. Gurbel, B. D. Horne, J. S. Hulot, A. Kastrati, G. Montalescot, F. J. Neumann, L. Shen, D. Sibbing, P. G. Steg, D. Trenk, S. D. Wiviott and M. S. Sabatine, *JAMA*, 2010, **304**, 1821.
47. L. Wallentin, S. James, R. F. Storey, M. Armstrong, B. J. Barratt, J. Horrow, S. Husted, H. Katus, P. G. Steg, S. H. Shah, R. C. Becker and P. Investigators, *Lancet*, 2010, **376**, 1320–1328.
48. FDA, *Label and Approval History–Coumadin*, 2015.
49. FDA, *Label and Approval History–Plavix*, 2015.
50. G. Englund, P. Hallberg, P. Artursson, K. Michaelsson and H. Melhus, *BMC Med.*, 2004, **2**, 8.
51. A. Seelig, *Eur. J. Biochem.*, 1998, **251**, 252.
52. A. Seelig, *Int. J. Clin. Pharmacol. Ther.*, 1998, **36**, 50.
53. V. K. Gombar, J. W. Polli, J. E. Humphreys, S. A. Wring and C. S. Serabjit-Singh, *J. Pharm. Sci.*, 2004, **93**, 957.
54. R. Didziapetris, P. Japertas, A. Avdeef and A. Petrauskas, *J. Drug Targeting*, 2003, **11**, 391.
55. A. H. Schinkel and J. W. Jonker, *Adv. Drug Delivery Rev.*, 2003, **55**, 3.
56. E. Gatlik-Landwojtowicz, P. Aanismaa and A. Seelig, *Biochemistry*, 2006, **45**, 3020.
57. L. Homolya, Z. Hollo, U. A. Germann, I. Pastan, M. M. Gottesman and B. Sarkadi, *J. Biol. Chem.*, 1993, **268**, 21493–21496.
58. A. B. Shapiro, A. B. Corder and V. Ling, *Eur. J. Biochem.*, 1997, **250**, 115.

59. B. L. Shneider, *Pediatr. Transplant.*, 2004, **8**, 609.
60. P. Matsson, J. M. Pedersen, U. Norinder, C. A. S. Bergström and P. Artursson, *Pharm. Res.*, 2009, **26**, 1816.
61. J. M. Pedersen, P. Matsson, C. A. S. Bergström, J. Hoogstraate, A. Noren, E. L. LeCluyse and P. Artursson, *Toxicol. Sci.*, 2013, **136**, 328.
62. M. Karlgren, A. Vildhede, U. Norinder, J. R. Wisniewski, E. Kimoto, Y. Lai, U. Haglund and P. Artursson, *J. Med. Chem.*, 2012, **55**, 4740.
63. M. Karlgren, G. Ahlin, C. A. S. Bergström, R. Svensson, J. Palm and P. Artursson, *Pharm. Res.*, 2012, **29**, 411.
64. T. De Bruyn, G. J. van Westen, A. P. Ijzerman, B. Stieger, P. de Witte, P. F. Augustijns and P. P. Annaert, *Mol. Pharmacol.*, 2013, **83**, 1257.
65. L. Liu, Y. Cui, A. Y. Chung, Y. Shitara, Y. Sugiyama, D. Keppler and K. S. Pang, *J. Pharmacol. Exp. Ther.*, 2006, **318**, 395.
66. G. Ahlin, J. Karlsson, J. M. Pedersen, L. Gustavsson, R. Larsson, P. Matsson, U. Norinder, C. A. S. Bergström and P. Artursson, *J. Med. Chem.*, 2008, **51**, 5932.
67. D. Bednarczyk, S. Ekins, J. H. Wikel and S. H. Wright, *Mol. Pharmacol.*, 2003, **63**, 489.
68. H. Koepsell, K. Lips and C. Volk, *Pharm. Res.*, 2007, **24**, 1227.
69. J. W. Jonker and A. H. Schinkel, *J. Pharmacol. Exp. Ther.*, 2004, **308**, 2.
70. G. Englund, F. Rorsman, A. Ronnblom, U. Karlbom, L. Lazorova, J. Grasjo, A. Kindmark and P. Artursson, *Eur. J. Pharm. Sci.*, 2006, **29**, 269–277.
71. C. Hilgendorf, G. Ahlin, A. Seithel, P. Artursson, A. L. Ungell and J. Karlsson, *Drug Metab. Dispos.*, 2007, **35**, 1333.
72. K. M. Giacomini, S. M. Huang, D. J. Tweedie, L. Z. Benet, K. L. Brouwer, X. Chu, A. Dahlin, R. Evers, V. Fischer, K. M. Hillgren, K. A. Hoffmaster, T. Ishikawa, D. Keppler, R. B. Kim, C. A. Lee, M. Niemi, J. W. Polli, Y. Sugiyama, P. W. Swaan, J. A. Ware, S. H. Wright, S. W. Yee, M. J. Zamek-Gliszczynski and L. Zhang, *Nat. Rev. Drug Discovery*, 2010, **9**, 215.
73. C. Groer, S. Bruck, Y. Lai, A. Paulick, A. Busemann, C. D. Heidecke, W. Siegmund and S. Oswald, *J. Pharm. Biomed. Anal.*, 2013, **85**, 253.
74. S. Ekins, G. Bravi, J. H. Wikel and S. A. Wrighton, *J. Pharmacol. Exp. Ther.*, 1999, **291**, 424.
75. U. Norinder, *SAR QSAR Environ. Res.*, 2005, **16**, 1.
76. L. Afzelius, I. Zamora, C. M. Masimirembwa, A. Karlen, T. B. Andersson, S. Mecucci, M. Baroni and G. Cruciani, *J. Med. Chem.*, 2004, **47**, 907.
77. G. Cruciani, E. Carosati, B. De Boeck, K. Ethirajulu, C. Mackie, T. Howe and R. Vianello, *J. Med. Chem.*, 2005, **48**, 6970.
78. I. Zamora, L. Afzelius and G. Cruciani, *J. Med. Chem.*, 2003, **46**, 2313.
79. L. Olsen, P. Rydberg, T. H. Rod and U. Ryde, *J. Med. Chem.*, 2006, **49**, 6489.
80. P. Rydberg, D. E. Gloriam, J. Zaretzki, C. Breneman and L. Olsen, *ACS Med. Chem. Lett.*, 2010, **1**, 96.
81. P. Rydberg and L. Olsen, *ChemMedChem*, 2012, **7**, 1202.
82. P. Rydberg and L. Olsen, *ACS Med. Chem. Lett.*, 2012, **3**, 69.
83. D. F. Lewis, *Chem.-Biol. Interact.*, 1987, **62**, 271.
84. M. T. Cronin and T. W. Schultz, *J. Mol. Struct.*, 2003, **622**, 39.

85. M. P. Gleeson, A. M. Davis, K. K. Chohan, S. W. Paine, S. Boyer, C. L. Gavaghan, C. H. Arnby, C. Kankkonen and N. Albertson, *J. Comput.-Aided Mol. Des.*, 2007, **21**, 559–573.

86. I. Choi, S. Y. Kim, H. Kim, N. S. Kang, M. A. Bae, S. E. Yoo, J. Jung and K. T. No, *Eur. J. Med. Chem.*, 2009, **44**, 2354.

87. S. Ekins, J. Berbaum and R. K. Harrison, *Drug Metab. Dispos.*, 2003, **31**, 1077.

88. B. C. Jones, G. Hawksworth, V. A. Horne, A. Newlands, J. Morsman, M. S. Tute and D. A. Smith, *Drug Metab. Dispos.*, 1996, **24**, 260.

89. A. Mancy, P. Broto, S. Dijols, P. M. Dansette and D. Mansuy, *Biochemistry*, 1995, **34**, 10365.

90. M. J. de Groot, A. A. Alex and B. C. Jones, *J. Med. Chem.*, 2002, **45**, 1983.

91. M. Ramesh and P. V. Bharatam, *J. Mol. Model.*, 2012, **18**, 709.

92. M. J. de Groot, F. Wakenhut, G. Whitlock and R. Hyland, *Drug Discovery Today*, 2009, **14**, 964.

93. S. Sciabola, I. Morao and M. J. de Groot, *J. Chem. Inf. Model.*, 2007, **47**, 76.

94. N. Manga, J. C. Duffy, P. H. Rowe and M. T. Cronin, *SAR QSAR Environ. Res.*, 2005, **16**, 43.

95. S. Ekins, G. Bravi, S. Binkley, J. S. Gillespie, B. J. Ring, J. H. Wikel and S. A. Wrighton, *Drug Metab. Dispos.*, 2000, **28**, 994.

96. J. A. Goldstein and S. M. de Morais, *Pharmacogenetics*, 1994, **4**, 285.

97. J. Kirchmair, M. J. Williamson, J. D. Tyzack, L. Tan, P. J. Bond, A. Bender and R. C. Glen, *J. Chem. Inf. Model.*, 2012, **52**, 617.

98. T. A. Clarke and L. A. Waskell, *Drug Metab. Dispos.*, 2003, **31**, 53.

99. P. Savi, J. M. Pereillo, M. F. Uzabiaga, J. Combalbert, C. Picard, J. P. Maffrand, M. Pascal and J. M. Herbert, *Thromb. Haemostasis*, 2000, **84**, 891.

CHAPTER 2

Role of Solubility, Permeability and Absorption in Drug Discovery and Development

JIBIN LI[a], QING WANG[a], AND ISMAEL J. HIDALGO*[a]

[a]Absorption Systems, L.P., 436 Creamery Way, Suite 600, Exton, PA 19341, USA
*E-mail: ihidalgo@absorption.com

2.1 Solubility

2.1.1 Introduction

Solubility is one of the most important physicochemical properties to be considered when evaluating compounds as potential drugs candidates. Broadly, solubility can be defined as the maximum amount of a substance (solute) that dissolves in a given volume of liquid (solvent) at a specific temperature. Drug solubilization is a prerequisite for drug absorption because in most cases drug molecules must be in solution before traversing the intestinal epithelium, the major barrier to intestinal absorption. Since solubility is a key determinant of drug absorption from the intestinal lumen, it is difficult to obtain good oral bioavailability for compounds with poor solubility. Incomplete solubility or slow dissolution rates in the gastrointestinal (GI) tract cause low and variable bioavailability. Work by Amidon *et al.*[1] demonstrated that the solubility/dissolution of solid dosage forms in the GI fluids

RSC Drug Discovery Series No. 49
New Horizons in Predictive Drug Metabolism and Pharmacokinetics
Edited by Alan G. E. Wilson
© The Royal Society of Chemistry 2016
Published by the Royal Society of Chemistry, www.rsc.org

and the permeability of the drug through the GI membrane are the primary factors governing the extent of a drug's intestinal absorption. As a result of that work, solubility and permeability were selected as the two primary parameters for classifying drug substances based on a valuable system used in guiding oral drug development, the Biopharmaceutics Classification System (BCS).[2,3]

Recent advances in drug discovery have led to the generation of large chemical libraries and to the design of drug candidates that interact strongly with complicated biological targets. However, these chemical libraries often contain large numbers of new chemical entities (NCEs) with high hydrophobicity and intrinsically low aqueous solubility. In fact, according to some estimates, more than 50% of drug development candidates have low aqueous solubility.[4,5] This trend (*i.e.*, an increasing number of drug candidates with low solubility) has been attributed to multiple factors. For example, the application of combinatorial chemistry and high-throughput screening assays, often conducted in non-aqueous media, may have biased the generation and selection of lipophilic compounds. Pursuing compounds with higher binding affinity towards receptors or enzymes usually involves hydrophobic interactions, and favors the selection of lipophilic drug candidates. In addition, exploration of challenging therapeutic areas requiring drug interactions with ion channels or intracellular targets such as nuclear receptors requires compounds with increasing lipophilicity to reach and interact with the target. The absorption and bioavailability of poorly water-soluble drugs after oral administration is often low, variable, and susceptible to the presence of food in the stomach, and, as a result, the development of this type of compound exhibits high attrition rates and is more expensive.[6,7] On the other hand, highly hydrophilic compounds, *i.e.*, highly water soluble, such as proteins, peptides, aminoglycosides, bisphosphonates, and antiviral agents often suffer from poor intestinal permeability, which results in low systemic delivery after oral administration.[8,9] Clearly the challenges for designing and selecting drug candidates possessing adequate biopharmaceutical properties are multifaceted. Factors that need to be considered include the affinity towards the intended biological target, the balance between aqueous solubility and membrane permeability, stability in GI fluids, presystemic metabolism, biliary excretion, and systemic clearance. Despite the role of solubility in drug permeability and absorption, solubility and permeability are not correlated (Figure 2.1), both parameters need to be determined in discovery and development.

2.1.2 Methodology for Measuring Solubility

Within the pharmaceutical industry, typically, two types of solubility are measured: kinetic and thermodynamic. Kinetic solubility is a measure of the maximum amount of compound in solution at a given time; the measurements could start from solid form or a highly concentrated organic stock solution of the compound, typically dimethyl sulfoxide (DMSO). By contrast,

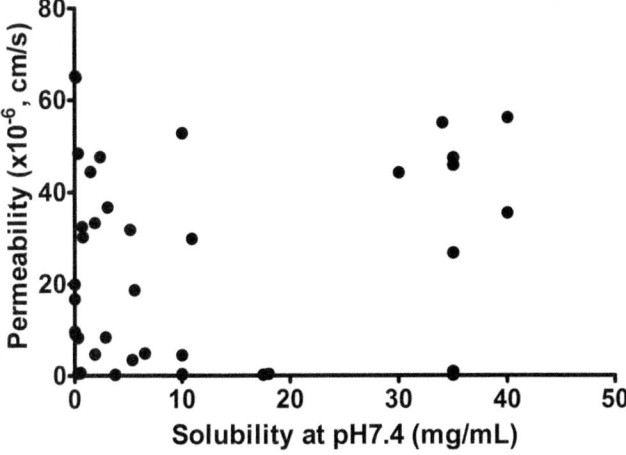

Figure 2.1   Caco-2 permeability *versus* equilibrium solubility at pH 7.4.

thermodynamic (equilibrium) solubility is the maximum amount of the most stable crystalline form of a compound that can remain in solution under equilibrium conditions.[10] The purpose of solubility measurements in drug discovery and development is different. In drug discovery, large numbers of NCEs are produced in limited quantities. Thus, solubility assays in discovery are routinely conducted using high-throughput methods for rank-ordering compounds, with the objective of identifying potential liabilities and validating hits with suitable apparent solubility. Solubility assays are often performed by diluting a highly concentrated DMSO stock solution into an aqueous solution; small aliquots of the DMSO solutions are incrementally added until precipitation occurs. As the content of organic solvent in the aqueous solution may affect compound solubility by changing the dielectric constant of the solution, it is desirable to maintain DMSO content to a minimum ($\leq$1%). Alternatively, in order to keep the DMSO content constant, a series of concentrations are prepared first in DMSO and then diluted in parallel into aqueous solutions to the same dilution ratio. Once precipitation has occurred and the target concentration has been reached, there are two common approaches to determine solubility: removing precipitates before measuring the concentration of compound in solution, or using the precipitates as an indication that a compound has reached the solubility limit. In the first approach, the precipitates are removed from the liquid phase by filtration, and then the concentration of the test compound in solution is measured in an ultraviolet (UV) plate reader or by liquid chromatography (LC)-UV or LC-mass spectrometry (MS) analysis. The second approach detects the formation of precipitates by measuring the light scattering signal using a nephelometric turbidity detector. Light scattering/turbidity solubility measurements are fast and economical but can be limited by interferences, impurities, particle size, and low sensitivity.[11] Kinetic solubility exhibits strong time dependence and, since it is commonly associated with supersaturation, it is typically higher than thermodynamic solubility.

In drug development, solubility measurements focus on the solid phase properties of active pharmaceutical ingredients, formulation development for clinical trials, and drug manufacturing strategies. Thermodynamic solubility is typically measured using the shake-flask method and often regarded as the gold standard for development needs. Because solubility is pH-dependent and the pH of the GI tract varies between regions, solubility values are typically determined at multiple pHs such as pH 1.2 (stomach), pH 6.5 (intestine), and pH 7.4 (blood). To measure the thermodynamic solubility, a solid drug substance is added, in excess, to a flask/vial containing an aqueous medium at an appropriate pH and the resulting suspension is incubated at 37 °C overnight or longer under shaking at a predetermined speed. Solubility samples are processed at one or several time points; residual solid is removed by filtration and drug concentration in the filtrate is determined by high-performance LC (HPLC) or LC-MS.[12,13] Bile salts increase solubility significantly for many drugs, especially lipophilic and basic compounds, where increases in solubility can be up to one or two orders of magnitude. Dissolution data obtained in simulated human intestinal fluids, especially for Class II drugs, provide a better correlation with *in vivo* oral drug absorption than data obtained using simple buffer solutions.[14] Potential food effects on solubility can be evaluated by determining solubility in fasted-state simulated intestinal fluid (FaSSIF) and fed-state simulated intestinal fluid (FeSSIF) solutions.[15]

2.1.3   Approaches to Increase Solubility

The solubility of a drug in solid state is primarily governed by two energy exchange events: (1) the energy required to extract molecules from the crystal lattice and bring them into solution; and (2) the energy generated from the interaction of solute and solvent molecules in solution. Drug molecules with strong intermolecular interactions in solid state and with low affinity for water (hydrophobic) tend to have low aqueous solubility. Therefore, aqueous solubility of poorly water-soluble drugs may be increased by weakening intermolecular interactions in solid state or enhancing drug–water interactions in solution. Intestinal drug absorption can be further enhanced by increasing the dissolution rate and inducing supersaturation.

In the solid state a compound can exist in multiple crystalline forms that differ only in the arrangement of drug molecules in the crystal lattice, a phenomenon known as polymorphism, and different crystalline forms of the same compound are described as polymorphs. Compounds that lack crystalline characteristics are referred to as amorphous. Molecular interactions within a crystal lattice include van der Waals forces, π–π stacking, electrostatic interactions, hydrogen bonding, and ionic interactions. The sum of the energies from all intermolecular interactions determines the total packing energy of a crystal or the crystal lattice energy. Stronger inter-molecular interactions minimize the mobility of the molecules within the crystal; high lattice energy increases the stability of a crystal, but decreases solubility and dissolution rate. The thermodynamic solubility of a compound is dictated by the most stable crystal form. By contrast, kinetic solubility depends on crystal forms, and different polymorphs of the same molecule can have different kinetic solubilities. Crystal modification can increase dissolution rate and kinetic solubility, but cannot change thermodynamic solubility; given sufficient time the undissolved solute will convert to the most stable polymorph and kinetic solubility will approach thermodynamic solubility. Therefore, dissolution rate and kinetic solubility can be improved by crystal engineering; however, improvement in thermodynamic solubility requires chemical modification of the structure of the drug molecule.

2.1.3.1   Chemical Structural Modification

One of the classical strategies for improving aqueous solubility through structural modifications by chemical means consists of incorporating hydrophilic group(s) into molecules of interest. However, this approach is not universally effective because the introduction of hydrophilic group(s) sometimes hinders the ability of the drug molecule to interact with the target protein. In addition, membrane permeability of small molecules is inversely related to hydrophilicity; highly hydrophilic compounds generally have low intestinal absorption unless uptake transporter(s) are involved.

A method recently used to increase solubility without a significant change in hydrophobicity consists of introducing inter-molecular forces between drug molecules by disrupting molecular planarity and symmetry.[16] The principle of this strategy is based on the fact that planar symmetric moieties of multiple conjugated aromatic structures favor the formation of tight crystal packing with strong π–π hydrophobic interactions and intermolecular hydrogen bonds. Disrupting molecular planarity/symmetry, in some cases, improved aqueous solubility several hundred-fold without increasing hydrophilicity.[16]

The use of prodrug strategies represents another approach to improving aqueous solubility.[17,18] For instance, phosphate ester prodrugs have been used to increase the oral bioavailability of poorly water-soluble drugs. Prodrugs are especially useful for drugs that require a high dose and exhibit dissolution rate limited absorption. In the GI tract, phosphate ester prodrugs are rapidly hydrolyzed to the parent drug by endogenous alkaline phosphatases at the apical (AP) surface of intestinal epithelial cells during the absorption phase, which results in a high concentration of the parent drug and low concentration of the prodrug in the systemic circulation. For instance, fosamprenavir, a phosphate ester prodrug of the HIV protease inhibitor amprenavir, showed improved water solubility and oral bioavailability compared with amprenavir.[19]

2.1.3.2 Solid State Engineering

Crystal engineering is a strategy for reducing the strength of the crystal lattice, and thus promoting solubility, dissolution rate, and absorption of poorly water-soluble drugs. In contrast to the stable crystal form, in which molecules have the maximum molecular interactions with adjacent molecules, high-energy polymorphs and amorphous forms have less than optimal intermolecular interactions. Since decreases in intermolecular attractive forces would inevitably lead to higher dissolution rates and higher apparent solubility, the initial drug concentrations of these metastable forms can be many times higher than that of the corresponding stable crystal, a phenomenon termed supersaturation. Drugs in a state of supersaturation are kinetically in solution at a concentration above their thermodynamic equilibrium solubility, and if the rate of recrystallization to the stable crystal is slow, relative to the GI transit time, or deliberately delayed, high initial drug concentrations may be sustained in the GI tract for a sufficient length of time to allow drug absorption across the intestinal mucosa. Several crystal structure techniques have been developed to enhance apparent solubility and, in turn, enhance oral absorption *in vivo*. Examples include the use of high-energy polymorphic and amorphous forms, particle salt formation, cocrystals, size reduction, and solid dispersion. In practice, the challenges of using high-energy polymorphs or amorphous forms are the long-term stability of formulated drugs and the stability of the supersaturated solution formed *in vivo*. Salt formation of weak acids or bases essentially converts neutral drug molecules into ionized species that have greater affinity for water, thus increases solubility by enhancing the degree of solvation. Counterions that are commonly used in pharmaceutical salt formation include sodium, potassium, and magnesium for acidic drugs, and chloride and maleate for basic drugs. Cocrystals improve solubility and dissolution by reducing the intermolecular interactions in the crystal lattice *via* complex formation between a drug and a water-soluble cocrystal former. Unlike the salt formation applied to weakly acidic or basic drugs, the cocrystal approach is more universal, not limited to ionizable drugs.

Particle size reduction increases the surface area of solid drugs available for solvation and thus enhances the rate of dissolution. Small particles can be produced by either crystallizing fine particles from supersaturated drug solution or fragmenting large particles *via* a milling process. Recent developments in sophisticated crystallization methods, and utilization of polymeric and surfactant stabilizers make it technically feasible to produce particles in the order of a few hundred nanometers. Nanoparticles comprise polymeric, liposomal, or solid lipid formulated nanoscale drug assemblies, and also include nanosized drug crystals and suspensions. Drug nanoparticles drastically increase the ratio of surface area to mass compared with simple drug powders, and have the potential to provide significant increases in the rate of dissolution. As a result, nanoparticles may also enhance oral bioavailability of poorly water-soluble drugs.

Solid dispersions increase drug dissolution and solubility *via* several mechanisms, including stabilization of the more soluble amorphous drug, reduction in effective particle size, improved wetting, and enhanced solubilization. The term solid dispersion refers to a range of solid products consisting of at least two different components, generally a hydrophobic drug dispersed within an inert hydrophilic carrier matrix. The carrier can exist in crystalline or amorphous form; typically water-soluble sugars, polymers, or surface active emulsifiers. Solid dispersions comprise a drug in either an amorphous or crystalline form dispersed in a carrier. In most cases, suspended drug particles have smaller sizes than traditional solid dosage forms, the reduction in particle size provides for an increase in effective surface area for dissolution. When exposed to aqueous media, the highly water-soluble carrier dissolves and the dispersed drug is released as fine colloidal particles. The enhanced surface area produces a higher dissolution rate that may lead to an increase in the bioavailability of poorly water-soluble drugs. The early generation of solid dispersions used low molecular weight, highly water-soluble carriers such as urea, sucrose, trehalose, sorbitol and mannitol, and the new generation of solid dispersions utilize polymeric carriers, including polyvinylpyrrolidone (PVP), polyethylene glycol (PEG), hydroxypropyl methylcellulose (HPMC), and surface-active excipients that promote emulsification of the formulation and solubilization of the dispersed drug. Despite the potential benefits of solid dispersions, they have only been used successfully in a few commercial products since the development of this technology several decades ago. This limited success reflects the difficulties associated with solid dispersions, including the complexities of preparation and manufacturing scale-up, the reproducibility of physicochemical characteristics, and the thermodynamic instability of drug and carrier in amorphous form. Common methods to manufacture solid dispersions include hot melting, solvent evaporation, supercritical antisolvent processing, electrospinning, and microwave irradiation. Among the various methods, the electrospinning technique holds particular potential for the preparation of solid dispersions and controlled release of biomedicines, as it is a simple and economical way to produce polymeric nanofibers.[20] In the preparation of solid dispersions by electrospinning, a charged drug–polymer melt or solution is passed through a nozzle and subjected to a high voltage to generate long nanofibers with uniform diameters (~100 nm) and high surface area to mass ratios.

2.1.3.3   *Solubilization Enhancement*

The solubility of poorly water-soluble substances may be enhanced by solubilization enhancement strategies, such as the uses of cosolvents, surfactants, cyclodextrins (CDs), and lipid based formulations.[21] Cosolvents are organic solvents that are miscible with and less polar than water. Cosolvents enhance the solubility of nonpolar drugs by lowering the polarity of the aqueous solution closer to the polarity of the drugs. Cosolvent formulations are used routinely at the preclinical stage for parenteral drug administration and are widely used in marketed parenteral products. Commonly used cosolvents include ethanol, propylene glycol, glycerol, dimethylacetamide (DMA), DMSO, and low molecular weight PEG. Cosolvents are also used in formulations for oral drug delivery, but normally as minor ingredients while other excipients play major roles in solubilization enhancement, and are often used in combination with other solubilization agents such as surfactants, CDs, and lipids. A caveat of using cosolvent formulations is a potential dilution effect. As cosolvents enhance aqueous solubility of drugs in a nonlinear fashion, a drug may be very soluble at higher concentrations of cosolvents, but poorly soluble at lower concentrations. Thus, once diluted with aqueous fluids (such as blood after intravenous administration), the solubilization power of cosolvents may decrease drastically, resulting in a nonlinear decrease in drug solubility, typically drug precipitation.

Surfactants are amphiphilic organic molecules, containing both hydrophilic (head) and hydrophobic (tail) groups. The hydrophobic tail groups of most surfactants are fairly similar, consisting of a hydrocarbon chain in various lengths. Surfactants are commonly classified according to the electrical composition of the hydrophilic head groups: nonionic, anionic, cationic, or zwitterionic. Nonionic surfactants, with no charge in the head group, are more commonly used in drug formulations owing to their better safety profile, superior capacity in solubilizing nonpolar drugs at lower concentrations, and compatibility with other pharmaceutical excipients. In the bulk aqueous solution surfactants form aggregates where the hydrophobic tails form the core of the aggregate and the hydrophilic heads remain in the water phase. Above a critical concentration, frequently referred to as the critical micelle concentration (CMC), the amphiphilic nature of surfactants promotes and facilitates the formation of micelles. Surfactants may act as detergents, wetting agents, emulsifiers, foaming agents, and dispersants. Surfactants are commonly used to enhance aqueous solubility of poorly water-soluble drugs, largely by incorporating drugs into the hydrophobic micelle core. Above the CMC, increasing the surfactant concentration leads to a linear increase in the solubility of poorly water-soluble drugs, thus creating a minimal dilution effect. In addition to the function of solubilizing drug molecules, several surfactants have been reported to inhibit efflux transporters including P-glycoprotein (P-gp), breast cancer resistance protein (BCRP), and MRP2,[22–24] thus having the potential to enhance the intestinal absorption and tumor cellular access of drugs that are substrates of efflux transporters.

The CDs are a family of compounds composed of sugar molecules joined together in a ring formation (cyclic oligosaccharides); naturally occurring CDs consist of six, seven, or eight dextrose units (α-, β- and γ-CDs, respectively). CD molecules have a torus macro-ring shape, like a truncated cone, with a hydrophobic inner cavity and a hydrophilic outer surface. CDs have utility for solubilizing and stabilizing a variety of drugs by forming inclusion complexes within the hydrophobic cavity; therefore, CDs have been extensively studied to improve drug properties, such as aqueous solubility, dissolution rate and oral bioavailability.[25] Although natural CDs are widely used for drug complexation, the relatively poor water solubility (19 mg mL^{-1} or less) of unmodified CDs limits their clinical use. Furthermore, α-CDs, β-CDs, and a number of alkylated CDs are known to be nephrotoxic.[26] In order to improve solubility and reduce nephrotoxicity, β-CD derivatives, such as hydroxypropyl-β-cyclodextrin (HP-β-CD) and sulfobutylether-β-cyclodextrin (SBE-β-CD), have been introduced. HP-β-CD and SBE-β-CD have significantly higher aqueous solubility and appear to be much safer than the parent β-CD. The toxicity of modified CDs appears to be similar to or lower than that of common surfactants or cosolvents, and is further reduced after oral administration as a result of the limited absorption of the vehicle. The ability of CDs to increase aqueous solubility of poorly water-soluble drugs may lead to improved oral bioavailability. For example, 20 mM HP-β-CD increased the solubility of diosgenin, a steroid saponin effective in treating hyperglycemia and hyperlipidemia, by more than 6000-fold (from 24 nM diosgenin alone to 144 μM diosgenin in HP-β-CD), and increased the oral bioavailability of diosgenin in rats by 11-fold (from 4.5% to 50%).[27] Unlike the nonlinear solubility issues associated with the use of cosolvents, CDs enhance drug solubility in a fairly linear fashion, similar to surfactants when concentrations are above CMC, and thus dilution of CD formulations is less problematic. CDs have been reported to enhance the stability of supersaturated drug solutions, suggesting that CDs are able to both promote the isolation of the amorphous form and stabilize the supersaturated solutions that form upon dissolution.[28] For instance, HP-β-CD has been used as a drug precipitation inhibitor to enhance the solubility and oral bioavailability of poorly water-soluble drugs.[29]

Lipid-based formulations incorporate poorly water-soluble drugs into inert lipid vehicles such as oils, surfactant dispersion, solid dispersions, solid lipid nanoparticles, emulsions, self-emulsifying formulations, and liposomes. Among the various approaches, self-emulsifying drug delivery systems (SEDDS) have gained much attention; the systems commonly include combinations of glyceride lipids, surfactants, and cosolvents, which spontaneously emulsify in contact with GI fluids. Lipid-based formulations may increase oral bioavailability *via* several mechanisms, such as enhancing dissolution rate and solubility, inducing supersaturation at the absorptive membrane, promoting intestinal lymphatic drug transport, and directly inhibiting intestinal efflux transporter systems.[30]

2.1.4 Role of Solubility in Drug Discovery

In the drug discovery stage, solubility plays crucial roles in bioassays as well as in studies of *in vitro* absorption, distribution, metabolism, excretion, and toxicity (ADMET). *In vitro* assays are conducted to evaluate biological properties with an assumption that a test compound is fully dissolved in solution under experimental conditions. Compounds with low solubility tend to give erratic or erroneous assay results, and usually result in artificially weak potency in high-throughput screening assays; thus, some compounds with therapeutic potential may fall through unnoticed. Conversely, cross-screens for off-target binding may show low hit rates; thus, compounds may be erroneously thought to have good selectivity, and be selected and advanced in discovery programs. Therefore, early solubility information helps identify potential issues in ADMET and bioassays, playing a critical role in lead compound selection. For *in vivo* animal studies, new drug candidates with low aqueous solubility present challenges for dose formulations, and possess the risk of precipitation after dosing, thus decreasing the reliability of measurements of pharmacokinetic or pharmacodynamic parameters, and potentially leading to adverse events. In *in vivo* toxicity studies, the quality of toxicological evaluation also could be compromised because higher doses are usually required to achieve higher exposure to assess drug safety. Overall, poor aqueous solubility is one of the major obstacles in the selection and development of highly potent therapeutics; therefore, NCE solubility should be determined in the early stages of the drug discovery process to assess if it is sufficient for the subsequent testing assays and the intended product profile.

2.1.5   Role of Solubility in Drug Development

Oral administration is the most common and preferable route of drug delivery in the market because it is more convenient than other routes of administration and this leads to better patient compliance. Factors that influence the extent of systemic absorption after oral administration include solubility, dissolution rate, GI stability, membrane permeability, pre-systemic metabolism, and drug transporters. Solubility is an important parameter for oral absorption because compounds with low aqueous solubility are often associated with poor oral absorption. In addition, they are more susceptible to food effects and tend to exhibit large inter-subject variability in oral bioavailability. Solubility not only affects oral absorption by the means of dissolved molecules available for intestinal absorption, but also dictates the dissolution rate by the balance between intermolecular interactions in solid form and solution. Drugs in formulations with slow dissolution rates might not be fully dissolved during the period of intestinal absorption (1.5–4 hours post-dosing depending on the species), thus resulting in only a fraction of the total drug available for absorption. Therefore, improved solubility can help enhance the oral absorption of dissolution rate-limited compounds. This implies that technologies that increase solubility can be beneficial for the development of Class II (low solubility, high permeability) compounds. Early formulation development of poorly water-soluble compounds is essential to facilitate *in vivo* pharmacokinetics, efficacy, and toxicity studies.

   Although solubility data in simple buffer are heavily used at the drug discovery stage, solubility measurements in biologically relevant media, such as FaSSIF, FeSSIF, and fasted-state simulated gastric fluid (FaSSGF), are more useful in establishing *in vitro–in vivo* correlation (IVIVC). FaSSIF, FeSSIF, and FaSSGF mimic the human intestinal fluids before and after a meal, and gastric content in an empty stomach, respectively. These media have been developed by taking into consideration vital properties of GI fluids such as pH, osmolality, presence of bile, buffer capacity, and surface tension; they contain bile salts, phospholipids, and physiologically relevant surfactants, thus representing the conditions in the small intestine and stomach more accurately. For example, one study showed that the prediction of *in vivo* performance using *in vitro* solubility data obtained in aqueous buffer tends to underestimate the true absorption of low solubility compounds compared with solubility data in simulated intestinal fluids.[14] Compounds with high permeability/lipophilicity and low solubility (*i.e.*, Class II) tend to undergo positive food effects, whereas compounds with low permeability and high solubility (*i.e.*, Class III) often show negative food effects.[31] Food effects can be the result of several factors such as delayed gastric emptying, increased gastric pH, drug solubilization by food components (*e.g.*, fats), slower input into the intestine, stimulation of bile salt secretion, increased blood flow, and competition for metabolizing enzymes. Solubility measured in FaSSIF and FeSSIF may help predict food effects *in vivo*; and accordingly, formulations may be developed to minimize food effects and inter-individual variability of systemic exposure.

In addition, it would be beneficial for the overall discovery and development process if formulations used in preclinical PK studies could be translated to the development of clinical dosage forms, with minimal modifications. Thus, for the development of potential clinical dosage forms, solubility and dissolution should be evaluated in various candidate formulations to identify the best possible approach(es). This evaluation includes aqueous solubility in multiple pH buffers and solubility in various excipients, such as cosolvents, CDs, surfactants, and lipids. For some projects, special techniques can be used to formulate insoluble compounds depending on their physicochemical properties. Amorphous solid forms, cocrystals, solid dispersions, SEDDS, micronization, and nanoparticle approaches are examples of these techniques.

Under certain conditions, *in vitro* solubility studies can be used to support requests to the US Food and Drug Administration (FDA) to waiver *in vivo* bioavailability and/or bioequivalence studies (biowaivers). The BCS, described in the 'Guideline for Industry' by the FDA, is a framework for classifying drug substances according to their aqueous solubility and intestinal permeability. Exemption from clinical bioequivalence studies can be requested for highly soluble and highly permeable (*i.e.*, Class I) drug substances in immediate-release solid oral dosage forms. As indicated in the current guidelines of the FDA, a drug substance is considered highly soluble when the highest dose strength is completely soluble in 250 mL or less of aqueous medium throughout the pH range of 1–7.5. A drug substance is considered highly permeable when the extent of absorption in humans is determined to be at least 90% of the administered dose. Alternatively, *in vitro* systems capable of predicting the extent of drug absorption in humans can be used (*e.g.*, human colon carcinoma-derived Caco-2 cells) to determine drug permeability class. If a product meets the criteria for solubility, *in vitro* permeability, *in vitro* dissolution profile, stability in the GI tract, quality of excipients, and therapeutic range, among others, it is considered bioequivalent to the reference product and can be exempted from the requirement to conduct human pharmacokinetic studies. It is expected that in the new guidelines, BCS biowaivers will be extended to Class III drugs, thus increasing the importance of solubility and permeability determination in late discovery or early drug development.

2.2   Permeability

2.2.1   Introduction

For orally administered drugs, a number of events take place during intestinal drug absorption. First of all, drug products need to disintegrate and dissolve in the GI tract, and then drug molecules need to permeate the cellular wall of the GI tract. It is also possible for the drug to undergo metabolism not only as it crosses the intestinal epithelium but also during the first pass through the liver. In the phase of discovery of NCEs intended for the oral route of administration, drug candidates must exhibit, in addition to sufficient solubility and suitable permeability, other "drug-like" properties such as adequate metabolic stability and lack of toxicity. Because NCEs with "drug-like" properties have a much greater potential of being developed as drugs, these properties are often assessed, using *in vitro* assays, early in the discovery phase. *In vitro* permeability assays have been widely used in pharmaceutical research. Some of the applications include qualitative prediction (*e.g.*, ranking order) of oral absorption potential, determination of mechanism(s) of transport, evaluation of pH effect on drug absorption, and assessment of the effect of excipients on drug permeability. Drug permeability, which is correlated with the rate of drug absorption, is one of the most important factors considered in drug discovery and development.

2.2.2   Methodology for Measuring Permeability

The ideal *in vitro* absorption model should closely mimic the physical and biochemical qualities of the intestinal epithelial barrier. Various systems have been developed that successfully recapitulate the relevant barrier properties of the intestinal mucosa. The techniques established to study intestinal permeability range in complexity, reliability, and physiological relevance.

2.2.2.1   Intestinal Models

This description of intestinal models will focus on perfused intestinal segments and excised intestinal mucosa (stripped or unstripped). The general approach used in experiments with perfused intestinal segments consists of applying a dosing solution of the compound to the mucosal side of the intestine and then measuring the disappearance of the drug from the dosing solution or its appearance on the serosal side to determine the rate of absorption. In the case of the excised tissues, a segment of intestine is opened and the ensuing sheet of intestinal mucosa, sometimes stripped from the underlying muscle layer, is mounted between the two halves of an Ussing chamber. The compound is applied, in solution, to one side and the rate of permeation is used to predict the absorption potential of the compound. An important difference between perfused intestinal segments and excised intestinal mucosa is that, in the case of the former, absorption rate is determined based on compound disappearance from the lumenal buffer solution, while with excised intestinal mucosa, permeability is calculated from the actual amount of compound that reaches the receiver chamber, after traversing the isolated intestinal mucosa. Together, perfused intestinal segments and excised intestinal mucosa have three clear advantages over other *in vitro* models: (a) they preserve the architectural integrity of the intestinal mucosa; (b) they can be used to determine absorption across different GI regions; and (c) they facilitate the comparison of intestinal permeability across different species.

2.2.2.2   Perfused Intestinal Segment

The perfused intestinal segment technique allows the measurement of the apparent permeability coefficient (P_{app}) in viable tissue under conditions that mimic the *in vivo* environment. One advantage of perfused intestinal loops over *in vivo* drug absorption models is that the technique can be applied to the study of segmental differences in drug absorption and metabolism without interference from physiological factors, such as gastric emptying and/or small intestinal transit time. There are two major drawbacks of this model compared with *in vitro* systems: first is the skills and time required in the surgical preparation of the model, and lengthy preparation precludes its use for large numbers of compounds; and second is that it requires relatively large amounts of compound. In early drug discovery, and even during the lead optimization phase, medicinal chemists commonly produce large numbers of compounds in small quantities rather than fewer compounds in large quantities. This is understandable because, before a drug candidate is selected it is preferable to run a few key screening tests on a larger number of analogs than running many tests on a few analogs. This strategy implies that as the funnel of chemical diversity is narrowed based on the results of current tests, in subsequent phases smaller numbers of analogs are synthesized in larger quantities as they show promising properties. Since the normal length of the intestinal segment used in perfusion experiments is 5–10 cm, the number of replicates that can be obtained from a rat is very limited. Unlike cell models, where the difference in permeability coefficient values between well-absorbed and poorly absorbed compounds are substantial, the dynamic range for permeability values in the perfused rat intestine model is fairly narrow.[32] This limitation not only increases uncertainty in the estimation of absorption potential, but also makes attempts to rank order permeability not very reliable.

As is the case with other *in situ* preparations, the viability of perfused intestinal segments must be monitored closely. As a result of these limitations, this technique is not widely used as a screening tool; instead, it is more valuable in drug formulation development, because of its greater adaptability than cellular or artificial systems for screening drug formulations, and in biopharmaceutical investigation. For example, it may be useful to investigate the absorption of drugs whose poor solubility requires the use of complex dosing vehicles, that can not be presented to other *in vitro* systems, such as culture cells, which tend to be very sensitive to organic solvents and formulations.[33]

2.2.2.3   Intestinal Mucosa Mounted on Ussing Chambers

The Ussing chamber technique is based on the excision of intestinal segments, which are cut open to make a flat sheet, whose muscle layer may be stripped or not, and then it is mounted on Ussing chambers. Two major concerns with this technique are the need to ensure that the receiver concentration of the compound does not exceed 10% of the donor concentration, to maintain sink conditions, and that proper oxygenation is achieved. The tissue is oxygenated by infusing a mixture of air/CO_2 (95%/5%) into buffer solutions and using this to bathe both sides of the tissue. This gas infusion not only oxygenates the tissue but also mixes the buffer solutions to homogenize the concentration of drug in the bulk phase of the chamber solution and decrease the unstirred thickness of the aqueous boundary layer adjacent to the tissue.

Since the viability and integrity of the tissue segments are critical to ensure the validity of the data, it essential to closely monitor the viability of the tissue segment during the course of the assay. Often tissue viability is verified based on the potential difference, short circuit current, and the value of transepithelial electrical resistance (TEER).[34] Tissue viability may also be verified by measuring the permeation rate of marker compounds that are known to cross the intestinal epithelial mucosa through passive paracellular diffusion. Examples of compounds commonly used for monitoring tissue integrity are mannitol, Lucifer yellow, and fluorescein 4000.[35,36]

2.2.2.4   Artificial Membranes

Parallel artificial membrane permeation assay (PAMPA) is a method used to measure the permeation of a compound through both a lipid-infused artificial membrane and an aqueous layer, in parallel.[37] The general experimental setting is as follows: a hydrophobic multiwell filter is placed on a microtiter plate containing buffer solution. Half of the wells in the filter are coated with mixtures of lecithin/phospholipids that are supposed to mimic the lipid bilayer of the intestinal cell membrane and the other half are coated with buffer, and the receiver compartments for all of the wells contain buffer only. At the beginning of the test, drug solution is added to the donor compartment, and the receiver compartment is drug free. After an incubation period, which may involve stirring, the filter is removed and the amount of drug is measured in each compartment. Mass balance allows calculation of the amount of drug that remains in the membrane.

Early models utilized iso-pH conditions in the compartments separated by a simple lipid membrane; subsequent products incorporate more sophisticated lipid membranes.[37] To date, PAMPA models have been reported to exhibit a good correlation with permeation across a variety of barriers, including Caco-2 monolayers,[38] the GI tract,[39] and the blood–brain barrier.[40] The popularity of PAMPA for early stage compound screening is due to the fact that the assay is run in microtiter plates, which achieve higher speeds than cell-based permeability assays at a relatively low cost per sample; desirable characteristics for pharmaceutical companies attempting to streamline operations as much as possible to contain costs. The major drawback of the PAMPA model is that it does not take into account transporter systems, drug metabolizing enzymes, and the potential role of the paracellular pathway, which is believed to be important for the intestinal absorption of small molecular weight, hydrophilic drugs such as ranitidine and atenolol.[41] In addition, the donor and/or receiver compartments may contain solubilizing agents, or additives that bind the drugs as they permeate.

2.2.2.5   Cell-Based Permeability Assays

Since the characterization of the Caco-2 cell line as an *in vitro* intestinal permeability model in 1989,[42] many different cell lines have been used to study various aspects of intestinal permeability. Cell-based permeability models have become critical tools in the current drug discovery paradigm within the pharmaceutical industry and academia.[43]

In principle, the study of intestinal drug absorption using cell-based methods involves several steps. First, the cells are grown on a microporous filter until they form monolayers that mimic, morphologically and functionally, the intestinal epithelial mucosa, a process that under standard culture conditions takes approximately 3 weeks.[43] Second, the monolayer is placed between the AP and basolateral (BL) chambers of a bi-chamber diffusion apparatus that represent the mucosal (lumen) and serosal (blood) surfaces of the intestine, respectively. Third, test compounds, in solution, are added to the AP or BL chamber, and their appearance on the opposite side is measured over time. Appearance in the BL chamber after AP dosing is indicative of absorption whereas appearance in the AP chamber after BL application reflects AP secretion, or efflux. The quantity of compound that reaches the receiver chamber, normalized to the filter surface area per time unit is known as flux. The P_{app} is obtained by dividing the flux by the initial drug concentration in the donor chamber. The directionality of transport provides insight into the potential absorption of a compound and the underlying processes that impact its overall transepithelial transport. For example, if the P_{app}(AP to BL) is greater than a value selected as the threshold for complete absorption, the compound might have a high absorption potential in humans; however, it is important to keep in mind that this threshold value exhibits large inter-laboratory variability.[44] Moreover, a P_{app}(BL to AP):P_{app}(AP to BL) ratio, known as the efflux ratio (ER), greater than 1 indicates that the compound undergoes net secretion, and an ER smaller than 1 reflects net absorption. Although, by definition, ER > 1 and <1 are both consistent with the involvement of a transport system (or systems) in the permeability of a test compound, in some practical situations the blind implementation of this definition can cause an undue amount of unnecessary work. For example, the FDA guidelines for drug–drug interactions (DDIs) state that an ER ≥ 2 can be considered a true indication of efflux. Although this is perfectly understandable for *in vitro* DDIs that will be used to make critical decisions about clinical DDIs, the application of this criterion to a discovery program, where scientists need to work with many compounds, often using simplified study protocols, would result in a large number of false positives. In the context of a drug discovery program, it may be more useful to set a higher threshold ER (*e.g.*, ≥3), as more definitive tests downstream will confirm or reject the preliminary classification. Due to the fact that cell-based models can provide a reliable prediction of absorption potential with a relatively low cost (compared with intestinal tissue preparations), and that they also maintain partially or complete functional systems of transporters/enzymes, which the artificial membrane systems lack entirely, cell models have become an essential tool for pharmaceutical scientists working on intestinal absorption. Various applications of cell-based systems are discussed below.

2.2.3 Applications of Cell-Based Models in Drug Discovery

2.2.3.1 *Absorption Prediction and BCS*

It is important to demonstrate a reliable correlation between *in vitro* permeability systems and drug absorption *in vivo* because the intended use of *in vitro* models is to predict *in vivo* (preferably in human) outcomes. The FDA has issued guidelines under which pharmaceutical companies can request a waiver from bioequivalence studies based on the BCS.[3] Two basic conclusions presented in the original study that led to the development of the BCS guidelines constitute the philosophical premises of the BCS:

(a) If two drug products, containing the same drug, have the same concentration–time profile at the intestinal membrane surface, then they will have the same rate and extent of absorption.

(b) If two drug products have the same *in vitro* dissolution profile under all luminal conditions, they will have the same rate and extent of drug absorption.

The difference in pH values along the GI tract may lead to variability in permeability values for drugs that exhibit pH-dependent solubility, because the pH can have an effect both in dissolution rate and permeability, but it should be kept in mind that the pH relevant to drug absorption is the pH in the local intestinal environment (*i.e.*, where absorption occurs). The FDA guidelines also list various *in vitro* methods acceptable for determining the permeability class of a drug substance. Among these, monolayers of cultured epithelial cells, across which drug transport can be measured, constitute the most employed systems. Specifically, the epithelial cell line most commonly used as a model system of intestinal permeability is Caco-2. However, as a result of large inter-laboratory variability in permeability results, the FDA guidelines indicate that cell monolayer transport assays must be validated in each individual laboratory before they can be used to determine the *in vitro* permeability class of drugs. The validation should include the establishment of a correlation between the rank order of the permeability values obtained from the test method and the extent of absorption in humans using a sufficient number of compounds spanning a relevant range of reported human fractional absorption. Based on the results obtained in our laboratory, the Caco-2 cell monolayer permeability method accurately identified all twenty-three tested compounds as having either low or high permeability (internal data).

Not only is there a correlation between the permeability coefficient of a drug and its reported fraction absorbed in humans, but a quick examination of the set of compounds used to validate the system revealed a clear separation between the permeability coefficients of high and low permeability compounds. Compounds with a P_{app} greater than 2×10^{-6} cm s^{-1} always had a high fraction absorbed (>90%) in humans, and compounds that exhibited low absorption in humans invariably had P_{app} values less than 1×10^{-6} cm s^{-1}, showing a wide separation between the two groups of compounds (unpublished data).

It is worth mentioning that for a number of these compounds, including fluvastatin, labetalol, pindolol, and timolol, the P_{app} values were pH dependent, most likely due to their different degrees of ionization at the two experimental pHs. To minimize the occurrence of false negatives (*i.e.*, that a compound with high permeability will be classified as poorly permeable), it is preferable to run the assay using two different AP pHs (*i.e.*, 6.5 and 7.4) to simulate the dynamic pH conditions in the intestinal luminal environment.

In addition, common practice when conducting a BCS assay with Caco-2 cells is to determine the directional (AP to BL) permeability of the test compound together with a low and high permeability control compound in the same cell monolayer. The purpose of the low permeability control compound is to verify the integrity of the cell monolayers. Thus, if the P_{app} value of the test compound is higher than that of the high permeability control compound, and the P_{app} of the low permeability marker is below an accepted threshold, it can be concluded that the intestinal permeation will not be an absorption rate limiting step, and that the fraction of the compound absorbed in humans should be nearly complete. As the BCS classification of the test compound is based on the comparison of its P_{app} value to that of the control compound, the selection of a suitable high permeability reference compound is of critical importance.

2.2.3.2 DDI Studies

Since efflux transporters expressed in the intestinal mucosa can attenuate drug absorption and transporters located on the bile canaliculi membrane can mediate the biliary excretion of drugs, the understanding of systemic drug absorption is incomplete without a thorough evaluation of the potential of drug candidates to interact with intestinal and hepatic membrane transporters. The specific impact of transporters in systemic drug absorption will depend on the level of expression, directionality of transport and anatomical location. The FDA requires data on potential interactions of NCEs with at least seven transporters (P-gp, BCRP, OATP1B1, OATP1B3, OAT1, OAT3, and OCT2) that have been shown to influence systemic drug absorption.[45] The European Medicines Agency (EMA) requires data on these seven plus two additional (OCT1 and Bsep) transporters.[46]

Although, understandably, the interest of regulatory agencies in these transporters stems from the potential risk to patients from transporter-mediated DDIs, other transporters [*e.g.*, peptide transporter 1 (PepT1), OATP2B1, and MCT1] have the potential to be exploited as delivery mechanisms for compounds that, due to their unfavorable physicochemical properties, would not be able to cross the cell membrane by simple diffusion, and thus are unsuitable for oral administration.[47,48]

The small intestinal mucosa expresses a large number of absorption transporters, which are responsible for the absorption of nutrients and vitamins. These transporters have been shown to mediate the absorption of nutrients, vitamins, and some drugs. Membrane transporters can play an important role in pharmacokinetics and drug exposure. To date, the vast majority of the well-known transporters belong to one of two superfamilies: ATP-binding cassette (ABC) and solute carrier (SLC). Multidrug resistance efflux transporters such as P-gp (or MDR1)[49] and BCRP[50] are members of the ABC transporter family, whereas PepT1[51] and organic anion transporting polypeptides (OATPs)[52] are members of the SLC family. These transporters regulate the transfer of solutes (*e.g.*, drugs and other xenobiotics) in and out of cells, are present in various tissues in the body, and are involved in drug absorption, distribution, tissue-specific accumulation, and elimination. Since the expression and function of some transporters in cells can be determined, and this information helps to predict drug absorption, cell-based models are widely regarded as valuable *in vitro* tools for investigating transporter-mediated DDIs.

Due to their participation in the active extrusion of numerous anti-cancer drugs out of cells, the ABC transporters were initially recognized for their role in chemotherapeutic resistance to cancer treatments. Many human cancers, particularly carcinomas, over-express P-gp, and as a result, exhibit resistance to chemotherapy.[53] Subsequent studies demonstrated that P-gp is not only present in tumors but is also widely distributed in normal human tissues, including the AP surfaces of epithelial cells of the liver, jejunum, colon, kidney, adrenal, and pancreas.[54] Additionally, P-gp is localized to the blood–brain barrier and other blood–tissue barriers such as the testes, skin, and placenta.[55,56] Although P-gp substrates are structurally diverse, they share certain physicochemical characteristics. For example, most P-gp substrates are lipophilic and, generally, either organic cations or neutral compounds with aromatic rings. In addition, P-gp substrates[57] not only include xenobiotics but also endogenous compounds.[58] Because of its well established pharmacokinetic significance, as indicated by its role in the excretion of xenobiotics (such as drugs and their metabolites) into urine, bile, and the lumen of the GI tract, the testing of potential DDIs of NCEs at the level of P-gp and other transporters continues to be recommended by regulatory authorities (the FDA and the EMA).

The FDA guidance on drug interaction studies lists bidirectional assays in Caco-2 cells or over-expressed cell lines (the most common being MDR1-transfected MDCK cells) as the preferred method for *in vitro* evaluation of the P-gp substrate potential of test compounds (Figure 2.2).[45] The ability of the efflux transporter P-gp to cause a substantial decrease in the absorptive flux of a prototypical P-gp substrate (*e.g.*, digoxin) demonstrates the potential impact of efflux transporters in drug absorption (Figure 2.3).

Despite great advances in transporter research in the last decade, the full potential impact on drug absorption of known transporters, and others not yet known, remains to be established. For example, SLCs mediate uptake processes and can increase intestinal drug absorption. This is the case for

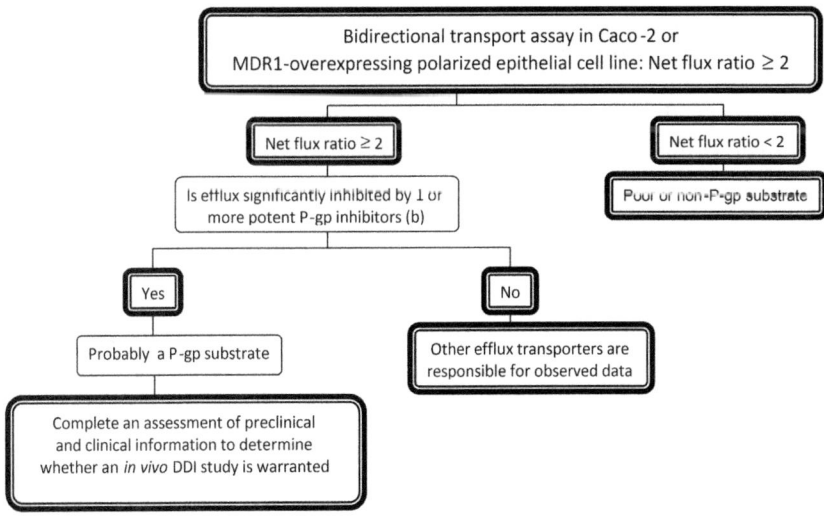

Figure 2.2   Decision tree to assess P-gp substrate potential. Reproduced with permission from Macmillan Publishers Ltd., Nature Publishing Group, K. M. Giacomini, S.-M. Huang, D. J. Tweedle, L. Z. Benet and K. L.R. Brouwer *et al.*, Membrane Transporters in Drug Development, *Nat. Rev. Drug Discovery*, 2010, **9**(3).

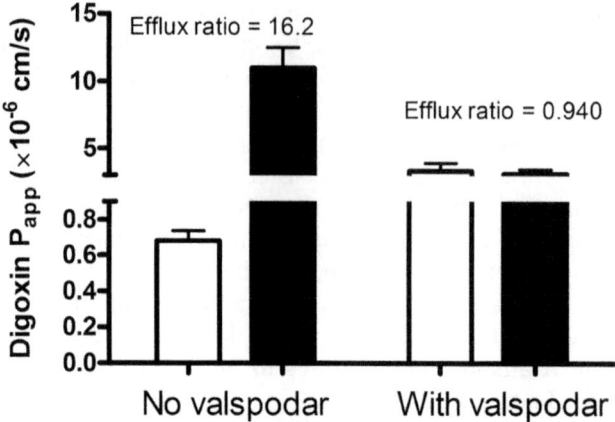

Figure 2.3   Bidirectional transport of digoxin (10 μM) in Caco-2 cell monolayers in the absence and presence of the P-gp inhibitor valspodar (1 μM). $N = 3$. Open bar: AP to BL; filled bar: BL to AP.

PepT1, which is involved in the transport of peptidomimetic drugs such as angiotensin converting enzyme inhibitors,[59] β-lactam antibiotics,[60] and renin inhibitors.[61] Thus, NCEs that are substrates for uptake transporters can achieve intestinal absorption higher than expected from their diffusion across cell membranes.

Although numerous studies have found a correlation between *in vitro* permeability and *in vivo* absorption, comparison of data from different laboratories is hampered by large inter-laboratory variability in P_{app} values. Such variability constitutes a challenge when data from multiple laboratories are pooled with the hope of increasing the size of databases from which models for *in silico* prediction of permeability or absorption potential could be developed. The combination of data obtained under different conditions in various laboratories, or resulting from high-throughput permeability screening, will most likely exhibit too much variability to be useful in trying to develop mathematical models truly predictive of intestinal absorption. Thus, in the absence of serious efforts either to normalize P_{app} values from different laboratories or to generate large databases within a single laboratory or a small group of laboratories that used the same cells and carefully standardized experimental protocols, the utility of *in silico* permeability or absorption models is likely to remain limited to small series of structurally related or carefully chosen compounds.

Such inter-laboratory variability has been widely recognized, and in some cases evaluated, by academia and industry scientists alike, yet efforts to harmonize procedures have not been undertaken. The pharmaceutical community would benefit greatly if laboratories made a serious attempt to harmonize their systems and procedures and establish consistent quality control criteria to help optimize the utility of these *in vitro* models and enhance the potential to predict pharmacokinetic performance.

Following oral drug administration, several events take place, some of them occur concomitantly and others sequentially. Thus, to enhance the probability of predicting human outcomes after oral drug administration, the various underlying processes (*i.e.*, dosage form and drug substance related) that influence drug dosage performance should be taken into account. Recently, some efforts have been made to modify *in vitro* assays with the aim of improving their correlation with *in vivo* outcomes. For instance, an experimental device that integrates drug dissolution and permeability assays *in vitro* has been introduced.[62] The attractiveness of the system is that it permits the evaluation of dissolution and permeability in the same experiment. The option to apply the drug or solid material *via* a macerated tablet or capsule directly into the mucosal chamber better re-creates the relationship between dissolution and permeation that occurs in the GI tract. Thus, by mimicking the *in vivo* drug absorption process, the drug reaching the BL chamber, which represents the total output of the dissolution and permeation processes, is expected to correlate with the fraction absorbed in humans. It has been proposed that this system is useful for the rapid evaluation of drug formulations during the development/optimization of novel formulations and for the evaluation of food effects on Class II drugs.[63] It is also easy to see how this approach could be used to optimize excipients for Class I and III drugs on the basis of the effect of excipients on the barrier properties of the monolayers.

The development of better IVIVC in oral drug absorption is of great interest because IVIVC can help streamline the drug development process and enhance the probability of success in the development of both innovator and generic drug products. However, due to the complexity of the processes involved in GI drug absorption, it is extremely challenging to achieve a perfect simulation of the *in vivo* absorption conditions in *in vitro* studies. The approaches described in the current chapter each have strengths and limitations and there is no substitute for the requirement that researchers should have a sound understanding of the purpose of the study and select or tailor the most effective approach(es) accordingly.

2.3 Absorption

Intestinal absorption is critical for the success of orally administered drugs, but it is very difficult to determine on a routine basis. Plasma drug concentrations alone cannot be used to calculate drug absorption unless it is known that the compounds does not undergo metabolism. Thus, it is necessary to administer radiolabeled drug, with the resulting plasma samples twice; total drug (unchanged + metabolites) is determined based on radioactivity counts, and unchanged drug must be analyzed by specific methods (*e.g.*, LC-MS or HPLC). Due to the need to synthesize radiolabeled material, which can be costly and time consuming, this type of evaluation is only done when a compound has been or is close to being selected as a drug candidate. Besides the synthesis of the radioactive drug, these studies also present several potential complications. For example, some drugs can undergo systemic absorption but can be secreted (from the systemic circulation) across the intestinal mucosa, and into the intestinal lumen or undergo enterohepatic recirculation. Since both of these processes involve membrane transporters, they are saturable, and the ensuing pharmacokinetics are dose dependent, the compound would have to be administered at a physiologically relevant dose to obtain a real insight into its *in vivo* absorption; however, this information is not available until the compound is in preclinical development. As a consequence of this difficulty, lead compounds are optimized for other endpoints, generally for biological activity with minimal information on absorption. Often *in vivo* pharmacological activity in an animal model is used as a surrogate of absorption, although it is known that: (a) absorption is different from bioavailability; and (b) the pharmacological activity may be elicited by a metabolite, which may not be produced in humans, rather than the parent compound.

Therefore, it is of great interest to assess the absorption potential of drug candidates during the initial life of discovery programs to ensure that absorption information is considered before synthesizing the next wave of analogs. Because of the serious limitations in trying to determine drug absorption *in vivo*, it is obvious that actionable absorption information in drug discovery will only be attainable through the use of simpler (*e.g.*, *in silico* or *in vitro*) tools. The approaches used to estimate oral absorption potential range from a simple calculation based on Lipinski's rule of 5 to perfused intestine,[64] some of which were discussed in previous sections.

One situation that limits the utility of *in vitro* measurements for the prediction of drug absorption is the lack of integration of the data. Identification of the permeability class of a drug candidate may be useful to design formulation development strategies; however, it would be much more useful if *in vitro* measurements could predict the comparative absorption of a drug following its administration in real dosage forms (tablet A *vs.* tablet B) containing different formulations. A recently characterized system, *In vitro* Dissolution Absorption System (IDAS), derived from a previously developed device,[62] permits the measurement of the dissolution and permeability of drug excipients applied in powder form to a modified Ussing chamber. Although in the initial studies we evaluated the dissolution and permeability of macerated tablets, an obvious application is to optimize the combination of excipients for a new formulation. Compounds from BCS Class I, II, and III were evaluated. There was a correlation between results in IDAS *versus* the fraction absorbed in humans (Table 2.1). For well-absorbed (≥80%) compounds at least 5% of the dose permeated to the receiver compartment in 2 h whereas for poorly absorbed (≤50%) compounds the fraction of dose that permeated in 2 h was less than 0.5%, a clear 10-fold separation. In addition, the simultaneous determination of dissolution and permeability showed that in the case of albendazole the poor absorption was due to low solubility, while in the cases of atenolol and ranitidine it was due to poor permeability.

Table 2.1   Potential utility of IDAS's drug dissolution and permeability data in predicting absorption in humans.

Clinical drugs	BCS class	Clinical dose (mg)	Applied dose (mg)	% Dissolved (in 2 h)	% Permeated (in 2 h)	% Absorbed in humans[a]
Albendazole	II	200	2.0	0.45	0.42	20
Amlodipine	I/III	5	0.05	100	6.78	64–90
Atenolol	III	50	0.5	100	0.23	50
Carbamazepine	II	100	1.0	86.1	10.2	83
Chlorpheniramine	I	6	0.06	100	5.49	80
Ketoprofen	II	50	0.5	98.2	22.8	85
Piroxicam	II	10	0.1	90	26.9	95
Propranolol	I	10	0.1	100	5.97	95
Ranitidine	III	150	1.5	100	0.15	50
Simvastatin	II	10	0.1	46.2	11.0	60–85
Warfarin	II	5	0.05	100	27.5	93.5

[a]Values obtained from ref. 62 or *Goodman & Gilman's the Pharmacological Basis of Therapeutics* (12th edn).

2.4   Closing Remarks

The oral route is the most convenient mode of drug administration and thus shows the highest patient compliance. Given the importance of solubility and permeability for drug absorption, several techniques have been developed to determine these parameters during the discovery and development phases. Although the methods used to measure solubility (*in vitro* or *in silico*) are fairly well established, the techniques used to determined permeability are not only numerous (*in silico*, artificial membranes, cell based, Ussing chamber, and perfused intestinal segments), but also exhibit a large degree of variability in how they are executed in different laboratories. Owing to the complexity of the mechanisms involved in intestinal drug absorption, computational methods are needed to integrate and analyze the various types of *in vitro* data, taking into account relevant cellular, kinetic and physiologic factors, to successfully predict *in vivo* drug absorption. A recent study used data from a carefully controlled protocol to develop cellular kinetics models to elucidate the mechanism of AP efflux transport and predict intracellular free drug concentration.[65] This strategy would greatly benefit from relatively large quantities of data generated under similar conditions to reduce variability. Such data can only be produced if there is a concerted effort to optimize and standardize the protocols used. Unfortunately, this task will not be easy because, although the merits are easily appreciated, in many discovery programs solubility and permeability data are produced using protocols optimized for speed and automation convenience, and not necessarily considering biological relevance.

References

1. G. L. Amidon, H. Lennernas, V. P. Shah and J. R. Crison, *Pharm. Res.*, 1995, **12**, 413–420.
2. R. Lobenberg and G. L. Amidon, *Eur. J. Pharm. Biopharm.*, 2000, **50**, 3–12.
3. US Department of Health and Human Services, Food and Drug Administration and Center of Drug Evaluation and Research (CDER), US FDA website, 2000, http://www.fda.gov/downloads/Drugs/.../Guidances/ucm070246.pdf.
4. C. A. Lipinski, *J. Pharmacol. Toxicol. Methods*, 2000, **44**, 235–249.
5. L. Di, E. H. Kerns and G. T. Carter, *Curr. Pharm. Des.*, 2009, **15**, 2184–2194.
6. S. Stegemann, F. Leveiller, D. Franchi, H. de Jong and H. Linden, *Eur. J. Pharm. Sci.*, 2007, **31**, 249–261.
7. C. A. Lipinski, F. Lombardo, B. W. Dominy and P. J. Feeney, *Adv. Drug Delivery Rev.*, 2001, **46**, 3–26.
8. J. M. Miller, A. Dahan, D. Gupta, S. Varghese and G. L. Amidon, *Mol. Pharm.*, 2010, **7**, 1223–1234.
9. B. J. Aungst, *AAPS J.*, 2012, **14**, 10–18.
10. S. N. Bhattachar, L. A. Deschenes and J. A. Wesley, *Drug Discovery Today*, 2006, **11**, 1012–1018.
11. L. Di, P. V. Fish and T. Mano, *Drug Discovery Today*, 2012, **17**, 486–495.
12. S. Nakashima, K. Yamamoto, Y. Arai and Y. Ikeda, *Chem. Pharm. Bull.*, 2013, **61**, 1228–1238.
13. A. Glomme, J. Marz and J. B. Dressman, *J. Pharm. Sci.*, 2005, **94**, 1–16.
14. E. Galia, E. Nicolaides, D. Horter, R. Lobenberg, C. Reppas and J. B. Dressman, *Pharm. Res.*, 1998, **15**, 698–705.
15. H. M. Jones, N. Parrott, G. Ohlenbusch and T. Lave, *Clin. Pharmacokinet.*, 2006, **45**, 1213–1226.
16. M. Ishikawa and Y. Hashimoto, *J. Med. Chem.*, 2011, **54**, 1539–1554.
17. V. J. Stella and K. W. Nti-Addae, *Adv. Drug Delivery Rev.*, 2007, **59**, 677–694.
18. J. Rautio, H. Kumpulainen, T. Heimbach, R. Oliyai, D. Oh, T. Jarvinen and J. Savolainen, *Nat. Rev. Drug Discovery*, 2008, **7**, 255–270.
19. M. B. Wire, M. J. Shelton and S. Studenberg, *Clin. Pharmacokinet.*, 2006, **45**, 137–168.
20. G. Yang, J. Wang, L. Li, S. Ding and S. Zhou, *Macromol. Biosci.*, 2014, **14**, 965–976.
21. T. R. Kommuru, B. Gurley, M. A. Khan and I. K. Reddy, *Int. J. Pharm.*, 2001, **212**, 233–246.
22. M. M. Nerurkar, P. S. Burton and R. T. Borchardt, *Pharm. Res.*, 1996, **13**, 528–534.
23. T. Yamagata, H. Kusuhara, M. Morishita, K. Takayama, H. Benameur and Y. Sugiyama, *J. Controlled Release*, 2007, **124**, 1–5.
24. U. Hanke, K. May, V. Rozehnal, S. Nagel, W. Siegmund and W. Weitschies, *Eur. J. Pharm. Biopharm.*, 2010, **76**, 260–268.
25. T. Loftsson and M. E. Brewster, *J. Pharm. Sci.*, 1996, **85**, 1017–1025.

26. T. Irie and K. Uekama, *J. Pharm. Sci.*, 1997, **86**, 147–162.
27. M. Okawara, Y. Tokudome, H. Todo, K. Sugibayashi and F. Hashimoto, *Biol. Pharm. Bull.*, 2014, **37**, 54–59.
28. M. E. Brewster, R. Vandecruys, J. Peeters, P. Neeskens, G. Verreck and T. Loftsson, *Eur. J. Pharm. Sci.*, 2008, **34**, 94–103.
29. M. S. Kim, *Int. J. Nanomed.*, 2013, **8**, 2029–2039.
30. H. D. Williams, N. L. Trevaskis, S. A. Charman, R. M. Shanker, W. N. Charman, C. W. Pouton and C. J. Porter, *Pharmacol. Rev.*, 2013, **65**, 315–499.
31. K. A. Lentz, *AAPS J.*, 2008, **10**, 282–288.
32. P. Zakeri-Milani, H. Valizadeh, H. Tajerzadeh, Y. Azarmi, Z. Islambolchilar, S. Barzegar and M. Barzegar-Jalali, *J. Pharm. Pharm. Sci.*, 2007, **10**, 368–379.
33. B. D. Rege, L. X. Yu, A. S. Hussain and J. E. Polli, *J. Pharm. Sci.*, 2001, **90**, 1776–1786.
34. P. Pinton, J. P. Nougayrede, J. C. Del Rio, C. Moreno, D. E. Marin, L. Ferrier, A. P. Bracarense, M. Kolf-Clauw and I. P. Oswald, *Toxicol. Appl. Pharmacol.*, 2009, **237**, 41–48.
35. M. Tomita, M. J. Menconi, R. L. Delude and M. P. Fink, *Gastroenterology*, 2000, **118**, 535–543.
36. D. A. Volpe, *AAPS J.*, 2010, **12**, 670–678.
37. X. Chen, A. Murawski, K. Patel, C. L. Crespi and P. V. Balimane, *Pharm. Res.*, 2008, **25**, 1511–1520.
38. M. Bermejo, A. Avdeef, A. Ruiz, R. Nalda, J. A. Ruell, O. Tsinman, I. Gonzalez, C. Fernandez, G. Sanchez, T. M. Garrigues and V. Merino, *Eur. J. Pharm. Sci.*, 2004, **21**, 429–441.
39. A. Avdeef, P. Artursson, S. Neuhoff, L. Lazorova, J. Grasjo and S. Tavelin, *Eur. J. Pharm. Sci.*, 2005, **24**, 333–349.
40. A. Avdeef, P. E. Nielsen and O. Tsinman, *Eur. J. Pharm. Sci.*, 2004, **22**, 365–374.
41. Z. S. Teksin, P. R. Seo and J. E. Polli, *AAPS J.*, 2010, **12**, 238–241.
42. I. J. Hidalgo, T. J. Raub and R. T. Borchardt, *Gastroenterology*, 1989, **96**, 736–749.
43. K. A. Lentz, J. Hayashi, L. J. Lucisano and J. E. Polli, *Int. J. Pharm.*, 2000, **200**, 41–51.
44. I. J. Hidalgo, *Curr. Top. Med. Chem.*, 2001, **1**, 385–401.
45. US Department of Health and Human Services, Food and Drug Administration and Center of Drug Evaluation and Research (CDER), US FDA website, 2012, http://www.fda.gov/downloads/Drugs/GuidanceComplianceRegulatoryInformation/Guidances/UCM292362.pdf.
46. European Medicinal Agency and Science Medicines Health, European Medicinal Agency website, 2012, http://www.ema.europa.eu/docs/en_GB/document_library/Scientific_guideline/2012/07/WC500129606.pdf.
47. M. E. Ganapathy, W. Huang, H. Wang, V. Ganapathy and F. H. Leibach, *Biochem. Biophys. Res. Commun.*, 1998, **246**, 470–475.
48. I. Tamai, *Adv. Drug Delivery Rev.*, 2012, **64**, 508–514.

49. R. L. Juliano and V. Ling, *Biochim. Biophys. Acta*, 1976, **455**, 152–162.

50. L. A. Doyle, W. Yang, L. V. Abruzzo, T. Krogmann, Y. Gao, A. K. Rishi and D. D. Ross, *Proc. Natl. Acad. Sci. U. S. A.*, 1998, **95**, 15665–15670.

51. M. J. Humphrey and P. S. Ringrose, *Drug Metab. Rev.*, 1986, **17**, 283–310.

52. H. Lennernas, *Clin. Pharmacokinet.*, 2003, **42**, 1141–1160.

53. L. J. Goldstein, H. Galski, A. Fojo, M. Willingham, S. L. Lai, A. Gazdar, R. Pirker, A. Green, W. Crist, G. M. Brodeur, *et al.*, *J. Natl. Cancer Inst.*, 1989, **81**, 116–124.

54. F. Thiebaut, T. Tsuruo, H. Hamada, M. M. Gottesman, I. Pastan and M. C. Willingham, *Proc. Natl. Acad. Sci. U. S. A.*, 1987, **84**, 7735–7738.

55. C. Cordon-Cardo, J. P. O'Brien, D. Casals, L. Rittman-Grauer, J. L. Biedler, M. R. Melamed and J. R. Bertino, *Proc. Natl. Acad. Sci. U. S. A.*, 1989, **86**, 695–698.

56. C. Cordon-Cardo, J. P. O'Brien, J. Boccia, D. Casals, J. R. Bertino and M. R. Melamed, *J. Histochem. Cytochem.*, 1990, **38**, 1277–1287.

57. F. J. Sharom, *Essays Biochem.*, 2011, **50**, 161–178.

58. T. Terasaki and S. Ohtsuki, *NeuroRx*, 2005, **2**, 63–72.

59. J. P. Bai, M. Hu, P. Subramanian, H. I. Mosberg and G. L. Amidon, *J. Pharm. Sci.*, 1992, **81**, 113–116.

60. S. Yamashita, Y. Yamazaki, M. Masada, T. Nadai, T. Kimura and H. Sezaki, *J. Pharmacobiodyn.*, 1986, **9**, 368–374.

61. W. Kramer, F. Girbig, U. Gutjahr, H. W. Kleemann, I. Leipe, H. Urbach and A. Wagner, *Biochim. Biophys. Acta*, 1990, **1027**, 25–30.

62. M. Kataoka, Y. Masaoka, Y. Yamazaki, T. Sakane, H. Sezaki and S. Yamashita, *Pharm. Res.*, 2003, **20**, 1674–1680.

63. R. Takano, M. Kataoka and S. Yamashita, *Biopharm. Drug Dispos.*, 2012, **33**, 354–365.

64. A. El-Kattan and M. Varma, in *Topics on Drug Metabolism*, ed. J. Paxton, InTech, Rijeka, Croatia, 2012, pp. 1–34.

65. K. R. Korzekwa, S. Nagar, J. Tucker, E. A. Weiskircher, S. Bhoopathy and I. J. Hidalgo, *Drug Metab. Dispos.*, 2012, **40**, 865–876.

CHAPTER 3

Models for Nonspecific Binding and Partitioning

KEN KORZEKWA*[a]

[a]Pharmaceutical Sciences, The School of Pharmacy, Temple University, 3307 N Broad St., Philadelphia, PA 19140, USA
*E-mail: korzekwa@temple.edu

3.1   Introduction

This chapter will describe predictive models for non-specific binding or partitioning. We will loosely define these processes as binding or partitioning into proteins or lipids that show very broad specificity and determine drug distribution. These include plasma protein binding, microsomal partitioning, non-specific binding to cells, and tissue binding. Together these processes describe the disposition of drugs at a cellular, tissue, and macro level.

At a cellular level, the free drug in the plasma, *i.e.* the drug not bound to plasma proteins, drives intracellular concentrations. If no transport or other active processes are involved, the free drug hypothesis states that the free drug in plasma equals the free drug in the cell at equilibrium.[1] Active processes such as transporter activity can shift the equilibrium, and drugs with poor membrane permeability may not reach equilibrium, and the free drug hypothesis will not hold. Extracellular and intracellular drugs can partition into membranes and neutral lipids, increasing the total cell concentration of the drug without affecting the unbound concentration at equilibrium.[2] Similarly, pH partitioning into lysosomes and mitochondria can also increase total

RSC Drug Discovery Series No. 49
New Horizons in Predictive Drug Metabolism and Pharmacokinetics
Edited by Alan G. E. Wilson

cellular concentration without increasing the unbound cytosolic concentration.[3-5] Differences between cytosolic pH and the pH of the interstitial fluid can result in increases or decreases of the intracellular concentration that do affect the unbound concentrations. Plasma protein binding decreases the concentration available to partition into the cell and thus decreases intracellular concentrations.

At the tissue level, the processes described above determine the amount of drug that partitions into the various tissues. Representations of these processes are used to construct physiologically based pharmacokinetic (PBPK) models. For perfusion-limited PBPK models, the tissue to plasma ratios are used to calculate the instantaneous distribution of a drug between the blood and various tissues. It is assumed that the unbound plasma concentration of the drug is available to distribute into tissues. Another tissue for which non-specific binding and partitioning processes play a key role is the brain. The presence of the blood–brain barrier can limit the distribution of a drug into the brain, and processes such as membrane partitioning and lysosomal partitioning can further decrease the unbound drug concentration.[3] Since the unbound concentration is the relevant concentration at the target, determination of brain distribution is important for CNS drugs and drugs with CNS side effects.

At a macro level, these processes ultimately determine the volume of distribution (V_D) parameters for a drug. By definition, V_D is the volume that relates the plasma drug concentration to the total amount of drug in the body. For most drugs, the V_D is determined by the competition between binding to plasma proteins and binding or partitioning into the tissues. Drugs that are highly bound to plasma proteins will have small V_D values when tissue binding is low and have large V_D values when tissue binding dominates. However, some drugs can bind tightly to plasma proteins and partition extensively into tissues. For example, tamoxifen is >99% bound to plasma proteins and yet has a very large V_D (60 L kg^{-1}).

Since it is generally the unbound concentration at the drug target that determines activity, and since V_D and clearance equally determine drug half-life, non-specific binding and partitioning processes will play a significant role in the distribution and therefore success of a drug candidate. Any predictive model that can help select candidates with the best distribution profile can be very useful in the drug discovery process.

3.2 Models for Plasma Protein Binding

The extent of plasma protein binding impacts almost all aspects of pharmacokinetics and pharmacodynamics.[6,7] Plasma proteins involved in nonspecific binding include, in order of importance, human serum albumin (HSA), α-acid glycoprotein (AAG), and lipoproteins.[8,9] All of these proteins show very broad substrate selectivity, with combinations of hydrophobic and ionic regions in their binding sites. Albumin primarily binds acidic and neutral hydrophobic compounds, but can bind hydrophobic bases as well[10] and is distributed in both plasma and the extracellular fluid (ECF). The ratio of HSA in the ECF to plasma is 0.116, but since there is more ECF than plasma, the majority of HSA is in the ECF. AAG is the protein to which most hydrophobic bases bind. Again the protein is present in both the plasma and ECF with an ECF to plasma ratio of 0.052. Lipoproteins are not as important as HSA and AAG for most drugs, but can bind some very hydrophobic molecules at levels similar to these proteins.[11,12]

Since the predictability of a model depends on the quality of the experimental data used to create the model, it is important to understand current and past methods to measure plasma protein binding. The two most common methods to measure protein binding are equilibrium dialysis and ultrafiltration. It is generally accepted that equilibrium dialysis is preferred, since ultrafiltration results can be greatly impacted by non-specific binding to the apparatus. Results from equilibrium dialysis can also be misleading if the pH of the plasma changes during the experiment. Using normal plasma exposed to air, the pH of plasma will rise from 7.4 to ~9 during the time required for a dialysis experiment.[13,14] This change in pH has a non-random effect on plasma protein binding, with fractions bound in plasma (f_{bp}) increasing by an average of 2- to 3-fold with unbuffered plasma.[14] Since CO_2 is used to buffer plasma *in vivo*, conducting the equilibrium dialysis experiment in the presence of 10% CO_2 prevents the increase in pH, leading to more reliable results. Another approach is to use plasma that has been dialyzed against phosphate buffer. Many laboratories now routinely conduct equilibrium dialysis experiments in a CO_2 incubator, but much of the historic plasma protein binding data will have higher fraction bound (f_b) values than would be measured with appropriately buffered plasma. This should be considered when building plasma protein binding models with historic data.

3.2.1 HSA Models

Due to its dominant role in plasma protein binding, the majority of modeling efforts have focused on predicting binding to HSA. These modeling efforts generally fall into two categories: quantitative structure activity relationship (QSAR) models and protein structure-based models. Models have been developed based on either the percent of plasma protein binding (%PPB) or the log of the binding constant ($\log K_b$). The association constant K_b can be calculated from the f_b by:

$$K_b[\text{HSA}] = \frac{f_b}{\left(1 - f_b\right)} \tag{3.1}$$

Linear free energy relationships suggest that the most appropriate method to model a binding event is to fit molecular parameters to $\log K_b$, since $\log K_b$ is proportional to Gibbs free energy (ΔG). In addition, there are some very practical reasons why $\log K_b$ should be used to predict %PPB. Predicting %PPB adequately represents the variance for compounds that bind plasma proteins in the low to moderate range. For compounds that are highly bound, a model with 10% error will not adequately distinguish between compounds with a fraction bound of 0.9, 0.99, and 0.999, even though the unbound fractions for the latter two are 10- and 100-fold lower than the first. When predicting the impact of plasma protein binding on many processes such as target activity, drug clearance, off-target activity (*e.g.* CYP inhibition or induction), and V_D for compounds with significant tissue distribution, $\log K_b$ models will be much more useful than %PPB models. For compounds that do not distribute greatly into tissues, %PPB models can adequately predict the impact of plasma protein binding on V_D since highly bound compounds will show V_D values equal to the V_D of the plasma protein to which they are bound (~0.1 L kg^{-1} for HSA).[15]

Models for HSA are complicated by both multiple binding sites and the broad substrate specificity of those sites.[16] Albumin contains two primary binding sites and several other secondary binding sites. Interactions at multiple sites can complicate datasets since different experimental conditions can result in different measured affinities. Albumin binding datasets are further complicated by partial overlap between binding sites, allosteric interactions between sites,[8,17] and altered protein properties in the presence of endogenous substrates such as fatty acids.[8]

Colmenarejo[18] *et al.* reported one of the first QSAR models for HSA. In this study, $\log K_b$ values for 95 drug-like molecules were estimated from retention times with high-performance HSA affinity chromatography. It was found that local models for most classes of compounds could be constructed with single, albeit different descriptors. For example, a model for β-adrenergic antagonists could be modeled with cLogP (cross-validated $q^2 = 0.74$). A global model was constructed for all compounds that could explain ~80% of the variance using six descriptors. It was found that hydrophobicity was the most important factor for HSA binding.

Using the dataset provided by Colmenarejo *et al.*,[18] Hall *et al.*[19] used a stepwise regression method and developed a model with six descriptors giving $q^2 = 0.7$ and a root mean square error (RMSE) of ~0.3 (2-fold error). Although neither $\log P$ nor $\log D$ were used as descriptors, the most important descriptors included aromatic, aliphatic, and halogen descriptors, suggesting that hydrophobicity is the most important component of this model.

Another modeling effort by Kratochwil *et al.*,[20] used topological pharmacophore and daylight fingerprint descriptors along with partial least squares to develop a model to predict $\log K_b$ for HSA. A dataset of 138 HSA binding values from the literature resulted in a model that could explain approximately 50% of the variance (cross-validated $q^2 = 0.48$). Better predictions could be obtained with local models, *i.e.* models built with data for similar compounds. The best predictive model was obtained for a local mode of 4-hydroxyquinolones ($q^2 = 0.71$).

It may be expected that building models for plasma protein binding will be more difficult than for HSA since, in addition to HSA, binding to AAG and lipoproteins are included in the measurement. Using internal plasma protein binding data from several internal GlaxoSmithKline lead optimization programs, Gleeson[21] developed local and global models using 30 descriptors and partial least squares regression. It was found that the models to predict $\log K_b$ for the individual programs had RMSEs that varied from 0.28 (2-fold error) to 0.56 (3.6-fold error). As expected, the global models had a greater RMSE (0.55 or 3.5-fold error) than the average of the individual models.

Votano *et al.*[22] used a large dataset (808 molecules in the training set and 200 compounds in the validation set) to model plasma protein binding. They used 115 topological descriptors along with four different modeling techniques to predict %PPB. The methods used for model development were multiple liner regression, *k*-nearest neighbor, artificial neural network, and support vector machine. The artificial neural network method provided the best model, with r^2 values for the training and validation sets of 0.90 and 0.70, respectively. The RMSEs were 11% and 19% for the training and validation sets, respectively. Since %PPB was modeled, this model can easily separate high binders from low binders, but cannot distinguish the degree of binding for highly bound compounds. Therefore the model will not be useful for most of the applications for which fraction unbound is used, *e.g.* clearance prediction, pharmacodynamics modeling, *etc.*, when protein binding is high (*e.g.* >90%).

Ghafourian and Amin[23] used most of the Votano dataset above and applied various modeling methods, including stepwise regression, regression tree, interactive tree, random forest, and boosted tree approaches. One of the boosted tree models gave the best predictive accuracy with $r^2 = 0.71$ and a mean absolute error of 13% for the test set, and $r^2 = 0.65$ and a mean absolute error of 15% for the validation set. Again, since %PPB was modeled, the model does not provide predictive capability for highly bound compounds.

Expanding the Votano dataset to 1200 compounds, Zhu *et al.*[24] modeled both %PPB and $\log K_b$ using *k*-nearest neighbor, random forest, and support vector machine methods. They concluded that modeling $\log K_b$ is superior for highly protein bound compounds.

To summarize the predictability of HSA and %PPB models, local models are often more predictive with fewer descriptors than global models. However, for some classes of compounds, predictive local models could not be obtained. For all modeling efforts, hydrophobicity appears to be the most important descriptor. When extensive datasets were used, most global models were limited in their predictive accuracy to RMSE values of approximately 0.5 for $\log K_b$ models and approximately 15% for %PPB models. None of the %PPB models are useful for accurately predicting the unbound fraction in plasma for highly bound compounds.

3.3 Models for Microsomal Membrane Partitioning

Microsomes are membrane vesicles prepared by differential centrifugation primarily consisting of the smooth endoplasmic reticulum subcellular fraction. Microsomes contain many drug metabolizing enzymes, including the cytochrome P450s (CYPs), UDP glucuronosyl transferases (UGTs), and microsomal esterases. Microsomes are used to characterize important metabolic properties including CYP metabolic stability and inhibition (both reversible and time-dependent). Metabolic stability assays are used to predict CYP mediated clearance by scaling up the observed *in vitro* clearance to human intrinsic clearance.[25-34] CYP inhibition is a major cause of drug interactions, and potent CYP inhibitors are generally not advanced into clinical trials. In order to correctly determine microsomal intrinsic clearances and inhibition constants it is necessary to measure the free fraction in a microsomal incubation. Therefore, non-specific binding to microsomes, or microsomal partitioning, has become an important component of *in vitro–in vivo* correlation. The term that is usually used to describe this binding is f_{um}, the fraction unbound in the microsomal incubation.

Microsomal partitioning, as well as any non-specific binding to the assay apparatus, will decrease the free fraction of the substrate or inhibitor, resulting in apparent intrinsic clearances that are lower than actual intrinsic clearances, and apparent inhibition constants that are higher than actual inhibition constants. Both of these errors can result in underestimating important metabolic liabilities. Since microsomal partitioning is unlikely to be saturated, errors in substrate concentration will be proportional to $1/f_{um}$, where f_{um} is the fraction unbound in the microsomal incubation. The standard clearance (CL) prediction equations can therefore be modified as follows:[32]

$$CL = \frac{Q \cdot f_{up} \dfrac{CL'_{int}}{f_{um}}}{Q + f_{up} \dfrac{CL'_{int}}{f_{um}}} \tag{3.2}$$

Any calculated K_m or K_i value can also be divided by f_{um} to give corrected values.

Since microsomes are essentially unsorted phospholipid vesicles, the partition constant for membrane partitioning will depend on both aqueous solubility and the ability to reside in an ordered phospholipid environment. The anionic phosphate groups in these membranes result in very different membrane affinities for neutral, acidic, and basic molecules. Neutral hydrophobic compounds can reside in the nonpolar region of the membrane. The partitioning of acids likely occurs for the neutral fraction and not the anionic fraction. Bases, on the other hand, can readily partition into membranes, presumably due to interactions between the cationic groups and the phosphate groups in the phospholipid. As a consequence, acidic molecules generally show high (approaching 1.0) f_{um} values and compounds with the lowest values tend to be hydrophobic amines.

The first model to predict f_{um} from physiochemical properties was provided by Austin *et al.*[29] Using $\log P$ for neutral and basic molecules and $\log D_{7.4}$

for acidic compounds, the following linear relationship was obtained for 40 compounds with $f_{um} < 0.9$:

$$\log\left(\frac{1 - f_{um}}{f_{um}}\right) = 0.53 \, \log P / D - 1.42 \tag{3.3}$$

Use of $\log D$ for acidic compounds and $\log P$ for basic compounds can be rationalized if it is primarily the neutral fraction of acidic molecules that partitions into the membrane, whereas both the neutral and cationic forms of bases can partition.

Hallifax and Houston[35] suggested that a quadratic relationship should be used to estimate f_{um} based on an extended dataset of reported and internal values. The fitted equation is given in eqn (3.4):

$$\log\left(\frac{1 - f_{um}}{f_{um}}\right) = 0.072\left(\log P / D\right)^2 + 0.0665\left(\log P / D\right) - 1.1256 \tag{3.4}$$

This equation is used frequently for the estimation of f_{um} for clearance predictions both using static and PBPK models.[36] It is not clear that the relationship between octanol/water partition coefficients and f_{um} should be quadratic,[2] and Austin pointed out that eqn (3.4) will result in increasing f_{um} values at $\log P$ values < -2, which is unlikely.[37] An analysis of the linear and quadratic models showed that both models can predict f_{um} accurately when $\log P/D < 3.0$ but both models show significant errors for highly lipophilic compounds.[38]

Using a descriptor-based approach, Li *et al.*[39] were able to build a model to predict f_{um} values. A total of 32 descriptors were generated for a combined training and test set of 86 drug molecules. Stepwise regression was used to select seven descriptors for a linear model for the microsomal binding constant. The training and validation sets resulted in models with r^2 values of 0.82 and 0.85, respectively.

3.4 Models for Partitioning into Hepatocytes

The use of hepatocytes is becoming common for a number of *in vitro* absorption, distribution, metabolism, and excretion (ADME) studies. Clearance prediction with hepatocytes is used when non-CYP enzymes are primarily responsible for hepatic clearance. UGT assays with microsomes are complicated by the location of the enzymes on the interior of the endoplasmic reticulum. Since both substrates and cofactors require access to the enzymes, kinetic characterization with microsomes can be unreliable. Hepatocytes provide the necessary components, *e.g.* transporters, to better represent the *in vivo* properties of hepatic tissue. As with microsomal assays, non-specific binding to hepatocytes can decrease the available substrate or inhibitor concentration, leading to an under-prediction of activity (*e.g.* clearance, inhibition, induction, *etc.*). Austin *et al.*

reported a linear relationship between $\log P/D$ and hepatocyte binding at 10^6 cells mL^{-1}:

$$\log\left(\frac{1 - f_{u,hep}}{f_{u,hep}}\right) = 0.4\log P / D - 1.38 \tag{3.5}$$

It was also found that microsomal binding was highly correlated with hepatocyte binding, with 1 mg microsomal protein giving similar binding to 10^6 hepatocytes per mL.

Kilford *et al.*[40] extended the quadratic relationship from Hallifax *et al.*[35] for hepatocytes and provided the following equation:

$$f_{u,hep} = \frac{1}{1 + 125V_R 10^{0.072\left(\log P/D\right)^2 + 0.0665\left(\log P/D\right) - 1.1256}} \tag{3.6}$$

This study confirmed that drug partitioning into 1 mg microsomal protein is similar to partitioning into approximately 10^6 hepatocytes per mL. Again, the errors are small (generally <2-fold) for compounds with $\log P/D < 3$, and higher for more lipophilic compounds. In general it appears that for molecules that are very hydrophobic, experimental determination of f_{um} and $f_{u,hep}$ may be necessary.

3.5 pH Partitioning

The free drug hypothesis[1] states that, at equilibrium, extracellular and intracellular unbound concentrations are equal for permeable compounds. However, if the drug is a transporter substrate or if the concentration is influenced by other active processes, this hypothesis may not apply. An important non-specific distribution process that occurs within cells is the partitioning of drugs due to differences in pH. For example, cytosolic pH is generally lower that that for the ECF (*e.g.* pH 7.1 *versus* 7.4 for hepatocytes and ECF, respectively). Active processes maintain this pH, and therefore, drug gradients can be observed with simple passive diffusion. For permeable compounds, expected differences in intracellular distribution can be modeled easily using pH partitioning equations obtained from the Henderson–Hasselbalch equation. The two most important applications of pH partitioning are: (1) the correction of unbound cytosolic concentrations relative to unbound extracellular concentrations; and (2) correction of total intracellular concentrations for lysosomal partitioning.

Berezhkovskiy[41] described the use of an ionization factor to correct various clearance models. For the well-stirred model for hepatic clearance, the ionization factor, F_I, is used to correct the intrinsic clearance for differences between intracellular and extracellular pH.

$$CL_h = \frac{Q \cdot f_{up} \dfrac{CL'_{int}}{f_{um}} F_I}{Q + f_{up} \dfrac{CL'_{int}}{f_{um}} F_I} \tag{3.7}$$

where F_I is the ionization factor defined as:

$$F_I = \frac{1 - f_p^i}{1 - f_{IW}^i} \qquad (3.8)$$

where f_p^i is the fraction ionized in the plasma, and f_{IW}^i is the fraction ionized in the intracellular water. For bases, $f^i = 1/(1 - 10^{pH-pKa})$ and for acids, $f^i = 1/(1 - 10^{pKa-pH})$. Given that plasma pH is ~7.4 and intracellular pH can be as low as 7.0, intracellular concentrations would be expected to be ~2.5-times lower than plasma concentrations for strong monoprotic acids and ~2.5-fold higher for monoprotic bases.

Another organelle in the cell that can sequester drug through pH partitioning is the lysosome. With a pH of 5, lysosomes can sequester bases at substantially higher concentrations than the cytosol. For a strong base, the concentration of drug in the lysosomes and can be 100-fold higher than the concentration in the plasma. Therefore, even a lysosomal volume of 1% of cell volume can double the apparent V_D of basic compounds in that cell. Fridén *et al.*[3] reported models for brain partitioning using homogenates and brain slices. It was found that the unbound V_D of the brain was under-predicted when pH partitioning was not included, with errors ranging from a 7.1-fold under-prediction to a 2.9-fold over-prediction. Including pH partitioning into the cytosol and lysosomes resulted in lower errors ranging between 2.2-fold under- and over-prediction. It should be pointed out that partitioning into compartments such as lysosomes will not alter the unbound cytosolic concentration at equilibrium, unless the amount of partitioning in the body is large enough to decrease the plasma concentration. These processes can change the total amount of drug in a tissue, but the unbound cytosolic concentration will still depend on the unbound plasma concentration and any active processes that alter cytosolic concentration (*e.g.* transporters).

3.6 Integrated Models for Predicting V_D

In addition to extrapolating *in vitro* activity and ADME data to predict *in vivo* properties, plasma protein binding and tissue partitioning are integral components of V_D. There are a number of descriptor-based V_D models reported. These include descriptor-based QSAR models,[42,43] more mechanistic equations, *e.g.* models based on the Oie-Tozer equation,[44,45] and tissue partitioning models used in PBPK approaches.[46–53]

A trend analysis on the relationship between V_D and several descriptors shows that much of the *in vivo* distribution process is determined by the physiochemical characteristics of the drug. Descriptor-based models could predict V_D values within 2-fold of the experimental values approximately 70% of the time.[42,43] High-performance liquid chromatography retention time data can be used to estimate binding constants when proteins or lipids are immobilized on the column solid phase.[54] Valkó *et al.* estimated the binding constant for phospholipids and HSA from retention times with immobilized phosphatidylcholine and HSA.[55,56] Models with these two binding constants were able to explain ~70% of the variance in V_D for 135 compounds from the literature and 300 in-house compounds. Sui *et al.* have published several models based on affinities to artificial immobilized membranes along with *in vitro* data such as plasma protein binding[57,58] or combinations of molecular properties, and *in vivo* preclinical data.[59] It was found that adding molecular descriptors such as molecular weight and fraction ionized to the measured preclinical V_D values improved the prediction of human V_D.

Within the PBPK approach, the V_D at steady state (V_{SS}) can be calculated as the sum of the individual tissue partition constants $(K_p s)$ times their tissue volumes plus the volume of the plasma. Methods to predict K_p values generally use experimental f_{up} values and relationships involving $\log P$ or $\log D$, pK_a, and tissue lipid composition.[46–50,52,53] In addition, the Rodgers method to calculate K_p values for bases uses an experimental blood to plasma ratio. A recent analysis to evaluate the accuracy of the various methods showed that 63–87% of the predicted volumes were within 3-fold of the experimental values.[53] All of the models currently implemented within the PBPK framework require some experimental data. This could be due to the relatively low accuracy of plasma protein binding models. As these models improve, it might be expected that V_D could be predicted from structure alone.

3.7 Conclusion

Nonspecific binding or partitioning plays a major role in the distribution and disposition of drugs. Plasma protein binding and partitioning into tissue membranes are two important processes that influence unbound concentrations and therefore most pharmacological and toxicological properties. Models for plasma protein binding are complicated by the presence of several binding proteins and multiple binding sites on these proteins. Computational models for plasma protein binding have been developed and several of these models can explain ~70% of the variance for diverse datasets. In general, local models are more accurate than global models. Models for membrane partitioning include microsomal membrane binding and nonspecific binding to hepatocytes. Accounting for these nonspecific binding processes is important when scaling up microsomal or cellular data to predict clearance and drug interactions. Models that include $\log P$ and $\log D$ can generally predict partitioning into microsomes and hepatocytes. Distribution into cells and organelles due to pH differences can be readily modeled by pH partitioning equations. Models for V_D can be constructed by integrating these processes. Models for V_D include descriptor-based models and mechanistic models. Within the PBPK framework there are integrated models to predict V_D that incorporate plasma protein binding, lipid partitioning, and pH partitioning. However, the current implementations of these of these models require some experimental data.

References

1. D. A. Smith, L. Di and E. H. Kerns, *Nat. Rev. Drug Discovery*, 2010, **9**, 929.
2. S. Nagar and K. Korzekwa, *Drug Metab. Dispos.*, 2012, **40**, 1649.
3. M. Fridén, F. Bergström, H. Wan, M. Rehngren, G. Ahlin, M. Hammarlund-Udenaes and U. Bredberg, *Drug Metab. Dispos.*, 2011, **39**, 353.
4. J. L. Chunta, K. S. Vistisen, Z. Yazdi and R. D. Braun, *PLoS One*, 2012, **7**, e37471.
5. N. Zheng, H. N. Tsai, X. Zhang and G. R. Rosania, *Mol. Pharm.*, 2011, **8**, 1619.
6. T. Bohnert and L. S. Gan, *J. Pharm. Sci.*, 2013, **102**, 2953.
7. X. Liu, M. Wright and C. E. Hop, *J. Med. Chem.*, 2014, **57**, 8238.
8. J. J. Vallner, *J. Pharm. Sci.*, 1977, **66**, 447.
9. G. Lambrinidis, T. Vallianatou and A. Tsantili-Kakoulidou, *Adv. Drug Delivery Rev.*, 2015, **5**, 583.
10. U. Kragh-Hansen, V. T. Chuang and M. Otagiri, *Biol. Pharm. Bull.*, 2002, **25**, 695.
11. H. Zahir, R. A. Nand, K. F. Brown, B. N. Tattam and A. J. McLachlan, *J. Pharmacol. Toxicol. Methods*, 2001, **46**, 27.
12. D. Colussi, C. Parisot, F. Legay and G. Lefèvre, *Eur. J. Pharm. Sci.*, 1999, **9**, 9.
13. H. Wan and M. Rehngren, *J. Chromatogr. A*, 2006, **1102**, 125.
14. C. J. Kochansky, D. R. McMasters, P. Lu, K. A. Koeplinger, H. H. Kerr, M. Shou and K. R. Korzekwa, *Mol. Pharm.*, 2008, **5**, 438.
15. M. Rowland and T. N. Tozer, *Clinical Pharmacokinetics and Pharmacodynamics: Concepts And Applications*, Wolters Kluwer Health/Lippincott William & Wilkins, 2010.
16. P. Ascenzi and M. Fasano, *Biophys. Chem.*, 2010, **148**, 16.
17. Q. Shen, L. Wang, H. Zhou, H. D. Jiang, L. S. Yu and S. Zeng, *Acta Pharmacol. Sin.*, 2013, **34**, 998.
18. G. Colmenarejo, A. Alvarez-Pedraglio and J. Lavandera, *J. Med. Chem.*, 2001, **44**, 4370.
19. L. M. Hall, L. H. Hall and L. B. Kier, *J. Chem. Inf. Comput. Sci.*, 2003, **43**, 2120.
20. N. A. Kratochwil, W. Huber, F. Müller, M. Kansy and P. R. Gerber, *Biochem. Pharmacol.*, 2002, **64**, 1355.
21. M. P. Gleeson, *J. Med. Chem.*, 2007, **50**, 101.
22. J. R. Votano, M. Parham, L. M. Hall, L. H. Hall, L. B. Kier, S. Oloff and A. Tropsha, *J. Med. Chem.*, 2006, **49**, 7169.
23. T. Ghafourian and Z. Amin, *Bioimpacts*, 2013, **3**, 21.
24. X. W. Zhu, A. Sedykh, H. Zhu, S. S. Liu and A. Tropsha, *Pharm. Res.*, 2013, **30**, 1790.
25. R. S. Obach, *Drug Metab. Dispos.*, 1997, **25**, 1359.
26. T. H. Tran, L. L. von Moltke, K. Venkatakrishnan, B. W. Granda, M. A. Gibbs, R. S. Obach, J. S. Harmatz and D. J. Greenblatt, *Drug Metab. Dispos.*, 2002, **30**, 1441.

27. J. M. Margolis and R. S. Obach, *Drug Metab. Dispos.*, 2003, **31**, 606.
28. R. S. Obach, A. E. Reed-Hagen, S. S. Krueger, B. J. Obach, T. N. O'Connell, K. S. Zandi, S. Miller and J. W. Coe, *Drug Metab. Dispos.*, 2006, **34**, 121.
29. R. P. Austin, P. Barton, S. L. Cockroft, M. C. Wenlock and R. J. Riley, *Drug Metab. Dispos.*, 2002, **30**, 1497.
30. R. S. Obach, R. L. Walsky, K. Venkatakrishnan, J. B. Houston and L. M. Tremaine, *Clin. Pharmacol. Ther.*, 2005, **78**, 582.
31. K. Grime and R. J. Riley, *Curr. Drug Metab.*, 2006, **7**, 251.
32. R. S. Obach, *Drug Metab. Dispos.*, 1999, **27**, 1350.
33. R. J. Riley, D. F. McGinnity and R. P. Austin, *Drug Metab. Dispos.*, 2005, **33**, 1304.
34. K. Venkatakrishnan, L. L. von Moltke, R. S. Obach and D. J. Greenblatt, *J. Pharmacol. Exp. Ther.*, 2000, **293**, 343.
35. D. Hallifax and J. B. Houston, *Drug Metab. Dispos.*, 2006, **34**, 724.
36. S. K. Quinney, X. Zhang, A. Lucksiri, J. C. Gorski, L. Li and S. D. Hall, *Drug Metab. Dispos.*, 2010, **38**, 241.
37. P. Austin, *Drug Metab. Dispos.*, 2006, **34**, 727.
38. M. Gertz, P. J. Kilford, J. B. Houston and A. Galetin, *Drug Metab. Dispos.*, 2008, **36**, 535.
39. H. Li, J. Sun, X. Sui, Z. Yan, Y. Sun, X. Liu, Y. Wang and Z. He, *AAPS J.*, 2009, **11**, 364.
40. P. J. Kilford, M. Gertz, J. B. Houston and A. Galetin, *Drug Metab. Dispos.*, 2008, **36**, 1194.
41. L. M. Berezhkovskiy, *J. Pharm. Sci.*, 2011, **100**, 1167.
42. G. Berellini, C. Springer, N. J. Waters and F. Lombardo, *J. Med. Chem.*, 2009, **52**, 4488.
43. F. Lombardo, R. S. Obach, F. M. Dicapua, G. A. Bakken, J. Lu, D. M. Potter, F. Gao, M. D. Miller and Y. Zhang, *J. Med. Chem.*, 2006, **49**, 2262.
44. F. Lombardo, R. S. Obach, M. Y. Shalaeva and F. Gao, *J. Med. Chem.*, 2002, **45**, 2867.
45. F. Lombardo, R. S. Obach, M. Y. Shalaeva and F. Gao, *J. Med. Chem.*, 2004, **47**, 1242.
46. P. Poulin and F. P. Theil, *J. Pharm. Sci.*, 2000, **89**, 16.
47. P. Poulin and F. P. Theil, *J. Pharm. Sci.*, 2002, **91**, 129.
48. T. Rodgers, D. Leahy and M. Rowland, *J. Pharm. Sci.*, 2005, **94**, 1259.
49. T. Rodgers and M. Rowland, *J. Pharm. Sci.*, 2006, **95**, 1238.
50. T. Rodgers and M. Rowland, *Pharm. Res.*, 2007, **24**, 918.
51. S. S. De Buck, V. K. Sinha, L. A. Fenu, R. A. Gilissen, C. E. Mackie and M. J. Nijsen, *Drug Metab. Dispos.*, 2007, **35**, 649.
52. P. Poulin and F. P. Theil, *J. Pharm. Sci.*, 2009, **98**, 4941.
53. H. Graham, M. Walker, O. Jones, J. Yates, A. Galetin and L. Aarons, *J. Pharm. Pharmacol.*, 2012, **64**, 383.
54. J. Turková, *J. Chromatogr. B: Biomed. Sci. Appl.*, 1999, **722**, 11.
55. F. Hollósy, K. Valkó, A. Hersey, S. Nunhuck, G. Kéri and C. Bevan, *J. Med. Chem.*, 2006, **49**, 6958.

56. K. L. Valkó, S. B. Nunhuck and A. P. Hill, *J. Pharm. Sci.*, 2010, **100**, 849.
57. X. Sui, J. Sun, X. Wu, H. Li, J. Liu and Z. He, *Curr. Drug Metab.*, 2008, **9**, 574.
58. X. Sui, J. Sun, H. Li, Y. Wang, J. Liu, X. Liu, W. Zhang, L. Chen and Z. He, *Eur. J. Med. Chem.*, 2009, **44**, 4455.
59. X. Sui, J. Sun, H. Li, Y. Pan, Y. Wang and Z. He, *Biopharm. Drug Dispos.*, 2010, **31**, 464.

CHAPTER 4

Cytochrome P450 Mediated Drug Metabolism

LARS OLSEN*[a], FLEMMING STEEN JØRGENSEN[a], AND
CHRIS OOSTENBRINK[b]

[a]Department of Drug Design and Pharmacology, University of Copenhagen,
Denmark; [b]Institute of Molecular Modeling and Simulation, University of
Natural Resources and Life Sciences, Austria
*E-mail: lo@sund.ku.dk

4.1 Function of Cytochrome P450

There are 57 genes in the human genome encoding for different Cytochrome
P450 (CYP) isoforms. The CYP 1A2, 2C9, 2C19, 2D6 and 3A4 isoforms contribute the most to the metabolism of drugs and other xenobiotics.[1] All CYP
isoforms contain a heme group that carries out oxidation reactions such
as aliphatic and aromatic oxidations, heteroatom oxidations, and N- and O-
dealkylations. A prerequisite for these CYP-mediated reactions to take place
is that the substrate has affinity for the CYP isoform, that the drug compound
adopts a proper orientation in the active site of the CYP enzyme and that the
reaction is energetically feasible.

Several CYP isoforms can be involved in the metabolism of a drug compound, catalyzing different reactions and thereby generating different
metabolites. There are numerous examples of different CYP enzymes
forming different metabolites from the same compound. For example,
four CYP isoforms (1A2, 2C9, 2C19 and 3A4) convert meclofenamic acid, a

RSC Drug Discovery Series No. 49
New Horizons in Predictive Drug Metabolism and Pharmacokinetics
Edited by Alan G. E. Wilson

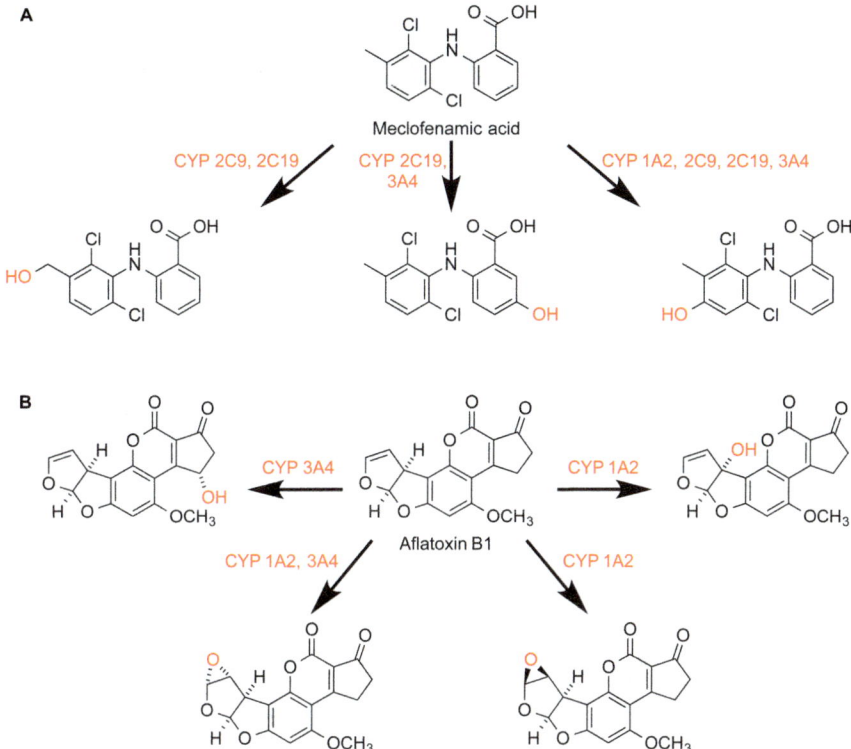

Figure 4.1 CYP mediated metabolism of meclofenamic acid (A) and aflatoxin B1 (B).

nonsteroidal anti-inflammatory drug, into three different metabolites[2] (see Figure 4.1A). As a result of the CYP reactions, aromatic hydroxylation in both aromatic rings and an aliphatic hydroxylation on the methyl occur. Another example is aflatoxin B1, a naturally occurring mycotoxin, which is converted into four different metabolites by the two CYP 1A2 and 3A4 isoforms (see Figure 4.1B).[3,4] For aflatoxin B1, epoxide formation and aliphatic hydroxylation reactions happen. In addition, it is noteworthy that the CYP enzymes perform stereoselective reactions as illustrated for the aflatoxin B1 substrate.

These examples show the challenge of understanding and predicting what metabolites are generated by the different CYP isoforms. To be able to predict the site of metabolism, both the binding and the reaction need to be considered. It is believed that the first step in the CYP reactions is the binding of the substrate to the enzyme, displacing a heme-bound water molecule (see structures **1** and **2** in Figure 4.2). Subsequently, a number of events occur, finally generating the active form of the enzyme, denoted compound **I** (structure **7** in Figure 4.2). Compound **I** very efficiently oxidizes drug compounds.

There are many different types of models for predicting the site of metabolism. Some are purely ligand-based and trained on series of compounds

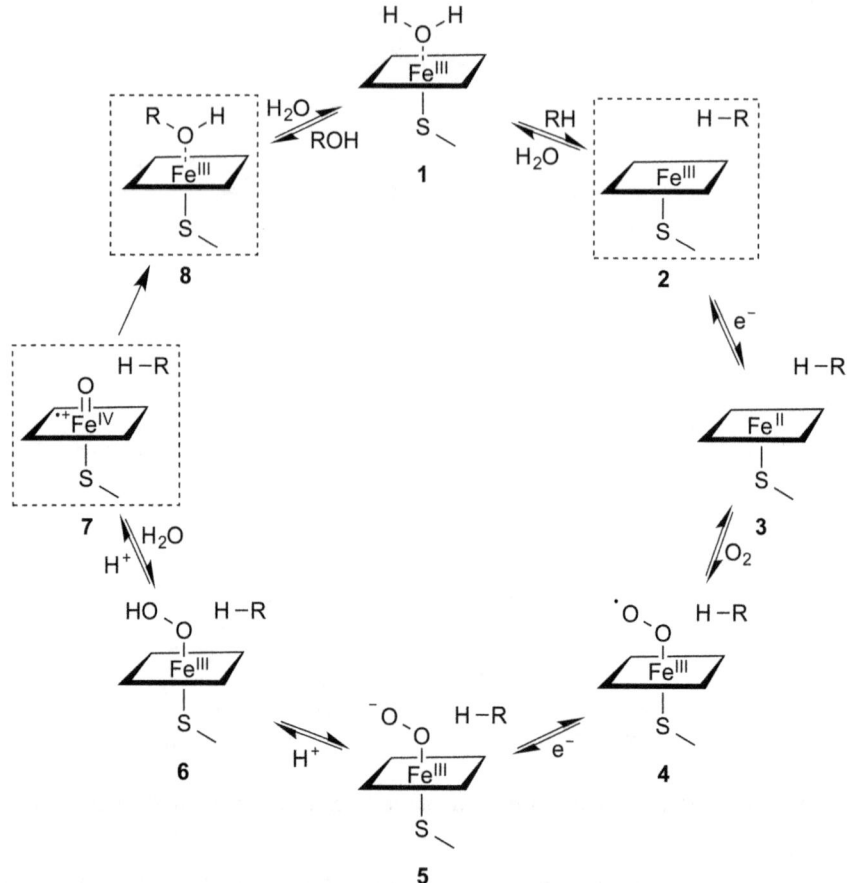

Figure 4.2   The CYP mediated catalytic cycle. R–H indicates the substrate.

with known metabolism, and subsequently evaluated on compounds with known metabolism that were not included in the training process. Other models use the characteristics of the active site of the CYP isoforms to predict the binding, and thereby the site of metabolism, by docking the compounds into the enzymes. The methods for ranking the different possibilities range from empirical scoring functions to advanced free energy calculations. Finally, models derived from the knowledge of the enzymatic/ oxidation reactions have been developed. In these models the reaction profile for the binding and subsequent oxidation reactions are calculated by quantum mechanical methods. Due to computational limitations, models of the reactive part of the enzyme, compound **I**, may replace the whole enzyme.

   In this review, the main focus will be on computational chemistry-based methods that determine what part of a compound is able to reach the oxygen of compound **I** and how easily the reaction occurs.

4.2 CYP Structures for Site of Metabolism Predictions

4.2.1 Structural Differences Between the CYP Isoforms

Although the CYP enzymes are promiscuous in nature, there are distinct differences in their active sites. The CYP 1A2 isoform has a relative flat and hydrophobic active site formed by a number of phenylalanines (F125, F226, F256 and F260) (see Figure 4.3A).[5] The CYP 2A6 isoform also has an active site formed by four phenylalanines (F111, F118, F206 and F207) as well as other hydrophobic residues (see Figure 4.3B),[6] but the orientations of the rather flat molecules metabolized by CYP 1A2 and CYP 2A6 are significantly different.[5,6] The CYP 2C9 isoform has a preference for acidic compounds due to the presence of an arginine (R108) in the active site. This arginine may adopt different orientations and accordingly the characteristics of the active size may change (see Figure 4.3C and D).[7–10] The CYP 2D6 isoform also has charged residues, two carboxylic acids (E216 and D301) in the active site, and accordingly this enzyme has a preference for basic compounds. CYP 2D6 may metabolize structurally rather different compounds, as shown by the superposition of the seven 3D structures of the CYP 2D6 complexes (see Figure 4.3E).[11,12] The CYP 3A4 isoform seems to have a very flexible active site and can accommodate many different types of compounds, as shown by the superposition of 14 different CYP 3A4 complexes (Figure 4.3F).[8]

4.2.2 Docking and Molecular Dynamics for Site of Metabolism Predictions

The CYP enzymes influence product formation by orienting the substrates in the active site, leading to regio- and stereospecific metabolism. The oxidation site of the substrate should be in the vicinity of the reactive center for the reaction to be able to take place.[13–15] Docking programs place the substrates in the active sites of proteins to predict how they bind. The distance between the site of metabolism in the substrate and the heme iron has been used as a very simple criterion to determine if a binding orientation agrees with the experimentally observed product formation. A distance of less than 6 Å has often been used, while larger distances indicate that this particular substrate orientation is incompatible with the experimental site of metabolism. In Figure 4.4A, the experimental orientation of flurbiprofen bound to CYP 2C9 is shown with a distance of 5 Å from the aromatic carbon atom being hydroxylated to the heme iron. Criteria taking into account whether the angles between the atoms involved in the reaction mimics well the subsequent transition state have also been proposed.

With the standard docking methods, the protein structure is kept rigid and water molecules in the active site are usually ignored. This is something to be aware of for docking into CYP enzymes, considering the flexibility of the CYP active sites shown in Figure 4.3.

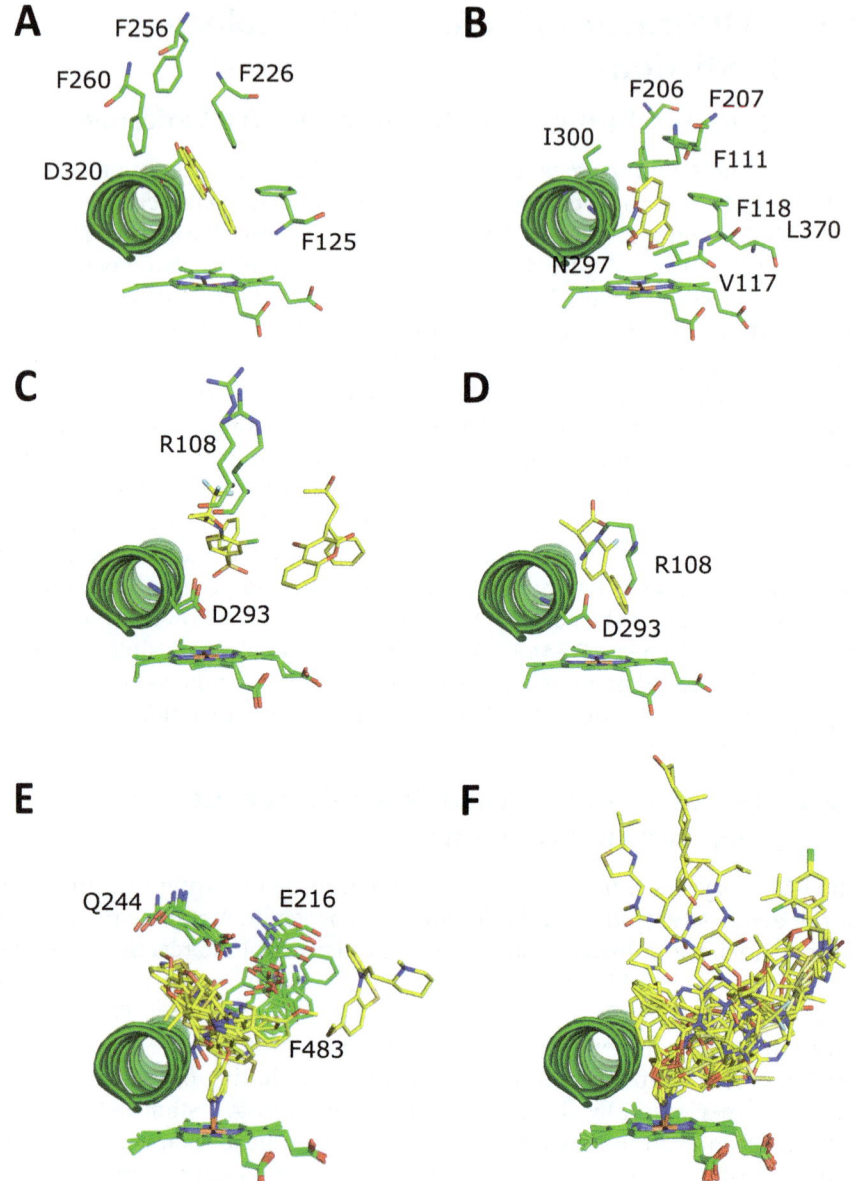

Figure 4.3 The active sites of selected CYPs. The heme group and helix I are displayed for all complexes to facilitate a direct comparison. (A) CYP 1A2 in complex with α-naphthoflavone (2HI4). (B) CYP 2A6 in complex with methoxsalen (1Z11). (C) CYP 2C9 in complex with warfarin (1OG5) and an inhibitor (2NZ2). (D) CYP 2C9 in complex with flurbiprofen (1R9O). (E) Seven CYP 2D6 complexes (3TBG, 3TDA, 3QM4, 4WNT, 4WNU, 4WNV and 4WNW). The 3TBG contains two thioridazine molecules, one of which is not binding close to the heme group. (F) Fourteen different CYP 3A4 complexes (1WOF, 1WOG, 2JOC, 2JOD, 2VOM, 3TJS, 3UA1, 4I4G, 4I4H, 4K9T, 4K9U, 4K9V, 4K9X and 4NY4).

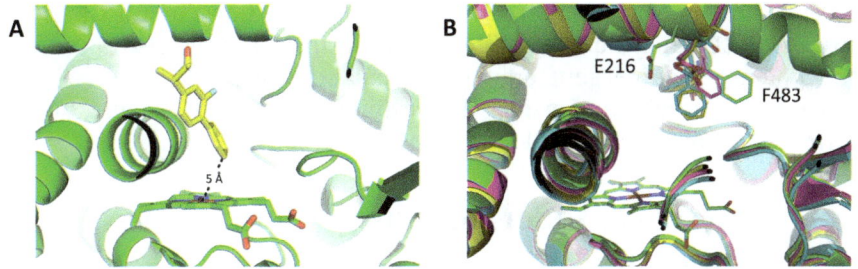

Figure 4.4 (A) The orientation of flurbiprofen in the crystal structure of CYP 2C9 (1R9O). (B) Four different crystal structures of CYP 2D6 (2F9Q, 3TBG, 3TDA and 3QM4).

For the CYP 1A2 isoform, 20 substrates were docked into the active site. It was tested whether the best-ranked substrate orientation was in agreement with the experimentally observed site of metabolism, *i.e.* whether the site in the substrate known to undergo a reaction was within 6 Å of the heme iron. Out the 20 substrates, 13 substrates of the best-ranked poses were in agreement with the experimentally observed site of metabolism. For four substrates the second ranked pose needed to be included to understand the metabolism, while three substrates could not be docked. Thus, most of the CYP metabolism can actually be explained by the binding to the enzyme using the docking program, without taking the subsequent reaction into account.[16]

The prediction of how the substrate binds to the CYP enzyme is probably more difficult for some of the more flexible isoforms such as CYP 2D6 and particularly CYP 3A4 compared with CYP 1A2. A lot of docking studies were done on the CYP 2D6 enzyme to study the site of metabolism, before the crystal structure was solved. To do this, various homology models of CYP 2D6 were constructed on the basis of X-ray structures of related CYP enzymes. Docking into a homology model of 2D6 gave agreement for 60% of the substrates with the experimentally observed metabolites. Interestingly, the prediction was improved further by including water molecules in the binding site, which is usually not done in a standard docking. After the X-ray structure of an *apo* form of CYP 2D6 became available, the same set of substrates were docked, but surprisingly, only 20% of the substrates could be docked with a site within 6 Å of the iron corresponding to the experimentally observed site of metabolism. Subsequently, 2500 CYP 2D6 structures were generated by molecular dynamics. Docking into this ensemble, the prediction rate increased to 52% and it was possible to identify a single structure of CYP 2D6 for which the prediction rate for the site of metabolism increased to 71%, while using three protein structures allowed an overall accuracy of up to 90% to be obtained. One of the reasons why an ensemble was needed is that certain residues, *e.g.* F483, seem to adopt different conformations in the active site. This flexibility of the active site residues was later also observed in three new crystal structures. Figure 4.4B demonstrates that F483 can adopt several different conformations, which will influence how the substrates bind to the CYP 2D6 enzyme. These different conformations were also observed in the protein structures generated by molecular dynamics.[17]

Thus, it is crucial to consider the flexibility of the CYP enzyme, but this introduces a significant challenge from an *in silico* point of view.

4.3 Reactivity Models for Site of Metabolism Predictions

4.3.1 CYP-Mediated Reactions

When using structure-based approaches as described in the previous section, it is assumed the oxidation reaction occurs if the atom in the substrate has the correct orientation compared with the heme group. This is probably a good assumption, because compound I oxidizes many different types of chemical group (see Figure 4.5). There are, however, computational chemistry-based methods for investigating how the reaction proceeds once the substrate is bound to the active site. These methods have been used extensively over the past decades for the CYP reactions.

Some of the first *in silico* studies were on the aliphatic hydroxylation reactions and were carried out by Shaik and coworkers[18] using density functional theory (DFT) calculations. For these types of calculation, a model system as shown in Figure 4.6 is used to determine the transition state and, thus, the activation energy. The initial hydrogen abstraction reaction in which the hydrogen atom on the aliphatic carbon atom is transferred from the substrate to the oxygen atom of compound I (see Figure 4.5 and 4.6) has the highest activation energy. The subsequent OH rebound that forms the hydroxylated product is without barriers on the doublet surface but has a barrier in the quartet spin state. The alkene and aromatic hydroxylation reactions and heteroatom reaction profiles were studied soon after. For the alkene and aromatic oxidations, the initial attack of the iron-bound oxygen atom on the sp^2-hybridized carbon atom is rate limiting and, subsequently, the epoxide, alcohol or ketone can be formed. Oxidations of heteroatoms such as sulfur and nitrogen containing groups can occur *via* direct insertion of the oxygen atom. For amines, except for tertiary amines, there can be competition between a hydrogen abstraction reaction (from the nitrogen atom) and a direct oxygen addition.

After the initial establishment of the reaction mechanism, many studies on substitution patterns followed. For example, it was established that activation energies in the following order are observed: primary carbons > secondary/tertiary carbons > carbons with adjacent sp^2 or aromatic groups > ethers/thioethers > amines.[19] Although the primary carbon atoms may have relatively high activation energies (see energy ranges for aliphatic hydroxylation and dealkylation in Figure 4.7), the CYP enzymes often do these reactions (as seen in the example in Figure 4.1).[20] The DFT-calculated activation energies just indicate that other reactions would occur more easily if the substrate could

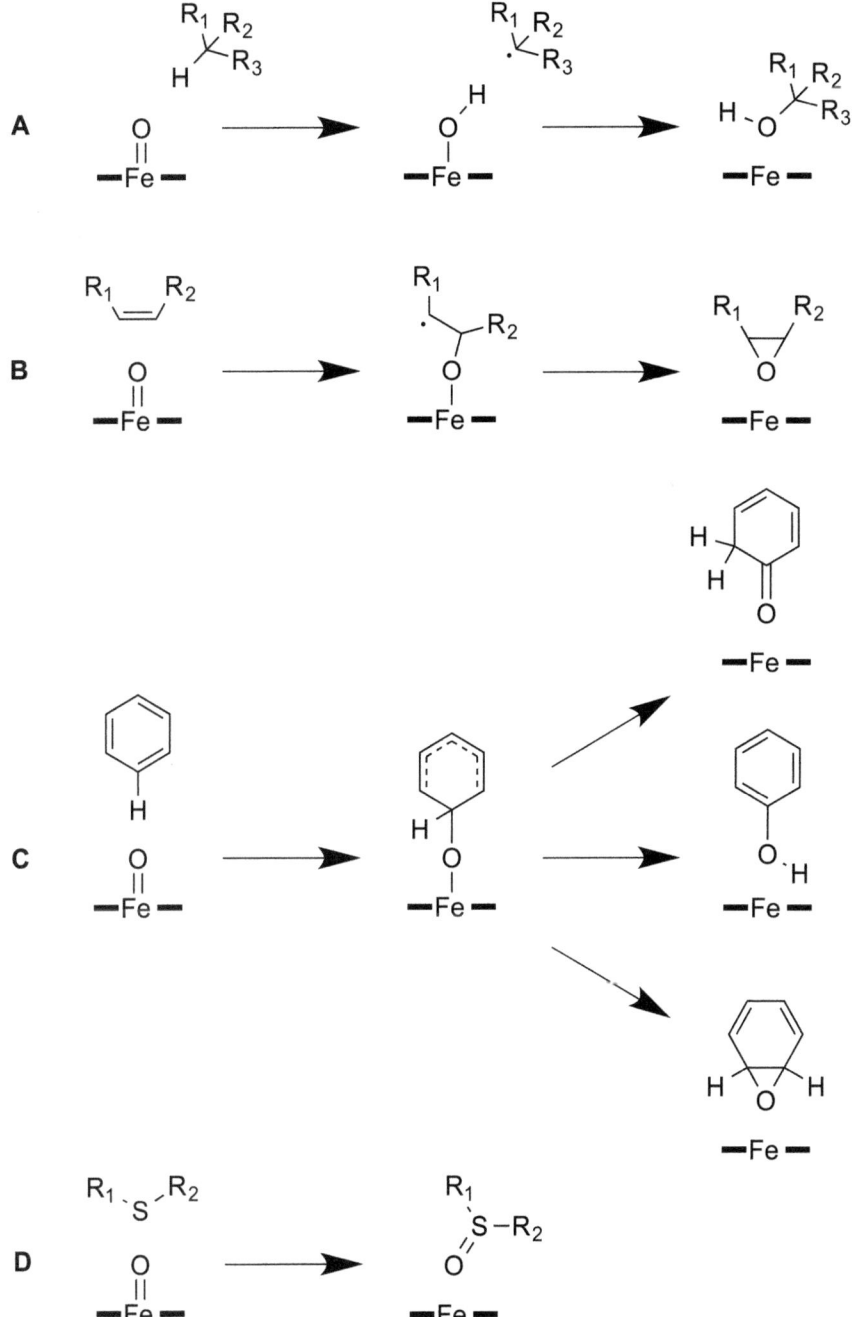

Figure 4.5 Aliphatic hydroxylation (A), epoxidation (B), aromatic hydroxylation (C), and heteroatom oxidations (D). The aliphatic hydroxylation reactions on amines and ethers/thioethers lead to dealkylation reactions.

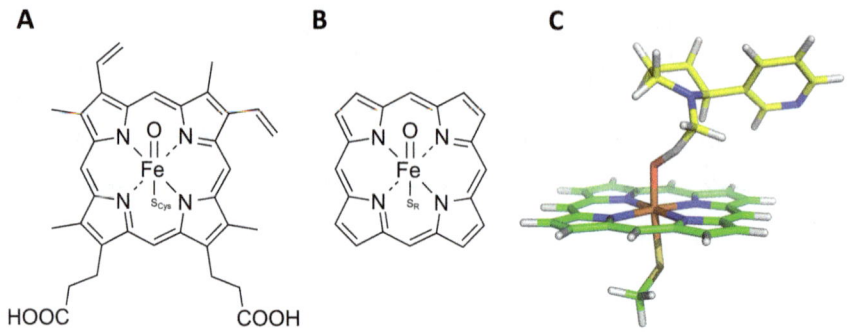

Figure 4.6 (A) Compound **I** with an axial cysteine residue coordinated by the iron atom. (B) Iron-oxo-porphine is typically used to model compound **I** in the DFT calculations (R = H/CH$_3$). (C) The transition state structure of the initial and rate-limiting step, hydrogen abstraction, in the aliphatic hydroxylation of nicotine.

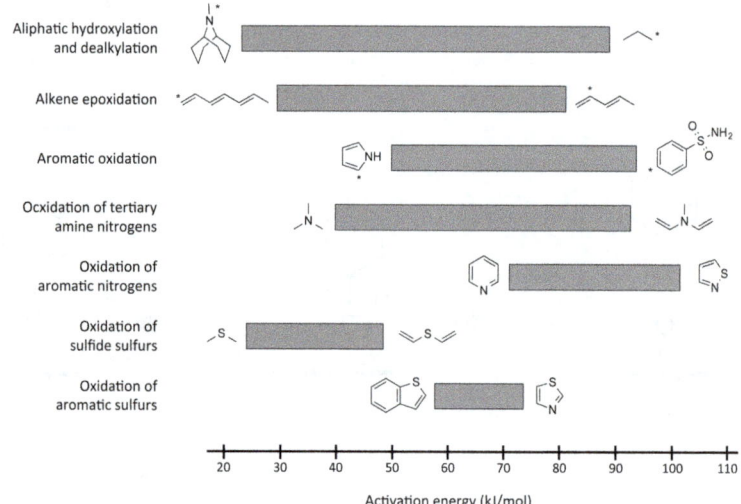

Figure 4.7 Ranges of the activation energies from DFT calculations.[20]

be oriented to make the reaction possible. On the other hand, the primary carbon atoms are quite accessible for the iron-bound oxygen of compound **I**, which is probably why they often undergo hydroxylation. The activation energies are often not affected much by the substitution on the chemical fragments. For example, many different aliphatic hydroxylation reactions on carbon atoms next to amine nitrogen atoms, often leading to *N*-dealkylation, have very similar activation energies (see Figure 4.8). This observation forms the basis for a simple and predictive model for the activation energies for aliphatic hydroxylation reactions. Similar studies for aromatic hydroxylations have been done[21] showing that substitutions have an effect as well.

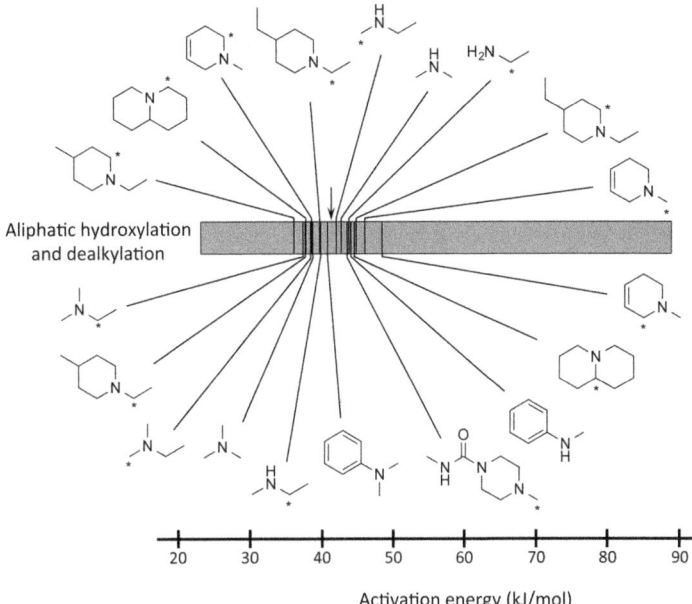

Figure 4.8 DFT-calculated activation energies for hydrogen abstraction from carbon atoms next to an amine. The arrow shows the average value used for prediction of the site of metabolism (41.1 ± 3.6 kJ mol⁻¹).[20]

In particular, electron donating chemical groups such as amines in the *ortho* or *para* position lower the activation barrier.[22]

4.3.2 Reactivity Models for Site of Metabolism Predictions

The DFT-calculated activation energies can be related to whether the site of metabolism is also observed experimentally. In principle, the reactions with the lowest activation energies would occur fastest. However, the binding to the enzyme is usually not taken into account in these types of studies, which is why the reactions with lowest activation energies are not necessarily the ones observed experimentally. The reason can be that the compound does not bind to the CYP isoform or it binds in a conformation where the transition state is too distorted for the reaction to be able to occur.

DFT calculations of activation energies on each possible site in a substrate are still quite time consuming. For example, there are more than 10 potential sites of metabolism to check in a small substrate such as meclofenamic acid or aflatoxin B1 (Figure 4.1). However, since similar fragments often have similar activation energies, the pre-computed ones can be used to assess how reactive a site in a substrate is (see Figure 4.7 and 4.8). The basis for the SMARTCyp algorithm is activation energies of chemical fragments derived from more than 200 DFT calculations.[23] As shown in Figure 4.7, there is quite a large range between the lowest and highest activation energies. However, similar fragments often have similar activation energies, as also illustrated in Figure 4.8 for hydrogen abstraction from aliphatic carbon atoms in amines. This makes it possible to make general rules for the activation energies. With these activation energy rules in combination with a simple accessibility measure applied to a set of CYP 3A4 substrates, the experimental sites of metabolism were identified within the two most reactive sites for 76% of the substrates. This observation, *i.e.* that the predicted reactive sites are often also seen experimentally as sites of metabolism for CYP 3A4, could be due to the large and flexible active site of CYP 3A4 (see Figure 4.3F).

Other CYP isoforms also seem to metabolize the sites with low activation energies. This could indicate that the binding to the enzyme cavity seems to be less important than one might expect judging from the significant differences in the 3D structures of the CYP isoforms (see Figure 4.3). This, however, is not the case for CYP 2D6 and 2C9 enzymes. This fits well with observations from the crystal structures of these enzymes that show that the E216 and D301 (see Figure 4.3E) residues in CYP 2D6 interact favorably with positively charged groups in substrates and the R108 residue in CYP 2C9 interacts favorably with negatively charged groups in substrates (see Figure 4.3C). A very simple correction to take this into account was applied to SMARTCyp, by adding a penalty for sites that are close to positively or negatively charged chemical groups, because this part of the substrate will never be in the proximity of the heme. This increases the agreement with the experimental sites of metabolism. Thus, without explicitly taking the enzyme into account, prediction rates of around 80% are achieved for the CYP 1A2, 2A6, 2B6, 2C8, 2C9, 2C19, 2D6, 2E1 and 3A4 isoforms.

The SMARTCyp activation energies have been used as a descriptor in other tools for prediction of the site of metabolism. Adding more descriptors has in some cases improved the predictions.[24] In addition, the docking scores of poses with a certain chemical group accessible to the heme have been corrected with these reactivities.[25]

4.4 Perspectives

Site of metabolism predictions for CYP enzymes is challenging to handle with *in silico* methods because the structures are flexible, the electronic properties of the heme are complex and there are many different relevant CYP isoforms to consider. The significant number of *in silico* studies carried out over the past decade on the binding to and reactions of CYP enzymes have contributed to the understanding of the function of these enzymes. In addition, this is a good example of knowledge derived from basic research that has later been applied by the experimental research community, both in academia and industry. There are still many things that can be studied and that could further improve our understanding. For example, ongoing issues being tackled by the scientific community include sampling of the protein introduced in molecular dynamics, the effect of the protein on the reactions (*e.g.* with the so-called combined quantum mechanical and molecular mechanics methods), and the effect of improved DFT or other quantum mechanical methods on the activation energies. However, it is encouraging that the quality of the *in silico* tools for site of metabolism detection has reached a level where they are useful in drug discovery. All the experience gained from the *in silico* studies on CYP enzymes will most likely make it a lot easier to study other drug-metabolizing enzymes and improve our understanding in this field.

References

1. F. P. Guengerich, *AAPS J.*, 2006, **8**, E101–E111.
2. H. Venkataraman, M. C. Verkade-Vreeker, L. Capoferri, D. P. Geerke, N. P. Vermeulen and J. N. Commandeur, *Bioorg. Med. Chem.*, 2014, **22**, 5613–5620.
3. E. P. Gallagher, K. L. Kunze, P. L. Stapleton and D. L. Eaton, *Toxicol. Appl. Pharmacol.*, 1996, **141**, 595–606.
4. H. Wang, R. Dick, H. Yin, E. Licad-Coles, D. L. Kroetz, G. Szklarz, G. Harlow, J. R. Halpert and M. A. Correia, *Biochemistry*, 1998, **37**, 12536–12545.
5. S. Sansen, J. K. Yano, R. L. Reynald, G. A. Schoch, K. J. Griffin, C. D. Stout and E. F. Johnson, *J. Biol. Chem.*, 2007, **282**, 14348–14355.
6. J. K. Yano, M. H. Hsu, K. J. Griffin, C. D. Stout and E. F. Johnson, *Nat. Struct. Mol. Biol.*, 2005, **12**, 822–823.
7. M. R. Wester, J. K. Yano, G. A. Schoch, C. Yang, K. J. Griffin, C. D. Stout and E. F. Johnson, *J. Biol. Chem.*, 2004, **279**, 35630–35637.
8. P. A. Williams, J. Cosme, D. M. Vinkovic, A. Ward, H. C. Angove, P. J. Day, C. Vonrhein, I. J. Tickle and H. Jhoti, *Science*, 2004, **305**, 683–686.
9. G. Branden, T. Sjogren, V. Schnecke and Y. Xue, *Drug Discovery Today*, 2014, **19**, 905–911.
10. P. A. Williams, J. Cosme, A. Ward, H. C. Angove, D. Matak Vinkovic and H. Jhoti, *Nature*, 2003, **424**, 464–468.
11. A. Wang, U. Savas, M. H. Hsu, C. D. Stout and E. F. Johnson, *J. Biol. Chem.*, 2012, **287**, 10834–10843.
12. A. Wang, C. D. Stout, Q. Zhang and E. F. Johnson, *J. Biol. Chem.*, 2015, **290**, 5092–5104.
13. E. Stjernschantz, N. P. Vermeulen and C. Oostenbrink, *Expert Opin. Drug Metab. Toxicol.*, 2008, **4**, 513–527.
14. G. Cruciani, E. Carosati, B. De Boeck, K. Ethirajulu, C. Mackie, T. Howe and R. Vianello, *J. Med. Chem.*, 2005, **48**, 6970–6979.
15. L. Afzelius, C. H. Arnby, A. Broo, L. Carlsson, C. Isaksson, U. Jurva, B. Kjellander, K. Kolmodin, K. Nilsson, F. Raubacher and L. Weidolf, *Drug Metab. Rev.*, 2007, **39**, 61–86.
16. P. Vasanthanathan, J. Hritz, O. Taboureau, L. Olsen, F. S. Jørgensen, N. P. Vermeulen and C. Oostenbrink, *J. Chem. Inf. Model.*, 2009, **49**, 43–52.
17. J. Hritz, A. de Ruiter and C. Oostenbrink, *J. Med. Chem.*, 2008, **51**, 7469–7477.

18. S. Shaik, D. Kumar, S. P. de Visser, A. Altun and W. Thiel, *Chem. Rev.*, 2005, **105**, 2279–2328.
19. L. Olsen, P. Rydberg, T. H. Rod and U. Ryde, *J. Med. Chem.*, 2006, **49**, 6489–6499.
20. P. Rydberg, M. S. Jørgensen, T. A. Jacobsen, A. M. Jacobsen, K. G. Madsen and L. Olsen, *Angew. Chem., Int. Ed. Engl.*, 2013, **52**, 993–997.
21. C. M. Bathelt, L. Ridder, A. J. Mulholland and J. N. Harvey, *Org. Biomol. Chem.*, 2004, **2**, 2998–3005.
22. P. Rydberg, U. Ryde and L. Olsen, *J. Phys. Chem. A*, 2008, **112**, 13058–13065.
23. P. Rydberg, D. E. Gloriam, J. Zaretzki, C. Breneman and L. Olsen, *ACS Med. Chem. Lett.*, 2010, **1**, 96–100.
24. J. D. Tyzack, M. J. Williamson, R. Torella and R. C. Glen, *J. Chem. Inf. Model.*, 2013, **53**, 1294–1305.
25. P. Rydberg, F. S. Jørgensen and L. Olsen, *Expert Opin. Drug Metab. Toxicol.*, 2014, **10**, 215–227.

CHAPTER 5

Non-Cytochrome P450 Enzymes and Glucuronidation

J. MATTHEW HUTZLER*[a] AND MICHAEL A. ZIENTEK[b]

[a]Q² Solutions, Bioanalytical and ADME Labs, 5225 Exploration Drive, Indianapolis, IN 46241, USA; [b]Pfizer Inc., Pharmacokinetics, Dynamics, and Metabolism, 10646 Science Center Drive CB4, San Diego, CA 92121, USA
*E-mail: matt.hutzler@Q2LabSolutions.com

5.1 Introduction

The metabolism of drug molecules has historically been dominated by the cytochrome P450 (CYP) super-family of enzymes, with CYP1A2, CYP2A6, CYP2B6, CYP2C8, CYP2C9, CYP2C19, CYP2D6, CYP3A4 and CYP3A5 being the most abundant in the liver.[1] Due to the positive impact of metabolic stability screening strategies early in drug discovery for optimization of drug molecules, as well as knowledge gained on lipophilicity correlating with promiscuous binding to unintended pharmacological targets,[2,3] the physicochemical properties that drug discovery chemists are exploring have evolved from lipophilic to more polar chemical scaffolds. This shift in the targeted chemical space has resulted in the emergence of non-CYP metabolic pathways (and transporters), which is forcing drug metabolism scientists to respond with a more complete understanding of the biochemistry of these drug-metabolizing enzymes. Critical methodologies necessary in the endeavor include how to identify the role of these enzymes in the metabolism of drug molecules *in vitro*, and how to integrate *in vitro* metabolism data

RSC Drug Discovery Series No. 49
New Horizons in Predictive Drug Metabolism and Pharmacokinetics
Edited by Alan G. E. Wilson
© The Royal Society of Chemistry 2016
Published by the Royal Society of Chemistry, www.rsc.org

with preclinical *in vivo* data to ultimately predict the disposition of drug molecules in humans, an undertaking that is extremely challenging.

Many non-CYP enzymes are known to be involved in the biotransformation (*i.e.* metabolism) of drug molecules, including alcohol/aldehyde dehydrogenases, monoamine oxidases (MAOs), esterases/amidases, aldehyde oxidase (AO), and conjugating enzymes (Table 5.1). It is critical to know how to characterize and identify the role of these enzymes in the metabolism of drug molecules, which starts with a fundamental understanding of where these enzymes reside within the cell. In addition, it is important to note that while the liver is considered the predominant drug-metabolizing organ that houses these metabolic enzymes, extrahepatic tissues such as the kidney and intestine also contain a plethora of metabolic enzymes.[4-6] Table 5.1 highlights the commonly used subcellular fractions that contain these drug-metabolizing enzymes, which include the cytosolic, microsomal, and mitochondrial fractions. Most metabolic screening paradigms involve incubating newly synthesized drug molecules in human liver microsomes (HLM), since the CYP enzymes have historically played a dominant role in drug metabolism. Unfortunately, examples are evident from the literature where a lack of complete understanding of non-CYP drug-metabolizing enzymes has led to unanticipated clinical failures, resulting from either poor drug exposure or toxicological outcomes.[7,8] Thus, for a comprehensive view on drug metabolism, the preferred *in vitro* system has become hepatocytes (fresh or cryopreserved), which contain the full complement of drug-metabolizing enzymes. Nonetheless, strategic use of specific subcellular fractions may aid in the ultimate identification and mechanistic understanding of non-CYP metabolic enzymes. In this regard, a proposed *in vitro* strategy for

Table 5.1 List of important drug metabolizing enzymes and their subcellular locations.

Reaction	Enzyme	Subcellular fraction
Oxidation	CYP	Microsomes
	Flavin monooxygenase (FMO)	Microsomes
	Prostaglandin H synthase (PGHS)	Microsomes
	Monoamine oxidase (MAO)	Mitochondria
	Alcohol dehydrogenase (ADH)	Cytosol
	Aldehyde dehydrogenase (ALDH)	Mitochondria, cytosol
	Aldehyde oxidase (AO)	Cytosol
	Xanthine oxidoreductase (XOR)	Cytosol
	Diamine oxidase (DAO)	Cytosol
Reduction	Aldo-keto reductases (AKR)	Cytosol
Hydrolysis	Carboxylesterase (CES)	Microsomes, cytosol, blood
Conjugation	Glucuronosyltransferase (UGT)	Microsomes
	Glutathione-*S*-transferase (GST)	Microsomes, cytosol
	Catechol *O*-methyl transferase (COMT)	Microsomes, cytosol, blood
	Amino acid transferase	Microsomes, mitochondria
	N-Acetyl transferase (NAT)	Mitochondria, cytosol
	Sulfotransferase (SULT)	Cytosol

demonstrating a potential role for non-CYP mediated metabolism of drug molecules is proposed in Figure 5.1.

Among the numerous phase I non-CYP drug-metabolizing enzymes, this chapter will focus attention on the flavin-containing monooxygenase (FMO) family of metabolic enzymes, and the molybdenum-cofactor (MoCo) containing AO, which has surged in interest in the drug development community. In addition, the uridine diphosphate (UDP) glucuronosyltransferase (UGT) family of conjugative enzymes, regarded as the second most important family of enzymes following CYP, will be discussed. The drug-metabolizing enzymes discussed have distinct characteristics from the more familiar CYP super-family of enzymes, and have been problematic when trying to extrapolate from *in vitro* and preclinical species to human metabolic clearance, due namely to either the lability of the enzyme in *in vitro* systems, extrahepatic expression, profound species differences, or a combination thereof. These aforementioned issues, as well as catalytic mechanism, tissue expression, and overall relevance to drug metabolism will be discussed in this chapter.

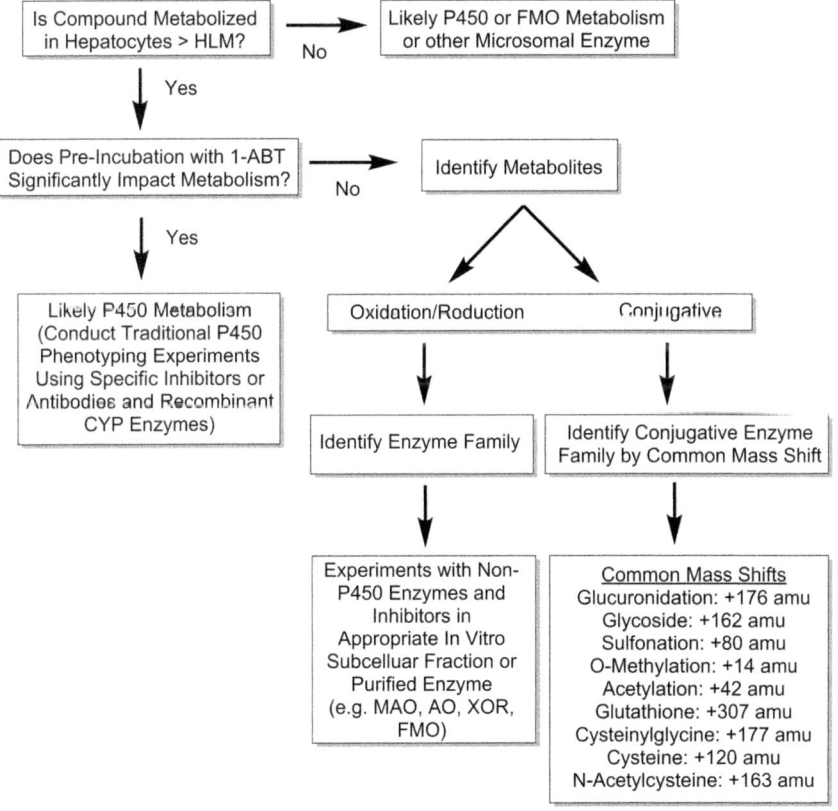

Figure 5.1 Proposed *in vitro* flow chart for identification of non-CYP enzyme involvement in the metabolism of a drug.

5.2   FMOs

Prior to the isolation and purification of FMO from pig liver in the early-1970s,[9] it was thought that oxidation of drug molecules to facilitate clearance by biosynthesis of more polar metabolites was predominantly the role of CYP enzymes, particularly in HLM. However, it is now recognized that the membrane-bound FMO enzymes, which are also located in the microsomal fraction, play an important role in drug metabolism. FMO enzymes are a family of nicotinamide-adenine dinucleotide phosphate (NADPH)-dependent and oxygen-dependent metabolic enzymes involved in the oxygenation of nitrogen-, sulfur-, phosphorous-, selenium-, and other nucleophilic heteroatom-containing small molecules.[10,11] The mammalian FMO gene family consists of five primary enzymes (FMO1, FMO2, FMO3, FMO4, and FMO5) that contain roughly 550 amino acid residues in their primary sequence. These five distinct forms have roughly 50–58% amino acid sequence identity and are apparently expressed in most mammalian species, although with substantial species and tissue expression differences.[12] It is likely that an under-appreciation for the role of FMO in drug metabolism exists today due to a lack of fundamental knowledge about the enzymology of this enzyme, including its thermal instability in the absence of NADPH, which is often not considered when conventional metabolic stability screening assays are conducted using pre-incubations with liver microsomes. Some of these confounding factors and recommended approaches in studying metabolism by FMO will be discussed in this chapter.

5.2.1   Characteristics and Catalytic Mechanism

The catalytic mechanism of FMO-mediated oxidation is complex and contains multiple steps (Figure 5.2). Each FMO enzyme contains two conserved glycine-rich regions: one that binds flavin adenine dinucleotide (FAD) non-covalently, and the other that binds NADPH.[13,14] The initial step in the FMO catalytic cycle involves reduction of the FAD cofactor by NADPH to $FADH_2$, a one-step hydride transfer to the flavin N5 atom. The reduced flavin readily reacts with molecular oxygen (O_2) to form the 4α-hydroperoxyflavin intermediate (FAD-OOH), a species that is reported to be stable due to the microenvironment around the prosthetic group,[15,16] which contributes to the high efficiency of FMO enzymes relative to CYP. Because the peroxyflavin intermediate is generated prior to substrate binding and is stable, it is able to wait until a soft nucleophilic substrate binds in proximity to the active oxygenating species.[17] This phenomenon has been described as the FMO enzyme being in a "cocked" position ready to oxidize any suitable substrate that becomes available.[18] Interestingly, $NADP^+$ stays bound to the FMO enzyme throughout the catalytic cycle, which helps promote the stability of the peroxyflavin,[19] thus minimizing reduction of the oxygen to H_2O_2 and the subsequent potential for extreme oxidative stress.[20] However, more recent work by Siddens *et al.* suggests that as much as 30–50% of consumed O_2 is released as H_2O_2

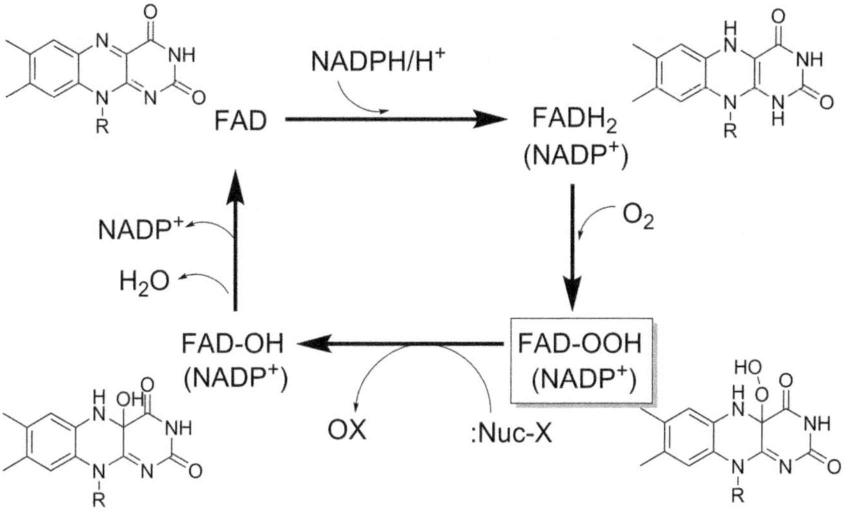

Figure 5.2 Catalytic mechanism of FMO.

in human FMOs 1, 2, and 3 expressed in Sf9 insect microsomes.[21] The next step involves binding of the soft nucleophilic substrate, which attacks the distal oxygen of the peroxyflavin intermediate, resulting in transfer of one atom of oxygen to generate the oxidized product metabolite that is released rapidly (typically, products from this mechanism include *N*-oxides and sulfoxide metabolites), along with a flavin hydroxy species (FAD-OH). Once the product metabolite is released, water and NADP⁺ are released to regenerate the flavin cofactor (FAD). It is believed that this last step (release of water to regenerate FAD and/or release of NADP⁺) is the rate-limiting step of the FMO catalytic cycle. Because binding of substrate is not rate limiting, this does not appear to impact the rate of catalysis. Thus, most reactions catalyzed by FMO tend to have similar maximal rates (V_{max} values).[22]

5.2.2 Tissue Expression, Polymorphisms, and Species Differences

In humans, there are five functional FMO enzymes (FMO1–FMO5) as well as six pseudogenes. Human FMO1 and FMO3 appear to play the most dominant role in xenobiotic metabolism, while the role of FMO2, FMO4, and FMO5 in xenobiotic metabolism is currently not as well understood.[23] A summary of the relative expression levels of the FMO enzymes in human tissues is shown in Table 5.2. FMO1 is the most highly expressed FMO in the adult kidney, but is also expressed in the small intestine and fetal liver, albeit much less compared with the adult kidney.[24] The high expression levels of FMO1 in human kidney coupled with high functional activity suggest that FMO1 may contribute to metabolic clearance of a diverse array of xenobiotics. FMO2 is the

Table 5.2 Tissue expression patterns of the human isoforms of FMO.[a]

Enzyme	Tissue expression
FMO1	Kidney > fetal liver > small intestine ~ lung
FMO2	Lung ≫ kidney > small intestine ~ liver
FMO3	Liver > lung > kidney ~ fetal liver > small intestine
FMO4	Liver > kidney > lung ~ intestine (all low)
FMO5	Liver > fetal liver > intestine ~ kidney ~ lung

[a]Adapted from Cashman and Zhang.[23]

dominant FMO in adult lung, but a premature stop codon renders the FMO2 enzyme inactive for most of the population.[25] This polymorphism is ethnically related, where all Caucasians and Asians genotyped have a mutation resulting in this premature stop codon and non-functional protein truncated at amino acid 472, whereas 26% of individuals of African descent carry at least one allele for full-length FMO2.[26] This may have implications for toxicity in individuals who express active FMO2, since this enzyme is responsible for the *S*-oxygenation of thiourea compounds, a known bioactivation pathway. FMO3 is the major FMO form in adult liver, while expression in other tissues such as lung, kidney, fetal liver, and small intestine are roughly 4.5%, 3.7%, 2.1%, and 1%, respectively, relative to the liver.[23] Interestingly, while FMO3 is the dominant FMO isoform in adult human liver, FMO1 is the major human FMO in fetal liver tissue. The FMO1/FMO3 switch and control mechanisms have been investigated by Koukouritaki *et al.*[27] In these studies, FMO1 and FMO3 were measured from microsomal fractions taken from 240 liver samples ranging in age from 8 weeks gestation to 18 years. FMO1 expression was high in the embryo, but was suppressed within 3 days postpartum. The onset of FMO3 expression was highly variable, but detectable in most individuals by 1–2 years of age.[27] This variability may be partly due to known genetic polymorphisms in the *FMO3* gene that code for either amino acid substitutions, or truncated forms that have little to no enzyme activity.[28,29] For example, FMO3 converts trimethylamine (TMA), an odorous tertiary amine by-product of choline and carnitine metabolism, to the non-odorous TMA *N*-oxide. TMA has an odor comparable to rotting fish, and people who are genetically deficient in FMO3 suffer from a condition called "fish-odor syndrome" caused by excretion of TMA in urine, sweat, and breath.[23] The cause of this condition involves a P153L amino acid substitution on the *FMO3* gene.[30] The numerous amino acid substitutions for FMO3 genetic variants have been summarized by Cashman.[31]

FMO4 mRNA is present in low abundance in several fetal and adult tissues and, thus, the corresponding gene appears to be expressed constitutively.[32] However, human FMO4 remains the least well-characterized isoform, and a clear role in drug metabolism is yet to be defined. While the abundance of FMO5 in human liver was once thought to be much less than FMO3, newer reports suggest that FMO5 expression is equal to or higher than FMO3 in liver, as determined by mRNA.[4,23] However, the role of FMO5 in drug metabolism pales in comparison to FMO3, as FMO5 demonstrates poor catalytic activity towards common FMO substrates. Recently, however, FMO5 was shown to selectively catalyze a Baeyer–Villiger oxidation of the ketone intermediate of E7016, an inhibitor of poly(ADP-ribose) polymerase.[33] At the time of this report, it was thought that this FMO5-catalyzed Baeyer–Villiger reaction was unique. However, a similar Baeyer–Villiger mechanism was more recently reported as being catalyzed by FMO5 for MRX-I, a novel analog of the antibacterial linezolid.[34] Thus, the role of FMO5 in the metabolism of drug molecules is continuing to emerge.

FMO isoforms also have distinct species-dependent, and in some cases, gender-dependent expression, which is important to consider when comparing FMO-mediated metabolism in preclinical species with humans.[35] For example, from a liver metabolism perspective, rats would be a poor model for human FMO drug metabolism, since the most abundant liver FMO enzyme for humans is FMO3, while that in rat liver is FMO1. Additional species differences and comparisons of metabolism by FMO1 and FMO3 in humans, rats, monkeys, and mini-pigs have been reported, and higher FMO1 levels in rat and mini-pig liver microsomes were demonstrated relative to monkey and human.[36] In addition, there are substantial gender differences in mice and rats. Ripp and colleagues reported that in addition to species differences, sex differences in FMO3 levels, as determined by methionine *S*-oxidation activity and immunoblotting, were observed for mice and dogs, with females displaying higher levels than males.[37] Thus, in general, when comparing metabolism across species for substrates of human FMO, caution is recommended, especially when clearance data from preclinical species are being utilized for human pharmacokinetic (PK) scaling purposes.

5.2.3 Substrate Specificities

FMO enzymes can oxidize hundreds of structurally diverse substrates in a very nonspecific manner, which include amines, hydrazines, thiols, sulfides, thioamides, thiocarbamides, and compounds possessing nucleophilic selenium and phosphorus atoms.[10] In general, FMO enzymes catalyze the oxidation of nucleophilic sp^3-hybridized tertiary amines to *N*-oxides, secondary amines to hydroxylamines and nitrones, and primary amines to hydroxylamines and oximes.[38] While the primary features of FMO substrates include being a soft nucleophile (typically a nitrogen or sulfur heteroatom), molecular size, charge, and even chirality play a role in recognition by the FMO enzymes. Examples of some of the well characterized substrates of FMO are depicted in Figure 5.3, with arrows indicating the site of oxygenation by FMO. Human FMO3 is primarily responsible for converting (*S*)-nicotine to its *N*-1'-oxide metabolite, according to *in vitro* data generated using cDNA-expressed adult human liver FMO3.[39] In addition, the stereoselectivity of the (*S*)-nicotine *N*-1'-oxide formation was investigated in healthy male smokers, and only the *trans* diastereomer was excreted into urine. Thus, the urinary metabolite of (*S*)-nicotine may be a useful *in vivo* probe for human FMO3

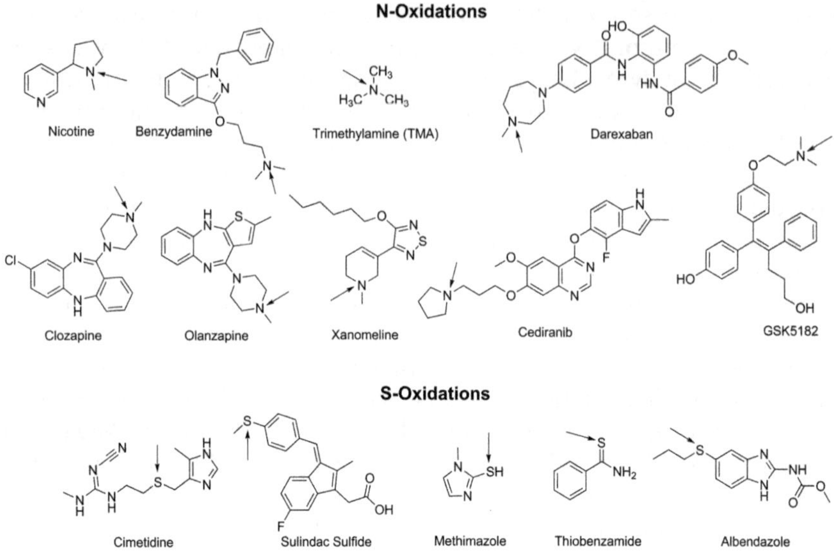

N-Oxidations

Nicotine Benzydamine Trimethylamine (TMA) Darexaban

Clozapine Olanzapine Xanomeline Cediranib GSK5182

S-Oxidations

Cimetidine Sulindac Sulfide Methimazole Thiobenzamide Albendazole

Figure 5.3 Structures of known substrates of FMO. Arrows indicate the primary sites of metabolism.

activity. Cimetidine is another substrate for FMO3 that is stereoselectively metabolized. It is sulfoxidated *in vitro* in HLM with a roughly 84:16 mixture of (−) and (+) enantiomers.[40] Interestingly, this ratio is fairly well predictive of the average urinary ratio reported from seven human subjects following a 900 mg oral dose [75:25 of (−):(+)],[40] and thus may also be a useful *in vivo* probe of human FMO3 activity. From an *in vitro* perspective, a useful FMO substrate is the anti-inflammatory drug benzydamine (Figure 5.3), which is extensively metabolized to benzydamine *N*-oxide.[41] Benzydamine was reported to undergo *N*-oxidation by recombinant human FMO1, FMO3, FMO4, and FMO5, with apparent K_m values of 60 μM, 80 μM, >3 mM, and >2 mM, respectively.[42] Thus, FMO1 and FMO3 catalyzed the *N*-oxidation of benzydamine most efficiently. Benzydamine *N*-oxidation kinetics in HLM were also characterized in the same time frame by a separate laboratory, with a reported K_m of 64 μM.[43] More recently, benzydamine was evaluated as an index reaction for FMO activity in liver microsomes from multiple species (rat, dog, monkey and human).[44] In this work, the FMO-mediated *N*-oxidation metabolic pathway, and the CYP-mediated *N*-demethylation pathway were compared under different *in vitro* conditions to separate and confirm FMO and CYP enzyme involvement. Actual methodologies for this will be discussed in more depth in the next section on differentiating FMO and CYP activity. Additional relevant drugs and endobiotics that have been characterized as substrates for FMO include clozapine,[45] olanzapine,[46] xanomeline,[47] and the endogenous substrate TMA.[48]

Some more recent drug candidates that were reported to be substrates of FMO include cediranib,[49] darexaban,[50] and GSK5182.[51] Cediranib was a vascular endothelial growth factor (VEGF) tyrosine kinase inhibitor in late-stage development by Astra Zeneca. The metabolism of cediranib was investigated to understand the species differences in metabolism and inform preclinical coverage of human metabolites. Following the observation that the general CYP inhibitor 1-aminobenzotriazole was unable to inhibit formation of the *N*-oxide metabolite in human hepatocytes, it was discovered that both FMO1 and FMO3 contributed to formation of the *N*-oxide. Meanwhile, FMO5 demonstrated no activity towards formation of the *N*-oxide.[49] Darexaban was a factor Xa inhibitor being developed by Astellas Pharma that inhibits prothrombin activation. In humans, darexaban was almost completely converted to a glucuronide metabolite. In addition, a 1:1 mixture of two *N*-oxide diastereomers of the glucuronide was detected in human plasma, representing ~10% of total radioactivity. *In vitro* in HLM, *N*-oxidation of darexaban glucuronide correlated with FMO marker activity (benzydamine *N*-oxidation) and was inhibited by methimazole, an inhibitor of FMO. In addition, recombinant FMO1 and FMO3 efficiently catalyzed the *N*-oxidation, while FMO5 did not. This represents one of the few examples of a glucuronide being a substrate of FMO.[50] GSK5182, a structural analog of 4-hydroxy-tamoxifen, is being evaluated in preclinical studies as an anti-diabetic agent. The *in vitro* metabolism in HLM was characterized, and a combination of co-incubation with specific CYP and FMO inhibitors, and incubation with recombinant enzymes provided results showing a role for FMO1 and FMO3 in the *N*-oxidation of GSK5182.[51] In addition, in 15 individual HLM preparations, a high correlation with benzydamine *N*-oxidation was observed ($r = 0.82$). A commonality in these aforementioned studies is the employment of cofactor manipulation (*e.g.* ±NADPH), specific inhibitors, recombinant enzymes, and correlation analysis to aid in identifying the role of FMO in the metabolism of these drugs.

5.2.4 Differentiation from CYP

Although FMO enzymes share a similar subcellular location (microsomes), demonstrate substrate overlap, and require the same cofactor (NADPH) for activity as the CYP enzymes, FMO enzymes are distinct from CYP in many ways (Table 5.3). For example, FMO reactions involve a one-step two-electron oxygenation of the substrate, whereas oxidation by CYP enzymes involves two sequential one-electron oxidations. Also, FMO does not require a coenzyme like CYP oxidoreductase to transfer electrons from NADPH since NADPH binds directly to FMO. For FMO enzymes, xenobiotic substrate is not required for oxygen activation, whereas for CYP, substrate binding precedes and is critical for dioxygen reduction.[18] Lastly, NADPH consumption for FMO is tightly coupled to product formation, in contrast to CYP, where the cycle often uncouples to form superoxide anion and/or hydrogen peroxide (H_2O_2)—reactive oxygen species (ROS). In addition, the pH optimum for FMO-catalyzed transformations is 8–10, whereas for CYP enzymes, activity is maximal around pH 7–8. Thus, higher activity of an oxidative pathway at

Table 5.3 Differentiation of FMO from CYP oxidative enzymes.

Characteristic	FMO	CYP
Subcellular location	Microsomes	Microsomes
Size	55–65 kDa	50–55 kDa
Reducing cofactor	NADPH	NADPH
Catalysis cofactor	FAD	Heme – protoporphyrin IX
Mechanism	One-step two-electron oxidation	Sequential one-electron oxidation
Tightly coupled	Yes	No
Typical substrates	Soft nucleophiles	Broad
Enantioselective	Yes	Yes
pH optimum	8–10	7–8
Antibodies	No	Yes
Selective inhibitors	No	Yes
Heat sensitive	Yes (45–50 °C for 5 minutes)[a]	No
Time-dependent inhibitors	No	Yes
DDI risk	Low	High

[a]Pre-incubation at 37 °C for 5–10 minutes may also lead to significant loss of FMO activity.

an elevated pH may indicate a role for FMO. FMO enzymes also display thermal instability in the absence of NADPH, although not all FMO isoforms are equally unstable. For example, FMO2 appears to be more thermally stable than FMO3.[52] Nonetheless, FMO activity can be substantially decreased by heat pre-treatment of microsomes (~45–50 °C for up to 5 minutes) in the absence of NADPH. In addition, the preparation of microsomes, with varying procurement and storage conditions, may also influence FMO activity, leading to potentially lower activity in liver microsomal preparations, and thus, underestimation of FMO contributions to metabolism.[53]

With the current information on FMO catalysis and enzymology, multiple approaches may be employed for diagnosing FMO-mediated oxidation, and differentiating it from CYP, including but not limited to: (1) heat inactivation of microsomes at 45–50 °C for 5 minutes; (2) protection from heat inactivation with NADPH; (3) pH effects; (4) inhibition using methimazole; and (5) metabolism using recombinant FMO enzyme. For example, benzydamine *N*-oxygenation in liver microsomes from rats, dogs, monkeys and humans was confirmed by demonstrating that *N*-oxygenation was extensively suppressed by pre-heating liver microsomes at 45 °C for 5 minutes in the absence of NADPH, and was also inhibited by co-incubation with methimazole. Benzydamine *N*-oxygenation activity was also demonstrated using recombinant human FMO1 and FMO3, and activity was observed in human kidney microsomes at pH 8.4. Collectively, these aforementioned studies helped to confirm the role of FMO in benzydamine *N*-oxygenation, and for CYP2D6 in *N*-demethylation.[44] Interestingly, for metabolic stability screens in microsomes, it is common for NADPH to be the last component added to initiate reactions following pre-incubation at 37 °C for 5–10 minutes.[54] A critical finding from the aforementioned studies with benzydamine was that pre-incubation at 37 °C for 5 and 10 minutes without NADPH yielded a loss of 30% and 50% of FMO activity, respectively.[44] A similar finding when using the traditional 37 °C pre-incubation methodology with benzydamine metabolism was reported by Fisher *et al.*[55] Thus, this common pre-incubation protocol may lead to a large underestimation of FMO involvement in the microsomal metabolism of a test compound, which should be avoided, in particular at later stages when characterizing the metabolic pathways of a drug candidate.

Lastly, in contrast to CYP enzymes, which a significant number of drug molecules inhibit in a reversible or time-dependent fashion (*e.g.* time-dependent inhibitors), inhibition of FMO is not a common phenomenon. In addition, FMO is not readily induced in humans, and thus, the risk for potential PK drug–drug interactions (DDIs) are minimized for drugs metabolized principally by FMO. Thus, increased involvement of FMO in the metabolism of a drug molecule may actually be advantageous to reduce the risk of victim DDIs, which further reinforces the importance of identifying non-CYP metabolic pathways such as FMO. In addition, examples of CYP enzymes bioactivating drug molecules to reactive electrophilic intermediates that can lead to covalent modification of critical proteins and toxicity are plentiful,[56] while examples of FMO being involved in metabolism that leads to toxicity pale in comparison to CYP. Examples exist linking FMO-mediated metabolism to bioactivation, and have been reviewed in a chapter by Hutzler and Cerny in the *Encyclopedia of Drug Metabolism and Interactions.*[57] For example, thiourea derivatives such as thiobenzamide (Figure 5.3) are excellent substrates for FMO-dependent *S*-oxidation, which leads to formation of sulfenic acids that can undergo redox cycling with glutathione (GSH) to form GSSG, undergo further oxidation to the sulfinic acid, bind to GSH, or covalently bind to proteins.[58,59] The generation of sulfenic acids as reactive intermediates and the resulting impact has been nicely reviewed by Mansuy and Dansette.[60] Lastly, generation of quinoneimine intermediates following *para*-hydroxylation of aniline-containing drugs has historically been viewed as CYP mediated. However, FMO1 was reported to catalyze the bioactivation of 4-fluoro-*N*-methylaniline *via* a carbon oxidation coupled with defluorination, leading to an electrophilic quinoneimine intermediate.[61] In closing, it is easy to assume the oxidative metabolic pathways in liver microsomes are CYP mediated. This conclusion is often made when metabolism is found to be NADPH dependent. However, the role of FMO in the metabolism should always be investigated for a complete understanding of metabolic pathways.

5.3 MoCo-Containing AO

AO is a MoCo-containing enzyme localized in the cytosolic subcellular fraction, and is related to xanthine oxidoreductase (XOR), although with a much broader substrate selectivity. AO catalyzes the oxidation of various aldehydes (as the name implies), to the corresponding carboxylic acid, but is also involved in oxidation of numerous heteroaromatic ring-containing drug

molecules,[62,63] as well as select reductive ring-opening pathways for zonis-
amide and ziprasidone.[64,65] Most recently, AO has even been implicated in
the amide hydrolysis of GDC-0834, a Bruton's tyrosine kinase (BTK) inhibitor.[66] Some common substrates of AO are shown in Figure 5.4, with arrows
indicating the primary site of metabolism. The liver is the primary site of
expression of AO (*AOX1*), although several other tissues, such as kidney, small
and large intestine, respiratory tissue, and adrenal gland, contain AO activity,
which may suggest physiological roles beyond xenobiotic metabolism.[4,67] AO
is active as a homodimer, with each monomer composed of two identical 150
kDa subunits divided into three conserved domains (linked by two non-con-
served hinge regions): a 20 kDa amino-terminal iron–sulfur (Fe–S) domain,
a 40 kDa FAD binding domain, and an 85 kDa carboxy-terminal domain
containing the MoCo and active site where the substrate binds.[68,69] To date,
only one mammalian crystal structure has been reported (mouse *AOX3*) that
depicts these domains in spatial relationship to each other.[70] In addition, a
three dimensional homology model of human AO has been reported, which
was utilized to better understand substrate interactions with phthalazine
and quinazoline derivatives.[71] Undoubtedly, a crystal structure for human
AO is being pursued, which would be a significant contribution to the understanding of binding interaction requirements for the human enzyme.

In recent years, the pharmaceutical industry has become more aware of
the potential clinical impact of AO-mediated metabolism due to a number of unfortunate failures of drug candidates. The halting of a number of
clinical programs has mostly been the result of rapid first-pass metabolism
and, thus, poor systemic exposure following an oral dose.[7,72–75] Toxicological findings due to AO-mediated metabolism have also been reported.[8]

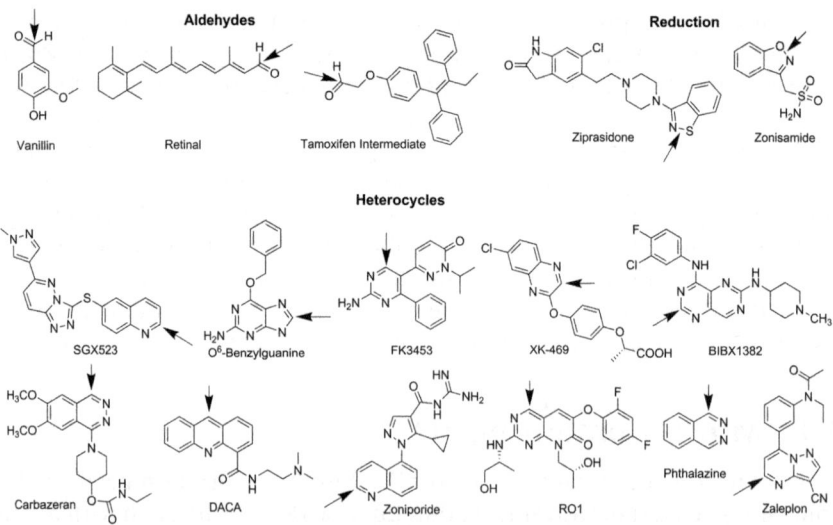

Figure 5.4 Structures of known substrates of AO. Arrows indicate the primary sites
of metabolism.

A summary of several examples is presented in Table 5.4. As described earlier in this chapter, clinical failures may have been averted if a more comprehensive understanding of the non-CYP metabolism mechanism was obtained during *in vitro* and *in vivo* characterization of these drug candidates. The reader is thus referred to several excellent reviews focused on this important metabolic enzyme.[76-80] The intent of this section is to highlight the most

Table 5.4 Summary of AO substrates that experienced clinical failure due to rapid metabolism, resulting in poor oral exposure or toxicity. Arrows indicate the site of metabolism by AO on each substrate.

Drug	Structure	Clinical finding
Carbazeran		Oral bioavailability <5%
BIBX1382		Mean oral bioavailability 5%
Zoniporide		High systemic clearance (and poor efficacy)
RO1		<1 Hour half-life
SGX523		Acute renal toxicity (poorly soluble metabolite)
FK3453		Unacceptably low exposure

important caveats of studying and understanding AO-mediated metabolism, including mechanism, species differences, donor variability, and considerations around prediction of human clearance.

5.3.1 Characteristics and Catalytic Mechanism

AO enzymes contain a MoCo and oxidize electron deficient carbons on substrates *via* a nucleophilic mechanism (Figure 5.5), which is distinct from the CYP mechanism. Substrate is oxidized to product at the MoCo center, with the initial step thought to involve a conserved active site glutamate (Glu) residue assisting with a base-catalyzed nucleophilic attack of the molybdenum-OH on an electrophilic sp^2-hybridized carbon of the substrate (a carbonyl carbon of an aldehyde or a carbon adjacent to an aromatic nitrogen atom). Concurrently, a hydride transfer from the substrate to the molybdenum-sulfur occurs, which is proposed to be the rate-limiting step. The overall mechanism is thought to occur by a concerted mechanism, but a step-wise mechanism with a tetrahedral intermediate cannot be ruled out.[81] The hydride transfer step is enabled by a post-translational sulfuration of the MoCo, which is critical for catalytic activity.[82,83] The oxygen that is then incorporated into the oxidized substrate originates from a nucleophilic attack by water, not molecular oxygen, a distinction from the CYP mechanism. Reducing equivalents are generated and shuttled *via* the iron–sulfur (Fe–S) centers to the FAD cofactor to form FADH$_2$. Molecular oxygen then re-oxidizes FADH$_2$ back to FAD, which generates H$_2$O$_2$ as a by-product. From work describing the crystal structure of mouse AOX3, it is proposed that the proton transfer from the hydroxyl ligand of molybdenum back to the conserved Glu-1266 disrupts the interaction of Glu-1266 with Lys-889, which enables product release from the active site.[70]

Supporting the hypothesis that the hydride transfer step from substrate to the molybdenum-sulfur is rate-limiting is the observation of large deuterium isotope effects.[84] Thus, one approach that may be effective in reducing the rate

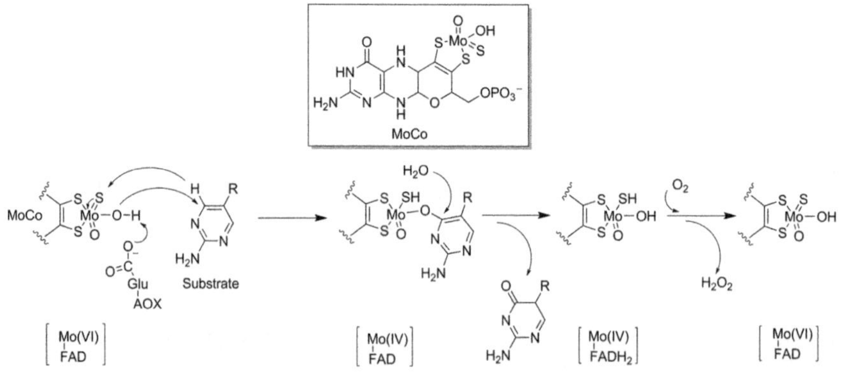

Figure 5.5   Catalytic mechanism of AO.

of metabolism and improving PK properties of AO substrates is selective deuteration on the carbon where oxidation occurs. In work published by Sharma and colleagues,[85] intra- and intermolecular kinetic deuterium isotope effects (KDIEs) were observed for oxidation of quinoxaline, phthalazine, quinoline, carbazeran, and zoniporide in human, rat, and guinea pig liver cytosol, as measured by differences in intrinsic clearance (CL_{int}) rates. Assuming AO is the predominant drug clearing mechanism, and clearance is low to moderate (*i.e.* not blood flow limited), this deuteration strategy may be used to improve the PK properties of AO substrates, particularly when this metabolic pathway cannot be eliminated with structural modification due to negative effects on potency for the intended pharmacology (*e.g.* kinase targets). A recently published novel chemical "litmus test" method that takes advantage of the AO nucleophilic mechanism is the use of bis(((difluoromethyl)sulfinyl)oxy) zinc (DFMS). With this approach, direct chemical addition of a $-CF_2H$ group (M + 50 peak) to the drug molecule of interest would indicate the susceptibility of heteroarenes to undergo an AO-mediated metabolic event.[86] This methodology may be used as an approach for developing a structure–activity relationship (SAR) for the AO metabolic pathway for a chemical series, in an effort to prioritize synthetic strategies in medicinal chemistry.

5.3.2 Differentiation from CYP

The primary difference between AO and CYP is that there is only one AO gene (*AOX1*) in humans, whereas CYP is a super-family of many enzymes with an extremely diverse range of substrates. In addition, the subcellular location is distinct, with CYP enzymes being present in the microsomal fraction, and AO in the cytosolic fraction. Thus, AO activity is not expected to be present in liver microsomes, unless there is contamination with the cytosol, which has been reported (unpublished observations). As previously described in Section 5.3.1, AO and CYP have an opposing preference for oxidizing carbon atoms. CYP enzymes prefer to oxidize carbons with high electron density, whereas AO prefers to oxidize carbons with low electron density due to its nucleophilic mechanism, with water being the source of the oxygen incorporated into the product. This mechanistic difference can be taken advantage of, particularly in an *in vitro* system where both CYP and AO are present (*e.g.* S-9 fraction or hepatocytes). By conducting incubations in the presence of isotopically labeled water ($H_2^{18}O$), the enzyme involved in the production of an oxidative metabolite (+16 mass units) can be narrowed down, rather than assuming the action of CYP enzymes. As shown in the mass spectra in Figure 5.6, when incubations are conducted in the presence of isotopically labeled water (50/50 mixture as one option), a characteristic isotope pattern is observed for the AO metabolite of carbazeran, with equally intense ions consistent with a +16 (m/z 377) and +18 (m/z 379) mass shift following incorporation of a roughly equal ratio of ^{16}O and ^{18}O from water into the substrate. Conversely, for midazolam (a substrate of CYP 3A), this pattern is not observed due to molecular oxygen being the source of oxygen

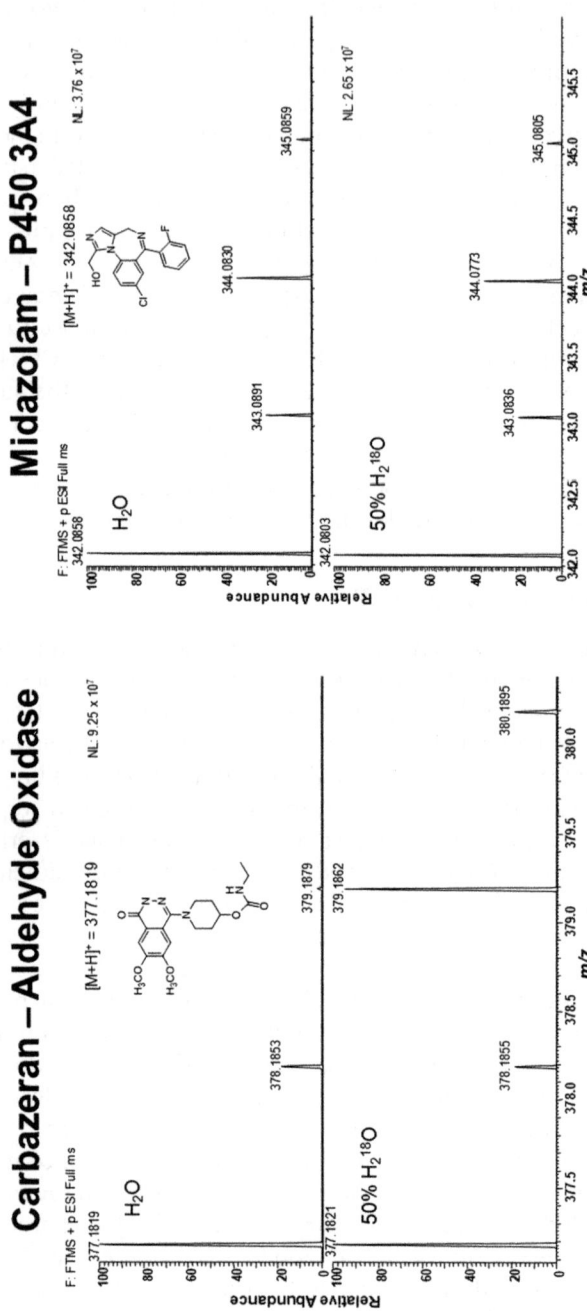

Figure 5.6 Mass spectrum demonstrating isotopic pattern of oxidative metabolites following *in vitro* incubation using 50% isotopically labelled water ($H_2^{18}O$). This approach can be employed to differentiate an AO from a CYP catalytic mechanism. Carbazeran is used as the probe substrate of AO where roughly a 50:50 ratio of ^{16}O:^{18}O is incorporated into the metabolite (from water), while midazolam is a probe for CYP 3A where only ^{16}O from molecular oxygen is incorporated into the metabolite.

in the metabolite (unpublished observations). It must be stated, however, that this experimental design alone does not differentiate AO from XOR, as both operate with a similar nucleophilic mechanism. Differentiation could be achieved by co-incubation of inhibitors specific to AO (*e.g.* raloxifene or menadione) and XOR (*e.g.* allopurinol). In addition, differentiation of CYP from FMO cannot be concluded from this experiment (see previous section on FMO). Another way to differentiate AO from CYP (or FMO) is by cofactor manipulation. For example, with incubations conducted in S-9 fractions, metabolite profiles following the addition of NADPH as the necessary cofactor for CYP and FMO could be compared to profiles from incubations devoid of this cofactor. If oxidative metabolites are observed in S-9 fractions devoid of NADPH, then the enzyme(s) involved can be identified (*i.e.* reaction phenotyping), which is an important exercise given the need to understand metabolic clearance mechanisms for drug molecules. A reported approach for differentiating AO from CYP-mediated metabolism in hepatocytes is the use of the AO-selective inhibitor hydralazine (25–50 μM), which does not cross over to the CYP enzymes, other than weakly inhibiting CYP2D6.[87] Employment of raloxifene or menadione as inhibitors of AO would be inappropriate in human hepatocytes due to their lack of selectivity over CYP enzymes.[88,89] Another mechanistic difference between AO and CYP enzymes is generation of ROS, such as H_2O_2. While both enzyme systems can generate H_2O_2 during their respective cycle, it is a normal step in the AO reaction cycle (following re-oxidation of $FADH_2$ by molecular oxygen), whereas the CYP reaction cycle has to "uncouple" to form ROS,[90] which partly explains the inefficiency and atypical kinetics often observed with CYP enzymes.[91]

In general, the strategy to mitigate AO-mediated metabolism as compared with CYP is in contrast. Again, with the mechanism being distinct, making a heterocyclic ring system less electron dense by the addition of electron-withdrawing substituents may function to reduce CYP-mediated metabolism, but will likely increase susceptibility to AO-mediated metabolism. Mitigating AO-mediated metabolism by decreasing lipophilicity (a common strategy for reducing CYP metabolism) will most likely not yield much success, as there is a weak relationship between lipophilicity and AO metabolism.[76] The best strategies for mitigating AO-mediated metabolism may include either directly blocking the site of oxidation by replacing the carbon or hydrogen atom at the site of oxidation with another group, bioisosteric ring replacement, or rearrangement of nitrogen atoms in the ring system.[79]

Regarding clinical DDI risk, it is well known that both perpetrator and victim DDIs for inhibitors and substrates of the CYP enzymes are a major area of concern, with regulatory guidance focused on strategies for identifying and addressing patient safety. Conversely, only one clinical PK DDI has been linked to inhibition of AO.[92] Following an 800 mg oral dose of cimetidine, the oral clearance of the AO substrate zaleplon was significantly decreased (to 56% of control), resulting in an increase in the area under the concentration–time curve (AUC) of zaleplon. In addition, it was discovered that the AO-derived 5-oxo metabolite of zaleplon was formed at a reduced rate after cimetidine administration. Retrospective *in vitro* experiments by Renwick demonstrated that cimetidine only weakly inhibited formation of the 5-oxo metabolite in human liver cytosol (K_i = 155 µM), and liver slices (K_i = 506 µM).[92] With these data, the actual mechanism of the observed DDI between cimetidine and zaleplon remains unclear. However, with the evolution of chemical matter in drug discovery and development efforts towards more heterocyclic-containing drug candidates, increased metabolic clearance by non-CYP drug-metabolizing enzymes such as AO is likely. This observation, coupled with a number of clinically used drugs being identified as inhibitors of AO,[93] suggests that this particular DDI mechanism may become more relevant in the future.[94,95] Most recently, diet-derived constituents such as catechins have been implicated as potent inhibitors of AO, a research area that still needs further attention.[96]

5.3.3 Species Differences

Among the issues associated with AO metabolism, profound species differences in expression and activity may drastically complicate early interpretation of PK behavior of drug candidates. The variable expression of AOX genes in humans and popular experimental animal species has been reviewed by Garattini and Terao.[77] AOX expression differences are a particular issue when coupled with the common drug discovery paradigm where PK studies are first conducted in rats and dogs, two species that generally have low to no AO activity.[97] This common *in vivo* discovery approach, in addition to early *in vitro* metabolic stability screening in HLMs (a subcellular fraction devoid of AO) may lead to a false positive view regarding the PK suitability of a drug candidate for humans (as indicated in Table 5.4). An additional risk associated with the striking species differences is the potential for a disproportionate or unique human metabolite for a drug that is metabolized by AO. As highlighted in the US Food and Drug Administration (FDA) guidance from 2008, and numerous publications,[98,99] the safety of metabolites observed in humans must be adequately tested, typically in one rodent and one non-rodent preclinical species, which tend to be rat and dog. An unfortunate example of an adverse outcome in a human clinical study due to an AO-derived metabolite was published by Diamond and co-workers.[8] SGX523 was an oncology drug candidate that progressed to clinical studies. Preclinically, SGX523 demonstrated a comparable metabolite profile in liver microsomes from rat, dog, monkey, and human. With these *in vitro* metabolism data, it was decided to conduct regulatory toxicology studies in rats and dogs to enable first in human (FIH) studies. However, despite an apparently favorable safety profile in those species, doses >80 mg administered to human subjects resulted in acute renal failure. Retrospectively, a major oxidative metabolite was observed when profiling human plasma that was not observed in the *in vitro* studies using liver microsomes. Additional metabolite profiling studies in human liver S-9 fraction conducted by Diamond and co-workers then revealed a predominant NADPH-independent metabolite (**M11**, 2-quinolinone-SGX523), which was subsequently proven to be AO derived. In addition, while the **M11** AO metabolite was not formed in rat and dog liver S-9, it was generated in liver S-9 from male cynomolgus monkey. Safety studies in monkey then recreated the adverse renal effects observed in humans.[100] The ultimate cause of the renal toxicity was proposed to be the extremely low solubility of the **M11** metabolite, which crystallized in the kidney. This example highlights the importance of comprehensive metabolite profiling studies using human *in vitro* systems that contain the full complement of drug-metabolizing enzymes (*e.g.* S-9 fraction with appropriate cofactors or hepatocytes). In addition, understanding metabolic mechanisms and species differences should enable an informed decision for the selection of a toxicology species that will most likely represent the human drug metabolism.

In a recent literature review by Garattini and Terao, it was stated that rhesus monkey and guinea pig represent the best *in vivo* proxy for PK studies with AO substrates.[77] Despite some evidence to suggest that these species may actually overestimate CL_{int} in humans,[101] there is precedence for the rhesus monkey. BIBX1382 was a clinical candidate being evaluated as an inhibitor of epidermal growth factor receptor (EGFR) in the treatment of cancer. Following the observation of extremely low oral exposure in humans (Table 5.4), it was found that the PK properties of BIBX1382 in rhesus monkey aligned with what was observed in humans.[72] When considering that the cynomolgus and rhesus monkey AOX1 enzymes are 96% homologous to human AOX1, and 99% homologous to each other (accession numbers for the AO genes: human, NP_001150; cyno, ACQ73553.1; rhesus, AFI36988.1), it is reasonable to suggest that perhaps cynomolgus monkeys would also represent a suitable surrogate species for human AO. In general, cynomolgus monkey is a preferred primate for PK/toxicokinetic assessment, and was recently reported to be a species that reproduced the high clearance and low oral exposure observed with BIBX1382.[102] Similar to this finding, the AO-mediated metabolism of SGX523 (as previously mentioned), zaleplon, SB-277011, and RS 8359 has been reported to be comparable between cynomolgus monkeys and humans.[102] With these examples, it is apparent that cynomolgus monkey may be a suitable and more practical primate compared with rhesus monkey, which requires more compound for dosing (rhesus monkeys weigh 2- to 3-fold more than cynomolgus monkeys), and is more expensive. It must be stressed, however, that there is no one species that will be a suitable surrogate for human AO for all substrates, and appropriate *in vitro* and *in vivo* studies need to be conducted to justify selection of species for toxicology testing. A more detailed strategy for toxicological considerations has been presented in a review by Hutzler and colleagues.[79]

5.3.4 Variability and Polymorphisms of Human AOX1

Further complicating AO-mediated metabolism is highly variable activity across multiple donors. For example, methotrexate 7-hydroxylase activity ranged 48-fold when assayed in liver cytosol from six different human donors.[103] Another report assessed AO activity in the cytosol using 13 donor livers, and an 18-fold range of CL_{int} was observed when using N-[(2-dimethyl-amino)ethyl] acridine-4-carboxamide (DACA) as a substrate, while a 5-fold range was reported with benzaldehyde as the probe substrate.[104] More recently, scientists at Pfizer published data demonstrating highly variable CL_{int} following incubation in liver cytosol from 20 donors, using three different probe substrates: carbazeran, zoniporide, and phthalazine.[105] Activity ranged 17- to 90-fold across the donors tested, and was substrate dependent. In addition, a liquid chromatography tandem mass spectrometry (LC-MS/MS) method was developed and employed to quantify AOX1 protein in human liver cytosol in an effort to correlate protein levels with observed activities across donors. Interestingly, a poor correlation between expression and activity was observed, with several donors having normal AOX1 protein levels, but low enzyme activity,[105] pointing towards other factors involved in regulating activity across donors.

Reports exist suggesting that the AO enzyme may be susceptible to instability, although the cause is unknown.[106] Hutzler and colleagues tested stability of AO activity in freshly prepared human hepatocytes, evaluating loss in activity over the first 24 hours following isolation of hepatocytes from 10 donor livers.[107] Findings from these studies included a substantial loss in activity over this time that was donor dependent (15–81%). In addition, cryopreserved hepatocytes prepared from those same donors appeared to maintain activity comparable to the fresh hepatocytes that were incubated within 2 hours of isolation (*i.e.* as fresh as possible), which suggests that cryopreserved human hepatocytes may be the ideal cell system for comparing activity across donors. Hutzler and colleagues expanded these findings to then assess variability in AO activity using O^6-benzylguanine in cryopreserved human hepatocytes prepared from 75 individual donors.[107] Overall, activity varied by at least 17-fold, with the lowest activity being unmeasurable by substrate depletion ($\leq$5.4 mL min^{-1} kg^{-1}) and the highest activity being 90 mL min^{-1} kg^{-1} (Figure 5.7). When evaluating donor demographics, no significant trends were noted when comparing ethnic background, gender, age, or body mass index of the donors.[107] Interestingly, a common finding with the aforementioned studies by Fu and colleagues was that donors with a recent history of heavy alcohol consumption appear to have extremely low AO activity,[105,107] a finding worthy of more focused research. Other contributing factors to variability may be molybdenum deficiency, different levels of AO enzyme dimerization, or single nucleotide polymorphisms (SNPs) for AOX1. In addition, diet-derived flavonoids, such as catechins from green tea beverages have been shown to be inhibitory towards AO activity,[96,108] which suggests that diet likely plays a role in the observed variability. Developmental expression of AO has also been studied, with one report demonstrating that neonates and infants (13 days to 4 months old) possess little to no AO activity, as determined in 16 human livers. However, activity increased rapidly and plateaued by 2 years of age.[109] Regarding clinical PK behavior of AO substrates, there appears to be a wide range of variability depending on the substrate. For example, the clearance of DACA across 28 individuals ranged from 5.2 to 35.8 mL min^{-1} kg^{-1} (about 7-fold).[110] Similarly, oral exposures (C_{max} and AUC) reported for FK3453[75] and BIBX1382[72]

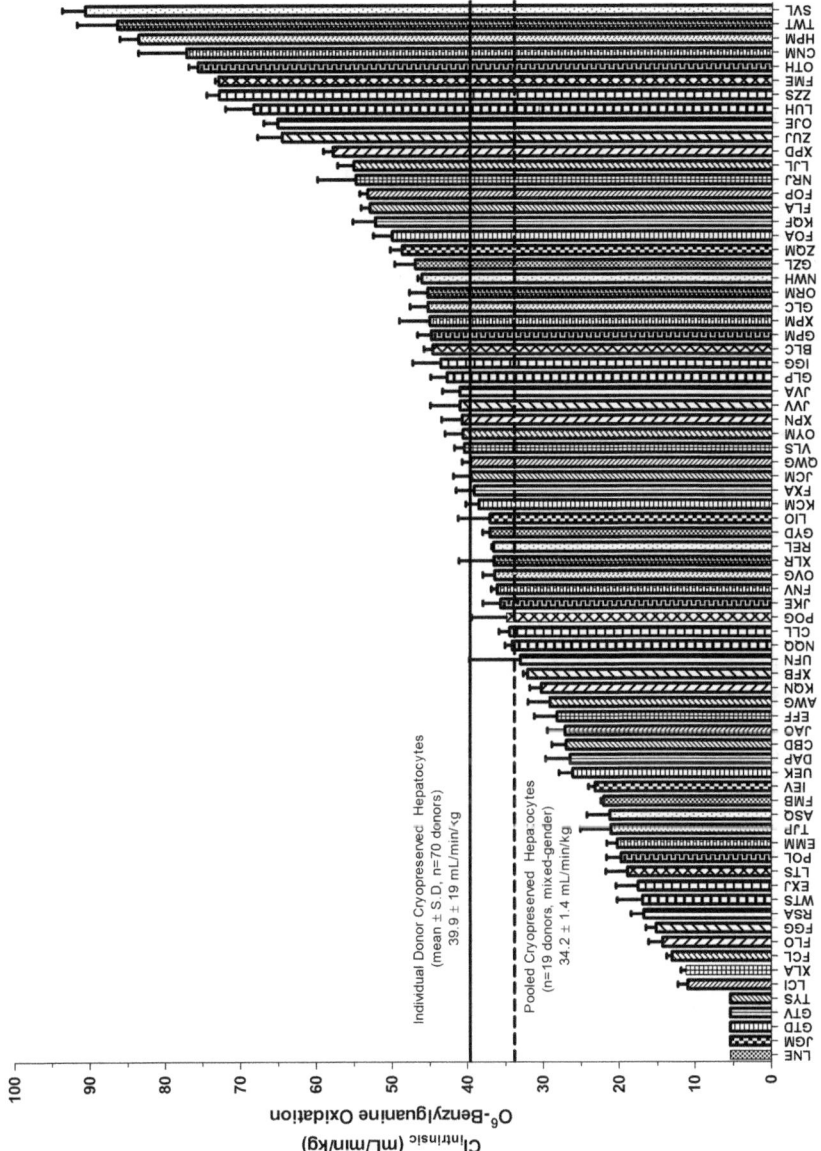

Figure 5.7 Variability in CL_{int} (mL min^{-1} per kilogram) for O^6-benzylguanine oxidation in cryopreserved hepatocytes from 75 individual donors. The dotted line represents observed CL_{int} for O^6-benzylguanine in a pooled cryopreserved hepatocyte lot consisting of 19 mixed-gender donors. Clearance values for all are the mean of $n = 4$ replicates, with error bars representing standard deviation (S.D.). Reprinted with permission from ref. 107 © ASPET 2014.

were notably variable, with ranges spanning ~23-fold, and 27-fold, respectively, indicating the potential for translation of *in vitro* variability to clinical variability in exposure for substrates of AO.

SNPs of the human *AOX1* gene are numerous, although the direct functional consequence of the majority of these SNPs has yet to be clearly determined.[77] A study in 180 volunteers from an Italian population was published where numerous synonymous, missense and nonsense SNPs in the coding region of *AOX1* were identified when sequencing the 35 coding exons of human *AOX1*.[111] Site directed mutagenesis of human AOX1 and protein purification were then performed to evaluate the functional consequence *in vitro* of selected mutations. It was found that SNPs rs55754655 (N1135S) and rs3731722 (H1297R) lead to higher catalytic activities relative to wild-type *AOX1* enzyme, which appears to agree with clinical findings related to the use of azathioprine where lack of azathioprine response was predicted by the rs55754655 SNP.[112] By contrast, Hutzler and colleagues found a lack of statistically significant effect on CL_{int} of O^6-benzylguanine relative to wild-type donors in cryopreserved human hepatocytes.[107] In addition, variability in clearance of XK469, a substrate eliminated mainly by AO, was unable to be linked to polymorphisms of *AOX1*.[113] Thus, based on the information to date, it seems likely that genotype is only one of many factors that regulate the phenotypic activity of AO activity. Nonetheless, targeted clinical studies need to be conducted in order to assess the true impact of polymorphisms of *AOX1*. The next section will describe how these knowledge gaps factor into the prediction of clearance in humans for substrates of AO.

5.3.5   Challenges in the Prediction of Human Clearance for AO Substrates

Prediction of clearance for the purposes of forecasting the PK behavior of drug candidates is perhaps the most important objective for any drug metabolism scientist, as it factors into projections of half-life and efficacious dose. A quantitatively successful method for predicting clearance for substrates of AO has proven elusive, as many reports show a general trend towards *in vitro* systems, such as liver cytosol, S-9 fraction, and hepatocytes, underpredicting clearance in humans.[114-116] There are several reasons that likely contribute to this phenomenon, one of which is the source of the enzyme. It was recently reported that there were substantial differences in AO activity in donor-matched liver cytosol and S-9 fraction from 3 different vendors.[117] This confounding issue is shown in Figure 5.8, which suggests that any laboratory conducting *in vitro* studies should test numerous lots of cytosol and/ or S-9 fractions with a range of AO substrates, and then use the one with the highest activity. Regarding the cause of the vendor differences in activity, it was proposed that the differences may be due mainly to the preparation process, as opposed the donor composition.[117] However, the extreme donor-to-donor variability highlighted earlier in the chapter should be considered. If AO activity of individual preparations can be measured prior to pooling,

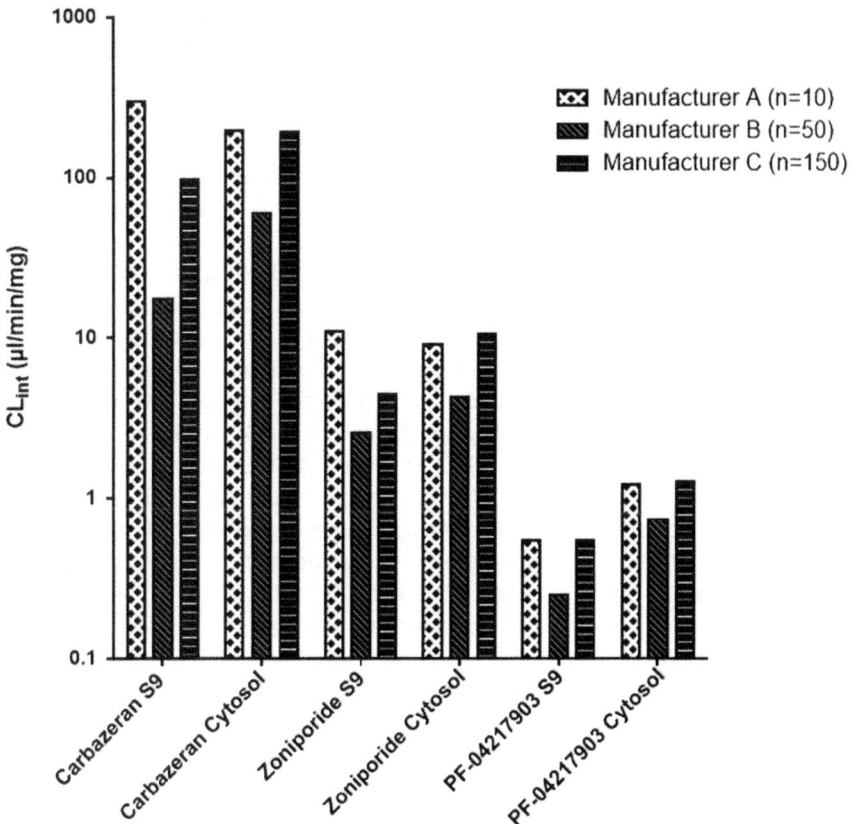

Figure 5.8 Comparison of AO enzyme activity (CL_{int}) from donor-matched cytosol and S-9 fractions obtained from three different manufacturers. The cross-hatched bars are from manufacturer A, the black and white diagonal lined bars are from manufacturer B, and the black and white horizontal bars are from manufacturer C. Reprinted with permission from ref. 117 © ASPET 2015.

then custom pools of cytosol, S-9 fraction, or cryopreserved hepatocytes composed of high activity donors should yield an *in vitro* system that will help to minimize under-predictions of metabolic clearance.[118] Unfortunately, most vendors do not routinely determine AO activity in their donors prior to preparing their pooled lots. Thus, this must be requested of the vendor if a suitable *in vitro* system is to be used for metabolism studies with AO substrates.

Additionally complicating the prediction of metabolic clearance by AO are data demonstrating expression in extrahepatic tissue. Expression of AOX1 has been reported in kidney, pancreas, intestine, and prostate, with high expression in the zona reticularis of the adrenal gland.[67] More recently, AO activity has also been determined in human skin.[119] All of these data suggest that only accounting for metabolism of AO substrates using liver tissue may lead to under-prediction of clearance, consistent with the aforementioned observations. It is likely that the liver and extrahepatic activity of AO, once quantitatively determined, may be used to develop some physiologically based PK (PBPK) models for the purpose of estimating PK profiles of drug candidates. In addition, an *in silico* model has been reported that factors in electronic and steric features of the substrate reaction, and CL_{int} can be predicted more accurately than with *in vitro* testing when assuming that 30% of AO activity is due to extrahepatic metabolism.[120] As demonstrated by Zhang and colleagues with a profound under-prediction of clearance for a p38 kinase inhibitor,[74] it is not advisable to employ traditional allometric scaling for the purposes of estimating human clearance for AO substrates due to the previously described species differences (the primary assumption with allometric scaling is no major species differences with respect to metabolic clearance mechanisms). However, with the rhesus and cynomolgus monkey shown to be potentially good proxies for AO activity in humans,[102] scaling clearance from these single species [*i.e.* single-species scaling (SSS)], which was reported as a reasonable approach in a retrospective analysis by scientists at Pfizer,[121] may be worth pursuing as a viable option for scaling clearance to humans. Research is needed to adequately test this approach, but it has been reported to be accurate for substrates of UGT.[122] Overall, it is clear that no one approach will be appropriate for all substrates of AO, but a combination of *in vitro* metabolism using pooled cryopreserved hepatocytes composed of high activity donors, as well as PK studies in a species that is representative of humans, such as rhesus or cynomolgus monkeys, from an AO metabolism standpoint, is advised as a practical approach for minimizing the noted under-predictions in the literature.

5.4 UGTs

UGT is a super-family of enzymes that catalyze the transfer of glucuronic acid to drug-like and endogenous substrates in the presence of the co-substrate UDPGA (uridine-5′-diphosphate-α-D-glucuronic acid), yielding a glucuronide conjugate (Figure 5.9). The nucleophilic substrates (aglycone) of UGT mediated reactions include those containing alcohols, phenols, carboxylic acids, amines, and occasionally, S-, and C-containing substrates.[123] This critical route of drug metabolism provides both a mechanism of increased solubilization of the substrate to facilitate renal or biliary excretion, and a route to prevent reactive nucleophiles from potentiating toxicological effects.[124,125]

The importance of the UGT family is second only to CYP as the initial pathway of metabolism, as the UGTs have been identified to be responsible for the metabolism of approximately 10% of the top 200 prescribed drugs.[126,127] More recently, UGTs were reported to play a role in the metabolism of 20–30% of all marketed drugs.[128] It has also been stated that UGTs are responsible for 40–70% of all drugs metabolized through conjugation reactions.[124,129–131] Examples of drug-like and endogenous compounds that are metabolized by UGTs are found in Figure 5.10.

The UGT super-family of enzymes has isoform nomenclature similar to those found with the CYP family. The general nomenclature has been

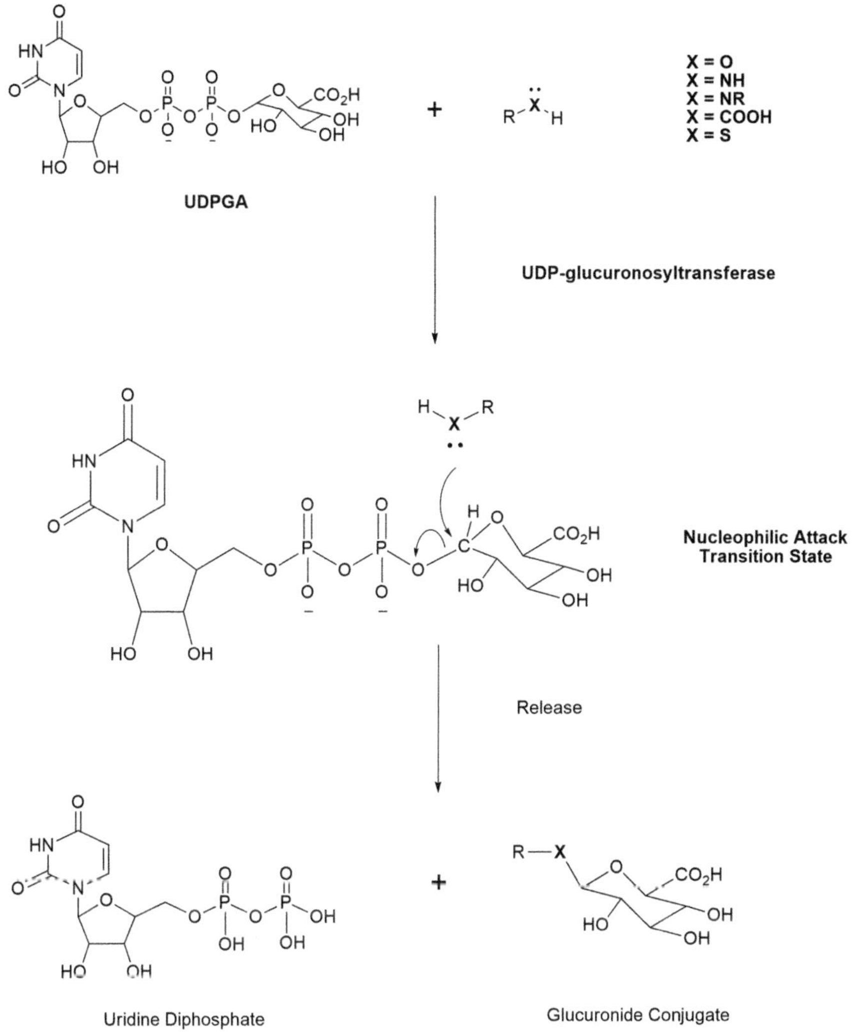

Figure 5.9 Catalytic mechanism of UGT.

standardized with the UGT family Arabic number (1, 2, 3, and 8), subfamily letter (A or B), and an Arabic number to denote the individual gene within that family or subfamily (*e.g.* UGT1A1). Based on homology there are 3 human functional subfamilies of UGTs, which comprise 19 different functional isoforms. The 1A subfamily includes 9 isoforms (1A1 and 1A3–1A10), the 2A subfamily is comprised of 3 isoforms (2A1–2A3), and the 2B subfamily has 7 members (2B4, 2B7, 2B10, 2B11, 2B15, 2B17, and 2B28).[132] There are two other UGT families that include UGT3 (3A1 and 3A2) and UGT8 (8A1), which are thought to be generally inactive as they do not use UDP-glucuronic acid as a sugar donor, but rather utilize a different sugar donor (UDP galactose ceramide, UDP glucose, or UDP-*N*-acetylglucosamine), which renders them unlikely to contribute to drug metabolism.[133–135] The UGTs that are

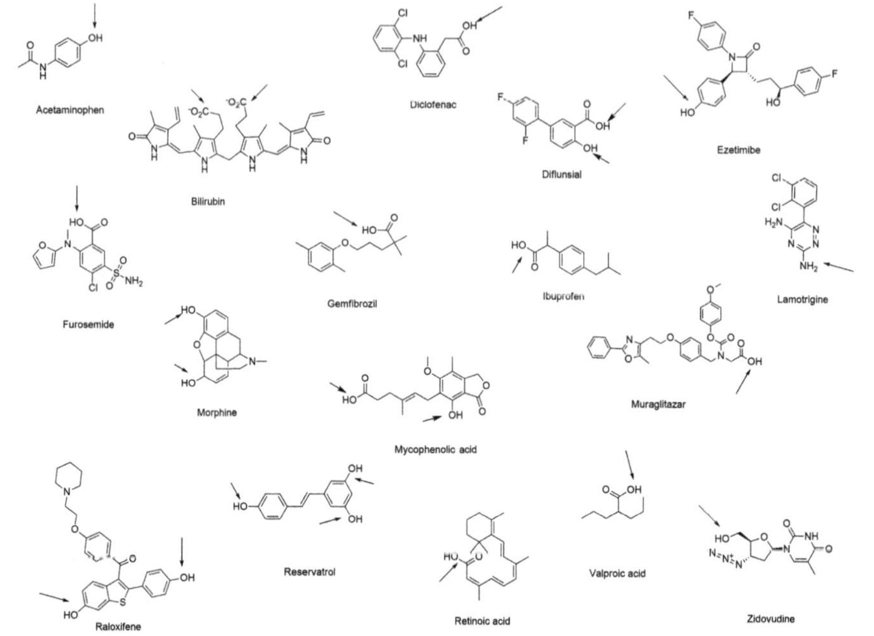

Figure 5.10   Structures of known substrates of UGTs. Arrows indicate the primary sites of metabolism.

known to metabolize xenobiotics are mainly found in the 1A and the 2B sub-families. The UGT isoforms of most interest to drug metabolism, due to their polymorphic nature and broad substrate specificity, according to the FDA and European Medicines Agency (EMA) are UGT1A1, 1A3, 1A4, 1A6, 1A9, 2B7, and 2B15.[136,137] Enzyme expression of the majority of these enzymes is found on the luminal side of the endoplasmic reticulum with a membrane-spanning region and a short cytoplasmic terminal tail.[138,139] As with all proteins, the UGT enzyme exists with an N- and C-terminal domain with each having specialized attributes for function. The variability of the N-terminal domain provides aglycone binding specificity, while the highly conserved C-terminus appears to be associated with cofactor binding across all family members.[140] Much of what is known about the folding of the enzyme and the vital amino acid residues of the active site for proton transfer and catalysis is based on the recently published crystal structure of UGT2B7[141] and the mutagenesis experiments that were inspired by this publication.[140,142]

5.4.1   Characteristics and Catalytic Mechanism

Glucuronidation of a substrate by UGTs can occur at any atom with enough nucleophilicity and is considered an S_N^2 reaction.[143] The site of glucuronidation is generally an electron-rich oxygen, sulfur, or nitrogen heteroatom, and occurs *via* a second-order nucleophilic substitution mechanism, where an inversion of the C_1 atom of glucuronic acid occurs, which reconfigures into the β-D configuration once the conjugate is formed (Figure 5.9). The resulting products are the glucuronide conjugate and UDP. The UGT binding pocket for the sugar donor (*i.e.* UDP-glucuronic acid) is comprised of 3 groups of residues for nucleotide binding, diphosphate interaction, and glucuronic acid interaction, all of which provide structure for the sugar cofactor to be utilized in conjunction with the substrate binding pocket to perform the conjugation reaction. The catalytic inner workings of the UGT active site were demonstrated using UGT2B7 mutagenesis[140] in conjunction with the published crystal structure of the C-terminal domain,[141] where the histidine residue (H35) of the UGT deprotonates the nucleophilic group on the substrate. The neighboring aspartic acid (D151) stabilizes the deprotonated substrate long enough for the substrate to attack the anomeric carbon of the sugar. This final attack step completes the covalent bond of the sugar to the substrate.

Although the glucuronidation pathway facilitates detoxification and elimination from the body, there are examples where UGTs generate a reactive conjugate metabolite that may covalently bind to macromolecules, particularly acyl glucuronides. This reactivity may either impact normal function of the protein or cause an immune response against the glucuronide-protein adduct. The carboxylate esterification seems to be of greater clinical significance due to the overall number of carboxylic acid containing endogenous and drug-like compounds that are metabolized by UGTs (Figure 5.10). There are two known mechanisms by which acyl glucuronides form protein adducts. The simplest mode is a direct displacement of the glucuronosyl group by a nucleophile in the target protein to produce acylation of the protein, referred to as a transacylation reaction (Figure 5.11). The second mechanism is more complex, going through multiple steps of acyl migration after nucleophilic attack from the initial C-1 position on the glucuronic acid to C-2, then to C-3 and C-4, followed by a ring opening, and ending with Amadori rearrangement to produce a protein adduct (Figure 5.11). There are multiple non-steroidal anti-inflammatory drugs (NSAIDs) on the market that have been found to undergo this migration and Amadori rearrangement mechanism, including benoxaprofen, diclofenac, ibufenac, ticrynafen, and tolmetin. Several reviews on the mechanism of acyl glucuronide-induced protein adducts have been presented in the literature.[144-148] The formation of acyl glucuronides, and links to reactions ranging from skin rash to renal and hepatic toxicities is believed to have led to the withdrawal of carboxylic acid containing drugs from the market, such as alcofenac, benoxaprofen, fenclofenac, ibufenac, indoprofen, pirprofen, suprofen, trovafloxacin, temafloxacin, ticrynafen, and zomepirac. Thus, approaches in early discovery to assess the stability of acyl glucuronides has become common, as buffer stability has been shown to correlate with reactivity.[144] Toward this effort, a novel rapid nuclear magnetic resonance method based on the disappearance of the anomeric resonance of the 1-*O*-acylglucuronide was reported, which enables rank ordering of acyl glucuronide forming drugs based on the potential reactivity of the

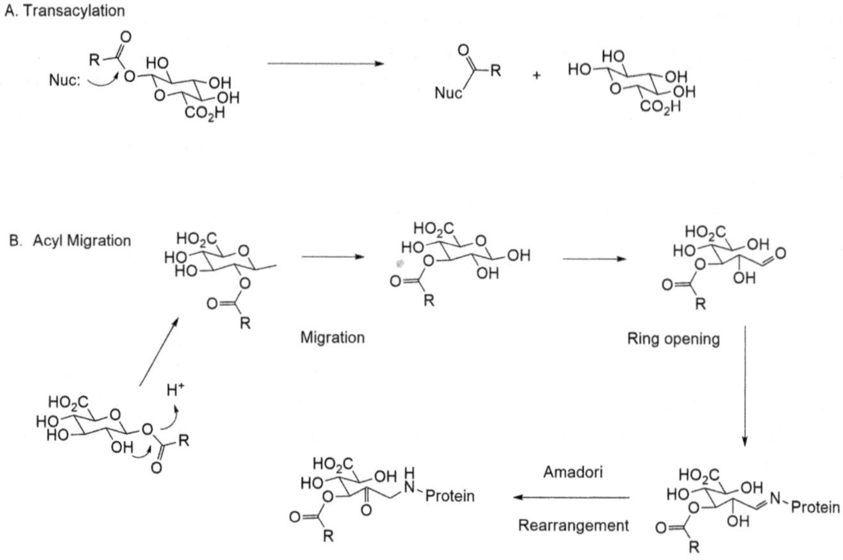

Figure 5.11 Mechanisms that may lead to covalent modification of proteins and toxicity by acyl glucuronide metabolites, including (A) transacylation and (B) acyl migration.

conjugates.[149] In general, the longer the half-life *in vitro* in buffer, the less reactive the acyl glucuronide is considered to be, with a half-life >4 hours a reasonable target. For example, the 1-*O*-acylglucuronide of telmisartan was reported to have an *in vitro* degradation half-life of 26 hours in pH 7.4 buffer, and consequently had very low covalent binding to human serum albumin.[150]

5.4.2 UGT Isoforms and Tissue Expression

Although there is substantial homology within the UGT family of enzymes, the differences among the UGT families and their isoforms begin at the gene location of family 1 and 2. Family 1 is found on human chromosome 2q37 and spans 200 kb with 13 individual promoters or first exons that share a set of exons numbered 2 to 5.[132,151] Alternate splicing of the 13 distinct first exons to the 4 exons in common provides 9 functional UGT1 enzymes (1A1, 1A3, 1A4, 1A5, 1A6, 1A7, 1A8, 1A9, and 1A10) with identical C-terminal and unique N-terminal domains. The remaining 4 proteins of the UGT1A family are pseudogenes (1A2p, 1A11p, 1A12p, and A13p), which are nonfunctional enzymes due to mutations that prevent the expression of active proteins. The UGT2 family is found on chromosome 4q13 and in humans the genes of this family span 1.45 Mb, where each isoform is comprised of 6 exons that are not shared among subfamily members, and thus, differ in sequence throughout compared with other family members. This family is then subdivided into 2 subfamilies (UGT2A and UGT2B). The UGT2A family is comprised of 3 members: 2A1, 2A2, and 2A3; while the UGT2B subfamily contains 7 functional members 2B1, 2B4, 2B7,

2B10, 2B11, 2B15, and 2B17. Five pseudogenes in the UGT2B subfamily have also been discovered (2B24P, 2B25P, 2B26P, 2B27P, and 2B28P).

A number of translational factors are involved in the regulation of UGT genes that may control the constitutive levels of UGTs in tissues.[152] These include hepatocyte nuclear factor (HNF) 1α[153] and HNF4β,[154] octamer transcription factor 1 (OCT-1),[155] CAAT-enhancer binding protein,[156] and pre-B cell homeobox factor 2 (Pbx2).[157] The translational factors that influence the activation of the promoter preceding the exon of each UGT or group of UGT exons are independently regulated in a tissue-specific and sequential manner, which may explain tissue dependent expression of each UGT isoform. UGT gene expression is also influenced by a number of members of the nuclear receptor super-family, such as pregnane X receptor (PXR),[158] constitutive androstane receptor (CAR),[159] farnesoid X receptor (FXR),[160] liver X receptor (LXR),[161] and the aryl hydrocarbon receptor (AhR),[162] all of which are modulated by endogenous compounds, such as hormones and drug-like compounds.[152] LXR is a good example of how a nuclear receptor can effect gene activation and expression of a UGT. Ligand-bound LXRα dimerizes with retinoid X receptor (RXR) and binds to direct repeats separated by a 4 bp (DR4) element in the *UGT1A3* promotor to activate *UGT1A3* transcription.[161] This process is thought to be triggered by cholestasis, where oxysterol accumulates. Oxysterol is a ligand of LXR, and thus activates the expression of UGT1A3, which in turn detoxifies bile acids through glucuronidation of chenodeoxycholic and lithocholic bile acid.

Expression levels of the UGT isoforms mirror those of the tissues that are mainly responsible for producing more water soluble compounds to clear them from systemic circulation, such as the liver and kidneys. There are a number of reports in the literature that have investigated quantifying UGT expression throughout the body, where large variability of expression levels has been observed between donors and within tissues in the body. The two most extensive analyses using multiple donors to quantifying tissue distribution throughout the body have used quantitative reverse transcript-polymerase chain reaction (qRT-PCR) for mRNA assessment.[163,164] In general, there is agreement in the literature as to which isoforms are most prevalent in certain tissues based on mRNA values. In both studies, the liver was identified as the organ with the most abundant complement of UGT isoforms. These isoforms include all of the UGT1 and UGT2 families except 1A5, 1A7, 1A8, 1A10, and 2A1. It is generally agreed that members of the UGT2B family are more abundant in the liver than members of the UGT1A family, and that UGT2B4 is the most abundant family member in the liver.[163,164] It has been speculated that UGT2B4 plays an important role in preventing accumulation of endogenous steroids and bile acids in the liver, thus the high relative abundance in the liver is warranted.

Renal UGTs have been shown to play a significant role in maintaining homeostasis in the kidney *via* limiting endogenous mediators that control electrolyte balance and renal blood flow.[165] Due to the physiological necessity provided by these UGTs the kidney has the ability to glucuronidate drug-like xenobiotics. The expression of UGTs in the kidneys has also been examined using the same RNA quantification techniques as those used for the liver, namely qRT-PCR. In both assessments, the mRNA levels were highest in the kidney for members of both the UGT1 and UGT2 families. The members that comprise 95% of all the UGTs expressed in the kidney are UGT1A6, UGT1A9, and UGT2B7, with the latter two being the most prevalent and with almost equal expression (~86%).[6,163,164]

The other major metabolizing organs of the gastrointestinal (GI) tract, stomach, small intestine and colon also show specificity for certain members of the UGT family. The studies by Ohno *et al.* and Court *et al.* provide general consensus as to which family members are expressed in each region of the GI tract. The major isoform expressed in the GI are UGT1A6, UGT1A8, UGT1A10, UGT2B15, UGT2B17, and most likely UGT2B7. The two family members UGT1A10 and UGT2B17 appear to be expressed predominately in the intestine and colon.[163,164] It has been shown that the general trends in the expression levels in the stomach mimic those of the kidney with rather few isoforms being expressed, albeit at high expression levels.[166] It is also worth noting that steroidogenic tissues such as the adrenal gland, breast, heart, and prostate express several members of the UGT family, however the levels are relatively low compared with the GI tract, kidneys and liver.

Estimating mRNA levels provides a general quantitative comparison among tissues. However, the issue with measuring mRNA levels is that high mRNA levels do not always translate to functional protein levels. Thus, multiple laboratories have undertaken the initiative to carry out absolute quantitative proteomics using either heavy atom standards in conjunction with LC/MS, or S-tag fusion proteins as recombinant standards.[167-174] The majority of the published UGT absolute abundance data in the literature have been attributed to The University of North Carolina at Chapel Hill in the USA and Tohoku University in Japan, both of which have used a heavy isotope internal standard to measure UGT abundance levels. For many of the isoforms tested in these two laboratories similar levels were observed, most likely because the same stable isotope-labeled peptides were used as internal standards. A summary of the quantification data available in the literature is presented in Table 5.5.

Recently, Achour and colleagues investigated another method to quantify hepatic UGT abundance.[175] Their study detailed the quantification of liver UGTs using the QconCAT (quantification concatemer) method. This technology quantifies multiple enzymes at once *via* an internal standard of concatenated peptide sequences, which are trypsinized to match the cleavage site of the native protein. Achour reported that, in general, abundance values were similar using the QconCAT method compared with those quantified *via* LC-MS/MS;[175] however, Achour's data indicated that UGT1A3 and UGT1A4 were expressed at much higher levels than previously reported using the heavy isotope LC-MS/MS methods (Table 5.5).

Consensus abundance values may be more attainable now that absolute quantification of protein levels is more common. With similar absolute

Table 5.5 Summary of literature derived UGT levels in the liver, intestine, and kidneys.

UGT	Mean liver abundance (pmols mg^{-1}) from human liver microsome samples	Mean intestinal abundance (pmols mg^{-1})	Mean kidney abundance (pmols mg^{-1})
1A1	20–35,[a] 18.3,[b] 21.5,[c] 22.4,[d] 33.5,[e] 120,[f] 0.133,[g] 36.2,[h] 33.6[i]	6–7[a]	7,[b] BLQ[g]
1A3	9.9,[b] 17.3,[e] 7.9,[h] 123.1[i]	BLQ[b]	BLQ[b]
1A4	4.6,[b] 5.4,[h] 58.0[i]	5.3[b]	11[b]
1A5	≥0.23[h]	NA	NA
1A6	3–5,[a] 4.6,[b] 114,[e] 0.452,[g] 9.7,[h] 107.1[i]	2.3[b]	2,[b] BLQ[g]
1A7	BLQ,[b] ≥0.23[h]	8.4[b]	14[b]
1A8	BLQ,[b] ≥0.23[h]	6.1[b]	8[b]
1A9	26.7,[b] 25.9,[e] 23.1,[h] 40.0[i]	6.6[b]	81[b]
1A10	BLQ,[b] ≥0.23[h]	4.7[b]	18[b]
2B4	70.8[i]	NA	NA
2B7	9.7,[c] 96,[d] 84.3,[e] 80.1,[h] 82.9[i]	NA	NA
2B10	6.5[h]	NA	NA
2B15	61.8,[e] 32.8,[h] 62.1[i]	NA	NA
2B17	8.1[h]	NA	NA

[a](n = 10 donors).[167]
[b](n = 9 donors).[169]
[c](n = 16 donors).[172]
[d](n = 3 donors).[174]
[e](n = 17 donors).[171]
[f](n = 15 donors).[173]
[g](n = 29 donors).[170]
[h](n = 60 donors).[168]
[i](n = 23–24 donors).[175]

abundance values coming from different internal standards and methods, confidence will establish average abundance values and also provide a range of values within a healthy volunteer or diseased population. Although the geometric mean levels are only determined from a small number of studies, UGT1A1, UGT1A3, UGT1A6, UGT1A9, UGT2B7, and UGT2B15 appear to have been assessed a number of times using multiple methods, thus providing usable abundance values. The geometric mean abundances estimated are approximately 17, 20, 9.5, 28, 55, and 50 pmol mg^{-1} of microsomal protein, respectively. However, scrutiny is warranted due to the consensus values coming from only relatively few assessments. Therefore, the most appropriate approach is to allow for a range of isoform-specific absolute abundance values obtained from Table 5.5 and to recognize the possibility of polymorphisms in the population for particular UGTs (*i.e.* UGT1A1).

5.4.3 *In vitro* Assay Optimization for UGTs

In vitro assay conditions have been shown to impact the efficiency of many UGTs. The utilization of albumin, alamethicin, MgCl$_2$, saccharolactone, uridine-diphosphate-glucuronic acid trisodium salt (UDPGA), and the appropriate buffer system have all been investigated.[176–184] There is universal agreement that the source of the transferred glucuronic acid to the substrate is UDPGA and it should be included in excess at a concentration of 5 mM to initiate the *in vitro* reaction.[183,185] Tris buffer has also been shown to be preferred to sodium phosphate buffer for the majority of UGTs to achieve the highest potential enzyme activity. It is thought that phosphorylation of UGTs adversely affects their selectivity and enzyme activity.[186] Thus, it is suggested that 100 mM Tris buffer, pH 7.5 at 37 °C be used for *in vitro* experiments. Saccharolactone has been shown to inhibit the ability of endogenous β-glucuronidases to remove the glucuronic acid from the substrate conjugate during incubation, and in some instances has been shown to preserve the glucuronide.[187] However, in other literature examples, saccharolactone did not preserve or increase glucuronide formation rates, and in fact, even lowered the glucuronide formation levels.[183,188,189] It is therefore thought that saccharolactone is not necessary in *in vitro* incubations due to its potential detrimental effects on enzyme activity.[117] However, Zientek and Youdim also qualified that a comparison of the cumulative metabolite formation rates with the parent depletion in a UGT cofactor fortified reaction is a good confirmation of the lack of need for saccharolactone, and if the rates are not complimentary, the incubation should be repeated with saccharolactone.[117] Another potential *in vitro* reagent addition to improve enzyme performance is divalent metal ions, such as MgCl$_2$.[176,177,183] Concentrations of MgCl$_2$ ranging from 4 to 5 mM have been shown to increase UGT activity in both recombinant UGTs and HLM by up to 4-fold.

A critical *in vitro* UGT reagent is alamethicin. Since most UGTs are found on the luminal side of the endoplasmic reticulum in *in vitro* experiments, and the location of expression is thought to impede the access of the UDPGA cofactor to the enzyme, pore forming reagents, such as alamethicin, have been used to increase accessibility. Alamethicin increases UGT enzyme activity significantly,[184] and is considered necessary to produce enough enzyme activity for adequate sensitivity. It has been noted that when optimizing alamethicin concentrations for superior enzyme activity, lower microsomal concentrations require a greater amount of alamethicin to activate the enzyme than at higher microsomal concentrations.[183] A concentration of 10 μg mL^{-1} alamethicin has been suggested to provide adequate levels of pore formation for microsomal protein levels from 0.01 to 0.5 mg mL^{-1}. Interestingly, no increase in activity has been observed with the addition of alamethicin to recombinant UGTs expressed in insect cell baculovirus,[183,188] and it has little to no effect on CYP activity in the limited examples in the literature.[190]

One of the most recent discoveries found to influence UGT activity is the addition of fatty acid-free bovine serum albumin (BSA) to the UGT reaction matrix. Rowland and colleagues were the first to indicate the *in vitro* enhancement of the clearance rates with the inclusion of BSA to UGT incubations. This first work using BSA details the use of propofol and zidovudine (AZT) to assess UGT1A9 and UGT2B7 CL$_{int}$.[181] Rowland *et al.* reported the observation of a decreased K_m without affecting V_{max}.[181] This "albumin-effect", has been described as albumin acting as a sink to bind free fatty acids released from the microsomal membranes during preparation. By removing the fatty acids, one avoids the competitive inhibition of the fatty acids on the UGTs. Additional studies confirmed the effects of BSA on UGT2B7, and also provided evidence that not only was the K_m decreased, but the V_{max} of UGT1A9 was also increased.[179,191] In experiments using recombinant human UGT1A7, UGT1A8, UGT1A10, UGT2A1, UGT2B15 and UGT2B17 expressed by baculovirus infected insect cells, each UGT was assessed with both selective and nonselective substrates in the presence and absence of fatty acid-free BSA.[192] Due to the use of two estradiol isomers as substrates and the observed high concentration-dependent binding of these isomers to BSA, the BSA concentration was reduced from the published 2% to 0.1%. The lower concentration of BSA has been shown to be sufficient to reduce the inhibitory effect of the free fatty acids.[179] The study concluded that each of the isoforms tested, with the exception of UGT2B17, showed a reduced K_m and an increased V_{max}. The increased V_{max} effects observed with certain substrates indicates more complex interactions than just the removal of competing free fatty acids. In a similar experiment, Shiraga and colleagues showed kinetic benefit from low levels of BSA with UGT1A9 when evaluating darexaban metabolism. At 0.1% BSA, similar kinetic parameters were observed when corrected for the free fraction to those obtained at 2% BSA.[193] However, the effects were most noticeable on the unbound K_m and not the V_{max}.

Certain UGTs have been found to be highly expressed in the kidneys and intestine, and consequently have been implicated as major contributors toward the total clearance of UGT cleared substrates.[194,195] As such, there has been particular interest in the effects of BSA on these enzymes, and whether their expression and the sequestration of free fatty acids liberated during microsomal preparation are affected similarly to that observed in the liver. UGT1A9 is an example of a highly expressed UGT isoform found in the kidney. It has been reported that the expression levels of UGT1A9, on a picomole per microliter basis, are 3–4-fold higher than in the liver.[169] It is not surprising that Gill and colleagues reported *in vitro* renal CL_{int} rates two-times higher on a per gram of tissue basis compared with liver for UGT1A9 when BSA was added to the incubation.[196] Furthermore, when the scaled renal UGT clearance from kidney microsomes was added to hepatic UGT clearance, an improvement in the *in vitro–in vivo* extrapolation of glucuronidation clearance was observed. Furthermore, the inclusion of BSA brought 50% of the drugs tested to within 2-fold of the clinically derived values when the *in vitro* data were scaled using tissue specific scaling factors. The magnitude of BSA effect on the clearance rates in each tissue was noted to possibly be influenced by the overall fatty acid content of that tissue.

The UGT isoforms that appear to kinetically benefit from the inclusion of fatty acid-free BSA in the incubation reaction include 1A7, 1A8, 1A9 1A10, 2A1, 2B7, and 2B15. UGT isoforms that do not appear to be affected are 1A1, 1A4, 1A6, and 2B17.[179,183,196] One consideration when incorporating fatty acid-free BSA into reactions to enhance UGT activity, as well as the clinical predictability of clearance, is to assess the free fraction of the compound in the BSA supplemented incubation reaction (fu_{inc}), regardless of the tissue investigated (*i.e.* kidney, liver, or intestine).[183,196] The resulting measurement should be incorporated into the mathematical method to calculate clearance associated with UGTs in the liver, kidney, and GI tract.[183,192] This mathematical correction of the free unbound clearance will then provide a better overall assessment of *in vivo* clearance prediction, and hence, a more thorough assessment of the fraction metabolized *via* the UGT route(s) in relation to other routes of metabolism. Regardless, highly bound compounds will suffer from unmeasurable clearance rates, due to being sequestered; therefore, utilizing the minimum amount of BSA to decrease the free fatty acids produced during microsomal preparation may be the best method to follow. The work of Manevski and colleagues provides a good compromise in keeping the concentration of BSA down and achieving the goal of reducing the concentration of detrimental free fatty acids that affect UGT, while still limiting the impact on the free concentration of the drug.[179]

One additional aspect, alluded to previously when deciding on the concentration of supplemental BSA in the UGT incubation reactions, is to consider the varying amount of free fatty acid in different enzyme sources. It has been reported that the levels of free fatty acids differ between enzyme sources (HLM > Sf9 cells > *Escherichia coli*), therefore the amount of BSA necessary for minimizing the detrimental free fatty acid effect may be pushed above the suggested 0.1%. Therefore, when optimizing a source of enzyme for the first time one should investigate multiple levels of BSA, and keep in mind that different UGT enzymes have different sensitivities to free fatty acid exposure.[197,198] The optimal conditions for each UGT isoform differ from isoform to isoform, and deciding on how much to optimize the conditions for each isoform is influenced by the degree of understanding needed to determine the metabolism or kinetic parameters of the single or multiple UGT isoform(s). However, with all the caveats, some general guidance can be provided for the UGT family and is summarized in Table 5.6. In short, the consensus conditions for preliminary studies that assure optimal UGT activity are 100 mM Tris buffer pH 7.5, 4 mM $MgCl_2$, 10 µg mL^{-1} alamethicin, 0.5 mg mL^{-1} HLM, and 1 µM substrate of interest, and finally the addition of 5 mM UDPGA to initiate the reaction. As the characterization of the enzymes responsible for the metabolism of the substrate become more apparent during the characterization process, the inclusion of an optimal amount of BSA is prudent.

5.4.4 UGT Phenotyping Strategies

In the discovery process of identifying the UGT isoforms responsible for the metabolism of a new chemical entity (NCE), there are three main strategies: (1) chemical inhibition using specific UGT isoform inhibitors; (2) the use of recombinant UGTs; and (3) correlation analysis based upon metabolite formation rates.[183,187,199] The *in vitro* correlation analysis utilizes verified specific

Table 5.6 Putative optimal reaction conditions for UGTs.

Purpose	Reagent	Concentration	Comments
Early discovery work	Tris buffer pH 7.5	100 mM	Putative buffer of choice
	MgCl$_2$	4 mM	Improves enzyme performance
	Alamethicin	10 µg mL^{-1}	Pore forming reagent to increase access of UDPGA to luminal side of endoplasmic reticulum
	Enzyme source	0.5 mg mL^{-1}	Pooled human liver microsomes for early discovery work
	UDPGA	5 mM	A co-substrate providing the sugar for conjugation, which can be used to initiate the reaction *in vitro*
Individual isoform, polymorphic enzyme, or kinetic assessments	Fatty acid free BSA	0.1 mg mL^{-1}	Isoforms affected by BSA: UGT1A7, UGT1A8, UGT1A9, UGT1A10, UGT2A1, UGT2B7, and UGT2B15
			Higher BSA levels may be necessary depending on enzyme source
			Protein binding correction necessary for intrinsic clearance characterization
	Enzyme source	Various	Recombinant UGTs, pooled or single polymorphic enzyme donor microsomes

substrates for each isoform of UGT with a characterized bank of donor HLM samples to compare with the metabolism rates of the NCE. The most precise utilization of the correlation analysis method is to monitor the rate of formation of a glucuronide metabolite of a known specific substrate and compare this linearly with the rate of formation of the glucuronide metabolite of the test substrate. The correlation assay is most useful as a companion to the other methods mentioned rather than a stand-alone phenotyping tool due to the need for previous metabolite identification and analytical method development for each glucuronide, in addition to having an authentic glucuronide standard for the test substrate. To aid in the utilization of the correlation analysis a list of some of the best understood specific substrates and metabolites for each isoform can be found in Table 5.7. Not all of the substrates listed in the table are completely specific for the isoform noted nor have they been completely vetted for all assay conditions (*i.e.* inclusion of BSA, buffer, optimal pH, and enzyme source); therefore, some caution or preparatory validation work is recommended.

More recently, optimized kinetic assay conditions have been identified for multiple UGT specific substrates. The work of Walsky *et al.* provided a 2-fold benefit for the advancement of UGT phenotyping: (1) specific UGT substrates

Table 5.7   List of specific substrates of UGT isoforms.[c]

UGT isoform	Specific substrate	Reported HLM unbound K_m or S_{50} in μM (V_{max}; pmol min^{-1} mg^{-1})
1A1	SN-38 (active metabolite of irinotecan), a small UGT1A7 contribution	1.4 (820) without 2% BSA
	β-Estradiol[a]	6.6 (1400) with 2% BSA (β-Estradiol-3-glucuronide)
1A3	Zolarsartan,[226] fulvestrant[227] hexafluoro-1α, 25-dihydroxyvitamin D$_3$[228]	
1A4	Imipramine[209]	11 (1500) without 2% BSA
	Trifluoperazine[a]	4.1 (870) with 2% BSA (Trifluoperazine-*N*-glucuronide)
1A6	Serotonin[204]	390 (66 000) without 2% BSA
	5-Hydroxytryptophol[a]	300 (47 000) with 2% BSA (5HTOL-*O*-glucuronide)
1A7 (extrahepatic)	Octylgallate	
1A8 (extrahepatic)	Dihydroxytestosterone metabolized to a diglucuronide[229]	
1A9	**Propofol**[a]	98 (1400) without 2% BSA
		7.8 (780) with 2% BSA (Propofol-*O*-glucuronide)
1A10 (extrahepatic)	Dopamine[230]	
2B7	**3′-Azido-3′-deoythymidine (AZT)**[a]	420 (2100) without 2% BSA
		100 (4700) with 2% BSA (AZT-5′-glucuronide)
2B15	**(S)-Oxazepam**[b]	54 (303) without BSA [(S)-Oxazepam glucuronide]

[a]Substrate and data acquired from Walsky *et al.*[183]
[b]Substrate and data acquired from Court *et al.*[231]
[c]**Bold print** under "specific substrate" indicates substrates that have been shown to be specific for each isoform, and are thus the preferred tool compounds for UGT phenotyping.

in optimized conditions; and (2) specific inhibitors of each UGT isoform.[183] The assay conditions optimized included the use of BSA, saccharolactone, alamethicin, MgCl$_2$, and the type of buffer used. The UGTs and substrates that were optimized were noted in bold type in Table 5.7 and have been shown elsewhere to be fairly specific for each isoform.[199–206]

Chemical inhibition phenotyping has provided sufficient understanding of the fraction metabolized by CYP and is widely accepted as one of the gold standards for reaction phenotyping. This method has also been acknowledged and accepted by both the FDA and EMA guidances.[136,137] The selectivity of a compound as an inhibitor is critical to its utility as a phenotyping tool. To be effective, the 90% inhibition concentration (IC$_{90}$) of a tool inhibitor should be selective enough to show very little, if any, effect on other enzymes responsible for metabolism. Phenotypic testing at the IC$_{90}$ allows for almost complete inhibition of the enzyme while providing an understanding of the fraction metabolized through the decrease in the rate of loss of the parent

Table 5.8 List of inhibitors of UGT isoforms.

UGT isoform	Inhibitor	Reported IC$_{50}$ (µM)	Inhibitor references
1A1	Atazanavir	1.9	Zhang *et al.*[208]
	Erlotinib	1.2 (K_i = 0.64)	Liu *et al.*[207]
1A3	Buprenorphine	40–50	Oechsler *et al.*[232]
1A4	Hecogenin	1.5	Uchaipichat *et al.*[209]
1A6	Troglitazone	20	Ito *et al.*[233]
1A7 (extrahepatic)	Phenylbutazone (nonselective)	3.9	Uchaipichat *et al.*[209]
1A8 (extrahepatic)	Emodin^a	15.6	Watanabe *et al.*[234]
1A9	Niflumic acid	0.0275	Mano *et al.*[214]
1A10 (extrahepatic)	Tacrolimus	0.034	Zucker *et al.*[235]
2B7	Fluconazole^b	146 (K_i = 73)	Uchaipichat *et al.*[203]
2B15	Ibuprofen	120	Sten *et al.*[236]

^{a}UGT1A10 interaction may influence specificity assessment.
^{b}Plus BSA in incubation.

versus time. While identification of specific UGT inhibitors has evolved slowly, there have been multiple publications in the literature that have identified specific inhibitors (Table 5.8). The most specific UGT inhibitors have been reported for four of the UGT isoforms: 1A1, 1A4, 1A9, and 2B7, and evidence for the inhibitors of these enzymes are discussed below.

UGT1A1, a highly polymorphic enzyme, accommodates a wide array of chemical substrates. A number of chemical inhibitors have been identified that are useful for UGT1A1 phenotyping purposes, and among these erlotinib and atazanavir stand out. Erlotinib has been reported to be a specific inhibitor of UGT1A1 with a K_i equal to 64 nM, and when tested at 100 µM, inhibited 4-methylumbelliferone glucuronidation by almost 90% and was 5-fold more selective than the other isoforms.[207] Atazanavir has also been identified as a potent and specific inhibitor of UGT1A1, with an IC$_{50}$ of 1.9 µM, and is mentioned as the UGT1A1 inhibitor of choice in regulatory guidances.[208]

The tendency of UGT1A4 to catalyze quaternary ammonium glucuronides helps to identify the utility and possible contribution of this isoform to the metabolism of compounds. This type of structural information also lends itself toward identifying potential high affinity UGT1A4 substrates that may out-compete other UGT1A1 substrates, causing an inhibitory effect. Through this method, hecogenin was identified and has been used successfully in phenotyping reactions to confirm the contribution of UGT1A4, with an IC$_{50}$ of 1.5 µM.[206,209] UGT1A9 is mainly expressed in the kidney, but is also found in other tissues such as the colon, liver, ovaries, and testis.[210–212] It is widely accepted that niflumic acid is a specific inhibitor of UGT1A9 with a potent K_i equal to 0.0275 µM.[213,214]

UGT2B7 is perhaps the most important UGT in drug metabolism due to its broad diversity of known substrates. UGT2B7 substrates include NSAIDs, opioids, and many other drug agents from many different therapeutic classes. Fluconazole is considered a competitive and specific inhibitor of UGT2B7. Unfortunately, when used in a fully fortified reaction for both UGTs and CYPs (*e.g.* supplemented with both UDPGA and NADPH), it is also a very good CYP3A4 inhibitor, which may create some ambiguity in experimental results. This lack of inhibitory specificity is a good example of the care that needs to be taken to isolate each route of metabolism by using the appropriate cofactors (UDPGA *vs.* NADPH) in HLM or human liver S-9 fractions. The competitive K_i of fluconazole has been reported to be 143 μM in HLM and 73 μM in rhUGT2B7. A concentration of fluconazole above 1.3 mM in a UGT chemical inhibition study should be enough to provide a good estimate of the fraction metabolized by UGT2B7 in HLM. For the other UGT isoforms not reported here, a more in-depth assessment is needed for generalized use. With the establishment of more optimized assay conditions across a number of laboratories, information on more specific inhibitors will inevitably be published in the near future.[183,206]

When recombinant enzymes are used to predict the fraction metabolized *via* a certain UGT, a mathematical correction is needed from the recombinant enzymes to those isolated directly from the organ of interest. When many of these recombinant human UGTs (rhUGT) are engineered they are forced with artificial factors, and high enzyme expression levels per milligram of microsomal protein are needed for them to perform similarly or superiorly to those isolated from the metabolizing organ. In this regard, two approaches have been adopted to help bridge the gap between drug catalytic rates observed in rhUGTs and HLMs. The first approach uses a relative activity factor (RAF), which defines the amount of rhUGT required to give an equivalent reaction velocity in a particular HLM sample, similar to what has been in place for recombinant CYP enzymes. However, this approach does not address inter-individual variability in UGT expression, or the apparent substrate specificity of RAFs. The second approach that has been used to overcome the difference in activity of rhUGTs and HLM as well as address inter-individual variability in UGT expression is the inter-system extrapolation factor (ISEF). The ISEF, a dimensionless correction factor, compares the intrinsic activities of rhUGTs *versus* liver microsomes and provides UGT abundance scaling by mathematical means through either V_{max} rates [eqn (5.1)] or CL_{int} [eqn (5.2)] normalization factors.

$$\text{VISEF}(V_{max}) = \frac{V_{max}(\text{HLM})}{V_{max}(\text{rhUGT})} \times \text{UGT abundance (HLM)} \qquad (5.1)$$

$$\text{CLISEF}(CL_{int}) = \frac{\dfrac{V_{max}}{K_m}(\text{HLM})}{\dfrac{V_{max}}{K_m}(\text{rhUGT})} \times \text{UGT abundance (HLM)} \qquad (5.2)$$

These methods have been used extensively and successfully when comparing recombinant CYP activity with HLM.[215,216] It has been pointed out that the advantage of one approach over the other seems very much dependent upon the laboratory conditions: HLM pools and expression systems used, experimental approach (*e.g.* metabolite formation or substrate depletion), and the probe substrate(s) used. To use the second approach one parameter that is needed is the accurate measurement of UGT abundance in tissue and recombinant enzymes in order to scale activity *in vitro* to organs responsible for metabolizing a drug agent of interest. Without this abundance information for tissues it is impossible to quantitatively extrapolate relative contributions of rhUGTs to human tissue, and thus provide projections and implications of population variability using an array of donor liver fractions. As the availability of UGT abundance data from numerous laboratories increases, putative abundance values can be applied to understand the relationship between recombinant enzymes and human liver, intestinal, and kidney microsomes on a per picomole basis.

The proteomics approaches have had particular utility with compounds that display extremely low clearance *in vitro* due to the now understood low abundance of the responsible enzymes in human liver homogenate and the inability to push the protein level high enough without encountering detrimental effects from protein and lipid binding. This realization has provided the unique opportunity to use rhUGTs to allow lower overall protein levels, with greater abundance of UGT enzyme per milligram of protein, and potentially greater activity on a picomole basis to push the reaction to measurable clearance rates. These results can then, in turn, be scaled to *in vivo* clearance using the appropriate scaling factors and applied to the variability in the population. Of course, this *in vitro* ISEF relationship is enzyme source specific for both the lot of recombinant enzyme and the corresponding pooled or single donor HLM. As such, caution should also be taken when using an ISEF from the multiple vendors of recombinant enzymes and liver microsomes.

With the current methods and reagents available, a preliminary ISEF can be established for these UGTs: 1A1, 1A6, 1A9, and 2B7. This ability to establish ISEFs for these enzymes is due to the combination of putative abundance values, the availability of both rhUGTs and hepatic liver fractions, matched with substrates and metabolite kinetics.

In lieu of enzyme abundance for UGTs, RAFs are still an option to connect the recombinant enzyme to those found in liver tissue fractions. Although, RAF scaling does not allow for relating the understanding of activity differences on the enzyme subunit level and the understanding of population variability, it allows for scaling of recombinant enzymes to whole organ clearance and provides a general prediction of clearance dictated by a particular lot of tissue fraction. Gibson *et al.* and Kato *et al.* have provided two examples of the use of RAF to extrapolate to whole body clearance for UGTs in the literature.[217,218] Gibson and colleagues used RAFs to scale rhUGT1A1, rhUGT1A9, and rhUGT2B7 to whole organ clearance of the liver and UGT1A9 and UGT2B7 in the kidney, while Kato and colleagues described RAFs for UGT1A4, UGT1A9, and UGT2B7 in the liver. Both groups describe their application of these derived RAFs to the quantitative involvement of each isoform to their respective compounds. Interestingly, Kato and colleagues found that the RAF using V_{max} or CL_{int} resulted in the overestimation of the contribution of a given enzyme if the probe substrates used were not specific for the enzyme. Furthermore, both studies could be expanded to derive ISEFs, if the enzyme abundance data presented in Table 5.5 represent those of the pooled microsomal lot, and if the corresponding recombinant lot of enzyme abundance had been measured.

On a broader scale, obtaining the abundances and the methods used to generate these data provides the ability to perform PBPK predictions, which can be expanded to polymorphic populations and even the effects that disease states have on enzyme expression. Moreover, abundance evaluations can be extended to extrahepatic tissue to provide a baseline for all enzyme expressing tissues, which currently are not well defined (*i.e.* individual sections of the intestine and colon, *etc.*). These data together will also help provide the ability to remedy the noted under-predictions observed from scaling from human liver fractions and hepatocytes alone. Additional work will have to be completed in the field to assess the most perfused tissues and the appropriate *in vitro* assay conditions to facilitate higher quality predictions of human UGT clearance.

5.4.5 Challenges in the Prediction of Human Clearance for UGT Substrates

The well documented under-prediction of *in vivo* hepatic clearance from *in vitro* human liver homogenates, and to a lesser extent human hepatocytes, has impeded a robust *in vitro* strategy to extrapolate human clearance from *in vitro* assessments.[176,185,200,219–221] Under-predictions may be attributed to any number of factors, including: the influence of incubation conditions; dependence on a consistent purified enzyme source; lack of an easy quantitation method to assess abundance of the enzyme; lack of specific substrates and/or identification of specific metabolites to establish RAF or ISEF calculations from HLM to rhUGTs; release of free fatty acids from the microsomal membrane that are potent inhibitors of certain UGT enzymes; extrahepatic contribution to total UGT metabolism; and the observation of atypical glucuronidation kinetics.

Where the science has advanced enough to provide a useful method of scaling *in vitro* clearance to *in vivo* is the utilization of BSA to improve *in vitro* activity for the most afflicted UGT isoforms. The data suggest fatty acid-free BSA "rescues" any detrimentally affected isoforms from long-chained free fatty acids and additionally helps to alleviate the under-prediction of clearance. Therefore, BSA helps to set the strategy for human clearance predictions. This strategy is illustrated in Figure 5.12. The strategy begins with an initial experiment utilizing either (1) rhUGTs or (2) human liver, intestinal, or kidney microsomes in the presence or absence of specific inhibitors. Either method provides information on which enzyme(s) contribute to the metabolism of the compound of interest. These initial experiments prepare for subsequent studies with human liver, intestinal, or kidney microsomes, which include or exclude BSA depending on the free fatty acid effect on the UGT isoform enzyme activity. These follow-up, enzyme specific experiments provide

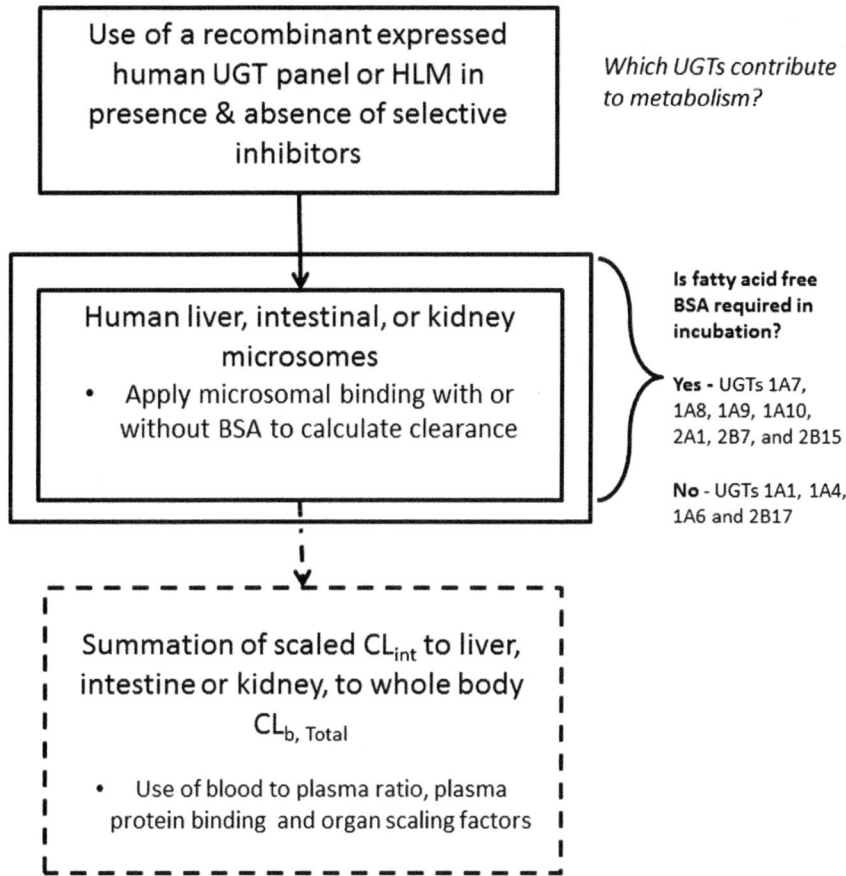

Figure 5.12 Proposed *in vitro* studies to identify UGT isoforms involved in the glucuronidation of a test drug, and approach to scale results to predict whole body clearance.

the basis for scaling to whole organ clearance based on the blood flow rates of each route of clearance. Much has been written about these scaling practices from organ microsomal homogenates.[176,185,196,219,222–225] Necessary information needed to scale to whole organs includes free fraction in the microsomal incubation (with or without BSA), the plasma protein binding, the blood to plasma ratio, organ blood flow rates, milligrams of microsomal protein per gram of organ tissue, and organ weight, as well as the body weight of the population being assessed. As an example of the appropriateness of this scaling using BSA bolstered incubation, Gill and colleagues have provided an *in vitro* to *in vivo* assessment of the use of fatty acid-free BSA to calculate intravenous UGT clearance.[196] Their work showed that the inclusion of BSA in microsomal (liver, kidney, or intestine) glucuronidation assays increased unbound CL_{int} in a tissue- and drug-dependent manner, altered the ratios of clearance between the tissues, and resulted in improved overall prediction accuracy of intravenous clearance (CL_{iv}). A summary equation for scaling CL_{iv} from liver and kidney is listed below. Since the intestine is believed to have little impact on CL_{iv}, Gill and colleagues did not include the unbound CL_{int} from the intestine into the total UGT CL_{iv} equation for comparison with the observed clinical value.

$$CL_{UGT} = \frac{CL_{int,u}\left(UGT,liver\right) \times fu_B \times Q_h}{CL_{int,u}\left(UGT,liver\right) \times fu_B + Q_h} + \frac{CL_{int,u}\left(UGT,renal\right) \times fu_B \times Q_r}{CL_{int,u}\left(UGT,renal\right) \times fu_B + Q_r}$$

(5.3)

The equation is based on the well stirred model and includes *in vitro* $CL_{int,u,UGT}$ data (per gram of tissue), corrected for the fraction unbound in the incubation (fu_{inc}), in HLM (liver) and HKM (renal) scaled to give $CL_{int,u,UGT}$ (per kilogram of body weight). This scaling uses the average organ weights of 21.4 g of tissue per kilogram and 4.5 g tissue per kilogram for liver and kidney, respectively. The fraction unbound in blood is represented by fu_B, Q_h is hepatic blood flow ($Q_h = 20.7$ mL min^{-1} kg^{-1}), and if applicable, Q_r (average renal blood flow of 16.4 mL min^{-1} kg^{-1}) and *in vitro* HKM data were used. CL_{UGT} represents the overall apparent intravenous *in vivo* glucuronidation clearance.

This strategy is still evolving due to the continued scientific advances being made in UGT enzymology and metabolism. However, quantitative scaling has shown some real promise. Further advances in UGT science with fully vetted optimized UGT protocols will continue to increase the precision and accuracy of *in vivo* clearance predictions, and will quite possibly increase the scalability of the recombinant enzymes to *in vivo* clearance by laying down a solid foundation for UGT optimal activity.

5.5 Future Perspective

While the CYP family of drug-metabolizing enzymes remains a primary focus in drug discovery and development, additional metabolic mechanisms are plentiful and should be understood. Changes to the targeted chemical space being explored by chemists, as well as successes in minimizing CYP-mediated metabolism by structural modification, have triggered the critical need to understand and identify these alternate metabolic clearance routes. In this regard, conventional metabolic stability screening assays utilizing HLMs have been both a blessing and a curse. While discovery teams have been able to rapidly assess SAR and address metabolic liability issues around CYP, not utilizing the appropriate *in vitro* system with the full complement of metabolic enzymes (*e.g.* hepatocytes), and not recognizing species differences in metabolism, has led to major misses and untoward outcomes in the clinic. FMO, AO, and UGT are three key enzyme families that fall into this category, and thus, their contribution to metabolism of drugs has often been missed. In some cases, this has been detrimental to the progression of a clinical program, and in other cases, the identification of these pathways has actually been of benefit, as the risk for DDIs is minimized by having a non-CYP route of clearance. As drug companies constantly work to refine and streamline their processes to enable faster discovery of drug candidates, it is critical that they do not attempt to replace basic science around drug metabolism. Additional academic research is needed for the enzymes discussed in this chapter, as well as the plethora of other non-CYP enzymes present in the liver and beyond, to ultimately improve the ability to predict human metabolic clearance for drugs moving towards the clinic, an effort that will be well worth the investment.

References

1. B. Achour, J. Barber and A. Rostami-Hodjegan, *Drug Metab. Dispos.*, 2014, **42**, 1349.
2. J. D. Hughes, J. Blagg, D. A. Price, S. Bailey, G. A. Decrescenzo, R. V. Devraj, E. Ellsworth, Y. M. Fobian, M. E. Gibbs, R. W. Gilles, N. Greene, E. Huang, T. Krieger-Burke, J. Loesel, T. Wager, L. Whiteley and Y. Zhang, *Bioorg. Med. Chem. Lett.*, 2008, **18**, 4872.
3. D. A. Price, J. Blagg, L. Jones, N. Greene and T. Wager, *Expert Opin. Drug Metab. Toxicol.*, 2009, **5**, 921.
4. M. Nishimura and S. Naito, *Drug Metab. Pharmacokinet.*, 2006, **21**, 357.
5. H. Komura and M. Iwaki, *Drug Metab. Rev.*, 2011, **43**, 476.
6. K. M. Knights, A. Rowland and J. O. Miners, *Br. J. Clin. Pharmacol.*, 2013, **76**, 587.
7. B. Kaye, J. L. Offerman, J. L. Reid, H. L. Elliott and W. S. Hillis, *Xenobiotica*, 1984, **14**, 935.
8. S. Diamond, J. Boer, T. P. Maduskuie, Jr., N. Falahatpisheh, Y. Li and S. Yeleswaram, *Drug Metab. Dispos.*, 2010, **38**, 1277.
9. D. M. Ziegler and C. H. Mitchell, *Arch. Biochem. Biophys.*, 1972, **150**, 116.
10. D. M. Ziegler, *Annu. Rev. Pharmacol. Toxicol.*, 1993, **33**, 179.
11. S. K. Krueger and D. E. Williams, *Pharmacol. Ther.*, 2005, **106**, 357.
12. M. P. Lawton, J. R. Cashman, T. Cresteil, C. T. Dolphin, A. A. Elfarra, R. N. Hines, E. Hodgson, T. Kimura, J. Ozols, I. R. Phillips, *et al.*, *Arch. Biochem. Biophys.*, 1994, **308**, 254.
13. M. P. Lawton and R. M. Philpot, *J. Biol. Chem.*, 1993, **268**, 5728.
14. A. Kubo, S. Itoh, K. Itoh and T. Kamataki, *Arch. Biochem. Biophys.*, 1997, **345**, 271.
15. L. L. Poulsen and D. M. Ziegler, *J. Biol. Chem.*, 1979, **254**, 6449.
16. N. B. Beaty and D. P. Ballou, *J. Biol. Chem.*, 1980, **255**, 3817.
17. K. C. Jones and D. P. Ballou, *J. Biol. Chem.*, 1986, **261**, 2553.
18. D. M. Ziegler, *Trends Pharmacol. Sci.*, 1990, **11**, 321.
19. A. Alfieri, E. Malito, R. Orru, M. W. Fraaije and A. Mattevi, *Proc. Natl. Acad. Sci. U. S. A.*, 2008, **105**, 6572.
20. B. A. Palfey and C. A. McDonald, *Arch. Biochem. Biophys.*, 2010, **493**, 26.
21. L. K. Siddens, S. K. Krueger, M. C. Henderson and D. E. Williams, *Biochem. Pharmacol.*, 2014, **89**, 141.

22. D. M. Ziegler, *Drug Metab. Rev.*, 1988, **19**, 1.
23. J. R. Cashman and J. Zhang, *Annu. Rev. Pharmacol. Toxicol.*, 2006, **46**, 65.
24. C. K. Yeung, D. H. Lang, K. E. Thummel and A. E. Rettie, *Drug Metab. Dispos.*, 2000, **28**, 1107.
25. V. Lattard, C. Longin-Sauvageon, S. K. Krueger, D. E. Williams and E. Benoit, *Biochem. Biophys. Res. Commun.*, 2002, **292**, 558.
26. S. K. Krueger, D. E. Williams, M. F. Yueh, S. R. Martin, R. N. Hines, J. L. Raucy, C. T. Dolphin, E. A. Shephard and I. R. Phillips, *Drug Metab. Rev.*, 2002, **34**, 523.
27. S. B. Koukouritaki, P. Simpson, C. K. Yeung, A. E. Rettie and R. N. Hines, *Pediatr. Res.*, 2002, **51**, 236.
28. M. Shimizu, S. Tomioka, N. Murayama and H. Yamazaki, *Drug Metab. Pharmacokinet.*, 2007, **22**, 61.
29. H. Yamazaki and M. Shimizu, *Curr. Drug Metab.*, 2007, **8**, 487.
30. C. T. Dolphin, A. Janmohamed, R. L. Smith, E. A. Shephard and I. R. Phillips, *Nat. Genet.*, 1997, **17**, 491.
31. J. R. Cashman, *Drug Discovery Today*, 2004, **9**, 574.
32. C. T. Dolphin, T. E. Cullingford, E. A. Shephard, R. L. Smith and I. R. Phillips, *Eur. J. Biochem.*, 1996, **235**, 683.
33. W. G. Lai, N. Farah, G. A. Moniz and Y. N. Wong, *Drug Metab. Dispos.*, 2011, **39**, 61.
34. J. Meng, D. Zhong, L. Li, Z. Yuan, H. Yuan, C. Xie, J. Zhou, C. Li, M. F. Gordeev, J. Liu and X. Chen, *Drug Metab. Dispos.*, 2015, **43**, 646.
35. N. J. Cherrington, J. G. Falls, R. L. Rose, K. M. Clements, R. M. Philpot, P. E. Levi and E. Hodgson, *J. Biochem. Mol. Toxicol.*, 1998, **12**, 205.
36. M. Yamazaki, M. Shimizu, Y. Uno and H. Yamazaki, *Biochem. Pharmacol.*, 2014, **90**, 159.
37. S. L. Ripp, K. Itagaki, R. M. Philpot and A. A. Elfarra, *Drug Metab. Dispos.*, 1999, **27**, 46.
38. A. Parkinson, in *Casarett and Doull's Toxicology, The Basic Science of Poisons*, ed. C. D. Klaassen, The McGraw-Hill Companies, Inc., 2001, ch. 6, pp. 133–224.
39. S. B. Park, P. Jacob, 3rd, N. L. Benowitz and J. R. Cashman, *Chem. Res. Toxicol.*, 1993, **6**, 880.
40. J. R. Cashman, S. B. Park, Z. C. Yang, C. B. Washington, D. Y. Gomez, K. M. Giacomini and C. M. Brett, *Drug Metab. Dispos.*, 1993, **21**, 587.
41. G. Ubeaud, C. D. Schiller, F. Hurbin, D. Jaeck and P. Coassolo, *Eur. J. Pharm. Sci.*, 1999, **8**, 255.
42. D. H. Lang and A. E. Rettie, *Br. J. Clin. Pharmacol.*, 2000, **50**, 311.
43. E. Stormer, I. Roots and J. Brockmoller, *Br. J. Clin. Pharmacol.*, 2000, **50**, 553.
44. T. Taniguchi-Takizawa, M. Shimizu, T. Kume and H. Yamazaki, *Drug Metab. Pharmacokinet.*, 2015, **30**, 64.
45. M. Tugnait, E. M. Hawes, G. McKay, A. E. Rettie, R. L. Haining and K. K. Midha, *Drug Metab. Dispos.*, 1997, **25**, 524.
46. B. J. Ring, J. Catlow, T. J. Lindsay, T. Gillespie, L. K. Roskos, B. J. Cerimele, S. P. Swanson, M. A. Hamman and S. A. Wrighton, *J. Pharmacol. Exp. Ther.*, 1996, **276**, 658.

47. B. J. Ring, S. A. Wrighton, S. L. Aldridge, K. Hansen, B. Haehner and L. A. Shipley, *Drug Metab. Dispos.*, 1999, **27**, 1099.
48. J. R. Cashman, *Curr. Drug Metab.*, 2000, **1**, 181.
49. T. Schulz-Utermoehl, M. Spear, C. R. Pollard, C. Pattison, H. Rollison, S. Sarda, M. Ward, N. Bushby, A. Jordan and M. Harrison, *Drug Metab. Dispos.*, 2010, **38**, 1688.
50. T. Shiraga, K. Yajima, T. Teragaki, K. Suzuki, T. Hashimoto, T. Iwatsubo, A. Miyashita and T. Usui, *Biol. Pharm. Bull.*, 2012, **35**, 413.
51. J. Joo, Z. Wu, B. Lee, J. C. Shon, T. Lee, I. K. Lee, T. Sim, K. H. Kim, N. D. Kim, S. H. Kim and K. H. Liu, *Biopharm. Drug Dispos.*, 2015, **36**, 163.
52. J. R. Cashman, *Expert Opin. Drug Metab. Toxicol.*, 2008, **4**, 1507.
53. J. R. Cashman, *Biochem. Biophys. Res. Commun.*, 2005, **338**, 599.
54. J. R. Cashman, *Chem. Res. Toxicol.*, 1995, **8**, 166.
55. M. B. Fisher, K. Yoon, M. L. Vaughn, T. J. Strelevitz and R. S. Foti, *Drug Metab. Dispos.*, 2002, **30**, 1087.
56. A. S. Kalgutkar, I. Gardner, R. S. Obach, C. L. Shaffer, E. Callegari, K. R. Henne, A. E. Mutlib, D. K. Dalvie, J. S. Lee, Y. Nakai, J. P. O'Donnell, J. Boer and S. P. Harriman, *Curr. Drug Metab.*, 2005, **6**, 161.
57. J. M. Hutzler and M. A. Cerny, in *Encyclopedia of Drug Metabolism and Interactions*, ed. A. V. Lyubimov, John Wiley & Sons, Inc., 1st edn, 2012, vol. 4, ch. 3, pp. 1–40.
58. C. J. Decker and D. R. Doerge, *Biochem. Pharmacol.*, 1992, **43**, 881.
59. M. C. Henderson, S. K. Krueger, J. F. Stevens and D. E. Williams, *Chem. Res. Toxicol.*, 2004, **17**, 633.
60. D. Mansuy and P. M. Dansette, *Arch. Biochem. Biophys.*, 2011, **507**, 174.
61. J. P. Driscoll, I. Aliagas, J. J. Harris, J. S. Halladay, S. Khatib-Shahidi, A. Deese, N. Segraves and S. C. Khojasteh-Bakht, *Chem. Res. Toxicol.*, 2010, **23**, 861.
62. C. Beedham, *Prog. Med. Chem.*, 1987, **24**, 85.
63. S. Kitamura, K. Sugihara and S. Ohta, *Drug Metab. Pharmacokinet.*, 2006, **21**, 83.
64. K. Sugihara, S. Kitamura and K. Tatsumi, *Drug Metab. Dispos.*, 1996, **24**, 199.
65. R. S. Obach, C. Prakash and A. M. Kamel, *Xenobiotica*, 2012, **42**, 1049.
66. J. K. Sodhi, S. Wong, D. S. Kirkpatrick, L. Liu, S. C. Khojasteh, C. E. Hop, J. T. Barr, J. P. Jones and J. S. Halladay, *Drug Metab. Dispos.*, 2015, **43**, 908.
67. Y. Moriwaki, T. Yamamoto, S. Takahashi, Z. Tsutsumi and T. Hada, *Histol. Histopathol.*, 2001, **16**, 745.
68. E. Garattini, M. Fratelli and M. Terao, *Cell. Mol. Life Sci.*, 2008, **65**, 1019.
69. E. Garattini and M. Terao, *Drug Metab. Rev.*, 2011, **43**, 374.
70. C. Coelho, M. Mahro, J. Trincao, A. T. Carvalho, M. J. Ramos, M. Terao, E. Garattini, S. Leimkuhler and M. J. Romao, *J. Biol. Chem.*, 2012, **287**, 40690.
71. S. Dastmalchi and M. Hamzeh-Mivehrod, *Daru, J. Fac. Pharm., Tehran Univ. Med. Sci.*, 2005, **13**, 82.
72. C. Dittrich, G. Greim, M. Borner, K. Weigang-Kohler, H. Huisman, A. Amelsberg, A. Ehret, J. Wanders, A. Hanauske and P. Fumoleau, *Eur. J. Cancer*, 2002, **38**, 1072.

73. D. Dalvie, C. Zhang, W. Chen, T. Smolarek, R. S. Obach and C. M. Loi, *Drug Metab. Dispos.*, 2010, **38**, 641.
74. X. Zhang, H. H. Liu, P. Weller, M. Zheng, W. Tao, J. Wang, G. Liao, M. Monshouwer and G. Peltz, *Pharmacogenomics J.*, 2011, **11**, 15.
75. T. Akabane, K. Tanaka, M. Irie, S. Terashita and T. Teramura, *Xenobiotica*, 2011, **41**, 372.
76. D. C. Pryde, D. Dalvie, Q. Hu, P. Jones, R. S. Obach and T. D. Tran, *J. Med. Chem.*, 2010, **53**, 8441.
77. E. Garattini and M. Terao, *Expert Opin. Drug Metab. Toxicol.*, 2012, **8**, 487.
78. E. Garattini and M. Terao, *Expert Opin. Drug Discovery*, 2013, **8**, 641.
79. J. M. Hutzler, R. S. Obach, D. Dalvie and M. A. Zientek, *Expert Opin. Drug Discovery*, 2013, **9**, 153.
80. S. Sanoh, Y. Tayama, K. Sugihara, S. Kitamura and S. Ohta, *Drug Metab. Pharmacokinet.*, 2015, **30**, 52.
81. J. F. Alfaro and J. P. Jones, *J. Org. Chem.*, 2008, **73**, 9469.
82. H. Peretz, M. S. Naamati, D. Levartovsky, A. Lagziel, E. Shani, I. Horn, H. Shalev and D. Landau, *Mol. Genet. Metab.*, 2007, **91**, 23.
83. K. Ichida, T. Matsumura, R. Sakuma, T. Hosoya and T. Nishino, *Biochem. Biophys. Res. Commun.*, 2001, **282**, 1194.
84. E. B. Skibo, J. H. Gilchrist and C. H. Lee, *Biochemistry*, 1987, **26**, 3032.
85. R. Sharma, T. J. Strelevitz, H. Gao, A. J. Clark, K. Schildknegt, R. S. Obach, S. L. Ripp, D. K. Spracklin, L. M. Tremaine and A. D. Vaz, *Drug Metab. Dispos.*, 2012, **40**, 625.
86. F. O'Hara, A. C. Burns, M. R. Collins, D. Dalvie, M. A. Ornelas, A. D. Vaz, Y. Fujiwara and P. S. Baran, *J. Med. Chem.*, 2014, **57**, 1616.
87. T. J. Strelevitz, C. C. Orozco and R. S. Obach, *Drug Metab. Dispos.*, 2012, **40**, 1441.
88. B. R. Baer, L. C. Wienkers and D. A. Rock, *Chem. Res. Toxicol.*, 2007, **20**, 954.
89. R. Nirogi, V. Kandikere, R. C. Palacharla, G. Bhyrapuneni, V. B. Kanamarlapudi, R. K. Ponnamaneni and A. K. Manoharan, *Xenobiotica*, 2014, **44**, 197.
90. P. J. Loida and S. G. Sligar, *Biochemistry*, 1993, **32**, 11530.
91. J. M. Hutzler, L. C. Wienkers, J. L. Wahlstrom, T. J. Carlson and T. S. Tracy, *Arch. Biochem. Biophys.*, 2003, **410**, 16.
92. A. B. Renwick, S. E. Ball, J. M. Tredger, R. J. Price, D. G. Walters, J. Kao, J. A. Scatina and B. G. Lake, *Xenobiotica*, 2002, **32**, 849.
93. R. S. Obach, P. Huynh, M. C. Allen and C. Beedham, *J. Clin. Pharmacol.*, 2004, **44**, 7.
94. J. T. Barr and J. P. Jones, *Drug Metab. Dispos.*, 2011, **39**, 2381.
95. J. T. Barr and J. P. Jones, *Drug Metab. Dispos.*, 2013, **41**, 24.
96. J. T. Barr, J. P. Jones, N. H. Oberlies and M. F. Paine, *Drug Metab. Dispos.*, 2015, **43**, 34.
97. C. Beedham, S. E. Bruce, D. J. Critchley, Y. al-Tayib and D. J. Rance, *Eur. J. Drug Metab. Pharmacokinet.*, 1987, **12**, 307.
98. D. A. Smith and R. S. Obach, *Chem. Res. Toxicol.*, 2009, **22**, 267.

99. H. Gao, A. Jacobs, R. E. White, B. P. Booth and R. S. Obach, *AAPS J.*, 2013, **15**, 970.

100. J. R. Infante, T. Rugg, M. Gordon, I. Rooney, L. Rosen, K. Zeh, R. Liu, H. A. Burris and R. K. Ramanathan, *Invest. New Drugs*, 2013, **31**, 363.

101. K. V. Choughule, J. T. Barr and J. P. Jones, *Drug Metab. Dispos.*, 2013, **41**, 1852.

102. J. M. Hutzler, M. A. Cerny, Y. S. Yang, C. Asher, D. Wong, K. Frederick and K. Gilpin, *Drug Metab. Dispos.*, 2014, **42**, 1751.

103. S. Kitamura, K. Sugihara, K. Nakatani, S. Ohta, T. Ohhara, S. Ninomiya, C. E. Green and C. A. Tyson, *IUBMB Life*, 1999, **48**, 607.

104. H. S. Al-Salmy, *IUBMB Life*, 2001, **51**, 249.

105. C. Fu, L. Di, X. Han, C. Soderstrom, M. Snyder, M. D. Troutman, R. S. Obach and H. Zhang, *Drug Metab. Dispos.*, 2013, **41**, 1797.

106. J. A. Duley, O. Harris and R. S. Holmes, *Alcohol.: Clin. Exp. Res.*, 1985, **9**, 263.

107. J. M. Hutzler, Y. S. Yang, C. Brown, S. Heyward and T. Moeller, *Drug Metab. Dispos.*, 2014, **42**, 1090.

108. Y. Tayama, K. Sugihara, S. Sanoh, K. Miyake, S. Morita, S. Kitamura and S. Ohta, *Drug Metab. Pharmacokinet.*, 2011, **26**, 94.

109. Y. Tayama, K. Sugihara, S. Sanoh, K. Miyake, S. Kitamura and S. Ohta, *Drug Metab. Pharmacokinet.*, 2012, **27**, 543.

110. P. Kestell, I. C. Dunlop, M. R. McCrystal, B. D. Evans, J. W. Paxton, R. S. Gamage and B. C. Baguley, *Cancer Chemother. Pharmacol.*, 1999, **44**, 45.

111. T. Hartmann, M. Terao, E. Garattini, C. Teutloff, J. F. Alfaro, J. P. Jones and S. Leimkuhler, *Drug Metab. Dispos.*, 2012, **40**, 856.

112. M. A. Smith, A. M. Marinaki, M. Arenas, M. Shobowale-Bakre, C. M. Lewis, A. Ansari, J. Duley and J. D. Sanderson, *Aliment. Pharmacol. Ther.*, 2009, **30**, 375.

113. J. Ramirez, T. W. Kim, W. Liu, J. L. Myers, S. Mirkov, K. Owzar, D. Watson, F. Mulkey, E. R. Gamazon, W. Stock, S. Undevia, F. Innocenti and M. J. Ratain, *Pharmacogenet. Genomics*, 2014, **24**, 129.

114. M. Zientek, Y. Jiang, K. Youdim and R. S. Obach, *Drug Metab. Dispos.*, 2010, **38**, 1322.

115. T. Akabane, N. Gerst, Y. Naritomi, J. N. Masters and K. Tamura, *Drug Metab. Pharmacokinet.*, 2012, **27**, 181.

116. J. M. Hutzler, Y. S. Yang, D. Albaugh, C. L. Fullenwider, J. Schmenk and M. B. Fisher, *Drug Metab. Dispos.*, 2012, **40**, 267.

117. M. A. Zientek and K. Youdim, *Drug Metab. Dispos.*, 2015, **43**, 163.

118. T. Akabane, N. Gerst, J. N. Masters and K. Tamura, *Xenobiotica*, 2012, **42**, 863.

119. N. Manevski, K. K. Balavenkatraman, B. Bertschi, P. Swart, M. Walles, G. Camenisch, H. Schiller, O. Kretz, B. Ling, R. Wettstein, D. J. Schaefer, F. Pognan, A. Wolf and K. Litherland, *Drug Metab. Dispos.*, 2014, **42**, 2049.

120. J. P. Jones and K. R. Korzekwa, *Mol. Pharm.*, 2013, **10**, 1262.

121. N. A. Hosea, W. T. Collard, S. Cole, T. S. Maurer, R. X. Fang, H. Jones, S. M. Kakar, Y. Nakai, B. J. Smith, R. Webster and K. Beaumont, *J. Clin. Pharmacol.*, 2009, **49**, 513.

122. T. Deguchi, N. Watanabe, A. Kurihara, K. Igeta, H. Ikenaga, K. Fusegawa, N. Suzuki, S. Murata, M. Hirouchi, Y. Furuta, M. Iwasaki, O. Okazaki and T. Izumi, *Drug Metab. Dispos.*, 2011, **39**, 820.

123. W. J. Richter, K. O. Alt, W. Dieterle, J. W. Faigle, H. P. Kriemler, H. Mory and T. Winkler, *Helv. Chim. Acta*, 1975, **58**, 2512.

124. A. Radominska-Pandya, P. J. Czernik, J. M. Little, E. Battaglia and P. I. Mackenzie, *Drug Metab. Rev.*, 1999, **31**, 817.

125. W. Lilienblum, B. S. Bock-Hennig and K. W. Bock, *Mol. Pharmacol.*, 1985, **27**, 451.

126. J. A. Williams, R. Hyland, B. C. Jones, D. A. Smith, S. Hurst, T. C. Goosen, V. Peterkin, J. R. Koup and S. E. Ball, *Drug Metab. Dispos.*, 2004, **32**, 1201.

127. L. C. Wienkers and T. G. Heath, *Nat. Rev. Drug Discovery*, 2005, **4**, 825.

128. J. C. Stingl, H. Bartels, R. Viviani, M. L. Lehmann and J. Brockmoller, *Pharmacol. Ther.*, 2014, **141**, 92.

129. K. W. Bock, W. Lilienblum, G. Fischer, G. Schirmer and B. S. Bock-Henning, *Arch. Toxicol.*, 1987, **60**, 22.

130. G. J. Mulder, *Annu. Rev. Pharmacol. Toxicol.*, 1992, **32**, 25.

131. R. H. Tukey and C. P. Strassburg, *Annu. Rev. Pharmacol. Toxicol.*, 2000, **40**, 581.

132. P. I. Mackenzie, K. W. Bock, B. Burchell, C. Guillemette, S. Ikushiro, T. Iyanagi, J. O. Miners, I. S. Owens and D. W. Nebert, *Pharmacogenet. Genomics*, 2005, **15**, 677.

133. S. Ichikawa, H. Sakiyama, G. Suzuki, K. I. Hidari and Y. Hirabayashi, *Proc. Natl. Acad. Sci. U. S. A.*, 1996, **93**, 12654.

134. P. I. MacKenzie, A. Rogers, D. J. Elliot, N. Chau, J. A. Hulin, J. O. Miners and R. Meech, *Mol. Pharmacol.*, 2011, **79**, 472.

135. P. I. Mackenzie, A. Rogers, J. Treloar, B. R. Jorgensen, J. O. Miners and R. Meech, *J. Biol. Chem.*, 2008, **283**, 36205.

136. USFDA, Guidance for Industry: Drug Interaction Studies-Study Design, Data Analysis, Implications for Dosing, and Label Recommendations, 2012.

137. EMEA, European Medicines Agency (EMA) Guideline on the Investigation of Drug Interactions, 2013.

138. K. W. Bock and C. Kohle, *Biochem. Pharmacol.*, 2009, **77**, 1458.

139. J. Magdalou, S. Fournel-Gigleux and M. Ouzzine, *Drug Metab. Rev.*, 2010, **42**, 159.

140. A. Radominska-Pandya, S. M. Bratton, M. R. Redinbo and M. J. Miley, *Drug Metab. Rev.*, 2010, **42**, 133.

141. M. J. Miley, A. K. Zielinska, J. E. Keenan, S. M. Bratton, A. Radominska-Pandya and M. R. Redinbo, *J. Mol. Biol.*, 2007, **369**, 498.

142. Y. Xiong, A. S. Patana, M. J. Miley, A. K. Zielinska, S. M. Bratton, G. P. Miller, A. Goldman, M. Finel, M. R. Redinbo and A. Radominska-Pandya, *Drug Metab. Dispos.*, 2008, **36**, 517.

143. H. Yin, G. Bennett and J. P. Jones, *Chem.-Biol. Interact.*, 1994, **90**, 47.

144. L. Z. Benet, H. Spahn-Langguth, S. Iwakawa, C. Volland, T. Mizuma, S. Mayer, E. Mutschler and E. T. Lin, *Life Sci.*, 1993, **53**, PL141.

145. U. A. Boelsterli, *Curr. Drug Metab.*, 2002, **3**, 439.
146. J. K. Ritter, *Chem.-Biol. Interact.*, 2000, **129**, 171.
147. M. J. Bailey and R. G. Dickinson, *Chem.-Biol. Interact.*, 2003, **145**, 117.
148. C. Skonberg, J. Olsen, K. G. Madsen, S. H. Hansen and M. P. Grillo, *Expert Opin. Drug Metab. Toxicol.*, 2008, **4**, 425.
149. G. S. Walker, J. Atherton, J. Bauman, C. Kohl, W. Lam, M. Reily, Z. Lou and A. Mutlib, *Chem. Res. Toxicol.*, 2007, **20**, 876.
150. T. Ebner, G. Heinzel, A. Prox, K. Beschke and H. Wachsmuth, *Drug Metab. Dispos.*, 1999, **27**, 1143.
151. Q. H. Gong, J. W. Cho, T. Huang, C. Potter, N. Gholami, N. K. Basu, S. Kubota, S. Carvalho, M. W. Pennington, I. S. Owens and N. C. Popescu, *Pharmacogenetics*, 2001, **11**, 357.
152. P. I. Mackenzie, P. A. Gregory, D. A. Gardner-Stephen, R. H. Lewinsky, B. R. Jorgensen, T. Nishiyama, W. Xie and A. Radominska-Pandya, *Curr. Drug Metab.*, 2003, **4**, 249.
153. P. Bernard, H. Goudonnet, Y. Artur, B. Desvergne and W. Wahli, *Mol. Pharmacol.*, 1999, **56**, 526.
154. D. A. Gardner-Stephen and P. I. Mackenzie, *Drug Metab. Dispos.*, 2007, **35**, 116.
155. Y. Ishii, A. J. Hansen and P. I. Mackenzie, *Mol. Pharmacol.*, 2000, **57**, 940.
156. A. J. Hansen, Y. H. Lee, E. Sterneck, F. J. Gonzalez and P. I. Mackenzie, *Mol. Pharmacol.*, 1998, **53**, 1027.
157. P. A. Gregory and P. I. Mackenzie, *Mol. Pharmacol.*, 2002, **62**, 154.
158. W. Xie, M. F. Yeuh, A. Radominska-Pandya, S. P. Saini, Y. Negishi, B. S. Bottroff, G. Y. Cabrera, R. H. Tukey and R. M. Evans, *Proc. Natl. Acad. Sci. U. S. A.*, 2003, **100**, 4150.
159. J. Sugatani, H. Kojima, A. Ueda, S. Kakizaki, K. Yoshinari, Q. H. Gong, I. S. Owens, M. Negishi and T. Sueyoshi, *Hepatology*, 2001, **33**, 1232.
160. O. Barbier, I. P. Torra, A. Sirvent, T. Claudel, C. Blanquart, D. Duran-Sandoval, F. Kuipers, V. Kosykh, J. C. Fruchart and B. Staels, *Gastroenterology*, 2003, **124**, 1926.
161. M. Verreault, K. Senekeo-Effenberger, J. Trottier, J. A. Bonzo, J. Belanger, J. Kaeding, B. Staels, P. Caron, R. H. Tukey and O. Barbier, *Hepatology*, 2006, **44**, 368.
162. M. F. Yueh, Y. H. Huang, A. Hiller, S. Chen, N. Nguyen and R. H. Tukey, *J. Biol. Chem.*, 2003, **278**, 15001.
163. S. Ohno and S. Nakajin, *Drug Metab. Dispos.*, 2009, **37**, 32.
164. M. H. Court, X. Zhang, X. Ding, K. K. Yee, L. M. Hesse and M. Finel, *Xenobiotica*, 2012, **42**, 266.
165. K. M. Knights and J. O. Miners, *Drug Metab. Rev.*, 2010, **42**, 63.
166. A. Rowland, J. O. Miners and P. I. Mackenzie, *Int. J. Biochem. Cell Biol.*, 2013, **45**, 1121.
167. J. K. Fallon, D. E. Harbourt, S. H. Maleki, F. K. Kessler, J. K. Ritter and P. C. Smith, *Drug Metab. Lett.*, 2008, **2**, 210.
168. J. K. Fallon, H. Neubert, T. Goosen and P. C. Smith, *Drug Metab. Dispos.*, 2013, **41**, 2076.

169. D. E. Harbourt, J. K. Fallon, S. Ito, T. Baba, J. K. Ritter, G. L. Glish and P. C. Smith, *Anal. Chem.*, 2012, **84**, 98.

170. A. M. Milne, B. Burchell and M. W. Coughtrie, *Drug Metab. Dispos.*, 2011, **39**, 2258.

171. S. Ohtsuki, O. Schaefer, H. Kawakami, T. Inoue, S. Liehner, A. Saito, N. Ishiguro, W. Kishimoto, E. Ludwig-Schwellinger, T. Ebner and T. Terasaki, *Drug Metab. Dispos.*, 2012, **40**, 83.

172. Y. Sato, M. Nagata, A. Kawamura, A. Miyashita and T. Usui, *Xenobiotica*, 2012, **42**, 823.

173. C. Sridar, I. Hanna and P. F. Hollenberg, *Xenobiotica*, 2013, **43**, 336.

174. O. Schaefer, S. Ohtsuki, H. Kawakami, T. Inoue, S. Liehner, A. Saito, A. Sakamoto, N. Ishiguro, T. Matsumaru, T. Terasaki and T. Ebner, *Drug Metab. Dispos.*, 2012, **40**, 93.

175. B. Achour, M. R. Russell, J. Barber and A. Rostami-Hodjegan, *Drug Metab. Dispos.*, 2014, **42**, 500.

176. S. Boase and J. O. Miners, *Br. J. Clin. Pharmacol.*, 2002, **54**, 493.

177. M. H. Court, in *Optimization in Drug Discovery*, ed. Z. Yan and G. W. Caldwell, Humana Press Inc., Totowa, N. J., 2004, ch. 12, pp. 185–202.

178. J. J. Engtrakul, R. S. Foti, T. J. Strelevitz and M. B. Fisher, *Drug Metab. Dispos.*, 2005, **33**, 1621.

179. N. Manevski, P. S. Moreolo, J. Yli-Kauhaluoma and M. Finel, *Drug Metab. Dispos.*, 2011, **39**, 2117.

180. A. E. Mutlib, T. C. Goosen, J. N. Bauman, J. A. Williams, S. Kulkarni and S. Kostrubsky, *Chem. Res. Toxicol.*, 2006, **19**, 701.

181. A. Rowland, K. M. Knights, P. I. Mackenzie and J. O. Miners, *Drug Metab. Dispos.*, 2008, **36**, 1056.

182. A. Rowland, K. M. Knights, P. I. Mackenzie and J. O. Miners, *Drug Metab. Dispos.*, 2009, **37**, 1395.

183. R. L. Walsky, J. N. Bauman, K. Bourcier, G. Giddens, K. Lapham, A. Negahban, T. F. Ryder, R. S. Obach, R. Hyland and T. C. Goosen, *Drug Metab. Dispos.*, 2012, **40**, 1051.

184. M. B. Fisher, M. F. Paine, T. J. Strelevitz and S. A. Wrighton, *Drug Metab. Rev.*, 2001, **33**, 273.

185. P. J. Kilford, R. Stringer, B. Sohal, J. B. Houston and A. Galetin, *Drug Metab. Dispos.*, 2009, **37**, 82.

186. N. K. Basu, M. Kovarova, A. Garza, S. Kubota, T. Saha, P. S. Mitra, R. Banerjee, J. Rivera and I. S. Owens, *Proc. Natl. Acad. Sci. U. S. A.*, 2005, **102**, 6285.

187. J. N. Bauman, T. C. Goosen, M. Tugnait, V. Peterkin, S. I. Hurst, L. C. Menning, M. Milad, M. H. Court and J. A. Williams, *Drug Metab. Dispos.*, 2005, **33**, 1349.

188. S. Kaivosaari, P. Toivonen, O. Aitio, J. Sipila, M. Koskinen, J. S. Salonen and M. Finel, *Drug Metab. Dispos.*, 2008, **36**, 1529.

189. L. Oleson and M. H. Court, *J. Pharm. Pharmacol.*, 2008, **60**, 1175.

190. Z. Yan and G. W. Caldwell, *Eur. J. Drug Metab. Pharmacokinet.*, 2003, **28**, 223.

191. N. Manevski, J. Yli-Kauhaluoma and M. Finel, *Drug Metab. Dispos.*, 2012, **40**, 2192.
192. N. Manevski, J. Troberg, P. Svaluto-Moreolo, K. Dziedzic, J. Yli-Kauhaluoma and M. Finel, *PloS One*, 2013, **8**, e54767.
193. T. Shiraga, K. Yajima, K. Suzuki, K. Suzuki, T. Hashimoto, T. Iwatsubo, A. Miyashita and T. Usui, *Drug Metab. Dispos.*, 2012, **40**, 276.
194. D. Dalvie, P. Kang, M. Zientek, C. Xiang, S. Zhou and R. S. Obach, *Chem. Res. Toxicol.*, 2008, **21**, 2260.
195. D. Takizawa, H. Hiraoka, F. Goto, K. Yamamoto and R. Horiuchi, *Anesthesiology*, 2005, **102**, 327.
196. K. L. Gill, J. B. Houston and A. Galetin, *Drug Metab. Dispos.*, 2012, **40**, 825.
197. A. Rowland, D. J. Elliot, K. M. Knights, P. I. Mackenzie and J. O. Miners, *Drug Metab. Dispos.*, 2008, **36**, 870.
198. A. Rowland, P. Gaganis, D. J. Elliot, P. I. Mackenzie, K. M. Knights and J. O. Miners, *J. Pharmacol. Exp. Ther.*, 2007, **321**, 137.
199. M. H. Court, *Methods Enzymol.*, 2005, **400**, 104.
200. M. G. Soars, D. M. Petullo, J. A. Eckstein, S. C. Kasper and S. A. Wrighton, *Drug Metab. Dispos.*, 2004, **32**, 140.
201. J. Lepine, O. Bernard, M. Plante, B. Tetu, G. Pelletier, F. Labrie, A. Belanger and C. Guillemette, *J. Clin. Endocrinol. Metab.*, 2004, **89**, 5222.
202. K. Itäaho, P. I. Mackenzie, S. Ikushiro, J. O. Miners and M. Finel, *Drug Metab. Dispos.*, 2008, **36**, 2307.
203. V. Uchaipichat, L. K. Winner, P. I. Mackenzie, D. J. Elliot, J. A. Williams and J. O. Miners, *Br. J. Clin. Pharmacol.*, 2006, **61**, 427.
204. S. Krishnaswamy, Q. Hao, L. L. Von Moltke, D. J. Greenblatt and M. H. Court, *Drug Metab. Dispos.*, 2004, **32**, 862.
205. M. H. Court, S. Krishnaswamy, Q. Hao, S. X. Duan, C. J. Patten, L. L. Von Moltke and D. J. Greenblatt, *Drug Metab. Dispos.*, 2003, **31**, 1125.
206. J. O. Miners, P. I. Mackenzie and K. M. Knights, *Drug Metab. Rev.*, 2010, **42**, 196.
207. Y. Liu, J. Ramirez, L. House and M. J. Ratain, *Drug Metab. Dispos.*, 2010, **38**, 32.
208. D. Zhang, T. J. Chando, D. W. Everett, C. J. Patten, S. S. Dehal and W. G. Humphreys, *Drug Metab. Dispos.*, 2005, **33**, 1729.
209. V. Uchaipichat, P. I. Mackenzie, D. J. Elliot and J. O. Miners, *Drug Metab. Dispos.*, 2006, **34**, 449.
210. C. P. Strassburg, M. P. Manns and R. H. Tukey, *J. Biol. Chem.*, 1998, **273**, 8719.
211. D. Wiener, D. R. Doerge, J. L. Fang, P. Upadhyaya and P. Lazarus, *Drug Metab. Dispos.*, 2004, **32**, 72.
212. M. D. Green, W. P. Bishop and T. R. Tephly, *Drug Metab. Dispos.*, 1995, **23**, 299.
213. P. Gaganis, J. O. Miners and K. M. Knights, *Biochem. Pharmacol.*, 2007, **73**, 1683.
214. Y. Mano, T. Usui and H. Kamimura, *Biopharm. Drug Dispos.*, 2006, **27**, 1.
215. C. L. Crespi, in *Advances in Drug Research*, ed. U. A. Meyer and B. Testa, Academic Press, New York, 1995, pp. 179–235.

216. N. J. Proctor, G. T. Tucker and A. Rostami-Hodjegan, *Xenobiotica*, 2004, **34**, 151.
217. C. R. Gibson, P. Lu, C. Maciolek, C. Wudarski, Z. Barter, K. Rowland-Yeo, M. Stroh, E. Lai and D. A. Nicoll-Griffith, *Xenobiotica*, 2013, **43**, 1027.
218. Y. Kato, M. Nakajima, S. Oda, T. Fukami and T. Yokoi, *Drug Metab. Dispos.*, 2012, **40**, 240.
219. J. O. Miners, K. M. Knights, J. B. Houston and P. I. Mackenzie, *Biochem. Pharmacol.*, 2006, **71**, 1531.
220. M. Mistry and J. B. Houston, *Drug Metab. Dispos.*, 1987, **15**, 710.
221. R. J. Riley, D. F. McGinnity and R. P. Austin, *Drug Metab. Dispos.*, 2005, **33**, 1304.
222. W. S. Al-Jahdari, K. Yamamoto, H. Hiraoka, K. Nakamura, F. Goto and R. Horiuchi, *Eur. J. Clin. Pharmacol.*, 2006, **62**, 527.
223. H. E. Cubitt, J. B. Houston and A. Galetin, *Pharm. Res.*, 2009, **26**, 1073.
224. D. Hallifax and J. B. Houston, *Drug Metab. Dispos.*, 2006, **34**, 724.
225. M. G. Soars, B. Burchell and R. J. Riley, *J. Pharmacol. Exp. Ther.*, 2002, **301**, 382.
226. A. Alonin, M. Finel and R. Kostiainen, *Biochem. Pharmacol.*, 2008, **76**, 763.
227. S. Chouinard, M. Tessier, G. Vernouillet, S. Gauthier, F. Labrie, O. Barbier and A. Belanger, *Mol. Pharmacol.*, 2006, **69**, 908.
228. N. Kasai, T. Sakaki, R. Shinkyo, S. Ikushiro, T. Iyanagi, M. Ohta and K. Inouye, *Drug Metab. Dispos.*, 2005, **33**, 102.
229. T. Murai, N. Samata, H. Iwabuchi and T. Ikeda, *Drug Metab. Dispos.*, 2006, **34**, 1102.
230. K. Itaaho, M. H. Court, P. Kostiainen, A. Radominska-Pandya and M. Finel, *Drug Metab. Dispos.*, 2009, **37**, 768.
231. M. H. Court, S. X. Duan, C. Guillemette, K. Journault, S. Krishnaswamy, L. L. Von Moltke and D. J. Greenblatt, *Drug Metab. Dispos.*, 2002, **30**, 1257.
232. S. Oechsler and G. Skopp, *Int. J. Legal Med.*, 2010, **124**, 187.
233. M. Ito, K. Yamamoto, H. Sato, Y. Fujiyama and T. Bamba, *Eur. J. Clin. Pharmacol.*, 2001, **56**, 893.
234. Y. Watanabe, M. Nakajima and T. Yokoi, *Drug Metab. Dispos.*, 2002, **30**, 1462.
235. K. Zucker, A. Tsaroucha, L. Olson, V. Esquenazi, A. Tzakis and J. Miller, *Ther. Drug Monit.*, 1999, **21**, 35.
236. T. Sten, M. Finel, B. Ask, A. Rane and L. Ekstrom, *Steroids*, 2009, **74**, 971.

CHAPTER 6

Metabolite Profiling

JAMES M. SCHMIDT*[a]

[a]ABC Laboratories, Inc., 4780 Discovery Drive, Columbia, MO 65201, USA
*E-mail: schmidtj@abclabs.com

6.1   Introduction

If a scientist can have a favorite quote on metabolite profiling, this would be the author's:

> *"In order to understand the actions of drugs it is an absolute necessity to have knowledge of the transformations they undergo in the body...we must not judge drugs according to the form and amount administered, but rather according to the form and amount which actually is eliciting the action."*[1]

From where did this sage advice arise? Another recent book on drug metabolism or metabolite profiling? No. A regulatory guidance document? No. In fact, this statement was written more than 150 years ago—in 1859—by Rudolph Buchheim (1820–79), a pioneer in experimental pharmacology.

The quote appeals to the author for several reasons; first, as someone interested in the history of chemistry and science; second, and more importantly, because it lays out as elegantly as any modern statement the very mission and importance of drug metabolism, pharmacokinetics (PK, "amount"), and pharmacology ("action"), especially the role of metabolite profiling and identification ("transformations" and "form").

Although the basic mission of metabolite profiling, as described by Buchheim, has not changed over the past 150 years, the strategies and tools that

RSC Drug Discovery Series No. 49
New Horizons in Predictive Drug Metabolism and Pharmacokinetics
Edited by Alan G. E. Wilson
© The Royal Society of Chemistry 2016
Published by the Royal Society of Chemistry, www.rsc.org

are employed have improved significantly. When and how those tools and strategies are used depends very much on the advancement of a new chemical entity through the continuum of thought experiment, synthesis, lead optimization, lead selection, development, and final product, and the iterations that are necessarily associated with the effort of drug discovery and development. Implementation of Buchheim's advice in the past quarter century has paid off in improved rates of drug attrition.

Metabolite profiling is an increasingly interdisciplinary field: minimally, it encompasses the intersection of experimental biology (with the *in vitro* and *in vivo* experiments that investigate drug metabolism, generally) and analytical chemistry; apart from that, it includes information science, organic synthesis, toxicology, regulatory and business considerations, and much more.

While it is hard to capture all of these aspects in a single chapter, the author has attempted to highlight strategies and tools of both general and special interest. Likewise, owing to the interdisciplinary nature of the subject, the reader will find that other chapters in this book will also provide new and interesting insights into metabolite profiling, and the author has endeavored to avoid significant overlap with the other subject matter.

6.2   Rationale

6.2.1   Attrition, Invention, and Diligence

The most practical reason for pursuing metabolite profiling efforts as early and as diligently as possible is attrition in the drug discovery process, in terms of rates, reasons for attrition, and in what phase of development attrition occurs. Industry "benchmarking" reports in the literature[2] demonstrate that, in 1991, 40% of attrition in drug development could be attributed to poor PK behavior. Owing, in no small part, to an increased focus on metabolite profiling in drug design, by 2000 poor PK had dropped to <10%. However, between those two periods, attrition due to safety issues rose from about 20% in 1991 to over 30% in 2000. Furthermore, factors that can presumably be controlled in preclinical evaluation (PK, toxicology, and formulation) that accounted for about 60% of the failures in 1991 were still responsible for nearly 50% of failures in 2000.

Readers are directed to an exceptional, unprecedented, and recent (2014) study[3] that provided a very transparent review of drug attrition in a corporate portfolio between 2005 and 2010. Poor PK behavior represented as little as 3% of drug failures in preclinical evaluation and safety represented >80% (efficacy and "strategy" each represented <10%), which would seem to point (if even indirectly) to the benefits of early metabolite profiling. That said, problems with PK actually increased from preclinical development to Phase I, and lack of efficacy increased to nearly 90% in Phase III. As will be demonstrated throughout this chapter, metabolite profiling can support troubleshooting of all aspects of drug attrition, and should not be limited simply to improving PK behavior as it was in the first part of the past two decades.

Early metabolite profiling and identification efforts can also be beneficial to intellectual property protection.[4] The worst cases are those in which an enterprise failed to file intellectual property on a drug metabolite that ultimately proved more active than its parent compound and lost protection on their invention. Likewise, the employment of the so-called "metabolite defense"[5] in the courts (with mixed results) further illuminates the importance of metabolite profiling in business decision-making. At a minimum, early understanding of the metabolism of a lead drug candidate provides drug makers with the necessary ammunition to determine whether metabolites merit intellectual property protection.

Another important rationale—and one the author has had the privilege of being involved with—and closely tied to the intellectual property considerations described above, is the due diligence process[6,7] that is necessarily associated with the process of acquisition of intellectual property and/or drug portfolios. While limited funding may result in a temptation to delay or minimize metabolite profiling efforts, that appeal should go unheeded. Scientific due diligence is every bit as essential as financial analysis in pharmaceutical and biotech acquisitions, and recent reviews and/or white papers confirm the importance of questions about metabolites and metabolite pathways as part of the process to minimize poor choices in investment decisions; likewise, groups should be prepared to answer these questions to improve the chances for desired investment.

6.2.2 Not Just a Good Idea

The aphorism applied to highway speed limits and (cheekily) applied to gravity—"It's Not Just a Good Idea. It's the Law."—can also be applied to metabolite profiling. Guidance documents, including—but not limited to—those from the US Food and Drug Administration (FDA)[8] and the European Medicines Agency (EMA)/ICH,[9] have formalized the regulatory framework and decision-making of metabolite profiling. The FDA guidance, properly published as "Safety Testing of Drug Metabolites," but colloquially known in the industry as "Metabolites in Safety Testing" (MIST), resulted in a significant amount of commentary before and after its publication.[10,11]

While one still sees commentary on the differences between the FDA and the EME/ICH guidance documents, specifically, the difference and/or debate of the merits of the threshold for a major metabolite: >10% of area under the concentration–time curve (AUC) of the parent drug at steady-state according to the FDA *versus* >10% of drug-related exposure according to the ICH, the debate has generally been settled by the FDA's subsequent adoption[12] of the ICH M3 threshold in 2010. Indeed, one report[13] concluded that while the guidelines seemed "to necessitate a paradigm shift to more thorough metabolite analysis during early development," their evaluation of best industry practices led to the conclusion that "the principles of the guidelines have always largely underpinned metabolism studies within the pharmaceutical industry."

This suggests that the most important consideration is a project-by-project assessment of metabolite profiling data and employment of appropriate analytical tools to make the best safety assessments.

6.2.3   Knowledge is Power

Apart from the important, more practical, aspects discussed above, metabolite profiling is a very intellectually satisfying exercise, owing in no small part to its interdisciplinary nature. The "detective work" of metabolite profiling contributes to medicinal chemistry, enzymology, pharmacology, toxicology, mechanistic chemistry, analytical chemistry, and many other fields. Among the more satisfying and exciting results of metabolite profiling is the discovery of novel and/or unexpected metabolites. Case studies are included throughout the chapter to illustrate particular points, but a few recent case studies of novel metabolites and/or pathways are presented below as evidence of important contributions to the scientific literature:

A report[14] on a proprietary compound detailed multiple biotransformations, among them cytochrome P450 (CYP)-mediated oxidations of its heterocycle pyrrolotriazine group. Two major metabolites resulted from the oxidation; one exhibited conventional hydroxylation of the heterocycle, but mass spectrometry (MS) and nuclear magnetic resonance (NMR) analyses confirmed that another metabolite exhibited an unusual rearrangement to form a hydroxypyridotriazine group. The team employed an isotopically labelled (deuterated and tritiated) parent compound in liver microsome experiments to examine the mechanism of the transformation.

The considerations of circulating metabolites in drug safety, as briefly described in Section 6.1.1, received attention in another recent report[15] in which the authors quantitatively examined the role of circulating metabolites in inhibitory drug–drug interactions (DDIs) *in vivo*.

Finally, getting back to "detective work" (literally and figuratively): metabolite profiling efforts—especially when combined with enzymology and/or enzymatics—can solve long-standing mysteries on metabolite pathways. One team recently (2015)[16] examined the mystery of which enzyme(s) are responsible for the formation of 3-hydroxydesloratadine, the major active human metabolite of loratadine, owing to the seeming inability of *in vitro* systems to generate this metabolite. In their study, they demonstrated that cryopreserved human hepatocytes form 3-hydroxydesloratadine and its corresponding O-glucuronide. Detailed mechanistic studies demonstrated for the first time that desloratadine glucuronidation by UGT2B10 followed by CYP2C8 oxidation and a deconjugation event are responsible for the formation of 3-hydroxydesloratadine.

6.3   Software-Assisted Metabolite Profiling and Prediction

Few aspects of metabolite profiling get to the heart of the mission of this volume—*New Horizons in Predictive Drug Metabolism and Pharmacokinetics*—more than software-assisted metabolite prediction. These *in silico* tools encompass a variety of research needs and outputs: *a priori* metabolite prediction, drug properties (virtual screening), DDIs (inhibition and induction), drug transport, and physiologically based PK (PBPK) models that predict the consequences of one or more of the aspects noted above.

Likewise, these tools have an equal variety of intended users in the drug discovery and development process: medicinal chemists looking to guide chemical synthesis towards desired properties; traditional drug metabolism scientists merging experimental biology (enzymology) and bio-analytical chemistry (metabolite characterization) data; and those responsible for preclinical and clinical development.

In terms of metabolite prediction, the tools may be further segmented: prediction of the identity of expected metabolites; predicted rate of metabolism; characterization of enzymes involved in metabolism; integration of predicted metabolite datasets with high-resolution MS data; and other outcomes.

It is a paradox that the time- and labor-intensive efforts needed for the elucidation of metabolite structures and pathways preclude the full implementation of metabolite profiling strategies for compounds under study in lead optimization, when in fact it is in this early stage that knowledge of structure–metabolism relationships would be the most useful. Yet, the economics of drug development dictate that a large number of candidates be examined in concert with the principles of minimizing costs and time. To that end, computer software provides a mechanism for earlier and faster prediction of the absorption, distribution, metabolism, and excretion (ADME) properties of candidates based on their chemical structure, including potential metabolites, hypothetical chemical structures, toxicity profiles, and other attributes.[17]

One team catalogued[17] a number of computational approaches that have been employed, including, but not limited to, rule-, ligand protein-, and ligand-based methods; as well as *ab initio*, classic pharmacophore, and three-dimensional quantitative structure–activity relationship (QSAR) pharmacophore-based methods.

A few of these tools are described below, with references to case studies. The author does acknowledge hand-on experience with some of the software described below and familiarity with others *via* the scientific literature or commercial/promotional literature; the reader will please note that the inclusion or exclusion of relevant software does not represent an endorsement or censure on the part of the author. Furthermore, software packages are in a constant state of refinement and improvement, and their features will almost certainly have changed after this was written. Reports of the use of metabolite prediction software packages in the scientific literature generally fall into several categories, including head-to-head comparisons, case studies of the use of a single software package (especially in comparison with experimental data as a validation set), and/or integration of two or more packages.

6.3.1 Meteor

Meteor (Lhasa, Ltd.)[18] has been described elsewhere[17] as:

> "A rule-based (empirical) software tool. Its algorithm involves three successive steps. First, Meteor checks whether the query structure contains substructures that are labile toward any of the biotransformations contained in its knowledge base. Second, absolute reasoning rules evaluate the likelihood of a biotransformation taking place based on five levels: probable, plausible, equivocal, doubted, and improbable. This classification depends on the $\log P$ of the query structure, whether the query structure is the unchanged drug or a metabolite, and in which species the metabolism is to be predicted. Third, relative reasoning then is used to rank those biotransformations that can occur concomitantly on the same compound, based on a set of relative precedences (*e.g.*, primary alcohols are oxidized in preference to secondary alcohols)."

Recent reports of the employment of Meteor include:

- Refinement of the Meteor knowledge base to improve predictions of certain pathways; the authors reported[19] updates to the knowledge base such as the exclusion of certain reactions (to minimize the over-prediction that is often associated with *in silico* metabolite profiling). A comparison between the updated and previous versions of the software was carried out using reference compounds, with the results demonstrating an improvement in predictive performance and selectivity for oxidative *N*-dealkylations and related biotransformations.
- A collaboration[20] with a regulatory agency (FDA) in which Meteor was employed for several hepatotoxic drugs to determine human-specific drug metabolites that might lead to chronic toxicity and possible DDIs. The authors suggest that *in silico* tools help both the development of therapeutics and also their safety assessment by the early identification of drug metabolites.
- In a particularly interesting study[21]—outside the realm of drug discovery, but a novel implementation of *in silico* metabolite prediction to environmental chemistry—the authors employed Meteor to predict the biotransformation mechanisms and products of polar contaminants in freshwater crustaceans, specifically the metabolites of biocides and pharmaceuticals formed in *Gammarus pulex* and *Daphnia magna*.

6.3.2 MetaSite

MetaSite (Molecular Discovery)[22] has been described[17] as:

> "An automated docking model with reactivity correction and is designed to predict phase I cytochrome P450 (P450) metabolism. Based on GRID

descriptors for the P450 enzymes and the potential substrate, metabolism is evaluated at all possible sites on the molecular structure, assigning every atom a likelihood of metabolism. Reactivity correction can be put in three different modes: (1) 'off'; (2) 'on for substrate'; and (3) 'on for substrate and CYP'."

Recent reports of the employment of MetaSite include:

- Validation[23] of MetaSite predictions with data generated from MS analysis of companion human microsomal incubations of marketed drugs and proprietary drug candidates. While MetaSite's "first rank" predictions were experimentally confirmed for only about 55% of the compounds, its second- or third-ranked predictions were consistent with the experimental data from another 30% of the compounds.
- The use of MetaSite to predict the skin metabolism of selected retinoids (retinol, retinaldehyde, retinoic acid, retinyl acetate, retinyl palmitate, acitretin, etretinate, adapalene, and bexarotene) employed in treatment of skin disorders and found in cosmeceuticals. The authors[24] found that MetaSite metabolism predictions for retinoic acid, acitretin, etretinate, adapalene, and bexarotene were in agreement with experimental findings. In the case of compounds being converted by enzymes other than CYP enzymes, the primary metabolites predicted by MetaSite differed from those reported previously. The authors concluded that MetaSite is a useful tool that can aid identification of the major metabolites of topically administered compounds.
- The *in silico* prediction of the main metabolic reactions of four proprietary synthetic cannabinoids using MetaSite.[25] Evaluation of the agreement between software prediction and experimental reactions was performed with *in vitro* experiments using rat liver slices and the obtained samples were analyzed by time-of-flight (TOF) liquid chromatography (LC)-MS. Comparison between the experimental findings and the *in silico* metabolism prediction using MetaSite showed a good correlation between experimental and *in silico* data.

6.3.3 StarDrop

The mechanics of StarDrop (Optibrium, Ltd.)[26] have been described:[17]

"StarDrop uses a quantum mechanical approach for the prediction of the relative involvement of CYP3A4, 2D6, and 2C9 of the query compound. Its mechanism is based on calculation of the energy barrier to the electron removal, which is considered to be the rate-limiting step in product formation. All of the modeled P450 isoforms use the same model for the calculation of electronic lability, but each isoform has a different model for steric accessibility and orientation effects (different regioselectivity)."

Recent reports of the employment of StarDrop include:

- Comparison of MetaSite and StarDrop[27] to test known probe substrates for CYP enzymes (twelve substrates of CYP3A4 and eighteen substrates of CYP2C9 and CYP2D6) by assigning a point system for each correct prediction; the total points assigned for each CYP isoform experimentally were compared as a percentage of the total points assigned theoretically for the first choice prediction for all substrates for each isoform. The authors' results demonstrated that MetaSite and StarDrop performed similarly in predicting the correct site of metabolism for CYP3A4, while StarDrop did slightly better in predicting the correct site of metabolism for CYP2C9 and CYP2D6 metabolism. The comparison was extended to a set of more than 30 proprietary compounds; overall the software were comparable in their first-rank predictions.
- Another team did a head-to-head comparison[17] of Meteor, MetaSite, and StarDrop using a chemically diverse test set of more than 20 compounds, for which metabolite profiles were well known (including *in vivo* human mass balance studies and metabolic schemes). Different settings within each software package were investigated to give the best prediction; the three different packages were combined using optimized settings to see whether a synergistic effect could be established for the overall metabolism prediction. Results varied in precision and sensitivity among the individual packages. The authors found that increased precision could be obtained by combining predictions from the different packages, suggesting that synergistic use of metabolite prediction software packages could prove useful.

6.3.4   Other Software and the Literature

While it may be argued that some of the exercises described above—especially *a priori* metabolite prediction in the absence of experimental or instrument data—fall outside the traditional definition of metabolite profiling, they do contribute to the same end. More importantly, some metabolite prediction software packages—including several of those noted above—show great promise in integrating *in silico* metabolite prediction with interrogation of high-resolution MS datasets.[28] Indeed, one report[29] concluded that these approaches offer "promising milestones toward an unsupervised process to metabolite identification and structural characterization moving away from a sample focused per-compound approach to a structure-driven generic workflow."

As noted above, there are other software packages—and no doubt will be more—to facilitate metabolite prediction or assist in metabolite profiling. A report[30] published as recently as this writing reviewed no less than 45 different packages, categorized by predictions of regioselectivity, metabolites, interactions of drugs with metabolizing enzymes, and toxicological effects of metabolites.

While reports of *in silico* metabolite prediction in support of metabolite profiling can be found in the traditional drug metabolism literature, the author points interested scientists to other recent and related publications, including those published in the *Journal of Computer-Aided Molecular Design*,[31] *Computers in Biology & Medicine*,[32] *Journal of Molecular Modeling*,[33] and other relevant journals.

Still, *in silico* approaches are a tool; not a panacea. As one team justly concluded,[34] "*In silico* studies cannot replace conventional *in vitro* or *in vivo* testing but it is likely that, in conjunction with other techniques, they will streamline the overall discovery process."

6.4 Metabolite Quantitation

Owing to the regulatory landscape associated with metabolite profiling mentioned earlier in this chapter, the quantification of metabolites—in addition to their characterization and identification—has become an early and important part of the drug development process, especially when the metabolite is toxic, pharmacologically active, and/or has circulating exposure that meets or exceeds the parent drug concentration. While advances in LC-MS technology have greatly improved the ability to detect and identify metabolites, obtaining quantitative metabolite profiles in preclinical or clinical studies can be challenging. Several alternatives, including direct quantitation, employment of radiolabeled material, the use of response factors, indirect quantitation, and NMR, are described below.

6.4.1 Direct Quantitation

Direct quantitation—using authentic reference standards—is obviously the preferred and most appropriate method, and makes best use of the specificity and sensitivity of LC-MS. However, authentic standards are typically not available early in the drug development process. Even when they are available, commercially or internally, their expense may preclude their use, especially in cost-conscious academic laboratories; likewise, limited quantities may preclude the extensive experiments and analyses required for proper method validation.

A seemingly natural and intuitive solution to this problem is to quantitate the metabolite concentration based on an LC-MS calibration curve of the parent compound, a standard of which is presumably more available. However, it has been demonstrated[35] that the structure modifications—even simple ones—that influence drug metabolism can result in significant changes in the ionization efficiency of the metabolite relative to the parent compound. In one case,[36] the response by positive ion electrospray ionisation (ESI)-MS for two isomeric oxidative metabolites differed by a factor of 25-fold. Even more confounding is when the metabolite requires detection using the opposite ionization mode as the parent compound.

A commonly used complimentary detection technique is ultraviolet (UV) detection—whether by fixed wavelength, variable wavelength, or photodiode array detection—which relies on a "chromophore" in the molecule for detection at one or more wavelengths in the UV spectrum. Metabolites often have the same chromophore as the parent drug, giving a similar response. Yet, as with LC-MS described above, there are many exceptions such that even minor changes in structure due to metabolism result in significant changes in absorbance. Even when absorption coefficients are conserved, UV detection often runs into practical limits on its utility, especially owing to insufficient sensitivity and/or lower selectivity when drugs/metabolites do not have UV absorption at wavelengths that can distinguish them from background levels.

Fluorescence and electrochemical detection offer great benefits in selectivity and sensitivity, but can also be subject to response changes concomitant with structural changes. Likewise, their very specificity limits their wider applicability.

So-called "universal detectors"—chemiluminescent nitrogen detector (CNLD), evaporative light scattering detector (ELSD), corona charged aerosol detection (CAD), refractive index (RI), and others—offer alternatives as well.[37] A typical strategy is to use the universal detector to calibrate the response factor ratio on a mass spectrometer generated from a parent compound and its metabolite(s) in a biological matrix; the response factor ratio can then be used to quantify the metabolite with the LC-MS/MS response obtained from the parent drug's standard curve.

In one study,[38] a team evaluated oxazepam and temazepam as a "drug/ metabolite" pair (with temazepam treated as the methylated metabolite of oxazepam). Fortified dog urine samples were analyzed by LC-CLND and LC-MS/MS to obtain a response factor ratio between the two analytes. From the ratio, temazepam was quantified using the oxazepam standard curve. The authors demonstrated that the difference between the concentration of temazepam obtained from the reconstructed standard curve and the concentration obtained directly from an authentic temazepam standard curve was within 13% (except at the lowest concentration). The methodology was then successfully applied to measuring the quantity of a metabolite of a proprietary compound in other *in vivo* studies.

6.4.2 Quantitation Using Radiotracer

The employment of radiolabeled (especially [14]C- or ^{3}H-labeled) material for *in vitro* or *in vivo* studies offers significant advantages in studying their metabolism, distribution, and or elimination, from either a mass balance perspective or in terms of metabolite profiling. Their detection by flow-through detectors or by fraction collection and liquid scintillation counting offers an equimolar response regardless of structural changes. When coupled with data from MS and/or UV detection, response ratios can be calculated between and among parent drugs and metabolites. Quantitation can be done using a standard curve of the parent compound. These efforts do require sufficient separation of the drug and metabolites.

Still, the employment of radiolabeled material in drug metabolism studies often does not happen until later in the drug development timeline, while efforts to conduct metabolite profiling are being pushed ever earlier (and justly so) in the timeline, thus reducing the utility of this response factor alternative.

6.4.3 Indirect Quantitation

Phase II metabolites (*e.g.*, glucuronides) can be quantified indirectly by cleavage of the conjugate by chemical or enzymatic hydrolysis to yield the parent drug. Both methods are subject to some limitations and/or efficiencies, including time-consuming sample preparation, incomplete hydrolysis, and uneven robustness of the methods.[39] Enzymatic hydrolysis can require optimization of incubation time, temperature, and enzyme concentrations, *etc.*; chemical hydrolysis is dependent on the chemical nature of the moiety that is conjugated: *O*- and *N*-glucuronides (primary and secondary amines) under acidic conditions, and acyl glucuronides and quaternary ammonium glucuronides under alkaline conditions. Despite these limitations, the methods can be useful for those metabolites—especially glucuronides—that are not readily accessible for traditional synthesis of authentic standards. Furthermore, the methods are similar to the often used and acceptable "common moiety" methods employed in pesticide residue analysis in raw agricultural commodities and/or animal tissues.

6.4.4 Quantitation by NMR

The use of nuclear magnetic resonance spectroscopy (NMR) as a tool for the quantitative determination of metabolites has received increasing attention in the literature.[40–42] Although there are some limitations, particularly in terms of the disadvantage of limited material that is often associated with isolated or low-abundance metabolites, the method does offer advantages in rank-ordering the concentration of metabolites in the absence of authentic standards, and where other methods, such as those described above, fail.

6.5 Metabolite Synthesis: The "Known Unknown"

It is difficult to denote a single ultimate goal of any particular metabolite profiling exercise, but a particularly satisfying one is the unequivocal identification of what once may have been referred to in the readers' laboratory as "Unknown *X*". Despite advances in LC/MS instrumentation, the results can still yield unsatisfactory ambiguity in the unequivocal structural elucidation of metabolites.

There are many avenues to success, but three major routes include chemical synthesis of a reference standard with subsequent chromatographic and/or spectral comparison; isolation from *in vitro* and/or *in vivo* samples with subsequent unequivocal identification by NMR; and a growing arsenal of nontraditional methods.

There are several drivers for synthesis of reference standards, including—but not limited to—avoiding the unsatisfying assumptions that are necessarily associated with semi-quantitative approaches to metabolite profiling, as discussed above; the need to screen metabolites for drug target activity in established assays; and the need for sufficient metabolite exposure in toxicity and other regulatory testing (drug transport, DDIs, *etc.*)

Chemical synthesis is often suitable for Phase I metabolites such as dealkylations, oxidations, and carbonyl reductions, *etc.* However, novel metabolites, especially Phase II metabolites, may not be synthetically accessible at the bench owing to difficult routes or cumbersome stereoselectivity, and other alternatives may need to be considered.

A standard alternative is to employ cell systems or purified enzymes for the *in vitro* production of metabolites. Examples include the use of liver homogenates, liver microsomal or S9 incubates, cell culture lines, and recombinant enzymes.[43,44]

6.5.1 Microbial Bioreactors

One team[45] identified several reasons for the employment of microbial bioreactors as a mechanism for metabolite production. Among the advantages they catalogued were: relatively low cost, mild conditions, ease of use, potential for efficient conversion with a high yield, scale up capability, and a potential to reduce the use of animals. The authors studied the metabolism of muraglitazar following a single oral dose in humans. No less than 16 metabolites were observed in plasma, urine, and/or feces, and the identification of several of the metabolites was precluded by low concentrations in the human samples.

The authors employed cultures of *Caenorhabditis elegans* and *Sororoditha hirsuta* (previously determined to produce oxidative metabolite profiles similar to those found in humans) and successfully bio-synthesized no less than six of the unknowns, which were produced in sufficient amounts for identification by NMR.

In a separate report,[46] members of the same team extended this successful strategy to the rapid screening of active strains of actinomycetes for the production of metabolites of both well-studied/marketed drugs and proprietary drug candidates.

6.5.2 Synthesis of Phase II Metabolites

The preparation of Phase II metabolites—especially glucuronide conjugates—can be challenging owing to their synthesis, purification, stability, isolation, and analysis. These challenges can be exacerbated when regioselectivity is a factor. For example, the author had the privilege of being associated with the study of a "-flozin" class drug, in which the principal biotransformation pathway involved glucuronidation of the glycoside hydroxyl groups to yield three possible regioisomeric metabolites. Interestingly, the regiospecificity was also species dependent. Bench synthesis of the glucuronide was achieved, but it favored production of the least abundant of the three regioisomers. Production of sufficient metabolite reference standard to support *in vitro* efficacy and DDI studies, as well as validations of quantitative bioanalytical methods was achieved by bulk incubation using recombinant UDP-glucuronosyltransferase (UGT) enzyme, followed by isolation by semi-preparative high-performance LC, and NMR confirmation (data not shown).

Similarly, one team described[47] the challenges of obtaining authentic standards of the conjugated metabolites of raloxifene. Raloxifene is metabolized to two distinct monoglucuronides and one diglucuronide. Attempts at glucuronide synthesis at the bench resulted in low yield and insufficient material for further study. Biosynthesis employing recombinant human UGT enzymes was successful in converting parent compound to both monoglucuronides.[48] Subsequently, all three metabolites were successfully prepared using a *Streptomyces* sp. bioreactor.[47]

Two recent reviews[49,50] describe the challenges and successes in the synthesis of Phase II metabolites.

6.5.3 Biomimetic Oxidation

Among the efforts to develop methods for metabolite synthesis to compliment metabolite profiling efforts is the employment of "biomimetic" techniques, including the use of metalloporphyrins (as surrogates for the active center of CYP enzymes), Fenton's reagent,[51] and electrochemical oxidation.[52] Recent reviews[53] of the techniques have concluded that they can be used during drug discovery and development of new drugs to "elucidate the structure of metabolites that are difficult to characterize in biological matrices" and that they show promise to "replace the classical chemistry strategy, especially when synthesis is complicated or too time-consuming in order to access metabolites for further testing."

Indeed, the techniques have been demonstrated to catalyze a wide variety of reactions, and in particular, most relevant oxidations. One recent review[53] catalogued some of the reactions that can be supported: the electrochemical oxidation systems successfully mimic benzylic hydroxylation, hydroxylation of aromatic rings containing electron-donating groups, *N*-dealkylation, *S*-oxidation, dehydrogenation, and others; the Fenton system is able to mimic aliphatic, benzylic, and aromatic hydroxylations, *N*- and *O*-dealkylations, *N*- and *S*-oxidations, and others; finally, the porphyrin systems can mimic all types of reactions, although the review cautioned that yields can be low for some of the reactions.

As an example, in one recent report[54] the authors combined microfluidic technology and electrochemistry by using a microfluidic electrochemical cell. They subjected several commercial drugs (chosen for various reactions based on reports of *in vivo* metabolism) to continuous-flow electrolysis and demonstrated that metabolites could be synthesized by flow electrolysis at the 10 to 100 mg scale, with subsequent full characterization. For example, they optimized the isolated yield of 5-OH-diclofenac (5-OH-DCF), such that it represented a reaction output of 85 mg of pure metabolite per hour of flow electrosynthesis. Of equal importance, they compared their efforts with the scheme and yields of traditional bench synthesis of 5-OH-DCF. Likewise, they demonstrated the successful electrochemical synthesis of metabolites resulting from alkyl oxidation, sulfoxidation, quinone imine formation, and glutathione conjugation—on a 10 to 100 mg scale (per hour of flow electrolysis)—for several other drugs, including tolbutamide, primidone, albendazole, and chlorpromazine.

In another recent report,[55] a team subjected phencyclidine (PCP) to chemical oxidation by a Fenton's reagent system, yielding several hydroxylated products, three of which were identical to metabolites derived from microsomal incubations. They also successfully employed the procedure to generate PCP–GSH adducts. The procedure was both a ready biomimetic system and a means to study the mechanism of inactivation of human CYPs by PCP.

Metalloporphyrins have long been employed for the purposes of biomimetic oxidation (BMO). A typical example is the report of the synthesis of major metabolites of dimethylaminoantipyrine[56] using iron *ortho*-nitrophenylporphyrin chloride as a catalyst. A more recent development is the commercialization of higher throughput BMO screening kits that afford more rapid authentication of produced metabolites by direct comparison with *in vitro* or *in vivo* reference samples. In one report,[57] the authors demonstrated the synthesis of multiple metabolites of dimethylaminopyridine, tolbutamide, tetrahydrofuran, and bupivacaine, as well as chemoselectivity, such that a single porphyrin promoted different oxidation reactions depending on the experimental conditions (oxidant, solvent, and ligand, *etc.*). Using the kits, the authors outlined a process of screening, optimization, and production of appreciable amounts (*i.e.*, hundreds of milligrams).

6.6   Enantioselective Metabolism

The author does lament a development concomitant with the increased routine use of MS detection in drug metabolite profiling: a de-emphasis on optimizing chromatographic separations. Although counterintuitive to the tendency towards high-throughput screening and "ballistic" mobile phase gradients, readers would do well to remind colleagues entering the field of metabolite profiling that the *real* chemistry takes place in the separation, not in the method of detection. The bottom line[58] is that "Good chromatographic separation is prerequisite for reliable and accurate quantification of metabolites in the biological samples."

This is especially true when LC is not coupled to an MS detector. While LC-MS/MS admittedly does not always require as extensive separation between and among the parent drug and metabolites, in many cases it is important in order to avoid interferences: different metabolites can share the same product ions or transitions; unstable metabolites may be converted to parent drug by in-source fragmentation or thermal degradation; and, most importantly, it helps to avoid interference of endogenous compounds, which can exert significant matrix effects on ionization.

While reverse-phase chromatography, employing the venerable C18 column, remains a mainstay of separations in metabolite profiling, attention should be given to other column chemistries, especially for those challenging instances of retention and/or separation of metabolites. These include hydrophilic interaction chromatography (HILIC), mixed-mode, normal phase, porous graphic carbon, or chiral columns.

Indeed, there are few aspects of metabolite profiling where chromatographic separations are more essential than in exploring enantioselective metabolism.

For the better part of a century, the consideration of chirality in drug metabolism was limited to academic study and/or to natural products, owing in no small part to the limits of separations chemistry. However, chirality has been earning ever-greater importance in drug discovery and development,[59-61] such that most of the new molecular entities reaching the market in the first decades of the 21st century are single enantiomers, rather than the racemic mixtures (or achiral drugs) that dominated the latter half of the 20th century.

While direct enantioselective effects on the physical–chemical aspects of adsorption, distribution, or elimination are minimal or are only now being studied, their effects on metabolism are the rule rather than the exception, as substrates or products, and on multiple enzyme systems. Examples include the prochiral/achiral metabolism (carbonyl reduction) of haloperidol (in humans, S-hydroxy-haloperidol is preferred); the chiral to chiral transformation of (S)-warfarin to (S)-7- or (S)-6-hydroxywarfarin; chiral to achiral transformations, such as those involving 1,4-dihydropyridine calcium antagonists to their pyridine analogs; chiral to diastereomer transformations such as the keto-reduction of warfarin, resulting in two pairs of diastereomeric alcohols; or chiral inversions (enzymatic and non-enzymatic) such as those that occur with 2-arylpropionic acid NSAIDS.

While it is not the mission of this chapter to generally describe the implications of DDIs, pharmacology, or drug safety, a few special cases reinforce the importance of considering the exploration of chirality in metabolite profiling exercises. The administration of racemic drugs, by definition, is polypharmacy; add in yet another drug, and the possibilities of DDIs can escalate when the induction or inhibition of one influences the PK behavior of the other(s). Examples include the interaction of warfarin with cimetidine (decreases the clearance of (R)-warfarin) or with sulfinpyrazone (decreases the clearance of (S)-warfarin).

Likewise, racemic mixtures can exert effects on pharmacodynamics and/or safety: the efficacy may be in a single enantiomer, the antipode being biologically inert; the pharmacological activity of each of the enantiomers may be different, such that each can be developed on its own merits; the enantiomers may have opposite effects at the same target; or the pharmacological activity lies in both enantiomers, but adverse safety is only associated with one. As stated earlier in this section, the increasing emphasis on single enantiomers rather than racemic mixtures should mitigate these potential impacts.

As mentioned from the start of this section, a driving factor in the increased appreciation of chiral-driven drug metabolism, PK, and pharmacodynamics has been an improvement in column chemistries to achieve the separations. Indeed, it has been stated[62] that the "development of complex PK models and plasma–concentration–effect relationships based on 'total' drug concentrations following administration of a racemate are of limited value and potentially useless." As with all quantitative analytical chemistry, the methods should aim for accuracy and reproducibility, with minimal sample preparation, and the employment of sample-friendly mobile phases or pH. However, special diligence in method development and validation is required for chiral separations. The preferred method is direct separation on a chiral stationary phase (*e.g.*, polysaccharide or immobilized protein). An alternative is an indirect method in which the enantiomers are derivatized with a chiral reagent to produce diastereoisomers, which can then be separated on conventional column chemistries.

The current movement towards single enantiomers as drug candidates, noted above, should result in mitigation of the DDIs that are potentially associated with racemic mixtures. This does not alleviate the concern or challenges that are associated with achiral-to-chiral transformations and/or chiral-to-chiral or chiral-to-diastereomer transformations.

6.6.1   Case Study: Enantioselective Metabolism LX6171

A case study of enantioselective metabolism and metabolite profiling, with which the author had the privilege to be closely associated, is described below.

LX6171 [63,64] ((3′-chlorobiphenyl-4-yl)-1-(pyrimidine-2-yl) piperidin-4-yl) methanone) is a small molecule drug candidate for cognitive disorders that demonstrated improved learning and memory in mice, and exhibited an acceptable safety and PK profile in preclinical and clinical studies. Early metabolite profiling efforts[65,66] indicated that the most significant metabolite pathway was keto-reduction to form the corresponding alcohol (similar to the example of haloperidol described above) with a chiral center; other metabolites resulted from oxidation of the pyrimidine, combinations of pyrimidine oxidation and keto-reduction, and other minor pathways.

Likewise, early attention was given to the possible enantioselective metabolism to the chiral alcohol. *In vitro* experiments (liver S9) in multiple species indicated that metabolism to the *S*-enantiomer of the keto-reduced metabolite was preferred (>90% in rat, dog, and human; >80% in mouse). It is interesting to note that the keto-reduced alcohol was not observed in monkeys, which would have had significant implications for selection of species for toxicological studies. PK experiments in mouse, rat, and dog were all consistent with the companion *in vitro* experiments; that is, the *S*-enantiomer was preferred over the *R*-enantiomer, consistent with the ratios observed in the *in vitro* experiments. Furthermore, plasma exposure of the keto-reduced metabolite in rats was several-fold higher than the parent compound. The *S*-enantiomer of the keto-reduced metabolite was also found to have significant efficacy against the target.

From a bio-analytical perspective, initial analyses employed an immobilized protein column that offered very good separation of the enantiomers of the keto-reduced metabolite, but required long (>60 minutes) run times, yielded suboptimal peak shapes and sensitivity, and was not robust enough to accommodate repeated injections of biological samples. Subsequent investigations resulted in the successful employment of a chiral column chemistry that allowed for shorter run times and good sensitivity so that the metabolite could be monitored in clinical studies.

The case study provides a good example of the need to consider possible enantioselective metabolism and its impact on PK, pharmacodynamics, toxicology, and bio-analytical chemistry; not to mention regulatory, intellectual property, business and product development, and other important considerations.

6.6.2 Other Recent Case Studies

There are many case studies of enantioselective metabolism in the literature. A handful of reports are briefly described below.

As mentioned above, enantioselective metabolism also extends to Phase II metabolism. In a recent report,[67] a team examined the profile, kinetics, and enzymology of the metabolism of ornidazole in humans. A total of 19 metabolites were identified in human urine and stereoselective glucuronidation was a principal metabolic pathway. The authors screened 12 available human recombinant UGTs and demonstrated that UGT1A9 was the predominant isoform involved in *R*-ornidazole glucuronidation, whereas *S*-ornidazole glucuronidation was predominantly catalyzed by UGT2B7. A chemical inhibition study with niflumic acid and flurbiprofen supported these findings. Furthermore, *in vitro* experiments demonstrated that the *S*-ornidazole glucuronidation was preferred in both liver and kidney microsomes.

Another recent study[68] encompassed many of the strategies discussed in this chapter—novel analytical techniques, novel metabolite synthesis techniques, consideration of enantioselective metabolism, and its impact on intellectual property. The authors studied the disposition of zopiclone (ZO), a chiral drug that undergoes metabolism to its *N*-desmethyl (*N*-Des-ZO) and *N*-oxide (*N*-Ox-ZO) products. Separate studies demonstrated that the (*S*)-*N*-Des-ZO metabolite has pharmacological (anxiolytic) activity and a patent for the metabolite was requested. The team employed fungi (*Cunninghamella*) to obtain *N*-Des-ZO and the novel technique of capillary electrophoresis (CE) and dispersive liquid–liquid microextraction (DLLME) to monitor its production.

Finally, another recent report[69] provides an excellent model for the diligence required in properly developing and validating quantitative analytical methods for enantiomeric drugs and/or their metabolites. The authors developed an enantioselective and sensitive LC-MS/MS method for determining morinidazole enantiomers in human plasma and employed it to interrogate the stereoselective PK of the compound. Chiral separation was optimized (a run time of <10 minutes) on a cellulose column with subsequent detection by MS, with good specificity, precision, dynamic range, and relevant limits of quantitation. The authors also investigated possible chiral inversion during sample storage, preparation, and analysis; none was observed.

6.7   Conclusion

What does the future hold for metabolite profiling? Some possible considerations include:

- Whether advances in analytical instrument sophistication and sensitivity may drive regulatory agencies to consider lower thresholds for identification of metabolites.
- The continued interdisciplinary nature of metabolite profiling seems certain and may accommodate additional sciences. One aspect is already both confounding and interesting: simple keyword searches for "metabolite profiling" in literature databases do provide some seemingly "false positive" hits from crossover with endobiotic metabolite profiling or "metabonomics" and "metabolomics." That said, there is a lot to be gained[70] from applying the tools and techniques of -omics to small molecule drug metabolite profiling. More importantly, the combination of metabolite profiling with biomarker profiling can provide insights into pharmacology and toxicology.
- We can certainly expect continued literature reports of interesting metabolites and solutions for long-standing mysteries of previously unidentified metabolites and pathways. For example, metabolite profiling of complex mixtures—especially of natural products, the diversity of which can make their separation and detection challenging—is gaining attention in the literature.

Most importantly, Buchheim's advice should continue to hold for the coming decades as it has for the past century plus, and guide a new generation of metabolite profiling scientists.

References

1. A. Conti and M. H. Bickel, *Drug Metab. Rev.*, 1977, **6**, 1–50.
2. I. Khola and J. Landis, *Nat. Rev. Drug Discovery*, 2004, **3**, 711–716.
3. D. Cook, D. Brown, R. Alexander, R. March, P. Morgan, G. Satterthwaite and M. Pangalos, *Nat. Rev. Drug Discovery*, 2014, **13**, 419–429.

4. C. P. Miller, *The Chemist's Companion Guide to Patent Law*, John Wiley & Sons, Hoboken, NJ, 2010.
5. F. Simon and P. Kotler, *Building Global Biobrands: Taking Biotechnology to Market*, Simon & Schuster, New York, NY, 2003, p. 194.
6. K. Burk, W. McCulloch, A. von Nieciecki and W. Meyer, *Beyond Financial Analysis – Scientific Due Diligence in Pharma and Biotech - Why is scientific due diligence essential in drug development?*, http://www.clindesc.com/pdf/ Scientific_Due_Diligence.pdf, accessed 23 September 2015.
7. R. Mandra, Eyes Wide Open: What you must do to see beyond the veil: FTO in the Wider Context - Due Diligence, *C5 4th International FTO Forum*, 2007.
8. U.S. Food and Drug Administration, Guidance for Industry Safety Testing of Drug Metabolites, 2008.
9. European Medicines Agency, Non-Clinical Safety Studies for the Conduct of Human Clinical Trials and Marketing Authorization for Pharmaceuticals, December 2009.
10. D. Smith and R. Obach, *Drug Metab. Dispos.*, 2005, **33**, 1409–1417.
11. A. Nedderman and P. Wright, *Bioanalysis*, 2010, **2**, 1235–1248.
12. U.S. Food and Drug Administration, Nonclinical Safety Studies for the Conduct of Human Clinical Trials and Marketing Authorization for Pharmaceuticals, December 2010.
13. H. Yu, D. Bischoff and D. Tweedie, *Expert Opin. Drug Metab. Toxicol.*, 2010, **6**, 1539–1549.
14. H. Hong, J. Caceres-Cortes, H. Su, X. Huang, V. Roongta, S. Bonacorsi, Y. Hong, Y. Tian, R. Iyer, W. Humphreys and L. Christopher, *Chem. Res. Toxicol.*, 2011, **24**, 125–134.
15. C. Yeung, Y. Fujioka, H. Hachad, R. Levy and N. Isoherranen, *Clin. Pharmacol. Ther.*, 2011, **89**, 105–113.
16. F. Kazmi, J. Barbara, P. Yerino and A. Parkinson, *Drug Metab. Dispos.*, 2015, **43**, 523–533.
17. H. T'jollyn, K. Bousscry, R. Mortishire-Smith, K. Coe, B. De Boeck, J. Van Bocxlaer and G. Mannens, *Drug Metab. Dispos.*, 2011, **39**, 2066–2075.
18. Lhasa Limited, http://www.lhasalimited.org.
19. E. Murray, T. Long and P. Rydberg, *In Silico Prediction of Metabolism: A Review of Oxidative N-Dealkylation Biotransformations*, European ISSX Conference, 2012, p. 146.
20. L. Valerio and A. Long, *Curr. Drug Discovery Technol.*, 2010, **7**, 170–187.
21. J. Jeon, D. Kurth and J. Hollender, *Chem. Res. Toxicol.*, 2013, **26**, 313–324.
22. Molecular Discovery, http://www.moldiscovery.com/.
23. M. Trunzer, B. Faller and A. Zimmerlin, *J. Med. Chem.*, 2009, **52**, 329–335.
24. K. Słoczyńska, A. Gunia-Krzyżak, D. Żelaszczyk, A. Waszkielewicz and H. Marona, *Acta Biochim. Pol.*, 2015, **62**, 201–206.
25. S. Strano-Rossi, L. Anzillotti, S. Dragoni, R. Pellegrino, L. Goracci, V. Pascali and G. Cruciani, *Anal. Bioanal. Chem.*, 2014, **406**, 3621–3636.
26. Optibrium, Ltd., http://www.optibrium.com/.

27. Y. Shin, H. Le, C. Khojasteh and C. Hop, *Comb. Chem. High Throughput Screening*, 2011, **14**, 811–823.
28. B. Bonn, C. Leandersson, F. Fontaine and I. Zamora, *Rapid Commun. Mass Spectrom.*, 2010, **24**, 3127–3138.
29. A. Pähler and A. Brink, *Drug Discovery Today: Technol.*, 2013, **10**, e207–e217.
30. J. Kirchmair, A. Göller, D. Lang, J. Kunze, B. Testa, I. Wilson, R. Glen and G. Schneider, *Nat. Rev. Drug Discovery*, 2015, **14**, 387–404.
31. T. Potter, R. Lewis, T. Luker, R. Bonnert, M. Bernstein, T. Birkinshaw, S. Thom, M. Wenlock and S. Paine, *J. Comput.-Aided Mol. Des.*, 2011, **25**, 997–1005.
32. D. Singh, D. Gawande, T. Singh, V. Poroikov and R. Goel, *Comput. Biol. Med.*, 2014, **47**, 1–6.
33. R. Braga, V. Alves, C. Fraga, E. Barreiro, V. Oliveira and C. Andrade, *J. Mol. Model.*, 2012, **18**, 2065–2078.
34. A. Nassar and R. Talaat, *Drug Discovery Today*, 2004, **9**, 317–327.
35. R. Ramanathan, J. Josephs, M. Jemal, M. Arnold, W. Humphreys, *Bioanalysis*, 2010, **2**, 1291–1313.
36. J. de Vlieger, M. Giezen, D. Falck, C. Tump, F. van Heuveln, M. Giera, J. Kool, H. Lingeman, J. Wieling, M. Honing, H. Irth and W. Niessen, *Anal. Chim. Acta*, 2011, **698**, 69–76.
37. P. Joshi, S. Bhoir, A. Bhagwat, *Sep. Sci.*, 2010, **2**, 12–14.
38. Y. Deng, J. Wu, H. Zhang and T. Olah, *Rapid Commun. Mass Spectrom.*, 2004, **18**, 1681–1685.
39. R. Ketola and K. Hakala, *Curr. Drug Metab.*, 2010, **11**, 561–582.
40. G. Walker, T. Ryder, R. Sharma, E. Smith and A. Freund, *Drug Metab. Dispos.*, 2011, **39**, 433–440.
41. R. Espina, L. Yu, J. Wang, Z. Tong, S. Vashishtha, R. Talaat, J. Scatina and A. Mutlib, *Chem. Res. Toxicol.*, 2009, **22**, 299–310.
42. G. Walker, J. Bauman, T. Ryder, E. Smith, D. Spracklin and R. Obach, *Drug Metab. Dispos.*, 2014, **42**, 1627–1639.
43. M. Soars, E. Mattiuz, D. Jackson, P. Kulanthaivel, W. Ehlhardt and S. Wrighton, *J. Pharmacol. Toxicol. Methods*, 2002, **47**, 161–168.
44. K. Cusacka, H. Koolmanb, U. Langec, H. Peltierb, I. Pielc and A. Vasudevanb, *Bioorg. Med. Chem. Lett.*, 2013, **23**, 5471–5483.
45. D. Zhang, H. Zhang, N. Aranibar, R. Hanson, Y. Huang, P. Cheng, S. Wu, S. Bonacorsi, M. Zhu, A. Swaminathan and W. Humphreys, *Drug Metab. Dispos.*, 2006, **34**, 267–280.
46. W. Li, J. Josephs, G. Skiles and W. Humphreys, *Drug Metab. Dispos.*, 2008, **36**, 721–730.
47. T. Trdan, R. Roškar, J. Trontelj, M. Ravnikar and A. Mrhar, *J. Chromatogr. B: Anal. Technol. Biomed. Life Sci.*, 2011, **879**, 2323–2331.
48. J. Trontelj, M. Bogataj, J. Marc and A. Mrhar, *J. Chromatogr. B: Anal. Technol. Biomed. Life Sci.*, 2007, **855**, 220–227.
49. A. Stachulski and X. Mengb, *Nat. Prod. Rep.*, 2013, **30**, 806–848.
50. J. Atzrodt, V. Derdau, W. Holla and M. Sandvoss, *ARKIVOC*, 2012, 257–278.

51. E. Nouri-Nigjeh, R. Bischoff, A. Bruins and H. Permentier, *Curr. Drug Metab.*, 2011, **12**, 359–371.
52. W. Lohmann and U. Karst, *Anal. Bioanal. Chem.*, 2008, **391**, 79–96.
53. T. Johansson, L. Weidolf and U. Jurva, *Rapid Commun. Mass Spectrom.*, 2007, **21**, 2323–2331.
54. R. Stalder and G. Roth, *ACS Med. Chem. Lett.*, 2013, **4**, 1119–1123.
55. M. Jushchyshyn, J. Wahlstrom, P. Hollenberg and L. Wienkers, *Drug Metab. Dispos.*, 2006, **34**, 1523–1529.
56. M. Bazin, H. Shi, J. Delaney, B. Kline, Z. Zhu, C. Kuhn, F. Berlioz, K. Farley, G. Fate, W. Lam, G. Walker, L. Yu and M. Pollastri, *Chem. Biol. Drug Des.*, 2007, **70**, 354–359.
57. M. Bazin and R. Buzdygon, Access to Drug Metabolites using Biomimetic Oxidation Systems, http://www.xenotechllc.com/posters/2014/hc-xt_poster.pdf, accessed 01 May 2015.
58. R. Roškar and T. Trdan Lušin, Analytical Methods for Quantification of Drug Metabolites in Biological Samples, in *Chromatography - The Most Versatile Method of Chemical Analysis*, ed. L. Calderon, 2012, InTech.
59. V. Campo, L. Bernardes and I. Carvalho, *Curr. Drug Metab.*, 2009, **10**, 188–205.
60. D. Brocks, *Biopharm. Drug Dispos.*, 2006, **27**, 387–406.
61. *Chirality in Drug Design and Development*, ed. I. Reddy and R. Mehvar, CRC Press, New York, 2004.
62. A. Hutt, *Metab. Drug Interact.*, 2007, **22**, 79–112.
63. P. Brown, X. Yu, K. Savelieva, M. Childers, K. Frazier, D. Walke, A. Wilson, W. Heydorn and T. Lanthorn, LX6171: A Novel Potential Treatment for Cognitive Disorders, *60th Annual Meeting, Am. Acad. Neurol.*, Chicago, 2008.
64. X. Yu, W. Zhang, A. Oldham, E. Buxton, S. Patel, N. Nghi, D. Tran, T. Lanthorn, C. Bomont, Z. Shi and Q. Liu, *Neurosci. Lett.*, 2009, **451**, 212–216.
65. J. Schmidt, A. Nouraldeen, L. Moran, L. Li and A. Wilson, Enantio-selective and Species-Dependent Carbonyl Reductase Metabolism of LX6171, *12th Annual Conference on Drug Metabolism and Applied Pharmacokinetics*, 2009.
66. L. Li, W. Heydorn, J. Kramer, A. Nouraldeen, J. Schmidt, J. Jiang, L. Moran and A. Wilson, Metabolism Mediated CYP2B Induction by LX6171 (3'-chlorobiphenyl-4-yl)-1-(pyrimidine-2-yl) piperidin-4-yl methanone in the Rat, *International Society for the Study of Xenobiotics (ISSX) Annual Meeting*, 2009.
67. J. Du, T. You, X. Chen and D. Zhong, *Drug Metab. Dispos.*, 2013, **41**, 1306–1318.
68. N. de Albuquerque, C. de Gaitani and A. de Oliveira, *J. Pharm. Biomed. Anal.*, 2015, **109**, 192–201.
69. K. Zhong, Z. Gao, Q. Li, D. Zhong and X. Chen, *J. Chromatogr. B: Anal. Technol. Biomed. Life Sci.*, 2014, **961**, 49–55.
70. F. Lia, F. Gonzalezb and X. Maa, *Acta Pharm. Sin. B*, 2012, **2**, 118–125.

Application of Humanised and Other Transgenic Models to Predict Human Responses to Drugs

C. ROLAND WOLF*[a], YURY KAPELYUKH[a], NICO SCHEER[b], AND COLIN J. HENDERSON[a]

[a]Cancer Research UK Molecular Pharmacology Laboratory, Jacqui Wood Cancer Centre, University of Dundee, Ninewells Hospital & Medical School, Dundee, DD1 9SY, UK; [b]Independent Consultant, Cologne, Germany
*E-mail: c.r.wolf@dundee.ac.uk

7.1   Introduction

All organisms have evolved complex metabolic networks to protect against the toxic and deleterious effect of chemicals to which they are exposed. In mammals the proteins involved have been classified on the basis of their functions as Phase 1, 2 and 3 enzymes. Phase 1 metabolism is predominantly mediated by the cytochrome P450 (CYP)-dependent mono-oxygenases;[1] Phase 2 metabolism is catalysed by enzymes such as the glutathione-transferases, glucuronyl-transferases and sulphotransferases[2] and Phase 3 pathways of disposition are mediated by drug transporters such as the ABC family of drug transporters.[3,4] These enzyme systems provide an adaptive response

RSC Drug Discovery Series No. 49
New Horizons in Predictive Drug Metabolism and Pharmacokinetics
Edited by Alan G. E. Wilson
© The Royal Society of Chemistry 2016
Published by the Royal Society of Chemistry, www.rsc.org

system to environmental challenge and are subject to tissue-specific patterns of gene expression predominantly located at portals of entry such as the liver, lungs, skin and gastrointestinal tract.[5] These enzyme systems provide an adaptive response to environmental challenges in that exposure to a compound often activates transcription factors that induce the expression of enzymes associated with the metabolism and or elimination of that compound. A number of transcription factors mediate this response, including the constitutive androstane receptor (CAR), the pregnane X receptor (PXR) and the aryl hydrocarbon receptor (AhR).[6–9]

As a consequence of the different environments in which mammalian species have evolved and their contrasting diets, the enzymes involved in chemical detoxification have diverged. Although Phase 1, 2 and 3 enzymes exist in all mammalian species the multiplicity and functionality of these enzymes is subject to marked species variability. These differences can affect the rates of metabolism and disposition of compounds, the metabolites produced and their toxicological and carcinogenic effects. In the context of drug development this factor makes the extrapolation of animal data to the human situation difficult with the result that drugs often fail once they reach the clinic for pharmacokinetic or safety reasons.[10–12]

Over the last few decades there have been major advances in identifying and characterising the enzymes involved in drug disposition, characterising genetic polymorphisms that affect the outcome of drug therapy and their mode of regulation.[9,13,14] This increase in knowledge is a major reason for the significant reduction in drug failure due to poor bioavailability.[15,16]

Our increased understanding of drug metabolism has resulted in *in vitro* and *in vivo* assays and the development of *in silico* models that are currently being used to predict human exposure and pharmacokinetics. These assays involve the use of recombinant enzymes, hepatic microsomal fractions, primary rodent and human hepatocytes or other cell based assays to obtain pharmacokinetic parameters for metabolism and drug transport. Primary human hepatocytes are commonly used to define human pathways of disposition; however, they have a significant number of limitations that include variability in quality and availability, the maintenance of gene expression in culture, and the variability in gene expression between individuals with each batch of cells having a different metabolic capacity and genetic background. Primary cells are also unsuitable for tests lasting more than a few days. In addition, because only primary human hepatocytes are available for such assays there are no *in vitro* tests, other than *in silico* modelling, to establish the role of extra-hepatic metabolism, for example by the gastrointestinal tract, on drug bioavailability. An experimental approach that allows a number of the current difficulties encountered in preclinical drug development to be addressed and provides further information that cannot be obtained from current approaches is through the use of transgenic animals.

The capacity to modulate patterns of gene expression by genetic manipulation in mice, and more recently in other species, has transformed our understanding of complex biochemical pathways *in vivo* and the pathogenesis of human disease. The ability to create mouse models carrying the genetic variants that are associated with human disease has provided new opportunities to understand disease processes and develop therapeutic interventions.

This review will focus predominantly on transgenic and humanised models for Phase 1 enzymes, although reference will be made to Phase 2 enzymes and drug transporters. There are a number of reviews on this topic to which the reader is referred.[7,17-19]

7.2 Transgenic Models

A variety of experimental technologies are available for the manipulation and measurement of gene expression in transgenic models.[18,20] Most of the studies in this area to date have been in the mouse. However, it is now possible to apply the technologies also to the rat[21] and although the rat remains the preferred species for preclinical drug development, the sophistication and genetics available in this species is at least a decade behind the mouse.

7.2.1 Experimental Approaches

The experimental approaches available include the deletion of specific genes by homologous recombination[22] (and increasingly by CRISPR technologies[23]) or conditional deletion in a cell type- or tissue-specific manner using Cre recombinase-based approaches (Figure 7.1).[24,25] This technology allows the role of specific proteins in complex biochemical pathways to be elucidated, and in a pharmacological context, the role of a protein or proteins in drug disposition, efficacy or toxicological response to be determined. The ability to knock out specific genes or gene clusters has also become of central importance for the interpretation of data using other transgenic lines such as humanised models where the mouse background needs to be eliminated.

In a second approach, transgenic models can be used to measure the transcriptional regulation of a gene both non-invasively in real time and in tissue sections by histochemistry. In this case a reporter such as luciferase (non-invasive: bioluminescent imaging) or human chorionic gonadotrophin (βhCG; non-invasive: secreted marker) or Lac Z (invasive: tissue histochemistry) is cloned into the promoter of the gene to be studied. This can be through random integration of the reporter construct (including promotor of choice) into the mouse genome or into a region of ubiquitous transcriptional expression (such as ROSA26[26]), or preferably through targeted integration into the endogenous gene locus. Recently, virus-derived peptides—2A sequences[27]—which can be used to create cassettes with multiple reporters (Figure 7.1) have been used to create a series of mouse models, utilising promotors reporting on DNA damage, apoptosis, inflammation and oxidative stress (Wolf, C. R. and Henderson, C. J., unpublished).

The activation of the promoter in such reporter models, either constitutively or as a consequence of exposure to drugs or environmental chemicals, can then be measured. In a drug development and toxicological context such reporters allow the capacity of drugs or environmental chemicals to activate

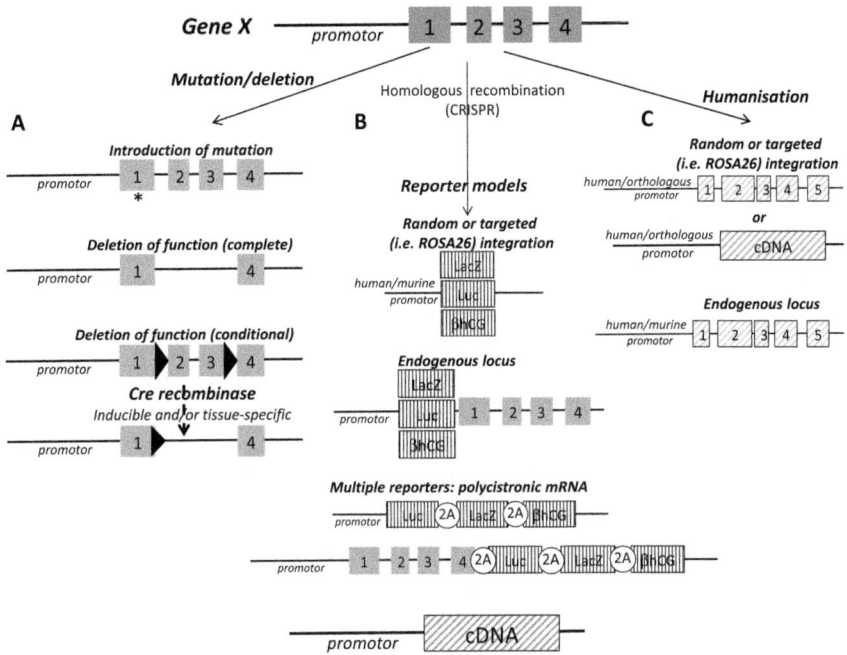

Figure 7.1 Experimental approaches to the generation of transgenic mouse models. A hypothetical 'Gene X' is illustrated. (A) Using homologous recombination or CRISPR, a mutation/mutations (∗) may be introduced, or all or part of the gene may be deleted. Alternatively, specific DNA sequences such as LoxP sites (black triangles) may be introduced to encompass either the entire gene or, as shown, a key region of the gene. Subsequent crossing of this mouse line with one expressing Cre recombinase in an inducible and/or tissue-specific manner allows deletion and inactivation of the gene in specific cells or tissue and/or in a temporal manner. (B) Reporter models may be generated by introducing genes such as LacZ, luciferase (Luc) or hCG, under the control of a promotor (orthologous, murine or human), and integrated randomly or targeted to a region of ubiquitous gene expression such as ROSA26.[26] Alternatively, the reporters can be targeted to an endogenous murine gene locus. Use may also be made of 2A sequences, for example from the foot and mouth disease virus,[27] that mediate 'ribosome skipping' and allow co-expression at equimolar amounts of multiple proteins, including endogenous proteins, from a single polycistronic mRNA under the control of a single promotor. (C) Human genes may be introduced into the murine genome, as a cDNA or genomic construct, either randomly or targeted to ROSA26, and with the associated human promotor or an orthologous promotor. Alternatively, the human gene (or gene cluster, for example generated from a bacterial artificial chromosome) may be inserted into the murine genome to replace the homologous mouse gene(s), utilising the murine promotor, or preferably retaining the human regulatory elements.

pathways that are considered precursors to toxicity such as oxidative stress, DNA damage or inflammation. They therefore serve as early biomarkers of toxic potential and also allow the *in vivo* effects of drugs on transcription factors, such as CAR or PXR for example, to be established.

7.2.2 Humanisation of Mouse Models

A further transgenic approach is the humanisation of mouse models thorough the introduction of human genes into the mouse genome. This can again be carried out by random integration of a gene or expression construct or by targeted integration into a specific gene locus. The expression of the transgene can either be off its own promoter, which is preferable, the murine promoter of the orthologous gene or by a heterologous promoter. All of these approaches have advantages and disadvantages (Table 7.1). In order to easily interpret experimental data obtained with the models it is important to minimise any contribution from the mouse background. This can be achieved through the concomitant deletion of murine genes. The most advantageous

Table 7.1   Experimental approaches in the generation of humanised mouse models.

Gene deletion	• Allows the function of a specific gene or gene cluster in drug metabolism or toxicological response to be evaluated *Caveats*: Possible that data are confounded by compensatory changes in other genes
Reporter models	• Defines the effects of endogenous or exogenous factors on gene expression • Suitable for studies into gene regulation, disease pathogenesis, cellular response to stress and for *in vivo* drug efficacy screening
Approaches	*Random integration*: • Easy to achieve *Caveats*: Reporter activity may be compromised by genomic positional effects. Reporter often silenced. Reporter may not contain all of the regulatory genomic elements *Targeted integration into the Rosa 26 locus*: • Avoids positional effects but still loses genomic context • Suitable for studying the regulation of human gene promoters *Targeted integration into the gene locus of interest*: • Retains genomic context • Expression of the endogenous gene can be retained at least in part by the use of 2A sequences *Humanised models*: • Generate *in vivo* data more relevant to the human situation • Mice humanised for specific genes or gene clusters on an orthologous null murine background improve the quality of the data generated • Genomic constructs retain intron/exon structure and enhancer elements, with high conservation of cellular splicing machinery allowing expression of splice variants • Allow the regulation of the human genes to be studied

approach for such models is where the orthologous gene or genes have been deleted in the mouse. This can be achieved concomitantly with humanisation or by crossing the humanised mouse with a mouse carrying a deletion of the heterologous genes. The former approach is preferable for many reasons, particularly when complex/compound transgenics are being created.[18]

Examples of how these different experimental models can be used to study drug metabolism and pathways of chemical toxicity are described below.

7.3 Defining Drug Interactions with Human Nuclear Receptors and Other Transcription Factors

As described above, the enzymes involved in chemical detoxification provide an adaptive response to drug or environmental chemical challenge. These enzymes are subject to complex patterns of regulation, which at the transcriptional level are controlled by a number of xenosensing receptors, such as CAR, PXR, peroxisome proliferator-activated receptor-α (PPARα) and AhR. A single compound can, for example, activate multiple receptors, and an activated receptor can induce the expression of an overlapping panel of downstream genes involved in drug disposition. These include CYPs, Phase 2 enzymes as well as drug transporters (Figure 7.2). Receptor activation can have profound effects on drug exposure, the rate of generation of pharmacologically active or toxic metabolites. These interactions become more complex when patients are given multiple drugs concomitantly. Being able to predict the consequences of such interactions is an essential component of drug development and clinical drug use. Studies into these systems are also complicated by the marked species differences in the capacity of compounds to activate these receptors, making it difficult to extrapolate animal data to man. In addition, although there are a number of *in vitro* assays that allow the capacity of compounds to activate these receptors to be measured, it is clear that such data cannot always be extrapolated, either qualitatively or quantitatively, to the *in vivo* situation.[28-31] This difficulty has been at least in part addressed through the development of transgenic mice where the receptors, either alone or in combination, have either been deleted or humanised. This powerful approach allows the complexity of drug receptor interactions and their downstream consequences to be evaluated *in vivo* allowing human responses to drugs, when administered alone or in combination with other compounds, to be evaluated.[32]

The models created to date have primarily focussed on three receptors. CAR, which is activated indirectly by compounds such as phenobarbital or by direct acting ligands; PXR, which is regulated by rifampicin, and in mice and rats by pregnenolone-16α-carbonitrile (PCN) and dexamethasone; and AhR, which is activated by ligands such as polycyclic aromatic hydrocarbons (PAH) and dioxins. A further receptor, Nrf2, which is activated by electrophiles, regulates the expression of a number of detoxification enzymes such as glutathione S-transferases (GSTs), aldo-keto reductases and certain CYPs.[33] Nrf2

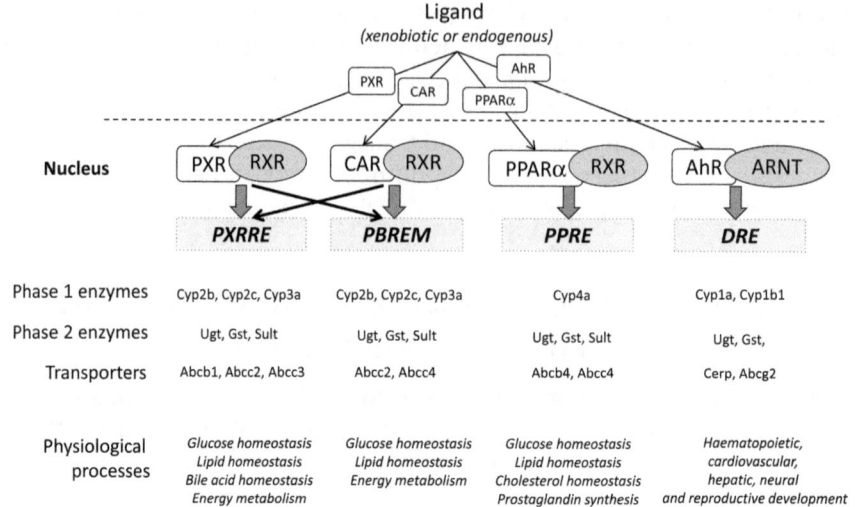

Figure 7.2   Nuclear receptors and regulation of Phase 1 and 2 drug metabolising enzymes, and drug transporters. Ligand-dependent activation of
nuclear receptors (and for CAR, also indirect activation) drives translocation to the nucleus and heterodimerisation with the retinoic
acid receptor (RXR) or arylhydrocarbon receptor nuclear translocator (ARNT), which binds to the corresponding response elements in
the promotors of target genes. In addition to inducing expression of
Phase 1 and 2 enzymes, and transporters, activated nuclear receptors
are also involved in regulating a number of physiological processes, a
selection of which are shown. Abcxx: ATP-binding cassette transporters;[119] DRE: dioxin response element; PBREM: phenobarbital response
element; PPRE: peroxisome proliferator response element; PXRRE: PXR
response; Sult: sulphotransferases. Adapted from Scheer and Wolf[17]
and Scheer *et al.*[18]

null mice have been created,[34] but humanised mice expressing this receptor
have not been reported.

   Receptor humanised or knockout mice have been used in a wide range of
studies, including drug induction, toxicological response and non-genotoxic
carcinogenesis, *etc.*[35–40] For example, a portfolio of knockout models has been
used to demonstrate that *in vivo* the activation of gene expression by phenobarbital is mediated almost exclusively by CAR in spite of the finding that
this compound can also activate PXR *in vitro*.[41,42] PXR humanised mice have
been used to demonstrate that the clinically observed hepatotoxicity of isoniazid when administered in conjunction with rifampicin is also observed in
humanised mice but not in wild-type animals.[43] Humanised receptor models
have also been used to study the ability of a range of anti-convulsive drugs
and non-genotoxic carcinogens to activate human CAR and or PXR (Henderson, C. J. and Wolf, C. R., unpublished). Non-genotoxic carcinogens cause
liver tumours in experimental animal models by a mechanism mediated by
nuclear receptors such as CAR, PPARα and possibly PXR.[44,45] In recent studies

it has been demonstrated that the non-genotoxic carcinogen phenobarbital can induce the same transcriptional, cell cycle and epigenetic changes in humanised CAR mice as in wild-type animals.[38] Indeed, long-term treatment of humanised CAR mice resulted in liver tumours, albeit at a reduced frequency to that observed in wild-type animals. These data provide evidence that the reported species differences in tumourigenicity are not due to the ability of phenobarbital to activate CAR.[35]

7.3.1 CAR and PXR

The transcription factors CAR and PXR control the expression of some key human drug metabolising enzymes such as CYP3A4 and CYP2B6, and the drug transporter ABCB1 (MDR1).[7] However, the extent to which different activators of CAR and PXR, or both, modulate the expression of these proteins and at what doses remains to a large degree undetermined. Mouse models humanised for both CAR and PXR as well as for the proteins regulated by them allows this to be established. Several mouse lines humanised for CYP3A4 have been created. Granvil *et al.* used random transgenesis with a bacterial artificial chromosome (BAC) containing the *CYP3A4* gene to create a mouse where hepatic expression was lacking but intestinal expression of CYP3A4 was robust, and both *in vitro* metabolism and *in vivo* pharmacokinetics of the CYP3A4 substrate midazolam were significantly changed compared with wild-type mice.[46] In a separate model, Cheung *et al.*, again using a BAC and a random transgenic approach, created a mouse model with both *CYP3A4* and *CYP3A7*, and ~10 kb of promotor sequence upstream of *CYP3A4* (including PXR regulatory elements),[47] which was further developed to include human PXR.[48] In this latter hPXR/CYP3A4 model, CYP3A4 expression was induced by the human-specific PXR ligand rifampicin, but not by the rodent-specific ligand PCN. More recently, another hCYP3A4 model has been made in which the *Cyp3a* gene cluster on chromosome 5 has been deleted and replaced with *CYP3A4* and *CYP3A7* from a BAC; this model has further been crossed with mice humanised for both CAR and PXR.[32] In addition to being subject to regulation by human transcription factors, this model has the additional advantage of a Cyp3a null background on which to investigate the role of CYP3A4 in drug metabolism and disposition.

In addition, a mouse has been made where the human *CYP2B6* gene containing ~20 kb of the promoter has been linked to the LacZ reporter. This model has been shown to be responsive to both CAR and PXR activators, and species specificity with regard to the nuclear receptors may also be determined. These experimental systems can be used for *in vivo* and *in vitro* experiments to establish whether a compound can activate CAR or PXR or both, and also the degree to which such activation changes the expression of these important drug metabolising enzymes in tissues such as the liver and gastrointestinal tract *in vivo*. These models can of course also be used to investigate other modes of *in vivo* regulation of these genes, for example by inflammation,[49,50] and in disease states such as diabetes and obesity (Figure 7.3).[51]

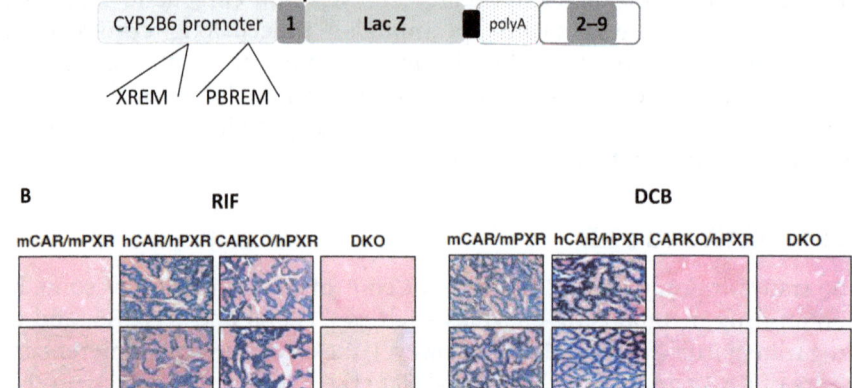

Figure 7.3 CYP2B6LacZ reporter. (A) A *lacZ* reporter gene construct (*lacZ* followed by a synthetic intron and polyadenylation motif) was cloned by Taconi-cArtemis GmbH (Cologne, Germany) onto the translational start ATG of exon 1 of *CYP2B6* in a BAC carrying the human *CYP2B6* gene locus (BAC RP11_203N14, ImaGenes GmbH, Berlin, Germany) by red/ET recombineering.[120] Approximately 20 kb of the *CYP2B6* promotor was present in the construct, including the xenobiotic response element module (XREM) at approximately −8.5 kb and the phenobarbital response element module at approximately −1.6 kb, which respond to PXR and CAR transcription factors, respectively.[121] CYP2B6LacZ reporter mice were generated by random transgenic insertion of the construct; heterozygous CYP2B6LacZ mice on a C57BL/6 background appeared indistinguishable from wild-type animals and had normal survival rates and fertility. (B) Liver sections stained for β-galactosidase activity from CYP-2B6LacZ reporter mice with endogenous CAR and PXR (mCAR/mPXR), a humanised CAR/PXR background (hCAR/hPXR), with CAR deleted and hPXR (CARKO/hPXR) or both CAR and PXR deleted (DKO) were treated with rifampicin (RIF; 10 mg kg⁻¹, intraperitoneal, 3 days) or 1,4-dichlorobenzene (DCB; 600 mg kg⁻¹, intraperitoneal, 3 days) (*Henderson, C. J. and Wolf, C. R., unpublished*).

A further model to measure CAR or PXR activation non-invasively has been developed where the luciferase reporter has been cloned into the CAR- and PXR-responsive murine *Cyp3a11* gene (Figure 7.4). This model allows the regulation of the reporters to be measured both invasively using Lac Z and non-invasively in real time by imaging.

An important species difference with CAR and PXR, and potential confounding factor, is that in humans these transcription factors are subject to alternative splicing, with splice variants being activated in response to different ligands.[52–54] Ross *et al.*, using double-humanised hCAR/hPXR mice, showed that the major CAR and PXR splice variants were not only generated in this model, but were found essentially in the same proportions as in human liver.[55]

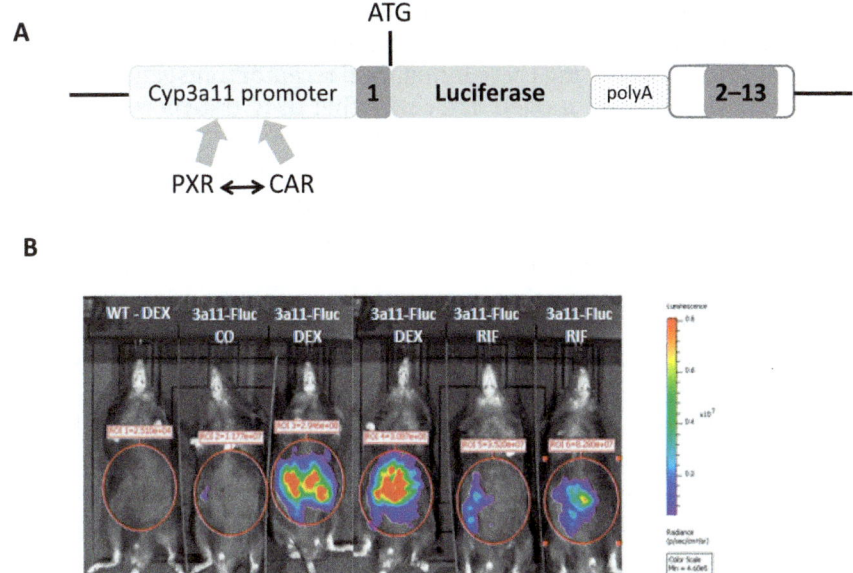

Figure 7.4 Cyp3a11Luc reporter. (A) A firefly luciferase gene was inserted into the *Cyp3a11* gene locus by homologous recombination, such that the reporter gene was fused to the transcriptional start ATG of the *Cyp3a11* gene. Exons 2–13 of the *Cyp3a11* gene are retained, but disruption of exon 1 results in inactivation of the endogenous *Cyp3a11* gene. Heterozygous Cyp3a11Luc mice bred and developed normally on a C57BL/6 background. (*Henderson, C. J. and Wolf, C. R., unpublished*). Both CAR and PXR have been shown to be involved in the regulation of Cyp3a11.[122,123] (B) Wild-type (WT) or Cyp3a11Luc (3a11-Fluc) mice were treated with vehicle [corn-oil (CO)] dexamethasone (DEX; 60 mg kg^{-1}, 3 days) or rifampicin (RIF; 60 mg kg^{-1}, 3 days) and imaged under anaesthesia for bioluminescence in an IVIS Caliper Lumina II according to the manufacturer's instructions (*Henderson, C. J. and Wolf, C. R., unpublished*). Scale on right-hand side illustrates relative bioluminescence, from blue (low) to red (high).

7.3.2 AhR

In the case of AhR, both null and humanised models have been described. AhR null mice are viable, but have early growth and hepatic defects, including reduced retinoic acid metabolism and hepatic accumulation of retinoids,[56–58] and AhR has also been implicated as a potential tumour suppressor gene.[59] More recent work has implicated AhR in the regulation of inflammatory responses.[60] A mouse line humanised for AhR was generated and exhibited a distinct response to TCDD in terms of gene regulation (including Cyp1a1/1a2 induction) compared with wild-type mice.[36,61–63]

One interesting recent finding is that in addition to regulating drug metabolising enzymes, AhR has been implicated in cardiac development and homeostasis,[64] and mediates the differentiation of T cells into Th17 cells.[65]

For further details of the role of AhR in T-cell biology and the immune system see the recent reviews by Ramsay and Cantrell[66] and Stockinger *et al.*[67]

In addition, mice carrying these humanised receptor transgenes have been crossed into humanised models carrying either drug transporters or CYPs, which has facilitated studies into whether drugs have the capacity to regulate the human genes associated with drug disposition (see below). The activation of both the nuclear AhR translocator and AhR, in addition to effecting drug disposition, can also play an essential role in pathways of chemical toxicity and carcinogenicity. For example, the induction of CYP enzymes responsible for the metabolic activation of chemicals can result in increased toxicity through AhR. On the other hand, activation of nuclear receptors such as CAR and possibly PXR results in epigenetic and hyperplastic responses in the liver that are a key factor in pathways of non-genotoxic carcinogenesis.[38,68] Therefore, mice that have been humanised for these receptors can be used to establish whether chemical compounds have the capacity to activate these pathways in a manner that may be indicative of potential harmful effects in man. This has been elegantly demonstrated in a paper by Moriguchi *et al.*, in which a hAhR knock-in mouse was used to investigate species differences in response to various AhR ligands, and the model was proposed as a platform to more confidently assess human responses to PAHs and related compounds.[63]

7.4   Defining the Role of CYPs in Drug Disposition

A range of *in vitro* methodologies is routinely used to establish the role of the CYP system, or indeed other pathways, in drug disposition. These include metabolic stability assays using rodent or human liver microsomal fractions, incubations with human hepatocytes and or recombinant human CYP enzymes, and drug transporter assays, *etc.* These data together with *in vivo* pharmacokinetic parameters in animals are used with *in silico* algorithms to predict pharmacokinetic parameters and levels of drug exposure in patients.

7.4.1   Transgenic Mouse Models with Deletion of POR

There are now a number of powerful *in vivo* transgenic models that can greatly increase the predictability of this paradigm and to make more informed predictions of drug exposure in man. These models also provide powerful genetically based models to define the role of the CYP system in pathways of chemical toxicity. In order to define the role of the CYP system a wide range of models have been developed were single or multiple CYP gene clusters have been deleted from the mouse (see below). In addition, a more general approach to this question has been achieved through the conditional deletion of CYP reductase (POR). This enzyme donates electrons to all of the CYPs involved in drug metabolism, and its deletion therefore inactivates all of the CYPs involved in drug disposition. Direct deletion of POR is embryonic lethal[69,70] so models have been developed where POR is inactivated in a tissue-specific manner postnatally using Cre recombinase-mediated gene excision. Tissue-specific and/or conditional POR deletions have been reported in the liver,[71,72] gastrointestinal tract,[73-75] cardiomyocytes[76] and renal proximal tubules.[77] Hepatic POR null mice have no overt phenotype and breed normally; however, they have enlarged, steatotic livers and increased expression of CYPs—inactive due to the absence of POR—regulated by unsaturated fatty acids *via* a CAR-dependent pathway.[73]

A number of methods for POR conditional deletion in the liver have been described, involving either the use of the albumin promoter to express Cre (constitutive deletion) or the *Cyp1a1* promoter[73,74] where Cre is activated by the administration of a Cyp1a1 inducing agent (conditional). The latter system has the advantage that the mice have functional POR until the *Cyp1a1* promotor is activated, adding an element of control to the system. These mouse models have been extensively used to define the role of hepatic CYP in drug disposition and chemical-induced toxicity.[78-85] A further strength of the Cyp1a1–Cre models is that depending on the Cyp1a1 inducing agent, or its dose, it is possible to obtain a POR deletion in either the liver or liver and gastrointestinal tract in the same animal model.[73,74] This provides a powerful approach to establish the role of hepatic or gastrointestinal metabolism in oral drug bioavailability.[74] By default, in the absence of CYP activity, these models also allow other pathways of drug disposition to be studied in a manner that is not confounded by Phase 1 metabolism. These models have also been used effectively to demonstrate the role of the CYP system in the metabolic activation of molecules to toxic products and also in pro-drug activation to pharmacological metabolites. Some applications of the POR null models in drug efficacy and preclinical drug development studies are listed in Table 7.2.

7.4.2 Transgenic Mouse Models with CYP Gene Deletions

More recently, further transgenic models have been developed where murine CYP genes or gene clusters have been deleted from the mouse genome. This provides an elegant approach to understand whether a particular CYP gene family is involved in drug disposition and also, in cases where multiple gene cluster knockouts have been created, whether the CYP *per se* is important in drug elimination. In this latter case the CYP system has been deleted in all tissues of the mouse and therefore there are no functional CYPs of the gene families involved in any tissue or cell type. A recent paper[86] described the deletion of all of the CYPs in the *Cyp2c*, *Cyp2d* and *Cyp3a* gene families, a total of 30 genes. A five drug cocktail of CYP isozyme probe substrates was used to demonstrate the utility of this model for the study of the CYP system in drug metabolism and efficacy, and chemical toxicity. Interestingly, these mice are viable and breed normally, suggesting that those CYPs involved in drug metabolism in the mouse have no critical housekeeping functions. A further model, which also includes the deletion of the *Cyp1a1* and *Cyp1a2*

Table 7.2   Applications of POR null models.

Example	Citation	Comment
Drug efficacy and toxicity	G. J. Pass, *et al.*, *Cancer Res.*, 2005, **65**, 4211–4217 [124]	Cyclophosphamide toxicokinetics
	C. J. Henderson, *Toxicol. Lett.*, 2006, **13**, 853–858 [125]	
	J. Gu, *et al.*, *J. Pharmacol. Exp. Ther.*, 2007, **321**, 91–97 [126]	
	Q. Y. Zhang, *et al.*, *Drug Metab. Dispos.*, 2007, **35**, 1617–1623 [127]	Role of small intestinal CYP in the bioavailability of oral nifedipine
	Q. Y. Zhang, *et al.*, *Drug Metab. Dispos.*, 2009, **37**, 651–657 [75]	
	Y. Weng, *et al.*, *Cancer Res.*, 2007, **67**, 7825–7832 [128]	Pulmonary CYP plays a major role in 4-(methylnitrosamino)-1-(3-pyridyl)-1-butanone (NNK)-induced lung cancer
	C. Fang, *et al.*, *Toxicol. Appl. Pharmacol.*, 2008, **227**, 48–55 [129]	Chloroform and renal toxicity
	C. Fang, *et al.*, *Drug Metab. Dispos.*, 2008, **36**, 1722–1728 [76]	Doxorubicin and cardiac toxicity
	A. Grimsley, *et al.*, *Biochem. Pharmacol.*, 2014, **92**, 701–711 [130]	Midazolam metabolism
	K. Pickup, *et al.*, *Xenobiotica*, 2014, **44**, 164–173 [131]	Fenclozic acid metabolism
	K. Pickup, *et al.*, *Xenobiotica*, 2012, **42**, 195–205 [132]	Diclofenac metabolism
	M. Stiborova, *Neuroendocrinol. Lett.*, 2013, **34**, 43–54 [85]	Role of hepatic CYPs in activation of the anti-cancer drug ellipticine
	V. Megaraj, *et al.*, *Chem. Res. Toxicol.*, 2014, **27**, 656–662 [133]	Bioactivation of azoxymethane
Preclinical drug development	A. Potega, *et al.*, *Drug Metab. Dispos.*, 2011, **39**, 1423–1432 [134]	Metabolism of an C-1311, imidazoacridinone anti-tumour drug
Safety	V. M. Arlt, *et al.*, *Toxicol. Res.*, 2015, **4**, 548–562 [79]	Metabolism, toxicity and carcinogenicity of environmental pollutants
Other	C. Kunne, *et al.*, *Lab. Invest.*, 2014, **94**, 1103–1113 [135]	Role of CYPs in hepatic steatosis and cholestasis
	C. Kunne, *et al.*, *Biochim. Biophys. Acta*, 2014, **1842**, 739–746 [136]	
	Y. Zhu, *et al.*, *J. Pharmacol. Exp. Ther.*, 2015, **354**, 10–17 [137]	Role of intestinal CYPs in dextran sulphate-induced colitis

genes, has recently been developed and is currently being characterised (Henderson, Scheer, Rode, Kapelyukh and Wolf, unpublished). In such models it is important to note that in certain cases, such as the *Cyp3a* gene cluster knockout, there are compensatory changes resulting in the increased expression of members of the *Cyp2c* gene cluster, *e.g. Cyp2c55*. For this reason, compound knockout or humanisations are often significantly more informative (see below).

7.4.3 Mice Humanised for CYP Enzymes

The species differences both in the functionality and multiplicity of CYP enzymes between rodents and humans complicates the extrapolation of rodent data to man. Whereas in mice 30–40 proteins appear to be involved in Phase 1 metabolism, in humans 5 enzymes account for more than 90% of CYP-mediated drug disposition[1,87] (Figure 7.5). This has the consequence that rates of metabolism, sites of drug oxidation and also the gene families involved are different between rodents and humans, both qualitatively and quantitatively. A large number of mouse lines have now been described that have been humanised for individual CYP enzymes or human CYP gene clusters. In early models mice were humanised for a particular CYP enzyme without concomitant deletion of their murine counterparts.[46,88,89] This made the interpretation of pharmacokinetic data using these models challenging. More recently the humanisations have involved the introduction of the human genes with concomitant deletion of the murine counterparts.[32,90–92] Table 7.3 shows the models that have been created to date. Some of these,

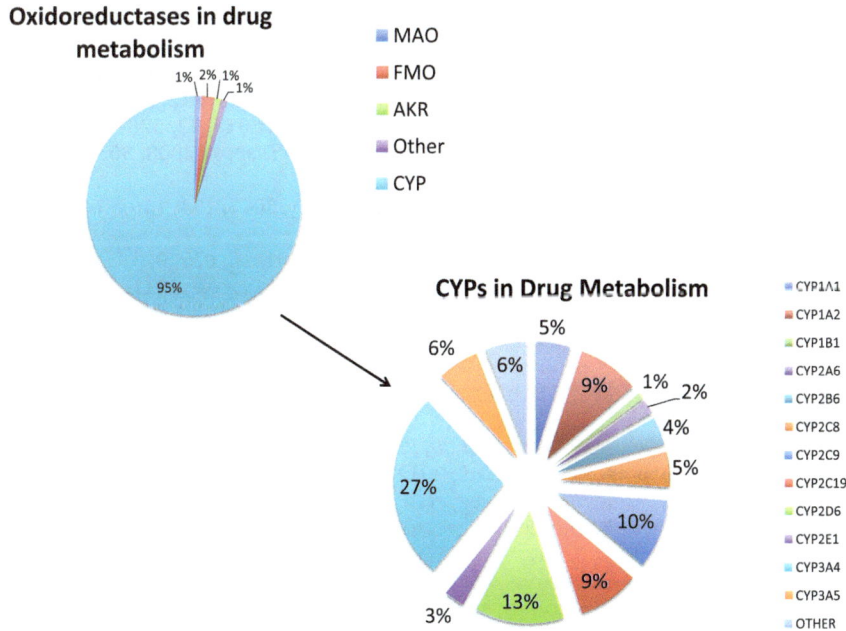

Figure 7.5 Involvement of human CYPs in drug metabolism. Involvement of human oxidoreductase enzymes in the metabolism of drugs (marketed and under development as at 2014), and further breakdown of CYP data into specific enzymes. Adapted and based on data from Rendic and Guengerich.[1]

Table 7.3 Humanised mouse models of drug metabolism and disposition.

Human gene	Recent selected references
Nuclear receptors	
AhR	C. A. Flaveny, & G. H. Perdew, *Mol. Cell. Pharmacol.*, 2009, **1**, 119–123 [36]
CAR	N. Scheer, *et al.*, *J. Clin. Invest.*, 2008, **118**, 3228–3239 [40]
PXR	J. Cheng, *et al.*, *J. Pharmacol. Exp. Ther.*, 2014, **351**, 559–567 [138]
CAR/PXR	R. Luisier, *et al.*, *Toxicol. Sci.*, 2014, **139**, 501–511 [38]
	A. Braeuning, *et al.*, *Toxicol. Sci.*, 2014, **240**, 259–270 [35]
	S. Y. Lee, *et al.*, *Toxicol. Lett.*, 2015, **235**, 107–115 [139]
PPARα	Y. Ito, *et al.*, PPAR Res., 2012, 201284
Phase 1 drug metabolising enzymes	
CYP1A1/1A2	S. Uno, *et al.*, *Toxicol. Appl. Pharmacol.*, 2011, **237**, 119–126 [140]
CYP1B1	D. Y. Hwang, *et al.*, *Int. J. Toxicol.*, 2007, **26**, 71–80 [141]
CYP2A6	Q. Y. Zhang, *et al.*, *Biochem. Biophys. Res. Commun.*, 2005, **338**, 318–324 [142]
CYP2A13	K. Jia, *et al.*, *Drug Metab. Dispos.*, 2014, **42**, 1341–1348 [143]
CYP2A13/2B6/2F1	Y. Wei, *et al.*, *Drug Metab. Dispos.*, 2012, **40**, 1144–1150 [144]
CYP2B6	Z. Liu, *et al.*, *Drug Metab. Dispos.*, 2015, **43**, 208–216 [145]
CYP2C9	N. Scheer, *et al.*, *Mol. Pharmacol.*, 2012, **82**, 1022–1029 [91]
CYP2C18/2C19	S. Löfgren, *et al.*, *Acta Vet Scand.*, 2008, **50**, 47 [146]
CYP2D6	C. J. Henderson, *et al.*, *Mol. Pharmacol.*, 2015, **87**, 733–739 [93]
	X. Pan, & H. Jeong, *Mol. Pharmacol.*, 2015, **88**, 106–112 [147]
CYP2E1	J. Cheng, *et al.*, *Int. J. Cancer*, 2013, **135**, 37–47 [148]
CYP3A4	M. Hasegawa, *et al.*, *Mol. Pharmacol.*, 2011, **80**, 518–528 [32]
	J. J. Hendrikx, *et al.*, *Int. J. Cancer*, 2013, **312**, 1649–1655 [148]
CYP3A4/3A5/3A7/3A43	Y. Kazuki, *et al.*, *Hum. Mol. Genet.*, 2013, **22**, 578–592 [149]
CYP3A4/2D6	M. A. Felmell, *et al.*, *Drug Metab. Dispos.*, 2008, **36**, 435–441 [150]
CYP3A7	X. Y. Pang, *et al.*, Endocrinology, 2012, **153**, 1453–1463 [151]
Phase 2 drug metabolising enzymes	
GSTP1	M. P. Vaughn, *et al.*, *PLoS One*, 2011, **6**, e25707 [108]
NAT2	K. S. Sugamori, *et al.*, *Drug Metab. Dispos.*, 2011, **39**, 882–890 [107]
UGT1A	Y. Kutsuno, *et al.*, *Pharmacol. Res. Perspect.*, 2013, **1**, e00002 [110]
UGT2B7	M. F. Yueh, *et al.*, *Mol. Pharmacol.*, 2011, **79**, 1053–1060 [105]
Drug transporters	
ABCB1	M. W. Sadiq, *et al.*, *PLoS One*, 2015, **10**, e0118638 [152]
ABCC2	N. Scheer, *et al.*, 2012, **40**, 2212–2218 [153]
OATP1A2/1B1/1B3	E. Van de Steeg, *et al.*, *Clin. Can Res.*, 2013, **19**, 821–832 [154]
OATP1B1	E. Van de Steeg, *et al.*, *Drug Metab. Dispos.*, 2009, **37**, 77–81 [155]
OATP1B3	S. Durmus, *et al.*, *Int. J. Cancer*, 2014, **135**, 1700–1710 [156]
OATP1B1/1B3	L. Salphati, *et al.*, *Drug Metab. Dispos.*, 2014, **42**, 1301–1313 [157]
Composite models	
PXR/CYP3A4	N. Holmstock, *et al.*, *Mol. Pharmacol.*, 2013, **10**, 1056–1062 [158]
CAR/PXR/CYP3A4/3A7	M. Hasegawa, *et al.*, *Mol. Pharmacol.*, 2011, **80**, 518–528 [32]
hCAR/hPXR/hCYP2C9/ hCYP2D6/ hCYP3A4/3A7	N. Scheer, *et al.*, *Drug Metab. Dispos.*, 2015, in press [94]

for example the *CYP2D6* humanisation combined with the *Cyp2d* gene cluster knockout, reflect the human genetic polymorphism at this gene locus.[92] Humanised models such as this have been used in a wide range of studies, including investigations into pathways of anti-cancer drug disposition,[93] drug–drug interactions,[32] as well as for research into pathways of drug-induced hepatotoxicity.[88]

Recently, more complex models of humanisation have been developed. These have involved the introduction of multiple human CYPs with concomitant deletion of the orthologous murine gene clusters on a humanised CAR and PXR background. A mouse model has recently been created expressing human CYP2C9/2D6/3A4 and CYP3A7 on a hCAR/PXR background, with the corresponding mouse orthologous genes or gene clusters deleted, *i.e.* where essentially all the major pathways of Phase 1 metabolism are human.[94] In a further development of this model, a mouse line has been generated that is additionally nulled for AhR and Cyp1a1/1a2, and humanised for these genes (unpublished). The significant advantage of such models is that essentially all of the murine CYP genes involved in drug disposition have been deleted and as a consequence the possibility that compensatory changes in murine Phase 1 enzymes confound data interpretation is greatly reduced. Also, the complex models allow the metabolism of drugs down multiple pathways by different CYPs *in vivo* to be investigated, including the generation of human-specific primary and secondary metabolites. In addition, because most of the CYPs are expressed off their own promoters, with the exception of *CYP2C9*, and the mice are humanised for CAR and PXR, the effects of drugs when administered alone or in combination on the level of expression of these enzymes and the possible consequences for drug–drug interactions or drug efficacy can be evaluated. It has recently been shown (2010 figures for the Tayside region of Scotland, UK) that almost 10% of patients over the age of 60 years take more than 10 drugs a day, rising to nearly 20% for the over-70s, and 24% for people aged 80 or above.[95] The potential for drug–drug interactions or loss of efficacy is therefore very high, with almost half of all patients aged 70 or over experiencing at least one drug–drug interaction, and those in their 80s with more than a 7-fold greater risk of experiencing a drug–drug interactions compared with patients aged 20–29 years. This clinical problem becomes even more important in the treatment of diseases such as cancer where the treatments can cause serious life-threatening side-effects. Indeed, many of the emerging anti-cancer drugs are substrates for both CYPs and drug transporters, or for example in the case of the new biological agents, have the potential to alter CYP gene expression. It is inconceivable to study the potential for complex drug–drug interactions of this nature in clinical trials; the humanised models will allow such complex interactions in relation to dosing regimen, exposure, *etc.*, to be investigated and used to identify where clinical problems are likely to occur. With the increase in polypharmacy there is an urgent need for such studies. These systems can also be employed to establish how the variability in drug exposure seen in patients may affect therapeutic outcome.

Table 7.4   Potential uses of complex humanised models.

Drug disposition	• The role of drug metabolizing enzymes in tissue distribution, drug bioavailability and clearance, without interference from murine enzymes • Opportunity to establish the effect of polymorphic variants on drug disposition
Drug–drug interactions	• Inhibition and induction studies in relation to drug–drug interactions
Safety assessment	• Generation of human-specific metabolite profiles from multiple metabolic pathways • Improved predictability and human relevance in short- or long-term assays for chemical toxicity or carcinogenicity
Regulation	• Expression of drug metabolising enzymes in relation to disease aetiology • Regulation of drug metabolising enzyme expression at mRNA and protein level • Role of human nuclear receptors, *i.e.* CAR, PXR and AhR, in the regulation of human drug metabolising enzymes *in vivo*
Efficacy screening	• More effective extrapolation of pharmacokinetic/pharmacodynamic relationships to man

Mouse models, including transgenic lines, are often used in drug development to establish the efficacy of new drug treatments. In these cases, the murine drug metabolising enzymes determine drug exposure. Also, chronic drug administration in such studies can induce drug disposition though the activation of Car or Pxr. This can significantly affect drug exposure, for example in anti-tumour xenograft studies, and therefore the outcome of the study. The use of humanised models will establish whether this might be a factor in the clinical use of the drug in man. One further potential application in cancer therapy is based on the current interest in using patient derived tumours grown in mice (patient-derived xenografts) to identify the therapies that are most likely to be efficacious. Based on the above discussion there is now the potential to improve the predictive value of this approach through the use of mice humanised for drug metabolism. Some of the potential uses of the complex humanised models are listed in Table 7.4.

7.5   Humanised and Null Mouse Models for Phase 2 Metabolising Enzymes

A number of mouse models have been generated where specific Phase 2 metabolising enzymes have been deleted from the mouse genome. This includes a number of GSTs (reviewed by Henderson and Wolf[96]), sulphotransferases,[97] *N*-acetyltransferase (NAT)[98–102] and UDP glucuronyl transferases (UGT).[103] However, to our knowledge the only models that have been humanised in this respect have been the *UGT1A* and *2B* gene families by the group led by Tukey;[104,105] NAT2 [106,107] and mice humanised for GSTP1 have also been reported.[108] In the case of the *UGT1* gene family a mouse model was created expressing a BAC encoding the entire human *UGT1* locus and validated using the anti-epileptic drug lamotrigine, metabolized primarily by UGT1A4 [109] and a number of other drugs that were subject to human-specific glucuronidation.[110,111] The Tukey laboratory went on to show that PXR is a key regulator of glucuronidation during pregnancy,[112] and developed a further humanised UGT model, for UGT2B7, also demonstrating a role for CAR in inhibiting UGT2B7 expression.[105] Humanisation for NAT2 was carried out on a murine Nat null background, using the albumin promotor to drive liver-specific expression of NAT2; metabolism of the NAT2-selective substrate sulfamethazine was 40–80-fold higher in the humanised mice compared with wild-type animals.[107] Vaughn *et al.*[108] generated a mouse line in which human GSTP1 was expressed on a Gstp1/p2 null background,[113] and not only showed that expression of the human enzyme was recapitulated in the liver and prostate, but also that patterns of methylation in the promotor were similar to those observed in humans.

7.6 Humanised and Null Mouse Models for Drug Transporters

As mentioned earlier in the text, animal models that have been nulled or humanised for drug transporters will not be covered in this chapter. Selected recent references to models that have been generated are given in Table 7.3, and further reading is recommended as follows: ABCB1,[114] ABCC2 [115] and OATP1A2/1B1/1B3.[116-118]

Acknowledgements

The authors gratefully acknowledge Taconic Biosciences for the generation of the humanised mouse models.

References

1. S. P. Rendic and F. P. Guengerich, *Chem. Res. Toxicol.*, 2015, **28**, 38–42.
2. P. Jancova, P. Anzenbacher and E. Anzenbacherova, *Biomed. Pap.*, 2010, **154**, 103–116.
3. B. Doring and E. Petzinger, *Drug Metab. Rev.*, 2014, **46**, 261–282.
4. F. Montanari and G. F. Ecker, *Adv. Drug Delivery Rev.*, 2015, **86**, 17–26.
5. P. Pavek and Z. Dvorak, *Curr. Drug Metab.*, 2008, **9**, 129–143.
6. P. Pavek and T. Smutny, *Drug Metab. Rev.*, 2014, **46**, 19–32.
7. L. A. Stanley, B. C. Horsburgh, J. Ross, N. Scheer and C. R. Wolf, *Drug Metab. Rev.*, 2006, **38**, 515–597.
8. J. Tian, Y. Feng, H. Fu, H. Q. Xie, J. X. Jiang and B. Zhao, *Environ. Sci. Technol.*, 2015, **49**, 9518–9531.

9. C. J. Omiecinski, J. P. Vanden Heuvel, G. H. Perdew and J. M. Peters, *Toxicol. Sci.*, 2011, **120**(Suppl 1), S49–S75.

10. L. Hutchinson and R. Kirk, *Nat. Rev. Clin. Oncol.*, 2011, **8**, 189–190.

11. I. Kola and J. Landis, *Nat. Rev. Drug Discovery*, 2004, **3**, 711–715.

12. M. J. Waring, J. Arrowsmith, A. R. Leach, P. D. Leeson, S. Mandrell, R. M. Owen, G. Pairaudeau, W. D. Pennie, S. D. Pickett, J. Wang, O. Wallace and A. Weir, *Nat. Rev. Drug Discovery*, 2015, **14**, 475–486.

13. C. R. Wolf, *Toxicol. Lett.*, 2002, **127**, 3–17.

14. S. C. Sim, M. Kacevska and M. Ingelman-Sundberg, *Pharmacogenomics J.*, 2013, **13**, 1–11.

15. L. Di, B. Feng, T. C. Goosen, Y. Lai, S. J. Steyn, M. V. Varma and R. S. Obach, *Drug Metab. Dispos.*, 2013, **41**, 1975–1993.

16. J. Yu, T. K. Ritchie, A. Mulgaonkar and I. Ragueneau-Majlessi, *Drug Metab. Dispos.*, 2014, **42**, 1991–2001.

17. N. Scheer and C. Roland Wolf, *Drug Metab. Rev.*, 2013, **45**, 110–121.

18. N. Scheer, M. Snaith, C. R. Wolf and J. Seibler, *Drug Discovery Today*, 2013, **18**, 1200–1211.

19. N. Scheer and C. R. Wolf, *Xenobiotica*, 2014, **44**, 96–108.

20. H. Bouabe and K. Okkenhaug, *Methods Mol. Biol.*, 2013, **1064**, 315–336.

21. T. Mashimo, *Dev., Growth Differ.*, 2014, **56**, 46–52.

22. R. Mortensen, *Current protocols in molecular biology*, ed. F. M. Ausubel, *et al.*, 2006, ch. 23, unit 23 21.

23. F. J. Sanchez-Rivera and T. Jacks, *Nat. Rev. Cancer*, 2015, **15**, 387–395.

24. S. Turan, C. Zehe, J. Kuehle, J. Qiao and J. Bode, *Gene*, 2013, **515**, 1–27.

25. G. D. Van Duyne, *Microbiol. Spectrum*, 2015, **3**, DOI: 10.1128/microbiolspec. MDNA3-0014-2014.

26. P. Soriano, *Nat. Genet.*, 1999, **21**, 70–71.

27. E. Minskaia and M. D. Ryan, *BioMed Res. Int.*, 2013, **2013**, 291730.

28. S. Alqahtani, L. A. Mohamed and A. Kaddoumi, *Expert Opin. Drug Metab. Toxicol.*, 2013, **9**, 1241–1254.

29. L. Di, *Expert Opin. Drug Metab. Toxicol.*, 2014, **10**, 379–393.

30. D. Hallifax and J. B. Houston, *Curr. Drug Metab.*, 2009, **10**, 307–321.

31. R. Li, H. A. Barton and M. V. Varma, *Clin. Pharmacokinet.*, 2014, **53**, 659–678.

32. M. Hasegawa, Y. Kapelyukh, H. Tahara, J. Seibler, A. Rode, S. Krueger, D. N. Lee, C. R. Wolf and N. Scheer, *Mol. Pharmacol.*, 2011, **80**, 518–528.

33. J. D. Hayes and A. T. Dinkova-Kostova, *Trends Biochem. Sci.*, 2014, **39**, 199–218.

34. K. Chan, R. Lu, J. C. Chang and Y. W. Kan, *Proc. Natl. Acad. Sci. U. S. A.*, 1996, **93**, 13943–13948.

35. A. Braeuning, A. Gavrilov, S. Brown, C. R. Wolf, C. J. Henderson and M. Schwarz, *Toxicol. Sci.*, 2014, **140**, 259–270.

36. C. A. Flaveny and G. H. Perdew, *Mol. Cell. Pharmacol.*, 2009, **1**, 119–123.

37. F. J. Gonzalez, P. Fernandez-Salguero, S. S. Lee, T. Pineau and J. M. Ward, *Toxicol. Lett.*, 1995, **82–83**, 117–121.

38. R. Luisier, H. Lempiainen, N. Scherbichler, A. Braeuning, M. Geissler, V. Dubost, A. Muller, N. Scheer, S. D. Chibout, H. Hara, F. Picard, D. Theil,

P. Couttet, A. Vitobello, O. Grenet, B. Grasl-Kraupp, H. Ellinger-Ziegelbauer, J. P. Thomson, R. R. Meehan, C. R. Elcombe, C. J. Henderson, C. R. Wolf, M. Schwarz, P. Moulin, R. Terranova and J. G. Moggs, *Toxicol. Sci.*, 2014, **139**, 501–511.

39. N. Scheer, J. Ross, Y. Kapelyukh, A. Rode and C. R. Wolf, *Drug Metab. Dispos.*, 2010, **38**, 1046–1053.

40. N. Scheer, J. Ross, A. Rode, B. Zevnik, S. Niehaves, N. Faust and C. R. Wolf, *J. Clin. Invest.*, 2008, **118**, 3228–3239.

41. J. M. Lehmann, D. D. McKee, M. A. Watson, T. M. Willson, J. T. Moore and S. A. Kliewer, *J. Clin. Invest.*, 1998, **102**, 1016–1023.

42. Z. Zhu, S. Kim, T. Chen, J. H. Lin, A. Bell, J. Bryson, Y. Dubaquie, N. Yan, J. Yanchunas, D. Xie, R. Stoffel, M. Sinz and K. Dickinson, *J. Biomol. Screening*, 2004, **9**, 533–540.

43. F. Li, J. Lu, J. Cheng, L. Wang, T. Matsubara, I. L. Csanaky, C. D. Klaassen, F. J. Gonzalez and X. Ma, *Nat. Med.*, 2013, **19**, 418–420.

44. V. Tamasi, P. Juvan, M. Beer, D. Rozman and U. A. Meyer, *Mol. Pharmaceutics*, 2009, **6**, 1573–1581.

45. Y. Yamamoto, R. Moore, T. L. Goldsworthy, M. Negishi and R. R. Maronpot, *Cancer Res.*, 2004, **64**, 7197–7200.

46. C. P. Granvil, A. M. Yu, G. Elizondo, T. E. Akiyama, C. Cheung, L. Feigenbaum, K. W. Krausz and F. J. Gonzalez, *Drug Metab. Dispos.*, 2003, **31**, 548–558.

47. C. Cheung, A. M. Yu, C. S. Chen, K. W. Krausz, L. G. Byrd, L. Feigenbaum, R. J. Edwards, D. J. Waxman and F. J. Gonzalez, *J. Pharmacol. Exp. Ther.*, 2006, **316**, 1328–1334.

48. X. Ma, C. Cheung, K. W. Krausz, Y. M. Shah, T. Wang, J. R. Idle and F. J. Gonzalez, *Drug Metab. Dispos.*, 2008, **36**, 2506–2512.

49. Y. Kusunoki, N. Ikarashi, Y. Hayakawa, M. Ishii, R. Kon, W. Ochiai, Y. Machida and K. Sugiyama, *Eur. J. Pharm. Sci.*, 2014, **54**, 17–27.

50. P. Shah, T. Guo, D. D. Moore and R. Ghose, *Drug Metab. Dispos.*, 2014, **42**, 172–181.

51. J. He, J. Gao, M. Xu, S. Ren, M. Stefanovic-Racic, R. M. O'Doherty and W. Xie, *Diabetes*, 2013, **62**, 1876–1887.

52. J. G. DeKeyser, E. M. Laurenzana, E. C. Peterson, T. Chen and C. J. Omiecinski, *Toxicol. Sci.*, 2011, **120**, 381–391.

53. J. K. Lamba, V. Lamba, K. Yasuda, Y. S. Lin, M. Assem, E. Thompson, S. Strom and E. Schuetz, *J. Pharmacol. Exp. Ther.*, 2004, **311**, 811–821.

54. V. Lamba, K. Yasuda, J. K. Lamba, M. Assem, J. Davila, S. Strom and E. G. Schuetz, *Toxicol. Appl. Pharmacol.*, 2004, **199**, 251–265.

55. J. Ross, S. M. Plummer, A. Rode, N. Scheer, C. C. Bower, O. Vogel, C. J. Henderson, C. R. Wolf and C. R. Elcombe, *Toxicol. Sci.*, 2010, **116**, 452–466.

56. F. Andreola, P. M. Fernandez-Salguero, M. V. Chiantore, M. P. Petkovich, F. J. Gonzalez and L. M. De Luca, *Cancer Res.*, 1997, **57**, 2835–2838.

57. F. J. Gonzalez and P. Fernandez-Salguero, *Drug Metab. Dispos.*, 1998, **26**, 1194–1198.

58. J. V. Schmidt, G. H. Su, J. K. Reddy, M. C. Simon and C. A. Bradfield, *Proc. Natl. Acad. Sci. U. S. A.*, 1996, **93**, 6731–6736.

59. Y. Fan, G. P. Boivin, E. S. Knudsen, D. W. Nebert, Y. Xia and A. Puga, *Cancer Res.*, 2010, **70**, 212–220.

60. P. Di Meglio, J. H. Duarte, H. Ahlfors, N. D. Owens, Y. Li, F. Villanova, I. Tosi, K. Hirota, F. O. Nestle, U. Mrowietz, M. J. Gilchrist and B. Stockinger, *Immunity*, 2014, **40**, 989–1001.

61. C. A. Flaveny, I. A. Murray, C. R. Chiaro and G. H. Perdew, *Mol. Pharmacol.*, 2009, **75**, 1412–1420.

62. C. A. Flaveny, I. A. Murray and G. H. Perdew, *Toxicol. Sci.*, 2010, **114**, 217–225.

63. T. Moriguchi, H. Motohashi, T. Hosoya, O. Nakajima, S. Takahashi, S. Ohsako, Y. Aoki, N. Nishimura, C. Tohyama, Y. Fujii-Kuriyama and M. Yamamoto, *Proc. Natl. Acad. Sci. U. S. A.*, 2003, **100**, 5652–5657.

64. V. S. Carreira, Y. Fan, Q. Wang, X. Zhang, H. Kurita, C. I. Ko, M. Natichioni, M. Jiang, S. Koch, M. Medvedovic, Y. Xia, J. Rubinstein and A. Puga, *Toxicol. Sci.*, 2015, DOI: 10.1093/toxsci/kfv138.

65. N. Gagliani, M. C. Vesely, A. Iseppon, L. Brockmann, H. Xu, N. W. Palm, M. R. de Zoete, P. Licona-Limon, R. S. Paiva, T. Ching, C. Weaver, X. Zi, X. Pan, R. Fan, L. X. Garmire, M. J. Cotton, Y. Drier, B. Bernstein, J. Geginat, B. Stockinger, E. Esplugues, S. Huber and R. A. Flavell, *Nature*, 2015, **523**, 221–225.

66. G. Ramsay and D. Cantrell, *Front. Immunol.*, 2015, **6**, 99.

67. B. Stockinger, P. Di Meglio, M. Gialitakis and J. H. Duarte, *Annu. Rev. Immunol.*, 2014, **32**, 403–432.

68. J. P. Thomson, J. G. Moggs, C. R. Wolf and R. R. Meehan, *Mutat. Res., Genet. Toxicol. Environ. Mutagen.*, 2014, **764–765**, 3–9.

69. D. M. Otto, C. J. Henderson, D. Carrie, M. Davey, T. E. Gundersen, R. Blomhoff, R. H. Adams, C. Tickle and C. R. Wolf, *Mol. Cell. Biol.*, 2003, **23**, 6103–6116.

70. V. Ribes, D. M. Otto, L. Dickmann, K. Schmidt, B. Schuhbaur, C. Henderson, R. Blomhoff, C. R. Wolf, C. Tickle and P. Dolle, *Dev. Biol.*, 2007, **303**, 66–81.

71. J. Gu, Y. Weng, Q. Y. Zhang, H. Cui, M. Behr, L. Wu, W. Yang, L. Zhang and X. Ding, *J. Biol. Chem.*, 2003, **278**, 25895–25901.

72. C. J. Henderson, D. M. Otto, D. Carrie, M. A. Magnuson, A. W. McLaren, I. Rosewell and C. R. Wolf, *J. Biol. Chem.*, 2003, **278**, 13480–13486.

73. R. D. Finn, A. W. McLaren, D. Carrie, C. J. Henderson and C. R. Wolf, *J. Pharmacol. Exp. Ther.*, 2007, **322**, 40–47.

74. C. J. Henderson, L. A. McLaughlin, M. Osuna-Cabello, M. Taylor, I. Gilbert, A. W. McLaren and C. R. Wolf, *Biochem. J.*, 2015, **465**, 479–488.

75. Q. Y. Zhang, C. Fang, J. Zhang, D. Dunbar, L. Kaminsky and X. Ding, *Drug Metab. Dispos.*, 2009, **37**, 651–657.

76. C. Fang, J. Gu, F. Xie, M. Behr, W. Yang, E. D. Abel and X. Ding, *Drug Metab. Dispos.*, 2008, **36**, 1722–1728.

77. S. Liu, Y. Yao, S. Lu, K. Aldous, X. Ding, C. Mei and J. Gu, *Toxicol. Appl. Pharmacol.*, 2013, **272**, 230–237.
78. V. M. Arlt, C. J. Henderson, C. R. Wolf, H. H. Schmeiser, D. H. Phillips and M. Stiborova, *Cancer Lett.*, 2006, **234**, 220–231.
79. V. M. Arlt, C. J. Henderson, C. R. Wolf, M. Stiborova and D. H. Phillips, *Toxicol. Res.*, 2015, **4**, 548–562.
80. V. M. Arlt, M. C. Poirier, S. E. Sykes, K. John, M. Moserova, M. Stiborova, C. R. Wolf, C. J. Henderson and D. H. Phillips, *Toxicol. Lett.*, 2012, **213**, 160–166.
81. V. M. Arlt, M. Stiborova, C. J. Henderson, M. R. Osborne, C. A. Bieler, E. Frei, V. Martinek, B. Sopko, C. R. Wolf, H. H. Schmeiser and D. H. Phillips, *Cancer Res.*, 2005, **65**, 2644–2652.
82. K. Levova, M. Moserova, V. Kotrbova, M. Sulc, C. J. Henderson, C. R. Wolf, D. H. Phillips, E. Frei, H. H. Schmeiser, J. Mares, V. M. Arlt and M. Stiborova, *Toxicol. Sci.*, 2011, **121**, 43–56.
83. M. Stiborova, V. M. Arlt, C. J. Henderson, C. R. Wolf, V. Kotrbova, M. Moserova, J. Hudecek, D. H. Phillips and E. Frei, *Toxicol. Appl. Pharmacol.*, 2008, **226**, 318–327.
84. M. Stiborova, V. M. Arlt, D. H. Phillips, C. J. Henderson, C. R. Wolf, P. Hodek, J. Hudecek and E. Frei, *Proceedings of the 15th International Conference on Cytochromes P450-Biochemistry, Biophysics and Functional Genomics*, 2007, pp. 129–133.
85. M. Stiborova, V. Cerna, M. Moserova, V. M. Arlt and E. Frei, *Neuroendocrinol. Lett.*, 2013, **34**, 43–54.
86. N. Scheer, L. A. McLaughlin, A. Rode, A. K. Macleod, C. J. Henderson and C. R. Wolf, *Drug Metab. Dispos.*, 2014, **42**, 1022–1030.
87. F. P. Guengerich, *Chem. Res. Toxicol.*, 2008, **21**, 70–83.
88. C. Cheung, A. M. Yu, J. M. Ward, K. W. Krausz, T. E. Akiyama, L. Feigenbaum and F. J. Gonzalez, *Drug Metab. Dispos.*, 2005, **33**, 449–457.
89. J. Corchero, C. P. Granvil, T. E. Akiyama, G. P. Hayhurst, S. Pimprale, L. Feigenbaum, J. R. Idle and F. J. Gonzalez, *Mol. Pharmacol.*, 2001, **60**, 1260–1267.
90. C. Cheung, X. Ma, K. W. Krausz, S. Kimura, L. Feigenbaum, T. P. Dalton, D. W. Nebert, J. R. Idle and F. J. Gonzalez, *Chem. Res. Toxicol.*, 2005, **18**, 1471–1478.
91. N. Scheer, Y. Kapelyukh, L. Chatham, A. Rode, S. Buechel and C. R. Wolf, *Mol. Pharmacol.*, 2012, **82**, 1022–1029.
92. N. Scheer, Y. Kapelyukh, J. McEwan, V. Beuger, L. A. Stanley, A. Rode and C. R. Wolf, *Mol. Pharmacol.*, 2012, **81**, 63–72.
93. C. J. Henderson, L. A. McLaughlin, N. Scheer, L. A. Stanley and C. R. Wolf, *Mol. Pharmacol.*, 2015, **87**, 733–739.
94. N. Scheer, Y. Kapelyukh, A. Rode, S. Oswald, D. Busch, L. A. McLaughlin, D. Lin, C. J. Henderson and C. R. Wolf, *Drug Metab. Dispos.*, 2015, DOI: 10.1124/dmd.115.065656.
95. B. Guthrie, B. Makubate, V. Hernandez-Santiago and T. Dreischulte, *BMC Med.*, 2015, **13**, 74.

96. C. J. Henderson and C. R. Wolf, *Drug Metab. Rev.*, 2011, **43**, 152–164.
97. B. Sachse, W. Meinl, H. Glatt and B. H. Monien, *Carcinogenesis*, 2014, **35**, 2339–2345.
98. V. A. Cornish, K. Pinter, S. Boukouvala, N. Johnson, C. Labrousse, M. Payton, H. Priddle, A. J. H. Smith and E. Sim, *Pharmacogenomics J.*, 2003, **3**, 169–177.
99. L. Wakefield, V. Cornish, H. Long, W. J. Griffiths and E. Sim, *Biochem. Biophys. Res. Commun.*, 2007, **364**, 556–560.
100. L. Wakefield, H. Long, N. Lack and E. Sim, *Mamm. Genome*, 2007, **18**, 270–276.
101. K. S. Sugamori, D. Brenneman, O. Sanchez, M. A. Doll, D. W. Hein, W. M. Pierce and D. M. Grant, *Cancer Lett.*, 2012, **318**, 206–213.
102. K. L. Witham, N. J. Butcher, K. S. Sugamori, D. Brenneman, D. M. Grant and R. F. Minchin, *PLoS One*, 2013, **8**, e77923.
103. N. Nguyen, J. A. Bonzo, S. Chen, S. Chouinard, M. J. Kelner, G. Hardiman, A. Belanger and R. H. Tukey, *J. Biol. Chem.*, 2008, **283**, 7901–7911.
104. S. Chen, D. Beaton, N. Nguyen, K. Senekeo-Effenberger, E. Brace-Sinnokrak, U. Argikar, R. P. Remmel, J. Trottier, O. Barbier, J. K. Ritter and R. H. Tukey, *J. Biol. Chem.*, 2005, **280**, 37547–37557.
105. M. F. Yueh, P. L. Mellon and R. H. Tukey, *Mol. Pharmacol.*, 2011, **79**, 1053–1060.
106. M. A. Leff, P. N. Epstein, M. A. Doll, A. J. Fretland, U. S. Devanaboyina, T. D. Rustan and D. W. Hein, *J. Pharmacol. Exp. Ther.*, 1999, **290**, 182–187.
107. K. S. Sugamori, D. Brenneman and D. M. Grant, *Drug Metab. Dispos.*, 2011, **39**, 882–890.
108. M. P. Vaughn, D. Biswal Shinohara, N. Castagna, J. L. Hicks, G. Netto, A. M. De Marzo, T. J. Speed, Z. R. Reichert, B. Kwabi-Addo, C. J. Henderson, C. R. Wolf, S. Yegnasubramanian and W. G. Nelson, *PLoS One*, 2011, **6**, e25707.
109. U. A. Argikar, K. Senekeo-Effenberger, E. E. Larson, R. H. Tukey and R. P. Remmel, *Xenobiotica*, 2009, **39**, 826–835.
110. Y. Kutsuno, K. Sumida, T. Itoh, R. H. Tukey and R. Fujiwara, *Pharmacol. Res. Perspect.*, 2013, **1**, e00002.
111. Y. Kutsuno, T. Itoh, R. H. Tukey and R. Fujiwara, *Drug Metab. Dispos.*, 2014, **42**, 1146–1152.
112. S. Chen, M. F. Yueh, R. M. Evans and R. H. Tukey, *Hepatology*, 2012, **56**, 658–667.
113. C. J. Henderson, A. G. Smith, J. Ure, K. Brown, E. J. Bacon and C. R. Wolf, *Proc. Natl. Acad. Sci. U. S. A.*, 1998, **95**, 5275–5280.
114. S. Durmus, J. J. Hendrikx and A. H. Schinkel, *Adv. Cancer Res.*, 2015, **125**, 1–41.
115. S. C. Tang, J. J. Hendrikx, J. H. Beijnen and A. H. Schinkel, *Curr. Opin. Pharmacol.*, 2013, **13**, 853–858.
116. D. Iusuf, J. J. Hendrikx, A. van Esch, E. van de Steeg, E. Wagenaar, H. Rosing, J. H. Beijnen and A. H. Schinkel, *Int. J. Cancer*, 2015, **136**, 225–233.

117. D. Iusuf, E. van de Steeg and A. H. Schinkel, *Trends Pharmacol. Sci.*, 2012, **33**, 100–108.
118. L. Salphati, X. Chu, L. Chen, B. Prasad, S. Dallas, R. Evers, D. Mamaril-Fishman, E. G. Geier, J. Kehler, J. Kunta, M. Mezler, L. Laplanche, J. Pang, A. Rode, M. G. Soars, J. D. Unadkat, R. A. van Waterschoot, J. Yabut, A. H. Schinkel and N. Scheer, *Drug Metab. Dispos.*, 2014, **42**, 1301–1313.
119. R. Allikmets, B. Gerrard, A. Hutchinson and M. Dean, *Hum. Mol. Genet.*, 1996, **5**, 1649–1655.
120. Y. Zhang, F. Buchholz, J. P. Muyrers and A. F. Stewart, *Nat. Genet.*, 1998, **20**, 123–128.
121. H. Wang, S. Faucette, T. Sueyoshi, R. Moore, S. Ferguson, M. Negishi and E. L. LeCluyse, *J. Biol. Chem.*, 2003, **278**, 14146–14152.
122. S. Anakk, A. Kalsotra, Y. Kikuta, W. Huang, J. Zhang, J. L. Staudinger, D. D. Moore and H. W. Strobel, *Pharmacogenomics J.*, 2004, **4**, 91–101.
123. P. Wei, J. Zhang, D. H. Dowhan, Y. Han and D. D. Moore, *Pharmacogenomics J.*, 2002, **2**, 117–126.
124. G. J. Pass, *et al.*, *Cancer Res.*, 2005, **65**, 4211–4217.
125. C. J. Henderson, *Toxicol. Lett.*, 2006, **13**, 853–858.
126. J. Gu, *et al.*, *J. Pharmacol. Exp. Ther.*, 2007, **321**, 91–97.
127. Q. Y. Zhang, *et al.*, *Drug Metab. Dispos.*, 2007, **35**, 1617–1623.
128. Y. Weng, *et al.*, *Cancer Res.*, 2007, **67**, 7825–7832.
129. C. Fang, *et al.*, *Toxicol. Appl. Pharmacol.*, 2008, **227**, 48–55.
130. A. Grimsley, *et al.*, *Biochem. Pharmacol.*, 2014, **92**, 701–711.
131. K. Pickup, *et al.*, *Xenobiotica*, 2014, **44**, 164–173.
132. K. Pickup, *et al.*, *Xenobiotica*, 2012, **42**, 195–205.
133. V. Megaraj, *et al.*, *Chem. Res. Toxicol.*, 2014, **27**, 656–662.
134. A. Potega, *et al.*, *Drug Metab. Dispos.*, 2011, **39**, 1423–1432.
135. C. Kunne, *et al.*, *Lab. Invest.*, 2014, **94**, 1103–1113.
136. C. Kunne, *et al.*, *Biochim. Biophys. Acta*, 2014, **1842**, 739–746.
137. Y. Zhu, *et al.*, *J. Pharmacol. Exp. Ther.*, 2015, **354**, 10–17.
138. J. Cheng, *et al.*, *J. Pharmacol. Exp. Ther.*, 2014, **351**, 559–567.
139. S. Y. Lee, *et al.*, *Toxicol. Lett.*, 2015, **235**, 107–115.
140. S. Uno, *et al.*, *Toxicol. Appl. Pharmacol.*, 2011, **237**, 119–126.
141. D. Y. Hwang, *et al.*, *Int. J. Toxicol.*, 2007, **26**, 71–80.
142. Q. Y. Zhang, *et al.*, *Biochem. Biophys. Res. Commun.*, 2005, **338**, 318–324.
143. K. Jia, *et al.*, *Drug Metab. Dispos.*, 2014, **42**, 1341–1348.
144. Y. Wei, *et al.*, *Drug Metab. Dispos.*, 2012, **40**, 1144–1150.
145. Z. Liu, *et al.*, *Drug Metab. Dispos.*, 2015, **43**, 208–216.
146. S. Löfgren, *et al.*, *Acta Vet Scand.*, 2008, **50**, 47.
147. X. Pan and H. Jeong, *Mol. Pharmacol.*, 2015, **88**, 106–112.
148. J. J. Hendrikx, *et al.*, *Int. J. Cancer*, 2013, **312**, 1649–1655.
149. Y. Kazuki, *et al.*, *Hum. Mol. Genet.*, 2013, **22**, 578–592.
150. M. A. Felmell, *et al.*, *Drug Metab. Dispos.*, 2008, **36**, 435–441.
151. X. Y. Pang, *et al.*, *Endocrinology*, 2012, **153**, 1453–1463.
152. M. W. Sadiq, *et al.*, *PLoS One*, 2015, **10**, e0118638.
153. N. Scheer, *et al.*, *Drug Metab. Dispos.*, 2012, **40**, 2212–2218.

154. E. Van de Steeg, *et al.*, *Clin. Can Res.*, 2013, **19**, 821–832.
155. E. Van de Steeg, *et al.*, *Drug Metab. Dispos.*, 2009, **37**, 77–81.
156. S. Durmus, *et al.*, *Int. J. Cancer*, 2014, **135**, 1700–1710.
157. L. Salphati, *et al.*, *Drug Metab. Dispos.*, 2014, **42**, 1301–1313.
158. N. Holmstock, *et al.*, *Mol. Pharmacol.*, 2013, **10**, 1056–1062.

CHAPTER 8

Stem Cells and Drug Metabolism

EDWARD J. KELLY*[a] AND JENNA L. VOELLINGER[a]

[a]Department of Pharmaceutics, University of Washington, 1959 NE
Pacific Street, Box 357610, Seattle, WA 98105, USA
*E-mail: edkelly@uw.edu

8.1   Introduction

Stem cells have a high self-renewal capability and can give rise to any cell
in the body making them a very attractive target for researchers in regenerative medicine. While there is excitement surrounding the possibilities of
stem cell research, this field is still in its infancy. The field of human pluripotent stem cell research is centered on two cell sources, embryonic stem
cells (ESCs) and induced pluripotent stem cells (iPSCs). Research with ESCs
first began with mouse ESCs in the early 1980's,[1,2] and was followed by the
establishment of the first human ESC (hESC) lines in 1998.[3] Due in part to
ethical concerns regarding development of ESC lines, interest arose in ways
to develop pluripotent stem cells from somatic cells or other non-embryonic
sources. A breakthrough in this area occurred in 2006, when a group from
Kyoto University, led by Shinya Yamanaka, were able to demonstrate that
a combination of four retrovirally delivered factors, Oct4, Klf4, Sox2, and
cMyc, could reprogram mouse fibroblasts to pluripotency; they termed these
cells induced pluripotent stem cells, or iPSCs.[4] They shortly followed this
work a year later with a demonstration that the same four factors could also

RSC Drug Discovery Series No. 49
New Horizons in Predictive Drug Metabolism and Pharmacokinetics
Edited by Alan G. E. Wilson
© The Royal Society of Chemistry 2016
Published by the Royal Society of Chemistry, www.rsc.org

reprogram human fibroblasts to pluripotency.[5] Development of iPSCs now allows the possibility of generating cell lines matched to specific patients, which can be used to study genetic diseases or as a source for regenerative medicine.[6] Just 6 years after the publication of this work on cellular reprogramming, Shinya Yamanaka and Sir John Gurdon were awarded the 2012 Nobel Prize in Physiology or Medicine.[6] This demonstrates the robustness of this approach, its rapid acceptance in the stem cell field, and vast potential for research.[6]

Since the establishment of human pluripotent stem cells lines, both ESCs and iPSCs, there have been some forays into their use for regenerative medicine. For example, the use of ESC derived oligodendrocyte progenitor cells to treat spinal cord injury. Geron Corporation was the first to gain US Food and Drug Administration (FDA) approval for a Phase I clinical trial involving ESCs in 2009. This trial was to test GRNOPC1, their hESC derived oligodendrocyte progenitor cells for acute spinal cord injury.[7,8] This was viewed as an important milestone in the field of regenerative medicine. Unfortunately, Geron stopped their trial prematurely solely for business reasons.[9] Following Geron's pioneering trial, other clinical trials have been initiated to examine hESC-based therapies, most notably with ESC derived retinal pigmented epithelial cells. As of September 2014, there are 8 clinical trials involving hESC therapies listed with http://ClinicalTrials.gov (http://www.ClincalTrials.gov). Of these 8 trials, 7 involve hESC derived retinal pigmented epithelial cells for therapy in Stargardt's macular dystrophy, dry age-related macular degeneration, and wet age-related macular degeneration (http://www.ClincalTrials.gov). The eighth trial is set to examine hESC derived cardiac progenitor cells in patients with severe heart failure (http://www.ClinicalTrials.gov). While iPSCs offer the potential for patient-derived cell lines to be used in regenerative medicine, there have been concerns regarding their safety, namely the oncogenic potential of the factors used for reprogramming, once injected back into the patient. However, in September 2014, the first iPSC derived cells (retinal pigmented epithelium) were injected into a human patient with macular degeneration in Japan.[10] Results of this trial may hold implications for future approval of iPSC-based cell therapies.

Stem cells not only offer invaluable opportunities for regenerative medicine, but also have vast potential as *in vitro* assays in the drug discovery and development process. Since stem cells can theoretically differentiate into any cell type, they can be used as cell models in drug screening, for both efficacy and toxicity.[11] The advent of iPSCs also allowed the development of cell lines from individuals with diverse genetic backgrounds to study a specific disease etiology, or genetic effect on drug metabolism.[11] In addition, stem cells can be used to replace primary cell types in metabolism and toxicity testing; for example, stem cell derived hepatocytes (SCDHs) in drug metabolism screening and stem cell derived cardiomyocytes in toxicity screening. The purpose of this chapter is to provide an overview of the current state of stem cell technologies regarding their use in drug metabolism screening, with an emphasis on SCDHs.

8.2 Human Pluripotent Stem Cells

Stem cells are defined as cells that can self-renew and have the ability to generate cells of a specific tissue through the process of differentiation.[12] Within the genre of stem cells there are 4 main classification types based on the potency of the stem cell, or types of cells that can be produced upon differentiation. This includes the totipotent stem cell, pluripotent stem cell, multipotent stem cell, and unipotent stem cell.[13] Totipotent stem cells are the most versatile; they can differentiate into any and all cell types, including cell types necessary for implantation and development of the embryo, such as the placenta, referred to as extraembryonic cell types. Totipotent stem cells are the only type that can independently give rise to a complete organism. Pluripotent stem cells fall one step below totipotent cells; they can differentiate into any cell type but not the extraembryonic cell types. Pluripotent stem cells can form any cell type derived from the three embryonic germ layers, the ectoderm, mesoderm, and endoderm, as illustrated in Figure 8.1. Multipotent stem cells are a more specialized type of stem cell that can differentiate only into a limited range of cell types derived from a specific lineage. For example, hematopoietic stem cells give rise to all types of blood cells and are considered multipotent cells. Unipotent stem cells can differentiate only into one mature cell type. For example, spermatogenic stem cells are unipotent stem cells because they can only form sperm cells. The main sources

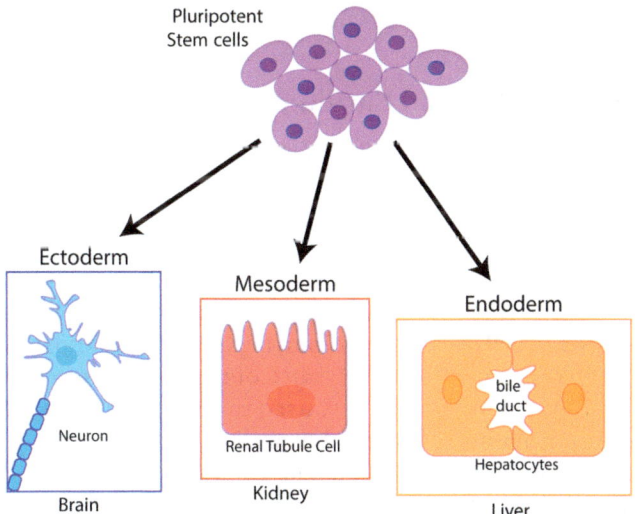

Figure 8.1   Pluripotent stem cells. Pluripotent stem cells can transform into cells from all three embryonic germ layers, the ectoderm, mesoderm, and endoderm. Representative tissue and cell types from each of these germ layers are illustrated here. Neurons of the brain are derived from the ectoderm lineage; renal tubule cells of the kidney are derived from the mesoderm lineage; and hepatocytes of the liver are derived from the endoderm lineage.

of pluripotent human stem cells in regenerative medicine include ESCs and iPSCs. In this chapter we will focus our discussion on the use and application of pluripotent stem cells.

The discovery of human pluripotent stem cells has resulted in an emerging field that holds promise for both bench top research to develop models of human disease and test new drugs in development, as well as in regenerative medicine to develop cells and tissues for transplant, and treatment of diseases.[14] While the discovery of mouse ESCs occurred in the early 1980's,[1,2] it was not until 1998 that the first hESCs were isolated.[3] These hESCs displayed the key characteristics of pluripotency, mainly they could be maintained and expanded in culture, and could generate derivatives from all three embryonic germ layers and form teratomas *in vivo*.[3] This was followed by the development of iPSCs, first from mouse embryonic fibroblasts in 2006, and then from human fibroblasts in 2007.[4,5] Formation of iPSCs was achieved through retroviral transduction of four factors, or pluripotency genes, Oct4, Sox2, c-Myc, and Klf4.[4,5] The resulting iPSCs morphologically resembled hESCs, were able to proliferate in culture, differentiate into cells from all three embryonic germ layers *in vitro*, and form teratomas *in vivo*.[4,5] A second group also published results on the generation of iPSCs in 2007 *via* lentiviral transduction of human fibroblast cells with the factors Oct4, Sox2, Nanog, and Lin28.[15] The development of these iPSC lines opens more doors for regenerative medicine, as well as medical research, with the possibility of creating iPSC lines from specific patients for autologous transplant, or patients with various disease or genetic backgrounds for study.

8.2.1 Stem Cell Derived Cardiomyocytes

Stem cells have a high self-renewal capability and can give rise to any cell in the body making them a very attractive target for researchers in regenerative medicine. While there is significant excitement surrounding the possibilities of stem cells in applications ranging from Parkinson's disease to spinal cord injury to organ transplants, this field is still in its infancy. One area with perhaps the most advanced research and application in terms of *in vitro* systems is the use of stem cell derived cardiomyocytes for cardiotoxicity screening such as QT prolongation, a leading cause of market withdrawal of prescription medications.[16,17] A common test used to screen for cardiotoxicity is the ability of the compound to inhibit the cardiac human ether-a-go-go related gene (hERG) channel, which is indicated by QT prolongation.[18] Currently used preclinical models for screening of cardiotoxicity do not accurately predict clinical outcomes.[16] These models include engineered cell lines expressing the hERG channel, isolated, arterially perfused rabbit ventricular wedge preparations, canine purkinje fibers, and arrhythmia rates in animals.[18,19] While human primary cardiomyocytes do make a good *in vitro* model, they are generally not used because of limited access and quality.[16,18] Due to these limitations for cardiotoxicity testing, there has been extensive work optimizing the differentiation of hESCs into cardiomyocytes. Stem cell derived cardiomyocytes exhibit functional synchronization of contraction allowing studies of cell-to-cell coupling, signal transduction, and repolarization characteristics.[18] They also survive for a prolonged period of time in culture, allowing for examination of both acute effects such as hERG channel inhibition and long-term effects such as ion channel trafficking.[18] Studies examining the potential of stem cell derived cardiomyocytes in safety testing found that, in general, stem cell derived cardiomyocytes exhibited similar responses to several drugs compared to mature cardiomyocytes, reviewed in Wobus and Loser (2011).[19] Although there are promising results for the utility of stem cell derived cardiomyocytes as an *in vitro* model, there are still concerns and reservations, including the purity of the stem cell derived cardiomyocyte population, maturity of the cells, and cost to produce large amounts of the cells.[18,19] Nevertheless, there are commercially available stem cell derived cardiomyocytes from companies such as Cellular Dynamics International.[20] A study conducted in 2013 utilizing stem cell derived cardiomyocytes from Cellular Dynamics was able to demonstrate relevant pharmacology and good correlations to current functional cardiac electrophysiological assays using 10 compounds with cardiovascular toxicity effects, justifying the use of stem cell derived cardiomyocytes for electrophysiological cardiac safety screening.[21] The potential of hESC derived cardiomyocytes in a regenerative medicine capacity has also been demonstrated using non-human primates. A study using a non-human primate model of myocardial ischemia showed that intra-myocardial delivery of hESC derived cardiomyocytes could remuscularize substantial amounts of the infarcted heart.[22] However, from a safety standpoint, they did observe non-fatal ventricular arrhythmias in the non-human primates that received the hESC derived cardiomyocytes.[22] Due to the extensive progress made with stem cell derived cardiomyocytes and insufficiencies with current preclinical models to predict cardiotoxicity, there is extensive interest in their routine use and application in drug safety screening. To this end, in July 2013 a meeting was held by the Cardiac Safety Research Consortium and the Health and Environmental Sciences Institute to discuss new approaches to assess drug-induced proarrhythmic risk, in which they included the use of electrophysiological tests with stem cell derived cardiomyocytes.[23,24] This demonstrates one application of a stem cell technology to enhance pharmaceutical development.

8.3 Drug Metabolism

Drug metabolism is an important area of study in drug development as metabolism is the main way drugs are eliminated from the body. Drugs can be eliminated from the body as either the unchanged parent compound or as metabolites.[25] Usually metabolism of drugs results in inactivation of the compound and renders the compound more water soluble to allow for easier excretion from the body; however, metabolism can also result in generation of a toxic metabolite. Because of this, preclinical screening of drug metabolism is a fundamental component of drug development and is used to aid in predicting drug bioavailability, drug–drug interactions, and toxicity. Pharmaceutically based drug–drug interactions occur when one drug affects the pharmacokinetics of another, or in other words, if one drug changes the absorption, distribution, metabolism, or excretion (ADME) of another.[26,27] Both inhibition and induction of drug metabolizing enzymes can alter the metabolism of a drug, representing two major reasons for such drug–drug interactions.[25]

The main family of enzymes responsible for drug metabolism is the cytochrome P450s (CYPs). The CYPs are a superfamily of hemoprotein enzymes that primarily catalyze oxidation reactions.[28] It is a large and diverse family of enzymes with 57 functional isozymes in humans. However, it is members of just three subfamilies (CYP1, CYP2, and CYP3) that are primarily responsible for most of the metabolic clearance of drugs.[29] They are expressed in numerous tissues with the main drug metabolizing CYPs being highly expressed in the primary tissues responsible for drug metabolism—the intestine, liver, and kidney. The liver is the most versatile of these organs and, thus, key to drug metabolism and clearance. Accordingly, when evaluating drug metabolism, the hepatic CYPs in particular are extensively studied. The liver, along with the intestine, also plays a crucial role in "first-pass metabolism" of orally administered compounds. Orally administered compounds are absorbed in the intestine into the portal system where they are delivered to the liver *via* the portal vein before entering the general blood circulation. This first-pass of compounds through the intestine and liver can result in extensive metabolism of the compound before it enters general circulation, having a major effect on a drug's bioavailability. This also means the liver may see high concentrations of orally dosed drugs and their metabolites, posing a risk for liver toxicity.[25] The CYPs are also highly polymorphic, and this genetic variation can play a role in therapeutic failure and drug toxicity risk.[26,30] Variation in the CYP genes can result in enzymes with no functional capacity, enzymes with altered functional capacity, or enzymes with altered expression levels. For each polymorphic gene these alterations result in a range of observed phenotypes classified as poor metabolizers (PMs), intermediate metabolizers (IMs), extensive metabolizers (EMs) and ultrarapid metabolizers (UMs).[26,30] The CYP with the most variation identified to date is CYP2D6, with more than 63 functional gene alleles (http://www.cypalleles.ki.se/cyp2d6.htm), including polymorphisms that result in gene deletion (PM status), defective splicing (PM status), and gene duplication (UM status).

Since metabolism plays a crucial role in both the efficacy and toxicity of drugs it is important to identify the metabolites formed and the enzymes responsible for metabolism.[25] Usually a drug is metabolized by several competing pathways, and the contributing fraction will depend on the relative rates of each parallel pathway. In particular, it's known that the fraction of dose metabolized by specific enzymes, such as the CYPs, is a major determinant in predicting drug–drug interactions and is important in understanding the impact of polymorphisms in metabolizing enzymes on total drug clearance.[25,26] Because blood drug or metabolite concentrations drive pharmacologic effect, the metabolic profile of a new chemical entity is determined *in vitro* and these data are now routinely included in regulatory documents, and are used to help determine the most appropriate follow up clinical studies to assess drug drug interactions.[26] This reaction phenotyping involves the use of multiple systems in combination to determine the major metabolic pathways responsible for drug metabolism and clearance. This includes purified recombinant proteins, microsomal membrane and other subcellular fractions, primary hepatocytes, coupled with selective chemical inhibitors, inhibitory antibodies, and substrate probes.[26,31] Probe substrates are useful in determining the inhibitory potential of a new chemical entity toward specific CYPs. CYP reaction phenotyping is used to estimate the fraction of a drug cleared by all of the CYPs (f_m) and the contribution of each individual CYP ($f_{m,CYP}$).[26] These data can then be used to predict the magnitude of a drug interaction and the impact of a CYP polymorphism on the pharmacokinetic profile of the drug. They can also be used to help design more effective clinical studies, so as to avoid therapeutic failure and unexpected toxicity.[26] In addition, the spectrum, reactivity, and abundance of a given metabolite is important, as defined by the FDA's Safety Testing of Drug Metabolites guidance, or MIST.[32] The goal of MIST is to assess circulating metabolite exposure, as the metabolites may have pharmacological activity or toxicity risks. This is determined in part from *in vitro* drug metabolism profiling in combination with animal studies and clinical trials. It is important to have a thorough understanding of the ADME properties of a new chemical entity, including the role of CYPs in the overall clearance of the drug, accurate *in vitro* CYP reaction phenotype data, metabolic clearance by non-CYP enzymes, renal clearance, and biliary clearance.[26] It's also known that the CYP enzymes are susceptible to induction. This induction has been observed primarily in the liver, although it has been observed in other tissues as well, notably the intestine.[26,33] Enzyme induction results in increased metabolic elimination of the drug and therefore reduced plasma concentration of the parent compound. In order to assess the potential for a drug interaction due to enzyme induction one needs knowledge of the enzymes and their contribution to the metabolic elimination of the drug candidate.[26]

While the CYP enzymes are the predominant family involved in drug metabolism, there are other families of enzymes that may play a significant role in the metabolic clearance of a drug. These include the flavin-containing monooxygenases (FMOs), monoamine oxidase, epoxide hydrolase, glutathione *S*-transferases (GSTs), sulfotransferases (SULTs), methyltransferases, *N*-acetyltransferases (NATs), and UDP-glucuronosyltransferases (UGTs).[31] Unlike with the CYPs, *in vitro* phenotyping experiments for these other enzymes are less well established and there are fewer selective probe substrates and inhibitors available.[26,31,34]

8.3.1 Tissues

Again, although the liver is the main organ responsible for metabolism there are other tissues with significant expression of the CYPs and other drug metabolizing enzymes that should also be considered when evaluating a drug's overall metabolic clearance, and may be particularly important in terms of localized toxicity.[26] The two other organs most commonly involved in drug metabolism along with the liver are the intestine and kidney. These three organ systems and their role in drug clearance are discussed below.

8.3.1.1 Liver

The liver possesses the highest expression levels of drug metabolizing CYPs, making it the most important organ for the metabolism, detoxification and elimination of drugs, and the focus of drug optimization and safety studies.[25,26] Metabolism in the liver plays a key role in determining plasma drug concentration and half-life.[25] Hepatocytes are the main cell type within the liver, comprising about 80% of the liver volume, and are the cell type where drug metabolizing enzymes, such as the CYPs, are found.[25] Hepatocytes are polarized cells with a blood-facing sinusoidal membrane and bile-facing canalicular membrane, as shown in Figure 8.2B. Each of these membranes expresses specific transporters that facilitate movement of drugs into and out of the cell. Transporters expressed on the sinusoidal membrane can affect access of the drug to the drug metabolizing enzymes within the hepatocyte, and transporters on the canalicular membrane affect biliary excretion. The drug metabolizing CYPs are found primarily in the endoplasmic reticulum (ER) of hepatocytes. CYP3A4 is the major hepatic microsomal CYP in humans in terms of both expression and role in metabolizing the majority of drugs.[26] CYP1A2, 2A6, 2B6, 2C8, 2C9, 2C19, 2D6, and 2E1 are also present in the liver ER and contribute to drug metabolism (Figure 8.2B).[26,28] With regards to screening for drug metabolism activity in the liver, *in vitro* systems include recombinant enzymes, human liver microsomes, S9 fractions, liver slices, and primary hepatocytes.[26] Each of these systems has their own advantages and disadvantages, so generally multiple different systems are used when evaluating the metabolic profile of a new chemical entity. The data from these various *in vitro* systems are then integrated to determine the overall metabolism profile.[26] Animal studies are also a useful complement to these *in vitro* human assays. However, they are not always an accurate model of human metabolic capacity because of inter-species differences in enzyme expression and function.[35] Ultimately, *in vivo* human ADME data are needed to both confirm the *in vitro* data and to help place the *in vitro* data in the appropriate clinical context.[26]

In vitro characterization of drug metabolism involves enzyme kinetic analysis of the metabolite formation rate. The enzyme kinetic model used most often was developed by Michaelis and Menten:[28,36]

$$v = \frac{V_{max} \times S}{K_m + S} \qquad (8.1)$$

in which v is the velocity, or rate of metabolism, and S is the substrate concentration. V_{max} is the maximal reaction velocity and is directly proportional to the total enzyme concentration. K_m is the Michaelis constant, it represents the affinity of the substrate for the enzyme and is mathematically

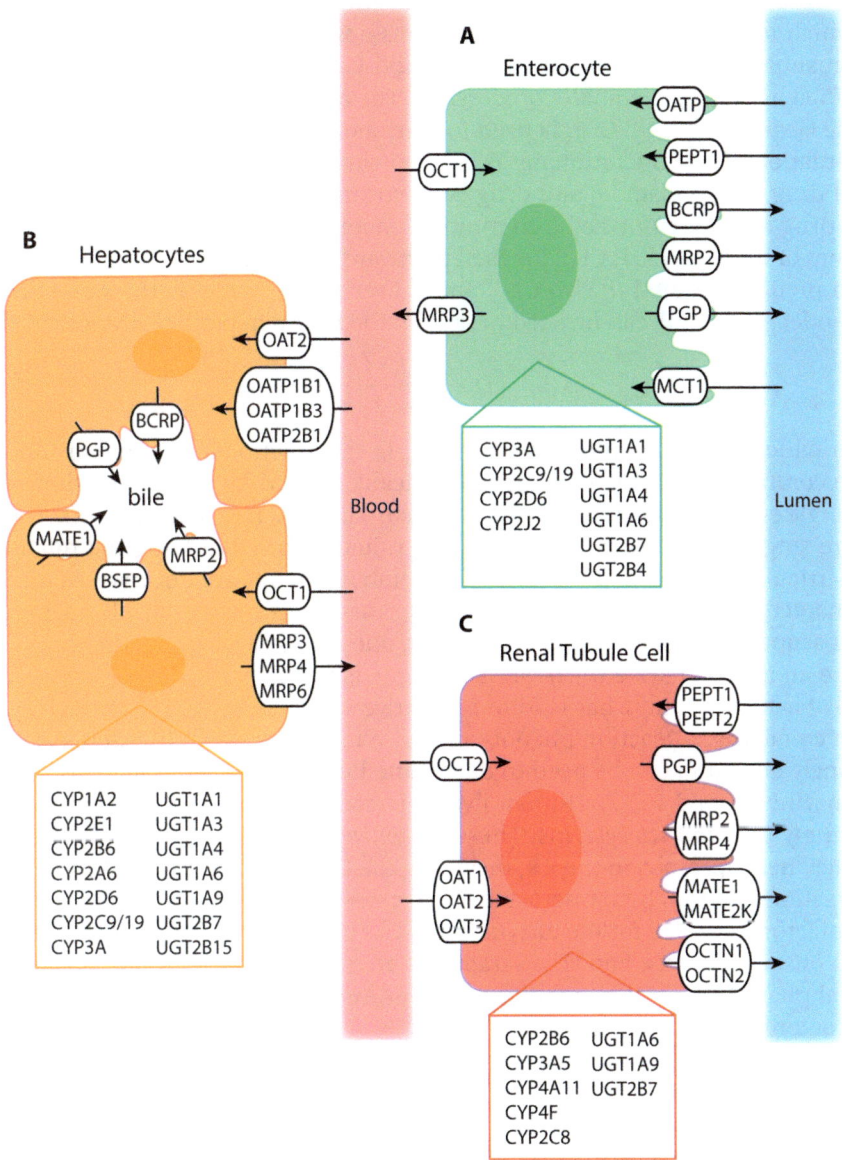

Figure 8.2 Cell types responsible for drug metabolism and transport. The three main organ systems considered important in drug metabolism are the intestine, liver and kidney. The cell types in each of these tissues where drug metabolizing enzymes and transporters are located are shown here. These include (A) enterocytes for the intestine, (B) hepatocytes for the liver, and (C) renal tubule cells for the kidney. For each cell type, the main transporters, CYPs and UGTs, are shown.

equated to the substrate concentration at which half maximal velocity (V_{max}) is attained.[28] When the substrate concentration is much smaller than K_m, which is true for most drugs *in vivo*, v is approximately linearly dependent on substrate concentration, and the ratio V_{max}/K_m represents the maximum efficiency of the metabolic process.[28,36] The ratio V_{max}/K_m is called the intrinsic clearance (CL_{int}). CL_{int} is used for extrapolating *in vitro* data to the *in vivo* situation, it acts operationally as a proportionality constant between the rate of drug metabolism (v) and drug concentration at the enzyme active site. If a drug is biotransformed into multiple metabolites then the net CL_{int} is the sum of the individual CL_{int} for each pathway.[28] The *in vitro* CL_{int} is then scaled to predict the total *in vivo* CL_{int} and a liver model, such as the well-stirred model [eqn (8.2)], can be used to predict the *in vivo* hepatic clearance.[28,36,37]

$$CL_h = Q \times \frac{f_u \times CL_{int}}{Q + (f_u \times CL_{int})} \qquad (8.2)$$

in which Q is liver blood flow and f_u is the fraction unbound in blood. Recombinant enzyme systems are typically created by over-expression of a single enzyme gene, most commonly in insect cells. Due to the fact that these are singly expressed enzymes they are valuable for identifying the role of a particular enzyme in a compound's metabolism, but are not that useful for characterizing the relative rates of drug metabolism *via* multiple pathways or sequential metabolism.[38,39] However, one needs to keep in mind that they are an artificial system where the enzyme is typically over-expressed at levels far higher than what is found in native tissue and requires the addition of co-factors.[26] Reaction phenotyping with recombinant CYP systems is routinely done and can be used to determine kinetic parameters such as single enzyme K_m and V_{max}.[26] Human liver microsomes are one of the most commonly used *in vitro* systems. These are ER vesicles and as such only contain enzymes expressed in the ER, including the CYPs, FMOs, and UGTs.[28,38,39] S9 fractions contain both microsomal and cytosolic fractions.[39] However, again, cofactors required for the enzymes must be added to the incubation in order to observe activity, and these fractions are not ideal for examining sequential phase I/phase II metabolism.[38,39] For example, to examine UGT activity, a detergent must be added to create pores in the membrane so the drug may access the active site of the enzyme, resulting in a non-physiological representation of UGT activity.[38,39] Hepatocytes are best for studying sequential and/or parallel oxidative and conjugative reactions.[28] While any of these systems can be used to study inhibition, cell systems such as hepatocytes are the only systems that can be used to study induction and its effects on the metabolic profile. This whole cell system is also ideally suited for evaluating the role of transporters and the potential for transporter-mediated drug interactions. Indeed, sandwich-cultured primary hepatocytes are considered the gold standard for determining liver CYP induction.[25] Hepatocytes cultured in the sandwich configuration, between collagen or collagen and Matrigel, morphologically resemble hepatocytes, maintain metabolism, and form canalicular membrane networks also providing a means to evaluate liver specific transporters (Figure 8.2B).[25,40,41] Along these lines, a US FDA draft Guideline to Industry recommends induction studies be performed with hepatocytes obtained from a minimum of three individuals in order to minimize inter-individual differences in responses.[42]

In summary, the metabolism of a drug by the liver is done using a combination of *in vitro* systems, such as recombinant enzyme systems, human liver microsomes, and primary hepatocytes. These results are then compared for an overall assessment of metabolic fate, in particular, the role of CYP-mediated metabolism.[26] The FDA guidance "Drug Interaction Studies—Study Design, Data Analysis, and Implications for Dosing and Labeling" highlights the use of human hepatocytes in determining the metabolic profile of a new chemical entity, and if the data indicate CYP enzymes contribute >25% to the total clearance of the compound then studies using human liver microsomes or recombinant enzymes should be performed to identify the individual CYP enzymes responsible for metabolism.[42] It is important in preclinical drug development to identify and understand the major pathways of metabolism in order to predict potential drug–drug interactions and potential for liver toxicity.[27]

8.3.1.2 *Intestine*

Although the liver is the main drug metabolizing organ, other tissues express drug metabolizing enzymes, and extra hepatic metabolism is thought to be important for some compounds; one such tissue is the intestine. Metabolism in the intestine in particular contributes to first-pass metabolism of orally administered compounds, and is thus a determinant of a drug's oral bioavailability. It is also important to have a clear understanding of the metabolites generated in specific tissues such as the intestine to predict potential toxicity in that tissue. Transcellular absorption of orally administered drugs occurs through enterocytes, the mature absorptive columnar epithelial cells that are part of the mucosal lining in the intestine. The enterocytes have an apical membrane that faces the lumen, which the intestinal villi face and where absorption from the gastrointestinal tract occurs, and a blood-facing basolateral membrane (illustrated in Figure 8.2A). Enterocytes also express significant levels of drug metabolizing enzymes, such as CYPs and UGTs (Figure 8.2A).

The main CYP enzyme expressed in the intestine is CYP3A, calculated to account for about 80% of the CYP content based on total immunoquantified CYPs, and interestingly is expressed in a gradient along the length of the small intestine, with expression being the highest in the duodenum, followed by the jejunum and lastly the ileum.[43-45] Other CYP enzymes expressed in the small intestine include CYP2C9, 2C19, 2D6, and 2J2.[26] Although CYP3A is the most abundant CYP in both the liver and small intestine, the total mass of CYP3A in the small intestine is estimated to be only about 1% of that in the liver.[45] This difference in total mass can be in part attributed to the low yield of microsomal protein from the small intestine compared with the liver, and because the localization of the CYPs in the small intestine is restricted to the enterocytes in the villus tip cells, which only account for a small fraction of the total intestinal cell population.[44] In addition, the liver is about twice as large as the small intestine by weight (about 1.5 kg *vs.* 0.7 kg).[44] Based on CYP content, levels of CYP3A4 have been estimated at 350 pmol mg^{-1} microsomal protein in the liver and 70–160 pmol mg^{-1} microsomal protein in the small intestine.[44,46] Comparison of two other studies show CYP3A content to be closer in range, at 96 pmol mg^{-1} microsomal protein in the liver and about 50 pmol mg^{-1} in the small intestine.[45,47] Although CYP3A content in the small intestine may be just a fraction of that in the liver based on total mass, the fact that CYP3A's contribution to total CYP content in the intestine is double that in the liver (80 *vs.* 40%), coupled with relatively similar microsomal content, substantiates the small intestine as an important site for first-pass drug metabolism.[45,47]

Similar to the process for determining metabolism in the liver, recombinant enzyme systems of the CYPs known to be expressed in the intestine are used to help understand their potential role in intestinal drug metabolism. In addition, several cell lines are used to study intestinal drug permeability and biotransformation, this includes primary enterocytes, and the immortalized human colon carcinoma cell lines Caco-2 and LS180 cells.[43] While primary enterocytes are metabolically competent, their viability is limited in culture.[48] Caco-2 cells are the more commonly used colon carcinoma cell line; although it should be noted that Caco-2 cells lack expression of most CYP enzymes, and particularly CYP3A4, which is the main CYP expressed in the small intestine.[48–50] However, Caco-2 cells can be induced to express low levels of CYP3A4 by treatment with vitamin D$_3$.[49] Alternatively, one can use CYP3A4-transfected Caco-2 cells, but this would be an artificial system. As in the liver, induction of drug metabolizing enzymes and drug transporters in the intestine may lead to drug interactions. LS180 cells have been shown to constitutively express the pregnane X receptor (PXR), which is a transcription factor responsible for induction of CYP3A4, and the efflux transporter P-glycoprotein (P-gp).[51,52] Therefore, LS180 cells can be used to study the effects of PXR-mediated induction of CYP3A4 and P-gp.[52] Another *in vitro* system used to study intestinal drug metabolism is precision-cut slices, these are very small intestinal cut slices of tissue from different species, allowing for evaluation of species differences in intestinal metabolism.[43,48,53] However, access to intestinal tissue for these slices is limited. Overall, there is a lack of robust intestinal cell-based models for assessing drug permeability, drug metabolism, DDIs and drug toxicity.[43] Generation of enterocytes from human pluripotent stem cells would in theory offer a human-based *in vitro* system to evaluate permeability as well as intestinal drug metabolism.

There has been limited work on developing protocols for differentiation of pluripotent stem cells to enterocyte or intestinal cells, although what has been attempted shows promising results. The small intestine is a unique organ with a highly regenerative luminal epithelium that turns over about once a week. This self-renewal is driven by intestinal stem cells (or adult stem cells) that reside in the crypt. These cells move up along the villi as they mature, essentially sloughing off the older cells at the tip of the villi.[54] These adult stem cells located in the intestinal crypt can be isolated from human surgical, or biopsy, specimens and used to develop *ex vivo* 3D enteroid cultures.[55–57] While this represents a promising preclinical model, it is limited by access to human intestinal tissue. For this reason, intestinal cells derived from hESCs and iPSCs may offer a more convenient solution. To date, most pluripotent stem cell derived intestinal work has been conducted by Dr Wells' group at Cincinnati Children's Hospital. This group has shown formation of human intestinal organoids (HIOs) from both hESCs and iPSCs that form mature human intestinal epithelium with crypt villus architecture.[58–60] Their HIOs express the intestinal markers CDX2, SOX9, and KLF5, and they develop crypt villus architecture with cells expressing LGR5 and ASCL2 (markers of the adult intestinal stem cell population).[58,59,61] The differentiation takes 35 days and involves the factors activin A, Wnt3a, fibroblast growth factor 4 (FGF4), Noggin, Rspondin1, and epidermal growth factor (EGF).[58,59] They were also able to show that taking the HIOs and then transplanting them under the kidney capsule of immune compromised mice for 6 weeks before removal allows them to further mature.[58] Additionally, these HIOs have been shown to support replication of a gastrointestinal virus, rotavirus, indicating that they are a biologically relevant model of the intestine.[62] While these organoids recapitulated many markers of the mature intestine, there has been no assessment to date of drug metabolizing enzyme functions. Thus, it is unclear, whether such a system would have utility for *in vitro* drug metabolism profiling. In conclusion, more work needs to be done on characterizing stem cell derived intestinal cells in terms of drug metabolizing enzymes and transporters in order for them to be a useful *in vitro* system for preclinical drug metabolism profiling.

8.3.1.3 Kidney

The kidney is a main route for drug excretion, but it can also play a key role in drug metabolism. Along with the intestine and liver, the kidney also expresses significant levels of various drug metabolizing enzymes, such as some of the CYPs and UGTs, as well as drug transporters (Figure 8.2C). The main cell type in the kidney where drug metabolism and transport occurs is the renal proximal tubule epithelial cells (PTECs). These cells have a polarized blood-facing basolateral membrane and an apical membrane that transports compounds into the collecting duct of the kidney to become part of the urine filtrate (illustrated in Figure 8.2C). In particular, PTECs are known to express CYP3A5 as opposed to CYP3A4 as in the liver.[43,63,64] However, CYP3A5 is a highly polymorphic enzyme, such that the majority of Caucasians (about 85%) do not express the functional CYP3A5 protein.[65] The primary variant responsible for this phenotype is *CYP3A5*3*, an intronic SNP that results in improperly spliced mRNA and a truncated protein.[65,66] To evaluate drug metabolism in the kidney, *in vitro* systems are used in combination with *in vivo* data from animal studies. For *in vitro* systems, immortalized cell lines such as LLC-PK1 (a pig kidney epithelial cell line) and MDCK (Madine Darby canine kidney) cells are commonly used; however, these are non-human cells and do not represent the true *in vivo* situation.[43,67] Some human renal epithelial cell lines are also available, including the HK-2 proximal tubule cell line.[68,69] However, the HK-2 cell line has been shown to lack expression of some key drug transporters, including OAT1, OAT3, and OCT2, limiting their use as an *in vitro* model of human kidney.[69]

There is a clear need to better understand the impact of kidney disease on drug disposition (including metabolism).[63] Not only does kidney disease affect renal drug clearance, but it also affects the clearance of drugs that are eliminated by the liver and intestine.[63] There is still a lack of *in vitro* models that accurately resemble the *in vivo* kidney. Development of protocols to generate various cells of the kidney from human pluripotent stem cells would have vast potential as an *in vitro* model to examine drug metabolism and transport within the kidney and also to study the effects of kidney disease on drug disposition. To gain a better understanding of the kidney's role in drug metabolism, disposition, and toxicity, development of 3D microphysiological systems (or a kidney-on-a-chip) would also be greatly beneficial.[70] For this type of system, stem cell derived renal tubular cells, along with the other cell types of the kidney, would provide a consistent human cell source for manipulation in 3D or microphysiological systems to more accurately model the kidney.

As with the intestine, there has been limited work to date on the development of stem cell derived renal cells. The kidney is one of the more complex organs in terms of lineage specification. Kidney formation involves an interaction between two different populations derived from intermediate mesoderm, metanephric mesenchyme, and ureteric bud.[71] The metanephric mesenchyme differentiates into the epithelial cells of the kidney (such as the renal tubule cells) and the ureteric bud forms the collecting duct system.[71] Studies examining the generation of kidney cells from human pluripotent stem cells have mostly utilized activin A, retinoic acid, and BMP7 in the differentiation process.[72–76] One study that classified the differentiated cells as being proximal tubular like cells utilized BMP2 and BMP7 in the differentiation protocol, followed by flow cytometry sorting for aquaporin1 positive cells.[76] More recent protocols have also employed the small molecule CHIR99021, a glycogen synthase kinase-3β inhibitor.[77–79] While these reports demonstrate generation of metanephric mesenchyme and renal proximal tubule like cells, more work needs to be done on developing protocols that definitively yield homogenous populations of renal tubule cells for evaluating the expression and activity of the drug metabolizing enzymes and transporters.

8.4   SCDHs

Primary human hepatocytes are isolated from liver organs deemed unsuitable for transplantation or *via* liver biopsy.[16] For *in vitro* screening, primary human hepatocytes are the most physiologically relevant model, given their expression of phase I and II drug metabolizing enzymes as well as transporters, under the right conditions. Thus, human hepatocytes have become an integral component for studying drug metabolism and toxicity.[16] While microsomes are still a favored model for high-throughput screening, they are increasingly being replaced or complemented by primary human hepatocytes.[80] However, the utility of human hepatocytes is hampered by donor availability, inter-donor variability, lack of cell proliferation, and a decline in characteristic hepatic functions over time.[16,81] Pluripotent stem cells have a high self-renewal capability and can give rise to any cell in the body, including hepatocytes. Hepatocytes derived from stem cells may provide a useful *in vitro* model for drug metabolism, pharmacogenetics, CYP inducibility, and toxicity studies to complement or replace currently available primary/cryopreserved human hepatocytes. In addition, there is a critical need to be able to accurately model human organ systems *in vitro*, such as the liver, to improve our understanding of drug efficacy and safety during drug development. SCDHs may provide a more readily available source of cells for manipulation in 3D or microphysiological systems to more accurately model the liver, or other organ systems.

8.4.1 Differentiation

Hepatocytes derived from hESCs or iPSCs represent an attractive alternative to bypass the limitations associated with primary hepatocytes. The aim of differentiation is to recapitulate natural development *in vitro* within a culture dish using various combinations of growth factors. For the liver this means directing the cells first towards the endoderm pathway, then to the hepatic lineage, and finally mature hepatocytes. There have been several groups reporting the differentiation of human pluripotent stem cells, hESCs, and more recently iPSCs into hepatocytes. One of the first able to demonstrate this were researchers from Geron Corporation in 2003.[82] While differentiation efficiencies (based on percentages of cells expressing hepatocyte markers such as albumin) were low to begin with there has been marked improvement in this area. Earlier protocols often relied on spontaneous differentiation of stem cells through formation of embryoid bodies (3D multicellular aggregates); a contributing factor to low differentiation efficiencies.[82,83] More recent protocols now rely on directed differentiation using set combinations of various factors, contributing to the increase in differentiation efficiency.[84–86] There have been a number of different factors used in differentiation protocols in an attempt to recapitulate normal liver development. This differentiation process is therefore broken down into a number of stages, with varying combinations of factors used. The total time to differentiate hepatocytes varies between protocols, ranging from 13 to 32 days.[82,83,86–98] A few factors that are common to most protocols include activin A, Wnt3, dimethyl sulfoxide (DMSO), hepatocyte growth factor (HGF), oncostatin M (OSM), and dexamethasone. In addition, other groups have reported transduction of transcription factors along with growth factor treatment as an efficient process for generating SCDHs.[90–92] Takayama *et al.* reported transduction of FOXA2 and HNF1α with an adenovirus vector in combination with a step-wise culture with growth factors including activin A, bone morphogenetic protein 4

(BMP4), FGF4, HGF, and OSM to generate SCDHs.[90,91] More recently, small molecules have also been used to generate SCDHs.[99] Other protocols have also investigated 3D culture of cells, such as spheroids and bioreactors, to enhance hepatocyte differentiation.[89,93,100,101]

In summary, there are various protocols available for generating SCDHs. While most of these protocols share common factors, there are differences in each. Protocols published in journals such as *Current Protocols in Stem Cell Biology* and *Nature Protocols* are an easy and convenient way to understand every step in a laboratory's differentiation process, especially to evaluate differentiation protocols side by side.[86,102] Before they can be used for *in vitro* metabolite profiling, the differentiation protocols that yield the most reliable, reproducible hepatocyte-like cells must be identified and thoroughly evaluated. In addition, these protocols must be easily scalable and cost-efficient to be implemented in an industry setting.

8.4.2   SCDHs for Studying Drug Metabolism

The biggest limitation in the field of SCDHs to date is the inability to reproducibly generate mature hepatocytes with high levels of functional drug metabolizing enzymes. It should be noted that the lack of mature differentiated cells is not unique to SCDHs, and a lack of functional maturity has been observed across various cell types, remaining a problem in the stem cell field in general.[103] For SCDHs to be used as an *in vitro* assay platform to determine metabolite profiles, this is something that must be overcome.

While there have been a number of publications addressing this issue, there is still an overall inability to obtain mature hepatocytes that possess fully functional CYP activity. Currently, to evaluate SCDH function, there is a repeating pattern of criteria used, including: gene expression profiling, immunocytochemistry, and western blotting of specific markers; indocyanine green staining; glycogen accumulation; and albumin secretion. While most groups acknowledge the importance of functional drug metabolizing enzymes, such as the CYPs, in hepatocytes, few groups have actually assessed functional activity, and not all using the gold standard of human primary hepatocytes (hPHs) as the comparator. Most groups generally utilize resorufin and P450-Glo™ assays to assess CYP activity; only a few studies have utilized liquid chromatography mass spectrometry (LC/MS) and compared CYP activity to primary hepatocytes.[85,88,91,104] There is also a large amount of variability between studies. For example, in studies reporting on CYP3A, activity levels vary from 0 to 90% of hPHs.[87,88,105–108] This wide range of results could be due to multiple factors, including the different stem cell lines used, the protocol used and/or the quality of primary hepatocytes used for comparison.[105] Selected studies examining functional drug metabolism are summarized in Table 8.1. In one example, LC/MS was utilized to assess activity of four major drug metabolizing CYPs (CYP1A2, 2C9, 3A4, and 2D6). Results from this study indicated CYP activity comparable to primary hepatocytes for CYP1A2 and 2D6, suggesting that the SCDHs obtained in this study did

Table 8.1 Summary of published metabolic activity in stem cell derived hepatocytes. 3-MC: 3-methylcholanthrene; BNF: β-naphthoflavone; HPLC:
high-performance liquid chromatography.

References	Assay	Evaluation	Result
Rambhatla *et al.*, 2003 [82]	EROD for CYP1A2	Basal activity compared with induced using 3-MC for SCDH and hPH	SCDHs exhibited 3–6-fold induction hPH exhibited 3-fold induction
Duan *et al.*, 2007 [83]	EROD for CYP1A2	Basal activity compared with induced using 3-MC for SCDH and hPH	SCDHs exhibited 11-fold induction hPH exhibited 32-fold induction
Ek *et al.*, 2007 [87]	EROD for CYP1A2	Basal activity	No activity detected in SCDHs
Hay *et al.*, 2007 [97]	HPLC	Incubated SCDHs with rifampin and testosterone with or without ketoconazole	No comparison with basal activity prior to rifampin incubation Peak detected that was absent in the presence of inhibitor
Hay *et al.*, 2008 [85]	LC/MS	Incubated cells with a cocktail of tolbutamide, bufuralol, phenacetin, and midazolam Compared with HepG with 2 cells	SCDHs metabolized phenacetin and bufuralol similarly to HepG2 cells; midazolam metabolism higher than HepG2 but not significant; tolbutamide metabolism in SCDHs but not HepG2 cells
Hay *et al.*, 2008 [84]	EROD for CYP1A2	Basal activity	CYP1A2 activity detected, no comparison with other cell lines
Basma *et al.*, 2009 [106]	EROD for CYP1A2 HPLC	CYP1A2 basal activity compared with induced using BNF	SCDHs exhibited inducible CYP1A2 activity at approximately 25–30% of that in hPHs
		CYP3A basal activity compared with induced using phenobarbital Compared with hPH	SCDHs form 6β-hydroxytestosterone comparable to hPHs

(*continued*)

Table 8.1 (*continued*)

References	Assay	Evaluation	Result
Brolen *et al.*, 2010[104]	LC/MS	Incubated cells with phenacetin, midazolam, or diclofenac Compared with HepG2 cells	Phenacetin metabolite levels similar to HepG2 cells; midazolam metabolite levels slightly higher than HepG2 cells; diclofenac metabolite levels higher than HepG2 cells, which exhibited no activity
Duan *et al.*, 2010[88]	LC/MS	Incubated cells with either phenacetin, midazolam, bufuralol, or diclofenac Compared with hPH	Phenacetin and bufuralol metabolite levels similar to hPH; midazolam and diclofenac metabolite levels lower than hPH
Sullivan *et al.*, 2010[98]	P450-Glo assay	CYP3A4 and CYP1A2 in SCDHs	Luminescent activity detected in SCDHs
Takayama *et al.*, 2012[91]	LC/MS	Incubated SCDHs with one of 9 substrates: phenacetin, bupropion, paclitaxel, tolbutamide, *S*-mephenytoin, bufuralol, midazolam, testosterone, or hydroxyl-coumarin (test for glucuronidation) Compared with hPH	Metabolite formation as follows, as percent compared with hPHs: acetaminophen: 6.7%, hydroxybupropion: 3.0%, 6α-hydroxypaclitaxel: 21.6%, hydroxytolbutamide: 15%, 4′-hydroxymephenytoin: 1.7%, 1′-hydroxybufuralol: 2.4%, 1′-hydroxymidazolam: 2.2%, 6β-hydroxytestosterone: 24%, 7-hydroxycoumarin glucuronide: 42%

express some functional CYP enzymes.[88] In addition, some published reports have characterized the metabolic capacity, as well as inductive potential of certain CYP enzymes, most using the ethoxyresorufin-*O*-deethylase (EROD) assay for CYP1A activity. However, when comparing SCDH CYP activity data using either resorufin assays[82,83,106] or LC/MS[88,91] to primary hepatocytes, all demonstrate lower activities in SCDHs than primary hepatocytes, further supporting the need to increase the efficiency of differentiation protocols.

At the heart of the situation is the fact that the majority of studies have reported SCDHs as still expressing α-fetoprotein (AFP), a protein that is highly expressed in fetal hepatocytes, but is dramatically down-regulated after birth such that healthy adult livers typically do not express it. Another marker for fetal liver is the preferential expression of CYP3A7, rather than the dominant adult isoform CYP3A4. Other commonly used markers include CYPs, transcription factors, albumin (ALB), α1-antitrypsin (AAT), CK18, and CK19 (a marker of biliary cells and hepatic progenitor cells). Results with these markers together indicate a mixed or immature population of cells. Overall, there is a significant need for improvement in generating and characterizing SCDHs, particularly with regards to their metabolic capacity compared with primary hepatocytes.

While there is evidence that SCDHs do express CYPs and other drug metabolizing enzymes, they still seem to be at immature levels (below hPHs). Additionally, the cells still express markers typical of fetal hepatocytes, such as AFP. Whether that poses a problem in terms of use in metabolite profiling and toxicity testing remains to be seen; indeed it could be one of the reasons for insufficient CYP activity. While it would be optimal for SCDHs to express functional drug metabolizing enzymes at the same level as cryopreserved and primary hepatocytes, as long as the expression and activity is reproducible and scalable, it may not be necessary. For example, if CYP3A4 content in SCDHs is consistently 50% of that of primary hepatocytes, this can be accounted for in the *in vitro* metabolite profile with a scaling factor.

Finally, significant work needs to be done to optimize a singular differentiation protocol for industry use that produces consistent and functional hepatocytes. To help in identifying and optimizing a protocol for SCDHs, there appears to be a need to develop standard endpoint assays for determining hepatocyte differentiation and function, and standard comparators such as primary hepatocytes (which should be validated on their own) to aid in comparing various differentiation protocols so that protocols that are efficient, reproducible, and robust for drug metabolism and toxicity screening can be further developed.[105]

8.5 Conclusions

Stem cells have a high self-renewal capability and can give rise to any cell in the body, making them a very attractive target for researchers in regenerative medicine, as well as drug discovery and development. As new chemical entities move into the lead optimization phase, ADME and drug–drug interaction data should be collected primarily from human models.[25] Stem cell derived culture systems offer a promising new tool for ADME studies, adding to our available human derived preclinical models. The three major organ systems involved in drug metabolism include the liver, intestine, and kidney. Tissue specific cells generated from pluripotent stem cells for all three of these organs would be very useful for drug metabolism screening. There has been extensive research on SCDHs for this purpose, and while there is evidence that SCDHs do express

CYPs and other drug metabolizing enzymes, they still remain at immature levels. Overall an improvement in generating and characterizing SCDHs is still needed, particularly with regards to their metabolic capacity compared with primary hepatocytes. While there has not been as much focus on stem cell derived enterocytes or renal proximal tubules, research in both of these areas shows promise. Overall, there is still a need to evaluate each of these cell systems for drug metabolizing enzyme and transporter activities before they could be used routinely for preclinical screening during drug development. In addition, there is a critical need to be able to accurately model these human organ systems *in vitro*, such as with 3D or microphysiological systems, to improve drug efficacy and safety assessment during drug development. Stem cells would be a consistent human cell source for manipulation in a 3D or microphysiological system that more accurately models organ function. Such systems have vast potential to advance the development of new therapeutic agents, enhancing the safety and efficacy of products approved for the market.

Acknowledgements

The authors would like to acknowledge Catherine Lockhart for her help generating the figures.

References

1. M. J. Evans and M. H. Kaufman, *Nature*, 1981, **292**, 154–156.
2. G. R. Martin, *Proc. Natl. Acad. Sci. U. S. A.*, 1981, **78**, 7634–7638.
3. J. A. Thomson, J. Itskovitz-Eldor, S. S. Shapiro, M. A. Waknitz, J. J. Swiergiel, V. S. Marshall and J. M. Jones, *Science*, 1998, **282**, 1145–1147.
4. K. Takahashi and S. Yamanaka, *Cell*, 2006, **126**, 663–676.
5. K. Takahashi, K. Tanabe, M. Ohnuki, M. Narita, T. Ichisaka, K. Tomoda and S. Yamanaka, *Cell*, 2007, **131**, 861–872.
6. M. W. Lensch and C. L. Mummery, *Stem Cell Rep.*, 2013, **1**, 5–17.
7. Geron Corporation, *Regener. Med.*, 2009, **4**, 161.
8. J. Alper, *Nat. Biotechnol.*, 2009, **27**, 213–214.
9. D. Brindley and C. Mason, *Regener. Med.*, 2012, **7**, 17–18.
10. S. Reardon and D. Cyranoski, *Nature*, 2014, **513**, 287–288.
11. R. E. Chapin and D. B. Stedman, *Toxicol. Sci.*, 2009, **112**, 17–22.
12. T. Reya, S. J. Morrison, M. F. Clarke and I. L. Weissman, *Nature*, 2001, **414**, 105–111.
13. A. Nagy, in *Essentials of Stem Cell Biology*, ed. R. Lanza, Elsevier, London, 2nd edn, 2009, pp. 429–436.
14. S. Irion, M. C. Nostro, S. J. Kattman and G. M. Keller, *Cold Spring Harbor Symp. Quant. Biol.*, 2008, **73**, 101–110.
15. J. Yu, M. A. Vodyanik, K. Smuga-Otto, J. Antosiewicz-Bourget, J. L. Frane, S. Tian, J. Nie, G. A. Jonsdottir, V. Ruotti, R. Stewart, I. I. Slukvin and J. A. Thomson, *Science*, 2007, **318**, 1917–1920.

16. J. C. Davila, G. G. Cezar, M. Thiede, S. Strom, T. Miki and J. Trosko, *Toxicol. Sci. Off. J. Soc. Toxicol.*, 2004, **79**, 214–223.
17. A. C. Need, A. G. Motulsky and D. B. Goldstein, *Nat. Genet.*, 2005, **37**, 671–681.
18. C. F. Mandenius, D. Steel, F. Noor, T. Meyer, E. Heinzle, J. Asp, S. Arain, U. Kraushaar, S. Bremer, R. Class and P. Sartipy, *J. Appl. Toxicol.*, 2011, **31**, 191–205.
19. A. M. Wobus and P. Loser, *Arch. Toxicol.*, 2011, **85**, 79–117.
20. S. Webb, *Nat. Biotechnol.*, 2009, **27**, 977–979.
21. K. Harris, M. Aylott, Y. Cui, J. B. Louttit, N. C. McMahon and A. Sridhar, *Toxicol. Sci. Off. J. Soc. Toxicol.*, 2013, **134**, 412–426.
22. J. J. Chong, X. Yang, C. W. Don, E. Minami, Y. W. Liu, J. J. Weyers, W. M. Mahoney, B. Van Biber, S. M. Cook, N. J. Palpant, J. A. Gantz, J. A. Fugate, V. Muskheli, G. M. Gough, K. W. Vogel, C. A. Astley, C. E. Hotchkiss, A. Baldessari, L. Pabon, H. Reinecke, E. A. Gill, V. Nelson, H. P. Kiem, M. A. Laflamme and C. E. Murry, *Nature*, 2014, **510**, 273–277.
23. K. R. Chi, *Nat. Rev. Drug Discovery*, 2013, **12**, 565–567.
24. P. T. Sager, G. Gintant, J. R. Turner, S. Pettit and N. Stockbridge, *Am. Heart J.*, 2014, **167**, 292–300.
25. J. M. McKim, in *New Horizons in Predictive Toxicology: Current Status and Application*, ed. A. G. Wilson, The Royal Society of Chemistry, Cambridge, 2012, pp. 157–214.
26. H. Zhang, C. D. Davis, M. W. Sinz and A. D. Rodrigues, *Expert Opin. Drug Metab. Toxicol.*, 2007, **3**, 667–687.
27. S. S. Singh, *Curr. Drug Metab.*, 2006, **7**, 165–182.
28. K. Venkatakrishnan, L. L. Von Moltke and D. J. Greenblatt, *J. Clin. Pharmacol.*, 2001, **41**, 1149–1179.
29. F. P. Guengerich, in *Cytochrome P450: Structure, Mechanism, and Biochemistry*, ed. P. R. O. d. Montellano, Kluwer Academic/Plenum Publishers, New York, 3rd edn, 2005, pp. 377–530.
30. M. Ingelman-Sundberg, S. C. Sim, A. Gomez and C. Rodriguez-Antona, *Pharmacol. Ther.*, 2007, **116**, 496–526.
31. A. Y. Lu, R. W. Wang and J. H. Lin, *Drug Metab. Dispos. Biol. Fate Chem.*, 2003, **31**, 345–350.
32. A. N. Nedderman, G. J. Dear, S. North, R. S. Obach and D. Higton, *Xenobiotica*, 2011, **41**, 605–622.
33. J. H. Lin and A. Y. Lu, *Pharmacol. Rev.*, 1997, **49**, 403–449.
34. J. O. Miners, K. M. Knights, J. B. Houston and P. I. Mackenzie, *Biochem. Pharmacol.*, 2006, **71**, 1531–1539.
35. S. A. Barros and R. B. Martin, *Methods Mol. Biol.*, 2008, **460**, 89–112.
36. J. B. Houston, *Biochem. Pharmacol.*, 1994, **47**, 1469–1479.
37. J. B. Houston and A. Galetin, *Curr. Drug Metab.*, 2008, **9**, 940–951.
38. S. A. Wrighton, B. J. Ring and M. Vandenbranden, *Toxicol. Pathol.*, 1995, **23**, 199–208.
39. E. F. A. Brandon, C. D. Raap, I. Meijerman, J. H. Beijnen and J. H. M. Schellens, *Toxicol. Appl. Pharmacol.*, 2003, **189**, 233–246.

40. P. Chandra, E. L. Lecluyse and K. L. Brouwer, *In Vitro Cell. Dev. Biol.: Anim.*, 2001, **37**, 380–385.

41. E. L. LeCluyse, *Eur. J. Pharm. Sci.*, 2001, **13**, 343–368.

42. S. M. Huang, J. M. Strong, L. Zhang, K. S. Reynolds, S. Nallani, R. Temple, S. Abraham, S. A. Habet, R. K. Baweja, G. J. Burckart, S. Chung, P. Colangelo, D. Frucht, M. D. Green, P. Hepp, E. Karnaukhova, H. S. Ko, J. I. Lee, P. J. Marroum, J. M. Norden, W. Qiu, A. Rahman, S. Sobel, T. Stifano, K. Thummel, X. X. Wei, S. Yasuda, J. H. Zheng, H. Zhao and L. J. Lesko, *J. Clin. Pharmacol.*, 2008, **48**, 662–670.

43. A. Costa, B. Sarmento and V. Seabra, *Expert Opin. Drug Metab. Toxicol.*, 2014, **10**, 103–119.

44. J. H. Lin, M. Chiba and T. A. Baillie, *Pharmacol. Rev.*, 1999, **51**, 135–158.

45. M. F. Paine, H. L. Hart, S. S. Ludington, R. L. Haining, A. E. Rettie and D. C. Zeldin, *Drug Metab. Dispos. Biol. Fate Chem.*, 2006, **34**, 880–886.

46. I. de Waziers, P. H. Cugnenc, C. S. Yang, J. P. Leroux and P. H. Beaune, *J. Pharmacol. Exp. Ther.*, 1990, **253**, 387–394.

47. T. Shimada, H. Yamazaki, M. Mimura, Y. Inui and F. P. Guengerich, *J. Pharmacol. Exp. Ther.*, 1994, **270**, 414–423.

48. G. M. Groothuis and I. A. de Graaf, *Curr. Drug Metab.*, 2013, **14**, 112–119.

49. R. B. van Breemen and Y. Li, *Expert Opin. Drug Metab. Toxicol.*, 2005, **1**, 175–185.

50. L. Z. Benet and C. L. Cummins, *Adv. Drug Delivery Rev.*, 2001, **50**(suppl. 1), S3–S11.

51. A. Pfrunder, H. Gutmann, C. Beglinger and J. Drewe, *J. Pharm. Pharmacol.*, 2003, **55**, 59–66.

52. A. Gupta, G. M. Mugundu, P. B. Desai, K. E. Thummel and J. D. Unadkat, *Drug Metab. Dispos. Biol. Fate Chem.*, 2008, **36**, 1172–1180.

53. E. G. van de Kerkhof, A. L. Ungell, A. K. Sjoberg, M. H. de Jager, C. Hilgendorf, I. A. de Graaf and G. M. Groothuis, *Drug Metab. Dispos. Biol. Fate Chem.*, 2006, **34**, 1893–1902.

54. S. A. Brugmann and J. M. Wells, *Stem Cell Res. Ther.*, 2013, **4**(suppl. 1), S1.

55. J. Foulke-Abel, J. In, O. Kovbasnjuk, N. C. Zachos, K. Ettayebi, S. E. Blutt, J. M. Hyser, X. L. Zeng, S. E. Crawford, J. R. Broughman, M. K. Estes and M. Donowitz, *Exp. Biol. Med.*, 2014, **239**, 1124–1134.

56. P. Jung, T. Sato, A. Merlos-Suarez, F. M. Barriga, M. Iglesias, D. Rossell, H. Auer, M. Gallardo, M. A. Blasco, E. Sancho, H. Clevers and E. Batlle, *Nat. Med.*, 2011, **17**, 1225–1227.

57. T. Sato, D. E. Stange, M. Ferrante, R. G. Vries, J. H. Van Es, S. van den Brink, W. J. Van Houdt, A. Pronk, J. Van Gorp, P. D. Siersema and H. Clevers, *Gastroenterology*, 2011, **141**, 1762–1772.

58. C. L. Watson, M. M. Mahe, J. Munera, J. C. Howell, N. Sundaram, H. M. Poling, J. I. Schweitzer, J. E. Vallance, C. N. Mayhew, Y. Sun, G. Grabowski, S. R. Finkbeiner, J. R. Spence, N. F. Shroyer, J. M. Wells and M. A. Helmrath, *Nat. Med.*, 2014, **20**, 1310–1314.

59. K. W. McCracken, J. C. Howell, J. M. Wells and J. R. Spence, *Nat. Protoc.*, 2011, **6**, 1920–1928.

60. J. R. Spence, C. N. Mayhew, S. A. Rankin, M. F. Kuhar, J. E. Vallance, K. Tolle, E. E. Hoskins, V. V. Kalinichenko, S. I. Wells, A. M. Zorn, N. F. Shroyer and J. M. Wells, *Nature*, 2011, **470**, 105–109.
61. A. Wang and M. Sander, *J. Mol. Med.*, 2012, **90**, 763–771.
62. S. R. Finkbeiner, X. L. Zeng, B. Utama, R. L. Atmar, N. F. Shroyer and M. K. Estes, *mBio*, 2012, **3**, e00159-12.
63. C. K. Yeung, D. D. Shen, K. E. Thummel and J. Himmelfarb, *Kidney Int.*, 2014, **85**, 522–528.
64. B. D. Haehner, J. C. Gorski, M. Vandenbranden, S. A. Wrighton, S. K. Janardan, P. B. Watkins and S. D. Hall, *Mol. Pharmacol.*, 1996, **50**, 52–59.
65. P. Kuehl, J. Zhang, Y. Lin, J. Lamba, M. Assem, J. Schuetz, P. B. Watkins, A. Daly, S. A. Wrighton, S. D. Hall, P. Maurel, M. Relling, C. Brimer, K. Yasuda, R. Venkataramanan, S. Strom, K. Thummel, M. S. Boguski and E. Schuetz, *Nat. Genet.*, 2001, **27**, 383–391.
66. Y. S. Lin, A. L. Dowling, S. D. Quigley, F. M. Farin, J. Zhang, J. Lamba, E. G. Schuetz and K. E. Thummel, *Mol. Pharmacol.*, 2002, **62**, 162–172.
67. J. W. Lohr, G. R. Willsky and M. A. Acara, *Pharmacol. Rev.*, 1998, **50**, 107–141.
68. M. J. Ryan, G. Johnson, J. Kirk, S. M. Fuerstenberg, R. A. Zager and B. Torok-Storb, *Kidney Int.*, 1994, **45**, 48–57.
69. S. E. Jenkinson, G. W. Chung, E. van Loon, N. S. Bakar, A. M. Dalzell and C. D. Brown, *Pflugers Arch.*, 2012, **464**, 601–611.
70. E. J. Kelly, Z. Wang, J. L. Voellinger, C. K. Yeung, D. D. Shen, K. E. Thummel, Y. Zheng, G. Ligresti, D. L. Eaton, K. A. Muczynski, J. S. Duffield, T. Neumann, A. Tourovskaia, M. Fauver, G. Kramer, E. Asp and J. Himmelfarb, *Stem Cell Res. Ther.*, 2013, **4**(suppl. 1), S17.
71. J. S. Uzarski, Y. Xia, J. C. Belmonte and J. A. Wertheim, *Curr. Opin. Nephrol. Hypertens.*, 2014, **23**, 399–405.
72. A. Q. Lam, B. S. Freedman and J. V. Bonventre, *Semin. Nephrol.*, 2014, **34**, 445–461.
73. C. A. Batchelder, C. C. Lee, D. G. Matsell, M. C. Yoder and A. F. Tarantal, *Differentiation*, 2009, **78**, 45–56.
74. S. A. Lin, G. Kolle, S. M. Grimmond, Q. Zhou, E. Doust, M. H. Little, B. Aronow, S. D. Ricardo, M. F. Pera, J. F. Bertram and A. L. Laslett, *Stem Cells Dev.*, 2010, **19**, 1637–1648.
75. B. Song, A. M. Smink, C. V. Jones, J. M. Callaghan, S. D. Firth, C. A. Bernard, A. L. Laslett, P. G. Kerr and S. D. Ricardo, *PLoS One*, 2012, 7, e46453.
76. K. Narayanan, K. M. Schumacher, F. Tasnim, K. Kandasamy, A. Schumacher, M. Ni, S. Gao, B. Gopalan, D. Zink and J. Y. Ying, *Kidney Int.*, 2013, **83**, 593–603.
77. A. Q. Lam, B. S. Freedman, R. Morizane, P. H. Lerou, M. T. Valerius and J. V. Bonventre, *J. Am. Soc. Nephrol.*, 2014, **25**, 1211–1225.
78. M. Takasato, P. X. Er, M. Becroft, J. M. Vanslambrouck, E. G. Stanley, A. G. Elefanty and M. H. Little, *Nat. Cell Biol.*, 2014, **16**, 118–126.
79. T. Araoka, S. Mae, Y. Kurose, M. Uesugi, A. Ohta, S. Yamanaka and K. Osafune, *PLoS One*, 2014, **9**, e84881.

80. N. J. Hewitt, M. J. Gómez Lechón, J. B. Houston, D. Hallifax, H. S. Brown, P. Maurel, J. G. Kenna, L. Gustavsson, C. Lohmann, C. Skonberg, A. Guillouzo, G. Tuschl, A. P. Li, E. LeCluyse, G. M. M. Groothuis and J. G. Hengstler, *Drug Metab. Rev.*, 2007, **39**, 159–234.

81. Claire N. Medine, S. Greenhough and D. C. Hay, *Biochem. Soc. Trans.*, 2010, **38**, 1033.

82. L. Rambhatla, C. P. Chiu, P. Kundu, Y. Peng and M. K. Carpenter, *Cell Transplant.*, 2003, **12**, 1–11.

83. Y. Duan, A. Catana, Y. Meng, N. Yamamoto, S. He, S. Gupta, S. S. Gambhir and M. A. Zern, *Stem Cells*, 2007, **25**, 3058–3068.

84. D. C. Hay, J. Fletcher, C. Payne, J. D. Terrace, R. C. J. Gallagher, J. Snoeys, J. R. Black, D. Wojtacha, K. Samuel, Z. Hannoun, A. Pryde, C. Filippi, I. S. Currie, S. J. Forbes, J. A. Ross, P. N. Newsome and J. P. Iredale, *Proc. Natl. Acad. Sci.*, 2008, **105**, 12301–12306.

85. D. C. Hay, D. Zhao, J. Fletcher, Z. A. Hewitt, D. McLean, A. Urruticoechea-Uriguen, J. R. Black, C. Elcombe, J. A. Ross, R. Wolf and W. Cui, *Stem Cells*, 2008, **26**, 894–902.

86. D. Szkolnicka, S. L. Farnworth, B. Lucendo-Villarin and D. C. Hay, *Curr. Protoc. Stem Cell Biol.*, 2014, **30**, 1G.5.1–1G.5.12.

87. M. Ek, T. Söderdahl, B. Küppers-Munther, J. Edsbagge, T. B. Andersson, P. Björquist, I. Cotgreave, B. Jernström, M. Ingelman-Sundberg and I. Johansson, *Biochem. Pharmacol.*, 2007, **74**, 496–503.

88. Y. Duan, X. Ma, W. Zou, C. Wang, I. S. Bahbahan, T. P. Ahuja, V. Tolstikov and M. A. Zern, *Stem Cells*, 2010, **28**, 674–686.

89. T. S. Ramasamy, J. S. L. Yu, C. Selden, H. Hodgson and W. Cui, *Tissue Eng., Part A*, 2013, **19**, 360–367.

90. K. Takayama, M. Inamura, K. Kawabata, K. Katayama, M. Higuchi, K. Tashiro, A. Nonaka, F. Sakurai, T. Hayakawa, M. Kusuda Furue and H. Mizuguchi, *Mol. Ther.*, 2011, **20**, 127–137.

91. K. Takayama, M. Inamura, K. Kawabata, M. Sugawara, K. Kikuchi, M. Higuchi, Y. Nagamoto, H. Watanabe, K. Tashiro, F. Sakurai, T. Hayakawa, M. K. Furue and H. Mizuguchi, *J. Hepatol.*, 2012, **57**, 628–636.

92. K. Takayama, K. Kawabata, Y. Nagamoto, K. Kishimoto, K. Tashiro, F. Sakurai, M. Tachibana, K. Kanda, T. Hayakawa, M. K. Furue and H. Mizuguchi, *Biomaterials*, 2013, **34**, 1781–1789.

93. S. Ogawa, J. Surapisitchat, C. Virtanen, M. Ogawa, M. Niapour, K. S. Sugamori, S. Wang, L. Tamblyn, C. Guillemette, E. Hoffmann, B. Zhao, S. Strom, R. R. Laposa, R. F. Tyndale, D. M. Grant and G. Keller, *Development*, 2013, **140**, 3285–3296.

94. N. Nakamura, K. Saeki, M. Mitsumoto, S. Matsuyama, M. Nishio, M. Hasegawa, Y. Miyagawa, H. Ohkita, N. Kiyokawa, M. Toyoda, H. Akutsu, A. Umezawa and A. Yuo, *Cell. Reprogramming*, 2012, **14**, 171–185.

95. N. L. Magner, Y. Jung, J. Wu, J. A. Nolta, M. A. Zern and P. Zhou, *Stem Cells*, 2013, **31**, 2095–2103.

96. J. Cai, Y. Zhao, Y. Liu, F. Ye, Z. Song, H. Qin, S. Meng, Y. Chen, R. Zhou, X. Song, Y. Guo, M. Ding and H. Deng, *Hepatology*, 2007, **45**, 1229–1239.

97. D. C. Hay, D. Zhao, A. Ross, R. Mandalam, J. Lebkowski and W. Cui, *Cloning Stem Cells*, 2007, **9**, 51–62.

98. G. J. Sullivan, D. C. Hay, I. H. Park, J. Fletcher, Z. Hannoun, C. M. Payne, D. Dalgetty, J. R. Black, J. A. Ross, K. Samuel, G. Wang, G. Q. Daley, J. H. Lee, G. M. Church, S. J. Forbes, J. P. Iredale and I. Wilmut, *Hepatology*, 2010, **51**, 329–335.

99. J. Shan, R. E. Schwartz, N. T. Ross, D. J. Logan, D. Thomas, S. A. Duncan, T. E. North, W. Goessling, A. E. Carpenter and S. N. Bhatia, *Nat. Chem. Biol.*, 2013, **9**, 514–520.

100. T. Miki, A. Ring and J. Gerlach, *Tissue Eng., Part C*, 2011, **17**, 557–568.

101. K. Subramanian, D. J. Owens, R. Raju, M. Firpo, T. D. O'Brien, C. M. Verfaillie and W. S. Hu, *Stem Cells Dev.*, 2014, **23**, 124–131.

102. N. R. Hannan, C. P. Segeritz, T. Touboul and L. Vallier, *Nat. Protoc.*, 2013, **8**, 430–437.

103. D. Zhao, S. Chen, S. Duo, C. Xiang, J. Jia, M. Guo, W. Lai, S. Lu and H. Deng, *Cell Res.*, 2013, **23**, 157–161.

104. G. Brolen, L. Sivertsson, P. Bjorquist, G. Eriksson, M. Ek, H. Semb, I. Johansson, T. B. Andersson, M. Ingelman-Sundberg and N. Heins, *J. Biotechnol.*, 2010, **145**, 284–294.

105. R. Kia, R. L. Sison, J. Heslop, N. R. Kitteringham, N. Hanley, J. S. Mills, B. K. Park and C. E. Goldring, *Br. J. Clin. Pharmacol.*, 2013, **75**, 885–896.

106. H. Basma, A. Soto-Gutiérrez, G. R. Yannam, L. Liu, R. Ito, T. Yamamoto, E. Ellis, S. D. Carson, S. Sato, Y. Chen, D. Muirhead, N. Navarro-Álvarez, R. J. Wong, J. Roy-Chowdhury, J. L. Platt, D. F. Mercer, J. D. Miller, S. C. Strom, N. Kobayashi and I. J. Fox, *Gastroenterology*, 2009, **136**, 990. e4–999.e4.

107. S. Zhang, S. Chen, W. Li, X. Guo, P. Zhao, J. Xu, Y. Chen, Q. Pan, X. Liu, D. Zychlinski, H. Lu, M. D. Tortorella, A. Schambach, Y. Wang, D. Pei and M. A. Esteban, *Hum. Mol. Genet.*, 2011, **20**, 3176–3187.

108. R. Yildirimman, G. Brolen, M. Vilardell, G. Eriksson, J. Synnergren, H. Gmuender, A. Kamburov, M. Ingelman-Sundberg, J. Castell, A. Lahoz, J. Kleinjans, J. van Delft, P. Bjorquist and R. Herwig, *Toxicol. Sci. Off. J. Soc. Toxicol.*, 2011, **124**, 278–290.

CHAPTER 9

Chemically Reactive Versus Stable Drug Metabolites: Role in Adverse Drug Reactions

THOMAS A. BAILLIE*[a]

[a]School of Pharmacy, University of Washington, Box 357631, Seattle, WA 98195-7631, U.S.A.
*E-mail: tbaillie@uw.edu

9.1 Introduction

Studies on the metabolic fate of candidate drugs, both in liver preparations from animal species, and humans *in vitro*, and in laboratory animals *in vivo*, are performed routinely at the preclinical stage of drug development for three primary reasons, namely: (1) to define clearance mechanisms; (2) to assess the formation of pharmacologically active or chemically reactive metabolites; and (3) to confirm that expected human metabolites are formed in the rodent and non-rodent species selected for safety assessment studies. In addition to these scientific drivers, an understanding of the metabolic fate of a new chemical entity, initially in animals and subsequently in humans, is necessary from a regulatory standpoint in terms of predicting possible inter-subject variability (due to pharmacogenomics or pathological conditions such as hepatic insufficiency, renal impairment, *etc.*) and drug interaction liabilities, in addition to assessing the adequacy of the preclinical toxicology program in terms of metabolite "coverage" (animal *versus* human exposure)

RSC Drug Discovery Series No. 49
New Horizons in Predictive Drug Metabolism and Pharmacokinetics
Edited by Alan G. E. Wilson
© The Royal Society of Chemistry 2016
Published by the Royal Society of Chemistry, www.rsc.org

according to current Metabolites in Safety Testing ("MIST") guidance.[1] The topic of pharmacologically active drug metabolites was covered by a recent comprehensive review[2] and will not be discussed here. Rather, the present chapter will focus on the role of drug metabolites as potential mediators of adverse drug reactions, and will discuss the approaches currently adopted in drug discovery and early development programs to minimize the likelihood that a new chemical entity will form toxic metabolites. For purposes of discussion, drug metabolites are divided into two distinct groups, chemically reactive intermediates and chemically stable metabolites, whose evaluation requires quite different approaches.

9.2 Chemically Reactive Metabolites and Drug-Induced Toxicity

Following the pioneering work of the Millers in the late 1940s on the metabolism of *N,N*-dimethylaminoazobenzene and related aminoazo dyes to reactive electrophiles that bind covalently to cellular macromolecules and cause liver damage,[3] Mitchell, Brodie, Gillette and co-workers at the National Institutes of Health applied similar concepts some 25 years later in their investigations into the hepatotoxic effects of the widely used non-prescription analgesic drug, acetaminophen (paracetamol; APAP). In what has now become a classic series of papers published back-to-back in the *Journal of Pharmacology and Experimental Therapeutics*,[4] it was shown that APAP undergoes cytochrome P450 (CYP)-mediated activation in liver tissue to a reactive intermediate that binds covalently to proteins and forms an *S*-linked conjugate with the endogenous tripeptide glutathione (GSH) (Figure 9.1). Based on the structure of this GSH conjugate, it was hypothesized that the reactive intermediate was

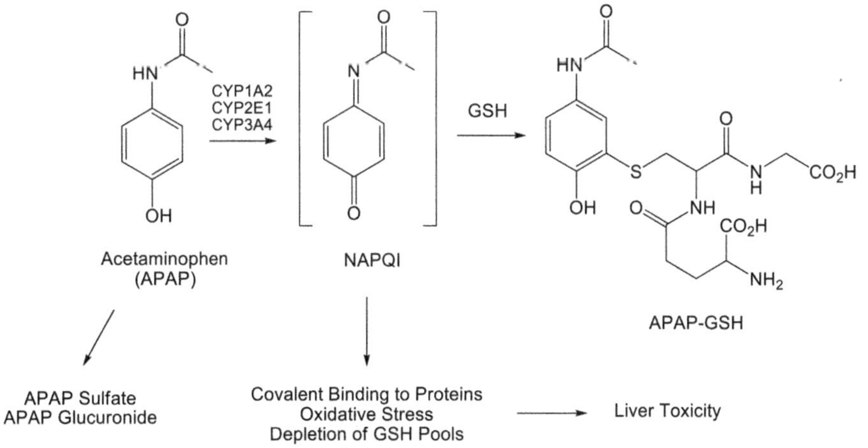

Figure 9.1   Metabolism of APAP, illustrating the metabolic activation pathway leading to NAPQI, believed to be the species responsible for the hepatotoxic effects of the drug. Reproduced with permission from Baillie and Rettie.[6]

N-acetyl-*p*-benzoquinoneimine (NAPQI), formed by two-electron oxidation of the parent drug.

At the time, this was a controversial proposal since CYP enzymes, which were well known to mediate the *oxygenation* of organic substrates, were not known to catalyze *dehydrogenation* across a substituted aromatic ring. However, the hypothesis proved to be correct, although it was not until 1984 that it was demonstrated that NAPQI could be generated from APAP *in vitro* using a reconstituted CYP system with cumene hydroperoxide as the oxidant.[5] Today, we recognize that many appropriately substituted aromatic compounds undergo metabolism by this dehydrogenation pathway, and that the resulting quinones, quinoneimines and quinonemethides, *etc.*, serve both as reactive electrophiles and as oxidizing agents that have the potential to cause cellular injury, especially once hepatic stores of GSH have been depleted.[6] In this regard, metabolic precursors of such quinoid species are now classified as "structural alerts" for toxicity (Figure 9.2).[7]

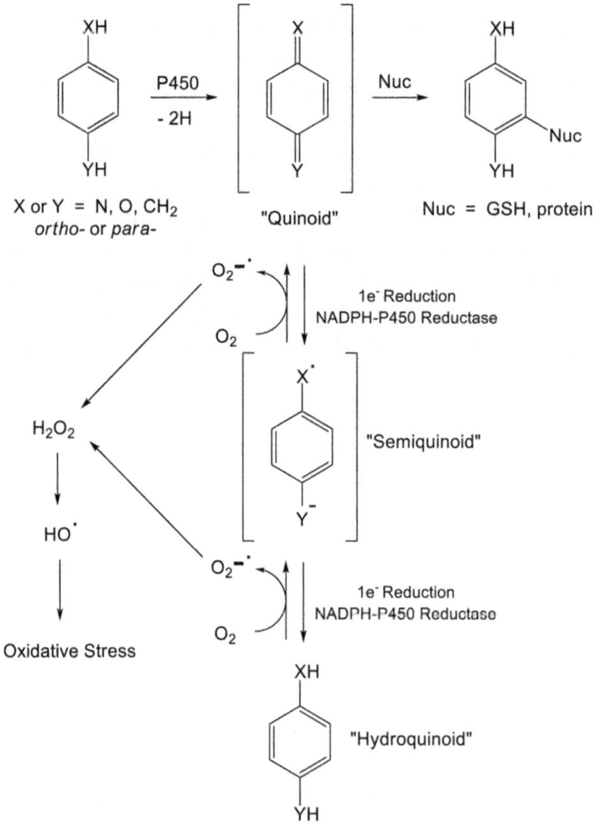

Figure 9.2   Quinoid precursors as structural alerts for toxicity. The quinoid intermediate can serve as both an electrophile that covalently binds to proteins or GSH, and as an oxidizing agent responsible for the formation of reactive oxygen species (superoxide anion, hydrogen peroxide and hydroxyl radical). Reproduced with permission from Baillie and Rettie.[6]

In contrast to major advances over the past 20 years in the instrumentation (notably liquid chromatography-tandem mass spectrometry [LC-MS/MS] systems) employed for the detection and structural characterization of GSH conjugates (from which the structures of electrophilic drug metabolites may be inferred), progress has been relatively slow in gaining an understanding of the molecular mechanisms by which exposure to reactive drug metabolites leads to toxicity. Early theories focused on the covalent binding of electrophilic metabolites to proteins as the causative event until it was shown that covalent binding *per se* frequently failed to correlate directly with toxicity. A striking example of such a disconnect is found with a positional isomer of APAP, namely 3'-hydroxyacetanilide (AMAP), which undergoes metabolism to a reactive quinone derivative analogous to NAPQI, and binds covalently to liver proteins in animals at levels similar to those observed following administration of APAP, yet it is not hepatotoxic.[8] This and related examples would suggest that the mere observation of covalent binding is an inadequate predictor of toxicity, but that additional factors must be important, such as the identities and subcellular locations of the target proteins of individual reactive intermediates. An intriguing observation in this regard is that APAP was found to alkylate predominantly mitochondrial proteins in mouse liver, whereas its non-hepatotoxic regioisomer AMAP was found to bind mainly to microsomal and cytosolic proteins.[9] Today, versatile proteomics LC-MS/MS techniques, coupled with novel methods for the isolation of covalently modified proteins from both *in vitro* and *in vivo* sources and powerful bioinformatics capabilities, provide the tools with which to address important questions regarding the nature of xenobiotic–protein adducts and their role in reactive metabolite-mediated toxicity.[10] Preliminary findings from such work have provided evidence that different reactive intermediates exhibit different degrees of selectivity, both in terms of their protein targets and the amino acid residues on these targets to which they bind.[11] Moreover, recent studies have revealed the existence of a hierarchy in the susceptibility of families of proteins towards alkylation damage, thereby providing an additional dimension to the element of selectivity.[12] While the protein targets of reactive electrophiles are known only for a limited number of drugs and other foreign compounds, currently available data on this topic suggest that it is unlikely that toxicity results from damage to a single protein, or even to a limited number of structurally or functionally important proteins, but rather results from damage to entire protein networks that are involved, for example, in intracellular signaling pathways, protein folding, unfolded protein response, or regulation of apoptosis.[13]

While much remains to be learned about the role of chemically reactive metabolites and associated covalent binding in drug-induced toxicities, experience over the past 40 years with the recall of marketed drugs and the failure of promising drug candidates in development have provided persuasive evidence that metabolic activation has been a contributing factor in many, if not most cases. Thus, in a survey of product withdrawals over the period 1980–2005 for reasons of toxicity, it was noted that most of the compounds formed reactive intermediates.[14] A high dosage (>50 mg per day) was also a characteristic of withdrawn drugs, suggesting that a high "body burden" of reactive metabolites may have played a role in their toxicity.[14,15] For those adverse drug reactions that appear to be mediated by the immune system—often referred to as "idiosyncratic" toxicities, affecting a very small number of patients with a delayed onset, and not predicted by animal models—it seems likely that haptenization of proteins by reactive drug metabolites is an underlying factor, although here again it is difficult to establish an unambiguous cause-and-effect relationship.[16] Consider the example of abacavir, a reverse transcriptase inhibitor employed in the treatment of HIV/AIDS, which causes a rare, but serious hypersensitivity reaction that bears the hallmarks of an immune drug reaction. Metabolism studies with abacavir demonstrated that the drug undergoes oxidation in animals and humans to an α,β-unsaturated aldehyde intermediate, which has the potential to serve as a Michael acceptor and react with protein sulfhydryls[17] (Figure 9.3). Indeed, a recent report describes the identification of novel cross-linked abacavir–albumin adducts in the serum of patients treated with the drug, with structures that are consistent with the formation of such a reactive intermediate.[18]

Interestingly, the incidence of hypersensitivity reactions to abacavir is markedly elevated in subjects who carry the B*57:01 variant in the human leukocyte antigen B (HLA-B) gene,[19] and it was hypothesized that peptide adducts formed *via* proteolysis of abacavir–protein conjugates may be presented more effectively to T-cell receptors in subjects carrying this HLA variant. However, it has now been shown that abacavir itself—and not a metabolite—induces a conformational change in HLA B*57:01 such that an abnormal suite of endogenous peptides are presented to the immune system, raising the possibility that this alternative (non-covalent) drug–protein interaction may underlie the hypersensitivity response to the drug.[20-22] Further studies will be required to establish which of the two mechanisms prevails, *i.e.* haptenization of proteins by a reactive metabolite of abacavir or modulation by the parent drug of the endogenous peptides that are displayed by antigen presenting cells. It is possible, of course, that both mechanisms play a role, or that some other, as yet unidentified factor is important, but this interesting example serves to highlight the danger in attributing a particular drug-induced toxicity to a reactive metabolite purely on the basis that the parent compound has been shown to undergo metabolic activation *in vitro* or *in vivo*.

Based on the foregoing discussion, it will be evident that the topic of chemically reactive metabolites is a challenging one in the context of drug discovery programs, since it is not possible at present to distinguish those reactive intermediates that may pose a significant toxicological risk from those that are likely to be benign. In some cases, serious adverse events in humans that are believed to be caused by reactive metabolite(s), *e.g.* APAP-induced hepatotoxicity, can be recapitulated in animal toxicology studies. In this situation, appropriate risk assessments can be performed based on a number of considerations, such as whether the toxicity is reversible and can

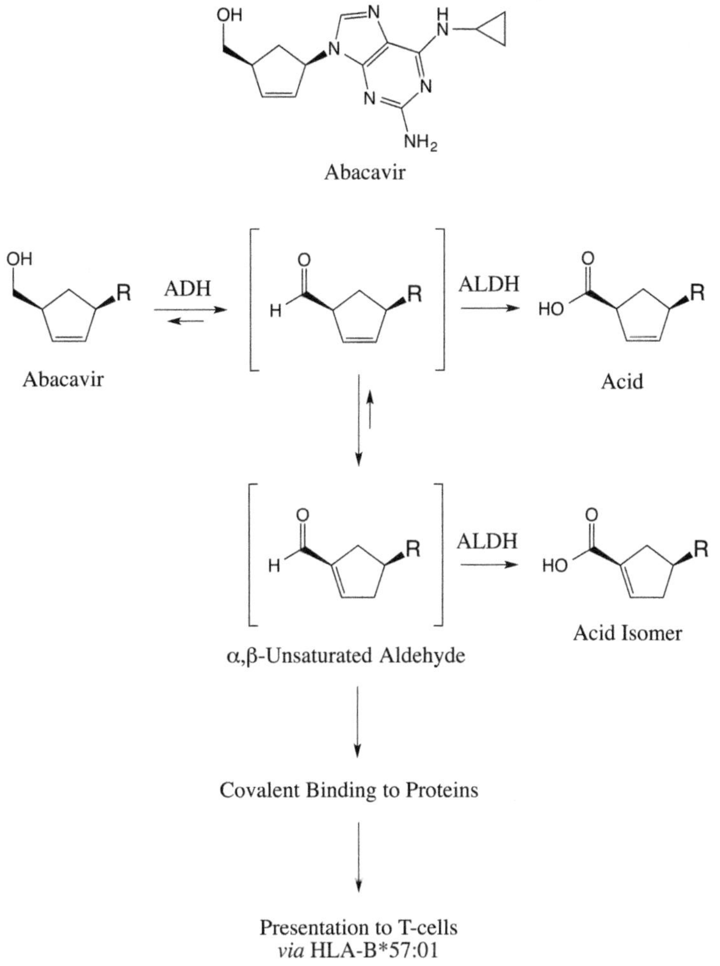

Figure 9.3 Structure of abacavir, and proposed metabolic activation pathway involving oxidation of the hydroxymethylcyclopentane moiety. Intermediates in brackets have not been isolated, but are inferred from the identities of the corresponding carboxylic acids that are excreted in urine. ADH: alcohol dehydrogenase; ALDH: aldehyde dehydrogenase.

be monitored and, if so, whether acceptable exposure margins can be established (animal area under the plasma concentration *versus* time curve [AUC$_p$] at the no observed adverse effect level [NOAEL] relative to the human AUC$_p$ at the maximum anticipated clinical dose). However, not all human toxicities are replicated in the animal species commonly employed in preclinical toxicology studies,[23] and this applies particularly to those adverse events mediated by the human immune system for which there is no generally applicable animal model.[16] The possibility that haptenization of proteins by a reactive metabolite may trigger a serious idiosyncratic reaction in a small number of recipients at a late stage of development, or even post-marketing, needs to be taken into consideration in the decision to advance a candidate drug that has been shown to form reactive metabolites. Hence, the dilemma for the pharmaceutical industry is how to place in context the observation that a lead candidate undergoes metabolic activation in animals *in vivo* or in animal/human liver preparations *in vitro*. The situation is complicated further by the fact that certain safe and highly effective therapeutic agents, such as omeprazole and clopidogrel, are converted to reactive sulfenic acid (–S–OH) species *in vivo*, and actually it is the covalent binding of these intermediates to their specific target proteins that has proven to be the basis of their pharmacological activity.[24]

Historically, industry has adopted one of two positions relative to metabolic activation of drug candidates: (1) ignore the issue, and rely on the accumulating body of safety data, initially from preclinical toxicology programs and subsequently from clinical trials, to assess the human safety characteristics of the drug candidate in question; or (2) identify the reactive metabolite(s) in question at an early stage and explore structural modifications designed to minimize, if not eliminate, metabolic activation of the lead candidate prior to entry into development. While the former approach predominated prior to the 1990s, most companies now have adopted strategies that, to varying degrees, endeavor to reduce potential metabolic activation liabilities in drug candidates at the lead optimization stage with a view to decreasing the risk of encountering reactive intermediate-induced toxicities in the course of drug development. Merck was the first company to implement such a strategy,[25] although many other major pharmaceutical manufacturers, such as GlaxoSmithKline[26] and AstraZeneca,[27] now have incorporated assessments of metabolic activation into their early risk assessment protocols. In general, three experimental approaches are employed to detect the formation of chemically reactive metabolites; in order of increasing resource requirements, these are: (a) observation of time-dependent CYP inhibition (TDI) *in vitro*,[28] (b) nucleophilic "trapping" experiments *in vitro* with agents such as GSH[29] or cyanide ion,[30] and (c) measurements of covalent binding of a radiolabeled analog of the drug candidate to liver proteins *in vitro* and/or *in vivo*[31]. These three methods have different end-points and provide different types of information. Thus, TDI reflects the formation of either highly reactive products of CYP catalysis that fail to escape from the enzyme's active site, or metabolic intermediate (MI) complexes that result from tight, non-covalent adducts to the CYP prosthetic heme iron.[32] In both cases, the consequence of TDI is a drug–drug interaction liability in which the CYP inhibitor serves as the perpetrator. Adducts from trapping experiments with GSH or cyanide can be characterized by LC-MS/MS techniques, and the resulting structural information used to provide valuable insight into the identities of the reactive intermediates themselves. By contrast, measurements of covalent binding provide no structural information, but reflect the portion of reactive metabolite formation that escapes capture by nucleophiles such as GSH (*i.e.* the reactive metabolite "cellular burden"). It is common for approaches (a) and (b) to be employed in a screening capacity during drug discovery programs, while the covalent binding studies of approach (c) are typically reserved for late-stage drug candidates where a decision is to be made between a limited number of compounds of the candidate to be taken forward into development. The following examples, all of which are drawn from drug discovery programs at Merck Research Laboratories, illustrate the application of each of the above methods to lead optimization efforts where the goal was to minimize the generation of reactive metabolites through rational structural redesign.

9.3 Elimination of CYP3A4 TDI

A promising lead compound from a melanocortin-4 agonist discovery program (Compound **1**, Figure 9.4), when incubated with recombinant CYP3A4, was found to generate an MI complex as evidenced by the characteristic Soret band at $\lambda = 355$ nm in the UV spectrum, which increased steadily in intensity during a 10 min incubation (Figure 9.4).[33] Further evidence pointing to an MI complex was obtained when potassium ferricyanide was added to the cuvette, which caused the peak at 355 nm to collapse, consistent with dissociation of the complex due to oxidation of the prosthetic heme to its Fe^{III} oxidation state.[32]

Since MI complexes often result from the association of nitroso functional groups with the Fe^{II} form of the CYP heme, suspicion centered on the primary amine in Compound **1** as the offending functionality, given that CYP enzymes can oxidize the $-NH_2$ moiety to the corresponding $-NO$ group. Based on these considerations, Compound **2** was synthesized by introducing a methyl group at the carbon atom adjacent to the primary amine in an effort to minimize oxidation of the latter due to steric hindrance. This strategy proved to be successful in that Compound **2** did not yield an MI complex *in vitro*, yet it retained the desirable pharmacological and pharmacokinetic properties of its predecessor. Hence, a simple structural change, based on an understanding of structural alerts for TDI, yielded a development candidate devoid of significant CYP inhibitory properties.

9.4 Use of GSH Trapping in Lead Optimization: The Discovery of Suvorexant

In this program, which was aimed at the identification of an antagonist of the orexin receptor for the treatment of sleep disorders, the lead compound contained the 6-fluoroquinazoline moiety depicted in Figure 9.5.[34] When this compound was incubated with human liver microsomal preparations fortified with GSH and the products were analyzed by LC-MS/MS, four thioether conjugates were detected, one of which had undergone oxidative defluorination (Figure 9.5). Based on MS/MS fragmentation pathways, it was concluded that these GSH conjugates resulted from metabolic activation of the fluoroquinazoline heterocycle to reactive isomeric arene oxide derivatives.

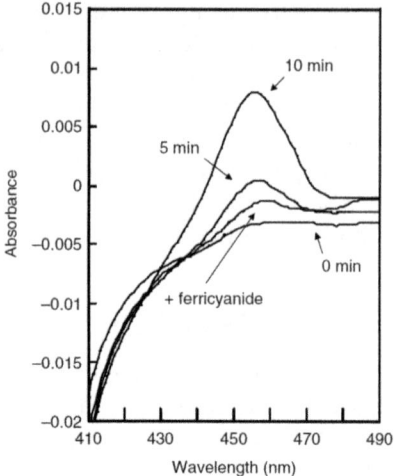

Figure 9.4 Optimization of a lead melanocortin-4 receptor agonist (Compound **1**) to eliminate the MI complex formed with recombinant CYP3A4. Formation of the MI complex, characterized by the appearance of the absorption with λ_{max} at 455 nm (inset) over a 10 minute incubation, was reversed by the addition of potassium ferricyanide. Metabolic activation of the primary amine in Compound **1** was blocked in Compound **2** due to the steric hindrance introduced by the methyl substituent α- to the primary amine. Reproduced with permission from Tang *et al.*[33]

This finding was supported by the results of parallel covalent binding studies in which an analog of the lead compound labeled with tritium in the phenyltriazole moiety was found to bind irreversibly to microsomal proteins in an NADPH-dependent manner, consistent with the generation of reactive metabolite(s). Furthermore, the covalent binding was reduced by ~90% when an excess of GSH was present in the incubation media, indicating that reactive species were being captured by the nucleophilic trap. Collectively, these results pointed to the 6-fluoroquinazoline ring as the locus of metabolic activation, as a result of which the medicinal chemistry program focused on identifying a replacement for this heterocycle that was refractory

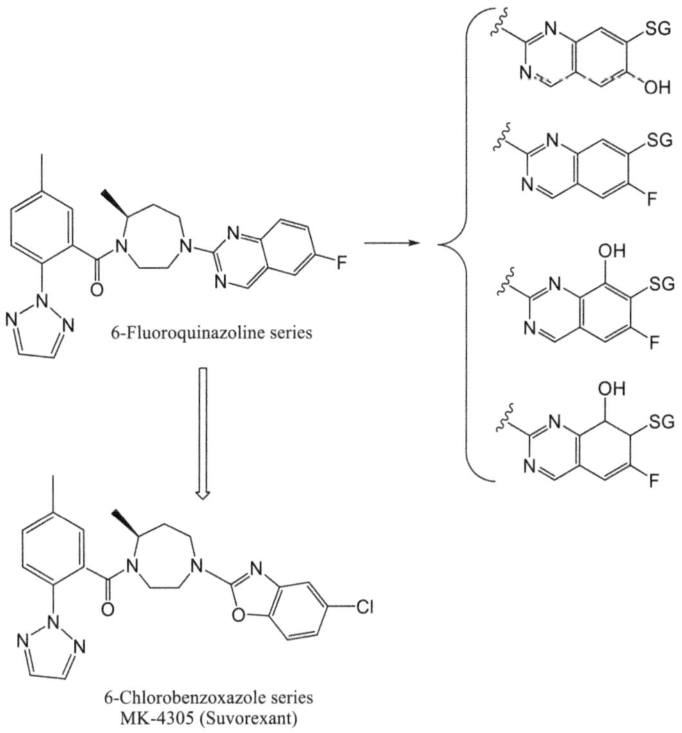

Figure 9.5 Metabolism of the lead orexin receptor antagonist in liver microsomal preparations fortified with GSH led to the formation of four GSH conjugates derived from oxidation of the 6-fluoroquinazoline ring system. This pathway of metabolic activation was blocked by the replacement of the quinazoline moiety with a 6-chlorobenzoxazole substituent, giving rise to MK-4305, which became suvorexant.

to bioactivation. These efforts were successful, with the preparation of the 6-chlorobenzoxazole analog (MK-4305) shown in Figure 9.5, which exhibited good potency and selectivity against the orexin receptor, had an excellent pharmacokinetic and safety profile in animals, and failed to generate detectable levels of GSH conjugates when incubated with animal or human liver microsomal preparations.[34] Accordingly, MK-4305 entered full development and ultimately gained US Food and Drug Administration (FDA) approval in August 2014, as the drug suvorexant (BELSOMRA®).

9.5 Covalent Binding as an Index of Metabolic Activation: The Discovery of Taranabant

Inverse agonists of the CB-1 receptor had been proposed as potential anti-obesity agents, and a lead compound was identified that exhibited good selectivity and high potency ($IC_{50} = 2.03$ nM) for this target. However, its oral

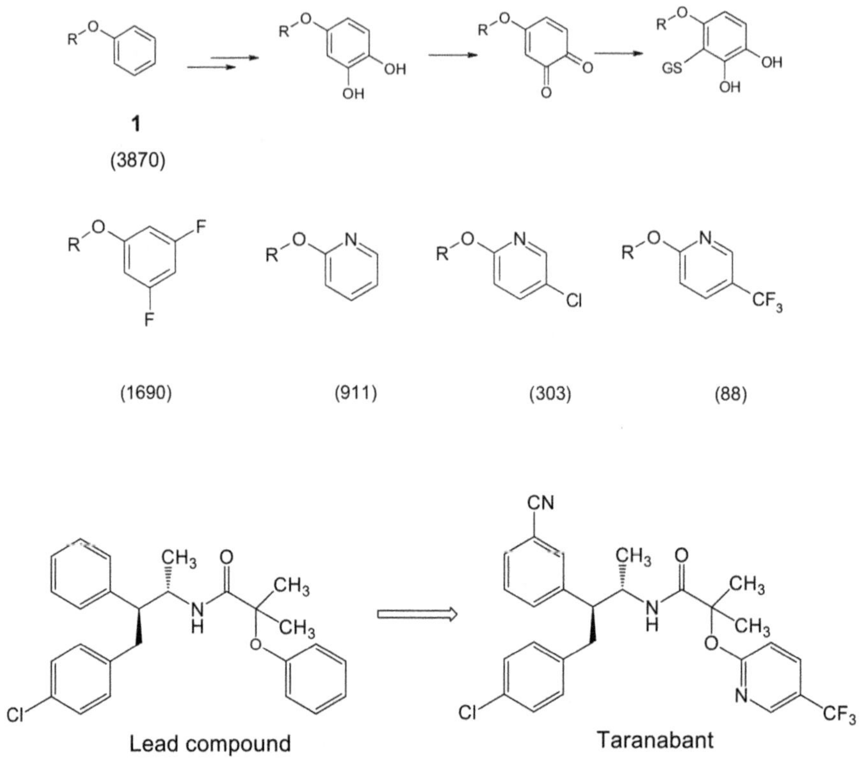

Figure 9.6 Use of covalent binding measurements *in vitro* (denoted in parentheses in units of pmol equiv. bound per mg protein) to assess the metabolic activation of a series of CB-1 inverse agonists in rat liver microsomal preparations. Upper portion: activation of the original lead, Compound **1**, *via* a catechol metabolite to the electrophilic *ortho*-quinone that could be captured by GSH. Lower portion: full structure of Compound **1** and the final development candidate that was essentially devoid of metabolic activation liabilities, and which became taranabant.

bioavailability in rats was low ($F = 9\%$), and when a radiolabeled analog was incubated with rat liver microsomal preparations, very high levels of covalent binding to protein were observed (3870 pmol equiv. mg^{-1} protein).[35] Studies on the metabolites formed in liver microsomes revealed that the phenoxy substituent was the likely site of bioactivation, based on the observation of a catechol derivative that could serve as a precursor of a reactive *ortho*-quinone (Figure 9.6).

Trapping experiments with GSH verified this hypothesis through the identification of the corresponding GSH adduct. It was concluded, therefore, that replacement of the phenoxy moiety with a functional group less prone to CYP-mediated oxidation represented a rational approach to the metabolic activation problem. Given that CYP enzymes activate molecular oxygen to an electron-deficient oxene-like species for insertion into the substrate, structural changes that decrease electron density at the site of metabolism generally suppress oxidation at that center. Based on this rationale, a number of analogs of the original lead compound were prepared in which the phenoxy substituent was replaced by functional groups rendered electron-deficient by halogenation (Figure 9.6). Since a radiolabel could be introduced readily into the structural scaffold (denoted as "R" in Figure 9.6), it proved relatively straightforward to synthesize radiolabeled derivatives of each of the new analogs for covalent binding studies. The results of these experiments demonstrated that covalent binding to liver microsomal preparations (expressed in units of pmol equiv. per mg protein) decreased markedly along the series with phenoxy being the highest (3870) > 3,5-diphenyloxy (1690) > 2-pyridyloxy (911) > 4-chloro-2-pyridyloxy (303) > 4-trifluoromethyl-2-pyridyloxy (88). In parallel with this work, the source of the poor oral bioavailability of the lead compound in rats was traced to facile hydroxylation of the "left-side" phenyl ring, which could be effectively blocked with a nitrile substituent. Combining this modification with the 4-trifluoromethyl-2-pyridyloxy replacement yielded a compound with remarkable properties, namely an IC_{50} at the CB-1 receptor of 0.29 nM (a 7-fold improvement over the original lead), an oral bioavailability in rat of 74% (an 8-fold improvement) and a protein covalent binding figure of 27 pmol equiv. mg^{-1} protein (a 143-fold improvement). This molecule, which was fully optimized in terms of its pharmacology, pharmacokinetics and metabolic characteristics, was taken forward into development and became the drug candidate taranabant.[36] Unfortunately, the CB-1 receptor ultimately proved to be a flawed target, inverse agonism of which led to adverse CNS effects in humans, and development of taranabant was discontinued when this became apparent. However, this example illustrates how covalent binding studies can complement other measures of metabolic activation in lead optimization programs.

9.6 The Role of Stable Drug Metabolites in Adverse Drug Reactions

The great majority of drug metabolites are chemically stable in nature, formed from their respective parent compounds by a combination of oxidation, reduction, hydrolysis and conjugation reactions. Of these, CYP-mediated oxidations tend to represent the major mechanism of drug clearance in humans,[37] leading to products of hydroxylation, dehydrogenation and heteroatom dealkylation, *etc.*, which ultimately are excreted *via* renal and/or biliary pathways. However, drug metabolites often enter the systemic circulation prior to being eliminated, where they can circulate at relatively high levels or accumulate over time with chronic dosing.[38] In some cases, drug metabolites exhibit biological activity, and there are numerous examples where a metabolite was found to exhibit pharmacological activity suitable for development as a therapeutic agent in its own right (often due to superior pharmacokinetics relative to its parent).[2] It is reasonable, therefore, to also ask whether chemically stable drug metabolites may possess any *toxicological* properties, either similar to or distinct from those of their respective parent compounds. However, as discussed by several authors,[39–41] there are relatively few published examples where the toxicity of a drug in laboratory animals or human subjects could be clearly ascribed to one or more of its metabolites. Cases where a metabolite has been identified as the cause of an adverse drug reaction include amygdalin and laetrile, which undergo CYP-mediated oxidation leading to the release of cyanide ion, a mitochondrial toxin,[42] acyl cyanamide derivatives that undergo hydrolysis to free cyanamide, which causes cataracts in rats,[43] and an experimental kinesin spindle protein (KSP) inhibitor that liberates fluoroacetaldehyde upon *N*-dealkylation of a 2-fluoroethylpiperidine moiety (Figure 9.7). In the latter example, administration of the drug to rats caused liver necrosis, and it was proposed that the fluoroacetaldehyde was further metabolized, *via* fluoroacetate, to 2-fluorocitrate, a tricarboxylic acid cycle poison.[44]

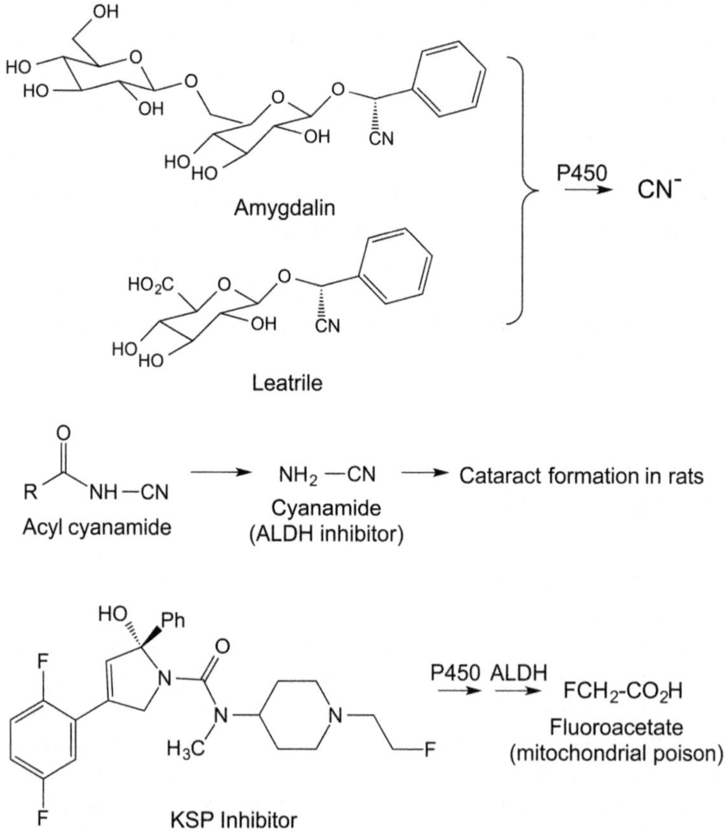

Figure 9.7   Compounds that undergo metabolism to stable, low molecular weight fragments that cause toxicity.

It should be noted that, in each of these cases, the toxic metabolite represented a small fragment of the original drug structure, and so it is not surprising that its biological activity differed markedly from that of the parent. However, a few examples do exist where an adverse drug reaction has been shown to reside in a stable metabolite whose structure is relatively close to that of its parent (Figure 9.8). For example, the neurotoxicity of MPTP in humans and non-human primates is due to accumulation of its pyridinium counterpart, MPP$^+$, formed by monoamine oxidase B (MAO-B)-catalyzed oxidation in dopaminergic neurons in the substantia nigra, leading to a Parkinson-like syndrome.[45] The sulfate conjugate of the PPARγ agonist troglitazone

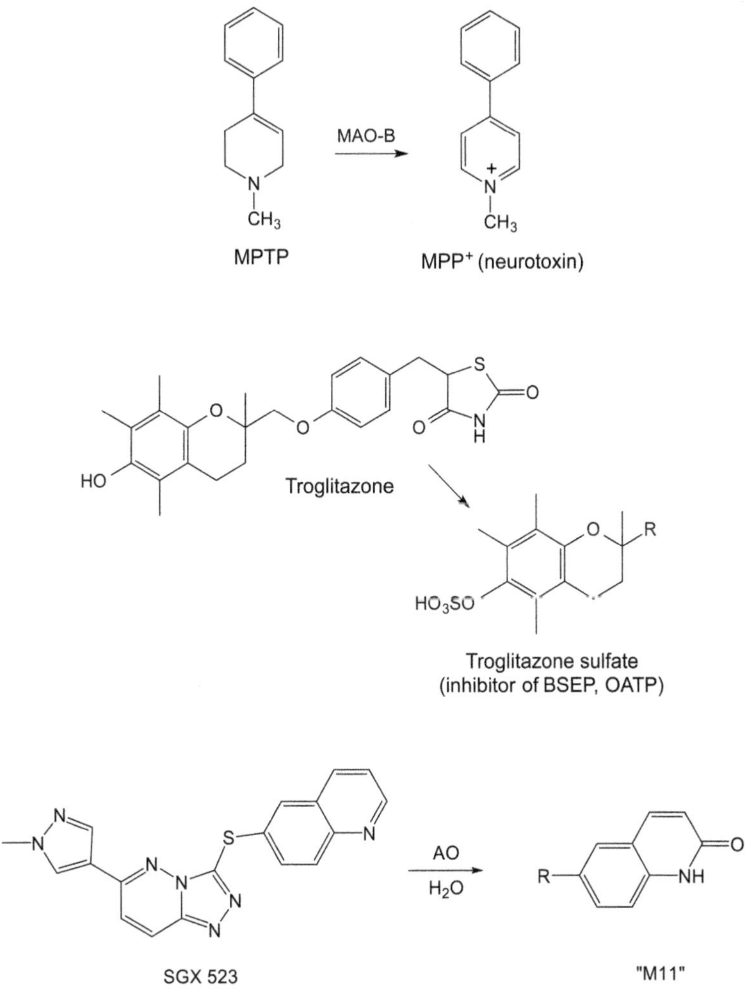

Figure 9.8 Compounds that undergo metabolism to stable metabolites that are structurally similar to their respective parents, but cause toxicity. AO: aldehyde oxidase.

proved to be an inhibitor of the transport proteins bile salt export protein (BSEP) and organic acid transport protein (OATP), and the hepatotoxicity of the drug in diabetic patients has been attributed, at least in part, to this property,[46,47] while the nephrotoxicity in monkeys of an experimental c-met inhibitor, SGX 523, resulted from crystallization of its sparingly soluble lactam metabolite in the kidney.[48]

As discussed by Smith and Obach,[41] the fact that relatively few cases are known in which stable metabolites have been shown to be sources of adverse drug reactions is consistent with the changes in physicochemical properties that accompany typical biotransformation reactions. Two of the key parameters in this regard are polar surface area (PSA) and lipophilicity (cLogP), as highlighted by an in-house analysis of the Pfizer database of compounds that had caused toxicities in preclinical studies.[49,50] In that survey, it was found that molecules with low PSA (<75 Å) and high cLogP (>3) values have a higher propensity to cause toxicity (regardless of end-point) and to exhibit greater "promiscuity" (lack of selectivity against the biological target). Since metabolic oxidation and conjugation processes invariably increase PSA and decrease $\log P$, it follows that metabolic transformations should decrease the likelihood that a compound will prove to be toxic. This can be rationalized in terms of lipophilicity considerations; more polar metabolites traverse cell membranes less effectively and interact less avidly with lipophilic binding sites on intracellular targets. These changes in PSA and $\log P$ also mean that polar metabolites will exhibit less promiscuity, *i.e.* they become more selective at their protein targets, which, in turn, suggests that they are less likely than the parent to elicit significant off-target effects. Therefore, as a general rule, a stable drug metabolite whose structure does not differ appreciably from that of the parent may be expected to exhibit decreased biological activity (both from a pharmacological and toxicological perspective) and greater selectivity than its parent molecule.[41] A caveat to this rule is when a metabolite is cleared slowly and accumulates following chronic administration to levels where biological effects are seen; however, these effects of the metabolite (both on- and off-target) usually will be similar to those caused by the parent drug when given at high doses.

9.7   MIST

Despite the theoretical argument presented above that stable drug metabolites should not be of undue toxicological concern, it is nevertheless important to demonstrate the safety of the collective suite of drug-related molecules that is generated following administration of a new chemical entity to humans. Prior to the publication of the FDA's first guidance on the conduct of drug–drug interaction studies in 1997,[51] which pointed to the need for information not only on parent drugs but also their metabolites, the focus of safety assessment programs was on exposure to parent molecules only. In 2002, a group of pharmaceutical companies belonging to the Pharmaceutical Research & Manufacturers Association of America (PhRMA) addressed the topic in a White Paper that became known as the *Metabolites in Safety Testing* ("MIST") paper.[52] The goal of this publication was to draw attention to the need to take into account drug metabolites, in addition to the parent drug, in safety assessment studies, and to propose an experimental approach for doing so. Over the ensuing years, numerous commentaries on the subject appeared in the literature,[39,40,53–55] many of which were driven by concerns that anticipated regulations dealing with drug metabolites would be overly burdensome from a resource perspective, and thus would be effectively detrimental to the drug development enterprise. However, as a result of this extensive debate, and the opportunity for widespread public comment, the FDA guidance on this subject, which finally appeared in 2008,[56] outlined a reasonable framework for addressing MIST issues.[57] Further discussion by regulatory agencies worldwide resulted in the publication of a consolidated position document by the International Conference on Harmonisation (ICH) in 2009.[1] Briefly, the ICH guidance recommends that those small molecule metabolites that circulate in human plasma at levels that exceed 10% of total drug-related AUC_p at steady-state should be shown to also be present in the plasma of at least one of the animal species used in the toxicology program. Moreover, systemic levels of such metabolites in animals should be sufficient to establish an adequate exposure margin (defined as the animal AUC_p being at least 50% of that seen in humans at the projected marketed dose[58]). In the absence of such an exposure margin, the metabolite is considered "disproportionate" in humans, and further studies may be required to establish its safety. Certain types of metabolite were exempt from these considerations, such as drug conjugates (other than acyl glucuronides, which the FDA guidance[56] refers to as "toxic molecules"), metabolites of oncology drugs, and chemically reactive metabolites. Aspects of the latter exemptions appear curious—for example, acyl glucuronides, some of which are weakly reactive, have long been suspected as contributing to the toxicity of a number of carboxylic acid-containing drugs,[59] but certainly insufficient evidence exists for the entire family to be branded as "toxic molecules".[60] Conversely, as discussed above, there is compelling evidence to implicate chemically reactive metabolites as the causative agents in a number of serious adverse drug reactions; presumably, they were excluded from the guidance since in most cases reactive intermediates cannot be measured in biological fluids, and regulatory agencies did not feel it appropriate to impose regulations dealing with species that could not be monitored directly. In terms of timing, the ICH guidance recommends that a comprehensive understanding of the metabolic fate of a drug candidate should be established prior to the initiation of large scale clinical trials, *i.e.* prior to the start of Phase 3 development.

Several key practical questions raised by the MIST guidance have generated considerable debate within the pharmaceutical industry, including the following: (1) the most straightforward means of establishing whether a circulating metabolite exceeds "10% of total drug-related AUC_p" would be through the administration of a radiolabeled analog of the parent drug, but radiotracers often are not available in early clinical development. Moreover, radiolabeled compounds typically are not dosed chronically, and so this approach cannot be used to establish metabolite exposure at steady state. How, then, does one determine whether a new chemical entity exceeds "10% of total drug-related AUC_p" in humans? (2) If "cold" (non-radioactive) methodology is to be used to detect, identify and quantify exposure to circulating metabolites, how is this achieved, particularly in the absence of validated bioanalytical methods using synthetic metabolite reference standards? (3) Since species differences are the rule, rather than the exception in drug metabolism,[6] there always will be cases where a metabolite will be abundant in humans but present at low levels in all of the commonly used laboratory species employed in toxicology studies. In light of this fact, how does one proceed in situations where it is simply not possible to achieve adequate exposure margins in animals? Related to this question is the issue that the marketed human dose may not be known until late in development, rendering ultimate exposure margins uncertain.

In response to the first two questions, a number of approaches using cold methodologies have been proposed for the assessment of circulating drug metabolites, most of which are based upon LC-MS/MS analysis of plasma samples and semi-quantitative determination of drug-related material using mass spectrometric responses that are calibrated by reference to an ancillary technique such as ultraviolet (UV) absorbance or nuclear magnetic resonance spectroscopy (or radioactivity where a radiotracer has been employed for preclinical metabolite profiling studies).[61-67] The goal here is to demonstrate that the metabolite in question does not represent more than 10% of the exposure to the *parent drug*, since if that criterion is met, then the metabolite cannot, by definition, represent more than 10% of *total drug-related material*. Another approach based on establishing relative, as opposed to absolute, metabolite exposures is to generate time-proportional pools from animal and human plasma that will reflect the metabolite AUC_p over the dosing interval, and then to compare the relative abundance of the metabolite of interest in the two samples to determine the animal-to-human exposure margin.[68,69] In those situations where a ^{14}C-labeled form of the drug is available for administration to humans, microdose studies using accelerator mass spectrometry afford yet another option for the detection and quantitation (but not direct structural characterization) of circulating drug metabolites.[70-72]

When it comes to the issue of not being able to generate an exposure margin in laboratory animals for a disproportionate human metabolite, the solution is less clear. Regulatory guidance recommends, as one option, administration of the preformed metabolite to animals to achieve adequate systemic exposures, but this approach is fraught with problems, not the least of which is that the disposition of a preformed metabolite given to an animal may well differ from that when the metabolite is formed endogenously from its parent.[73,74] If a toxicological response is elicited from such an experiment, it is unclear whether this would necessarily be relevant to the situation when the parent drug itself is administered. A related problem is that, in the case of drugs given by the oral route, the preformed metabolite may not be absorbed after an oral dose, and so intravenous administration may be required, further complicating the analysis of any biological response. A more reasonable approach to the problem, therefore, might be to conduct a limited series of toxicology studies with a synthetic sample of the disproportionate metabolite, *e.g.* using a battery of genotoxicity and *in vitro* cytotoxicity assays, in order to establish the absence of any significant toxicological potential. Ultimately, the safety profile of the drug in clinical trials will determine its suitability for late stage development.

In spite of the initial concern over the implementation of the MIST guidances, the pharmaceutical industry as a whole now appears to have adopted relatively standardized approaches to the challenge of demonstrating that both parent drug and circulating human metabolites have been adequately assessed for safety prior to the initiation of large scale clinical trials. Several thoughtful commentaries on the subject have appeared in the literature in recent years, and examples of individual company strategies have been published.[41,75-87] While there are many similarities in these strategies, it is clear that there is a need for flexibility in the application of the MIST guidance, and tiered, fit-for-purpose approaches have been widely advocated. Thus, each compound needs to be considered on its merits, since no two new chemical entities are identical when it comes to their metabolic and dispositional characteristics. In other words, the most appropriate studies to ensure the safety of both a new drug candidate and its human metabolites require the application of the most suitable methodologies for the case in hand together with sound scientific judgment.

9.8 Future Prospects

In recent years, the safety of human pharmaceuticals has become a topic that has received increasing attention from the general public, driven by enhanced reporting of adverse drug reactions and by some high profile product recalls. As a consequence, new candidate drugs have come under close scrutiny by regulatory agencies, which have a public responsibility to ensure, to the greatest possible extent, the safety, efficacy and cost effectiveness of new medicines. The recent inclusion of drug metabolites in assessments of the safety profile of a candidate drug is one manifestation of today's heightened regulatory environment, which for some time has mandated detailed information on the potential involvement of new drugs in pharmacokinetic drug interactions that can also have implications for drug safety. In looking to the future, it seems unlikely that the current focus on drug safety will diminish, nor should it, although there is an ongoing need to improve public awareness of risk–benefit considerations in the use of new medicines. From a scientific perspective, it is important to better understand the relationship between drug metabolism and drug-induced toxicities, both in the area of chemically reactive metabolites and chemically stable metabolites.

9.8.1   Chemically Reactive Drug Metabolites

In the field of chemically reactive metabolites, a key priority should be to establish which types of electrophiles we should be concerned about. Not all electrophiles are created equal—they exhibit a wide range of chemical reactivities and selectivity in binding to macromolecules in a biological milieu—yet they tend to be lumped together as a single group. Today, a number of major pharmaceutical companies have put in place preclinical drug candidate selection strategies that take into account metabolic activation and protein covalent binding, but often nothing is known about the reactive intermediates or the proteins to which they bind.[88,89] Intuitively, one might suspect that those reactive intermediates at the two extremes of the electrophilicity spectrum would be less likely to cause widespread damage throughout the cell, but a quantitative framework needs to be developed linking intrinsic reactivity to cellular toxicity. Similarly, much remains to be learned about the protein targets of reactive drug metabolites—what are they, and which ones are toxicologically relevant? Are certain protein *networks* more vulnerable to alkylation/oxidation damage than others? Could specific drug–protein covalent adducts serve as biomarkers of toxicity, in much the same way as Keap-1 serves as an electrophile sensor,[90] alkylation of which initiates the transcription of a series of cellular defense genes[91]? Answers to these questions will require a significant investment in resources, both from public/private granting agencies and the pharmaceutical industry, but the rewards will be considerable in terms of understanding (and predicting) the role of reactive metabolites in drug-induced toxicity.

9.8.2   Chemically Stable Drug Metabolites

Research opportunities in the area of stable drug metabolites lie in improving our ability to predict which products will be formed in humans and, more importantly, which metabolites will circulate in human plasma at significant levels.[79,84] Currently, *in silico* approaches to predictive drug metabolism remain somewhat rudimentary; potential pathways are identified, and in some cases suggestions are made (largely based on electronic considerations) as to which products may be significant. However, there is no substitute at present for *in vitro* and animal *in vivo* experimental data when quantitative projections of drug biotransformation are the goal,[92] and this situation is unlikely to change in the foreseeable future. Nevertheless, it is to be expected that marked improvements will be made in our ability to extrapolate *in vitro* data on drug metabolism to the *in vivo* situation through the use of physiologically based pharmacokinetic modeling approaches, which are becoming increasingly refined and widely used in drug development programs. The molecular basis for interspecies differences in drug metabolism, both in terms of the underlying genetics, enzymology and drug transport phenomena, will continue to evolve and aid in the extrapolation of drug metabolism in animals to that in humans. Similarly, continued development of "organ-on-a-chip" technology, in which the 3D architecture of the tissue is retained (with or without flow), will provide superior *in vitro* tools for the early study of drug metabolism and safety in both laboratory animals and humans. The advent of molecular imaging techniques, such as those based on matrix-assisted laser desorption ionization (MALDI) mass spectrometry,[93] will allow quantitative assessments to be made of the levels of both parent drug and metabolites in sections of tissue, which will be of great value in investigating the role of metabolites as contributors to both the pharmacological activity and toxicity of new chemical entities. As a consequence of the MIST guidance, there will be an ongoing need for reference samples of drug metabolites on the 10–100 mg scale, and alternative approaches to organic synthesis (*e.g.* use of metalloporphyrin CYP mimics, recombinant bacterial CYP enzymes with a broad range of substrate selectivities and electrochemical methods) will become commonplace. Lastly, continued development and validation of humanized animal models (*e.g.* transgenic mice) will lead to broader adoption of these *in vivo* tools for predicting the metabolism and toxicity of new chemical entities in man.[94]

9.9 Conclusions

Collectively, our knowledge accrued over the past four decades on the metabolism of drugs and other foreign compounds that cause toxicity in animals and humans indicates that metabolic activation plays an important role. However, the relationship between exposure to electrophilic drug metabolites and the expression of tissue damage is not always a linear one, and in some cases reactive metabolites appear to be relatively benign. Until we gain a true mechanistic understanding of the role of reactive intermediates in drug toxicity, a prudent approach appears to be to minimize the propensity of drug candidates to undergo metabolic activation through appropriate structural design and, as described in this chapter, methodologies currently exist to achieve this goal. Stable drug metabolites, in contrast, appear to have a low probability of causing adverse drug reactions, and this may be understood in terms of their physicochemical properties. However, on occasion, stable metabolites may differ appreciably from their respective parents in terms of molecular structure, and so it remains necessary to assess the safety of the full complement of metabolites of a candidate drug, as well as the parent compound itself, in the course of drug development activities. Advances in analytical methodology, combined with improved *in vitro* and *in silico* tools and the continued development of transgenic animal models, will greatly facilitate future extrapolation of animal metabolism data to humans, as well as *in vitro* to *in vivo* projections, leading to more confident predictions of drug metabolism and drug safety in man. However, the greatest challenge to predictive toxicology will be to develop a true mechanistic understanding of the factors—reactivity of the electrophile, selectivity of its covalent binding, and vulnerability of protein networks to oxidation or alkylation damage—that dictate a toxic response to a foreign compound and its metabolites. The tools to address these pressing questions are available today, and so the next 40 years are guaranteed to be exciting ones!

References

1. *Guidance on Nonclinical Safety Studies for the Conduct of Human Clinical Trials and Marketing Authorization for Pharmaceuticals*, ICH Harmonised Tripartite Guideline M3(R2), 2009, http://www.ich.org/fileadmin/Public_Web_Site/ICH_Products/Guidelines/Multidisciplinary/M3_R2/Step4/M3_R2__Guideline.pdf, accessed 15 January, 2015.
2. R. S. Obach, *Pharmacol. Rev.*, 2013, **53**, 167.
3. E. C. Miller and J. A. Miller, *Cancer Res.*, 1947, **7**, 468.
4. J. R. Mitchell, D. J. Jollow, W. Z. Potter, D. C. Davis, J. R. Gillette and B. B. Brodie, *J. Pharmacol. Exp. Ther.*, 1973, **187**, 185.
5. D. C. Dahlin, G. T. Miwa, A. Y. H. Lu and S. D. Nelson, *Proc. Nat. Acad. Sci. U. S. A.*, 1984, **81**, 3327.
6. T. A. Baillie and A. E. Rettie, *Drug Metab. Pharmacokinet.*, 2011, **26**, 15.
7. A. F. Stepan, D. P. Walker, J. Bauman, D. A. Price, T. A. Baillie, A. S. Kalgutkar and M. D. Aleo, *Chem. Res. Toxicol.*, 2011, **24**, 1345.
8. A. J. Streeter, S. M. Bjorge, D. B. Axworthy, S. D. Nelson and T. A. Baillie, *Drug Metab. Dispos.*, 1984, **12**, 565.
9. M. A. Tirmenstein and S. D. Nelson, *J. Biol. Chem.*, 1989, **264**, 9814.
10. H.-Y. H. Kim, K. A. Tallman, D. C. Liebler and N. A. Porter, *Mol. Cell. Proteomics*, 2009, **8**, 2080.
11. R. E. Connor, L. J. Marnett and D. C. Liebler, *Chem. Res. Toxicol.*, 2011, **24**, 1275.
12. S. G. Codreanu, J. C. Ullery, J. Zhu, K. A. Tallman, W. N. Beavers, N. A. Porter, L. J. Marnett, B. Zhang and D. C. Liebler, *Mol. Cell. Proteomics*, 2014, **13**, 849.
13. R. P. Hanzlik, Y. M. Koem and J. Fang, *Toxicol. Sci.*, 2013, **135**, 390.
14. D. A. Smith and E. F. Schmid, *Curr. Opin. Drug Discovery Dev.*, 2006, **9**, 38.
15. C. Lammert, S. Einarsson, C. Saha, A. Niklasson, E. Bjornsson and N. Chalasani, *Hepatology*, 2008, **47**, 2003.
16. J. Uetrecht and D. J. Naisbitt, *Pharmacol. Rev.*, 2013, **65**, 779.
17. N. A. Grilo, C. Charneira, S. A. Pereira, E. C. Monteiro, M. M. Marques and A. M. M. Antunes, *Toxicol. Lett.*, 2014, **224**, 416.
18. X. Meng, A. S. Lawrenson, N. G. Berry, J. L. Maggs, N. S. French, D. J. Black, S. H. Khoo, D. J. Naisbitt and B. K. Park, *Chem. Res. Toxicol.*, 2014, **27**, 524.
19. M. A. Martin and D. L. Kroetz, *Pharmacotherapy*, 2013, **33**, 765.
20. P. T. Illing, J. P. Vivian, N. L. Dudek, L. Kostenko, Z. Chen, M. Bharadwaj, J. J. Miles, L. Kjer-Nielsen, S. Gras, N. A. Williamson, S. R. Burrows, A. W. Purcell, J. Rossjohn and J. McCluskey, *Nature*, 2012, **486**, 554.

21. D. A. Ostrov, B. J. Grant, Y. A. Pompeu, J. Sidney, M. Harndahl, S. Southwood, C. Oseroff, S. Lu, J. Jakoncic, C. A. de Oliveria, L. Yang, H. Mei, L. Shi, J. Shabanowitz, A. M. English, A. Wriston, A. Lucas, E. Phillips, S. Mallal, H. M. Grey, A. Sette, D. F. Hunt, S. Buus and B. Peters, *Proc. Natl. Acad. Sci. U. S. A.*, 2012, **109**, 9959.
22. M. A. Norcross, S. Luo, L. Lu, M. T. Boyne, M. Gomarteli, A. D. Rennels, J. Woodcock, D. H. Margulies, C. McMurtrey, S. Verson, W. H. Hildebrand and R. Buchli, *AIDS*, 2012, **26**, F21.
23. H. Olson, G. Betton, D. Robinson, K. Thomas, A. Monro, G. Kolaja, P. Lilly, J. Sanders, G. Sipes, W. Bracken, M. Dorato, K. Van Deun, P. Smith, B. Berger and A. Heller, *Regul. Toxicol. Pharmacol.*, 2000, **32**, 56.
24. M. H. Potashman and M. E. Duggan, *J. Med. Chem.*, 2009, **52**, 1231.
25. D. C. Evans, A. P. Watt, D. A. Nicoll-Griffith and T. A. Baillie, *Chem. Res. Toxicol.*, 2004, **17**, 3.
26. M. Reese, M. Sakatis, J. Ambroso, A. Harrell, E. Yang, L. Chen, M. Taylor, I. Baines, L. Zhu, A. Ayrton and S. Clarke, *Chem.-Biol. Interact.*, 2011, **192**, 60.
27. R. A. Thompson, E. M. Isin, Y. Li, R. Weaver, L. Weidolf, I. Wilson, A. Claesson, K. Page, H. Dolgos and J. G. Kenna, *Chem.-Biol. Interact.*, 2011, **192**, 65.
28. S. W. Grimm, H. J. Einolf, S. D. Hall, K. He, H.-K. Lim, K.-H. J. Ling, A. A. Nomeir, E. Seibert, K. W. Skordos, G. R. Tonn, R. Van Horn, R. W. Wang, Y. N. Wong, T. J. Yan and R. S. Obach, *Drug Metab. Dispos.*, 2009, **37**, 1355.
29. A. V. Stachulski, T. A. Baillie, B. K. Park, R. S. Obach, D. K. Dalvie, D. P. Williams, A. Srivastava, S. L. Regan, D. J. Antoine, C. E. P. Goldring, A. J. L. Chia, N. R. Kitteringham, L. E. Randle, H. Callan, J. L. Castrejon, J. Farrell, D. J. Naisbitt and M. S. Lennard, *Med. Res. Rev.*, 2013, **33**, 985.
30. D. Argoti, L. Liang, A. Conteh, L. Liangfu Chen, D. Bershas, C. P. Yu, P. Vouros and E. Yang, *Chem. Res. Toxicol.*, 2005, **18**, 1537.
31. S. H. Day, A. Mao, R. White, T. Schulz-Utermoehl, R. Miller and M. G. Beconi, *J. Pharmacol. Toxicol.*, 2005, **52**, 278.
32. P. R. Ortiz de Montellano and J. J. De Voss, *Cytochromes P450: Structure, Mechanism and Biochemistry*, ed. P. R. Ortiz de Montellano, Kluwer Academic/Plenum Publishers, New York, 2005, ch. 6, pp. 183–230.
33. W. Tang, R. A. Stearns, R. W. Wang, R. R. Miller, Q. Chen, J. Ngui, R. K. Bakshi, R. P. Nargund, D. C. Dean and T. A. Baillie, *Xenobiotica*, 2008, **38**, 1437.
34. C. D. Cox, M. J. Breslin, D. B. Whitman, J. D. Schreier, G. B. McGaughey, M. J. Bogusky, A. J. Roecker, S. P. Mercer, R. A. Bednar, W. Lemaire, J. G. Bruno, D. R. Reiss, C. Meacham Harrell, K. L. Murphy, S. L. Garson, S. M. Doran, T. Prueksaritanont, W. B. Anderson, C. Tang, S. Roller, T. D. Cabalu, D. Cui, G. D. Hartman, S. D. Young, K. S. Koblan, C. J. Winrow, J. J. Renger and P. J. Coleman, *J. Med. Chem.*, 2010, **53**, 5320.
35. W. K. Hagman, *J. Med. Chem.*, 2008, **51**, 4359.
36. K. Samuel, W. Yin, R. A. Stearns, Y. S. Tang, A. G. Chaudhary, J. P. Jewell, T. Lanza Jr., W. K. Hagman, D. C. Evans and S. Kumar, *J. Mass Spectrom.*, 2003, **38**, 211.
37. L. C. Wienkers and T. G. Heath, *Nat. Rev. Drug Discovery*, 2005, **4**, 825.

38. D. A. Smith and D. Dalvie, *Xenobiotica*, 2012, **42**, 107.
39. F. P. Guengerich, *Chem. Res. Toxicol.*, 2006, **19**, 1559.
40. W. G. Humphreys and S. E. Unger, *Chem. Res. Toxicol.*, 2006, **19**, 1564.
41. D. A. Smith and R. S. Obach, *Bioanalysis*, 2010, **2**, 1223.
42. B. O'Brien, C. Quigg and T. Leong, *Eur. J. Emerg. Med.*, 2001, **12**, 257.
43. S. Sparrow, personal communication.
44. C. D. Cox, P. J. Coleman, M. J. Breslin, D. B. Whitman, R. M. Garbaccio, M. E. Fraley, C. A. Buser, E. S. Walsh, K. Hamilton, M. D. Schaber, R. B. Lobell, W. Tao, J. P. Davide, R. E. Diehl, M. T. Abrams, V. J. South, H. H. Huber, M. Torrent, T. Prueksaritanont, C. Li, D. E. Slaughter, E. Mahan, C. Fernandez-Metzler, Y. Yan, L. C. Kuo, N. E. Kohl and G. D. Hartman, *J. Med. Chem.*, 2008, **51**, 4239.
45. R. J. Smeyne and V. Jackson-Lewis, *Mol. Brain Res.*, 2005, **134**, 57.
46. C. Funk, M. Pantze, L. Jehle, C. Ponelle, G. Scheuermann, M. Lazendic and R. Gasser, *Toxicology*, 2001, **167**, 83.
47. T. Nozawa, S. Sugiura, M. Nakajima, A. Goto, T. Yokoi, J. Nezu, A. Tsuji and I. Tamai, *Drug Metab. Dispos.*, 2004, **32**, 291.
48. S. Diamond, J. Boer, T. P. Maduskuie, N. Falahatpisheh, Y. Li and S. Yeleswaram, *Drug Metab. Dispos.*, 2010, **38**, 1277.
49. J. D. Hughes, J. Blagg, D. A. Price, S. Bailey, G. A. DeCrescenzo, R. V. Devraj, E. Ellsworth, Y. M. Fobian, M. E. Gibbs, R. W. Gilles, N. Greene, E. Huang, T. Krieger-Burke, J. Loesel, T. Wager, L. Whiteley and Y. Zhang, *Bioorg. Med. Chem. Lett.*, 2008, **18**, 4872.
50. D. A. Price, J. Blagg, L. Jones, N. Greene and T. Wager, *Expert Opin. Drug Metab. Toxicol.*, 2009, **5**, 921.
51. *Guidance for Industry. Drug Metabolism/Drug Interaction Studies in the Drug Development Process: Studies In Vitro*, US Food & Drug Administration, 1997, http://www.fda.gov/downloads/AboutFDA/CentersOffices/CDER/UCM142439.pdf, accessed January 15, 2015.
52. T. A. Baillie, M. N. Cayen, H. Fouda, R. J. Gerson, J. D. Green, S. J. Grossman, L. J. Klunk, B. LeBlanc, D. G. Perkins and L. A. Shipley, *Toxicol. Appl. Pharmacol.*, 2002, **182**, 188.
53. D. A. Smith and R. S. Obach, *Drug Metab. Dispos.*, 2005, **33**, 1409.
54. K. L. Davis-Bruno and A. Atrakchi, *Chem. Res. Toxicol.*, 2006, **19**, 1561.
55. (a) D. A. Smith and R. S. Obach, *Chem. Res. Toxicol.*, 2006, **19**, 1570; (b) D. Luffer-Atlas, *Drug Metab. Rev.*, 2008, **40**, 447.
56. *Guidance for Industry. Safety Testing of Drug Metabolites*, US Food & Drug Administration, 2008, http://www.fda.gov/OHRMS/DOCKETS/98fr/FDA-2008-D-0065-GDL.pdf, accessed 15 January, 2015.
57. T. W. Robinson and A. Jacobs, *Bioanalysis*, 2009, **1**, 1193.
58. H. Gao, A. Jacobs, R. E. White, B. P. Booth and R. S. Obach, *AAPS J.*, 2013, **15**, 970.
59. E. M. Faed, *Drug Metab. Rev.*, 1984, **15**, 1213.
60. A. V. Stachulski and X. Meng, *Nat. Prod. Rep.*, 2013, **30**, 806.
61. G. J. Dear, C. Beaumont, A. Roberts, B. Squillaci, S. Thomas, M. Nash and D. Fraser, *Bioanalsis*, 2011, **3**, 197.

62. A. N. R. Nedderman, *Biopharm. Drug Dispos.*, 2009, **30**, 153.
63. D. Luffer-Atlas, *Expert Opin. Drug Metab. Toxicol.*, 2012, **8**, 985.
64. R. Espina, L. Yu, J. Wang, Z. Tong, S. Vashishtha, R. Talaat, J. Scatina and A. Mutlib, *Chem. Res. Toxicol.*, 2009, **22**, 299.
65. K. Vishwanathan, K. Babalola, J. Wang, R. Espina, L. Yu, A. Adedoyin, R. Talaat and J. Scatina, *Chem. Res. Toxicol.*, 2009, **22**, 311.
66. J. Caceres and M. D. Reily, *Bioanalysis*, 2010, **2**, 1263.
67. R. Ramanathan, J. J. Josephs, M. Jemal, M. Arnold and W. G. Humphreys, *Bioanalysis*, 2010, **2**, 1291.
68. H. Gao, S. Deng and R. S. Obach, *Drug Metab. Dispos.*, 2010, **38**, 2147.
69. H. Gao and R. S. Obach, *Curr. Drug Metab.*, 2011, **12**, 578.
70. G. Lappin and M. Seymour, *Bioanalysis*, 2010, **2**, 1315.
71. A. Nedderman, *Bioanalysis*, 2011, **3**, 2695.
72. G. Lappin, M. Seymour, G. Gross, M. Jørgensen, M. Kall and L. Kværnø, *Bioanalysis*, 2012, **4**, 407.
73. T. Prueksaritanont, J. H. Lin and T. A. Baillie, *Toxicol. Appl. Pharmacol.*, 2006, **217**, 143.
74. K. S. Pang, *Chem.-Biol. Interact.*, 2009, **179**, 45.
75. H. Yu, D. Bischoff and D. Tweedie, *Expert Opin. Drug Metab. Toxicol.*, 2010, **6**, 1539.
76. D. Walker, J. brady, D. Dalvie, J. Davis, M. Dowty, J. N. Duncan, A. Nedderman, R. S. Obach and P. Wright, *Chem. Res. Toxicol.*, 2009, **22**, 1653.
77. D. A. Smith and R. S. Obach, *Chem. Res. Toxicol.*, 2009, **22**, 267.
78. D. A. Smith, R. S. Obach, D. P. Williams and B. K. Park, *Chem.-Biol. Interact.*, 2009, **179**, 60.
79. S. Anderson, D. Luffer-Atlas and M. P. Knadler, *Chem. Res. Toxicol.*, 2009, **22**, 243.
80. A. N. R. Nedderman, G. J. Dear, S. North, R. S. Obach and D. Higton, *Xenobiotica*, 2011, **41**, 605.
81. D. A. Smith and D. Dalvie, *Xenobiotica*, 2012, **42**, 107.
82. C. Prakash, Z. Li, C. Orlandi and L. Klunk, *Drug Metab. Dispos.*, 2012, **40**, 1308.
83. T. Minagawa, K. Nakano, S. Furuta, T. Iwasa, K. Takekawa, K. Minato, T. Koga, T. Sato, K. Kawashima, Y. Kurahashi, H. Onodera, S. Naito and K. Nakamura, *J. Toxicol. Sci.*, 2012, **37**, 667.
84. C.-M. Loi, D. A. Smith and D. Dalvie, *Drug Metab. Dispos.*, 2013, **41**, 933.
85. R. Subramanian and J. G. Slatter, in *Encyclopedia of Drug Metabolism and Interactions*, ed. A. V. Lyubimov, John Wiley & Sons, New York, 1st edn, 2012, ch. 6, vol. 6, pp. 1–15.
86. J. Haglund, M. M. Haldin, Å. Brunnström, G. Eklund, A. Kautianen, A. Sandholm and S. L. Iverson, *Chem. Res. Toxicol.*, 2014, **27**, 601.
87. L. Leclerq, F. Cuyckens, G. S. J. Mannens, R. de Vries, P. Timmerman and D. C. Evans, *Chem. Res. Toxicol.*, 2009, **22**, 280.
88. R. A. Thompson, E. M. Isin, Y. Li, L. Weidolf, K. Page, I. Wilson, S. Swallow, B. Middleton, S. Stahl, A. J. Foster, H. Dolgos, R. Weaver and J. G. Kenna, *Chem. Res. Toxicol.*, 2012, **25**, 1616.

89. M. Z. Sakatis, M. J. Reese, A. W. Harrell, M. A. Taylor, I. A. Baines, L. Chen, J. C. Bloomer, E. Y. Yang, H. M. Ellens, J. L. Ambroso, C. A. Lovatt, A. D. Ayrton and S. E. Clarke, *Chem. Res. Toxicol.*, 2012, **25**, 2067.

90. F. Hong, K. R. Sekhar, M. L. Freeman and D. C. Liebler, *J. Biol. Chem.*, 2005, **280**, 31768.

91. I. M. Copple, C. E. Goldring, N. R. Kitteringham and B. K. Park, *Toxicology*, 2008, **246**, 24.

92. D. Dalvie, R. S. Obach, P. Kang, C. Prakash, C. M. Loi, S. Hurst, A. Nedderman, L. Goulet, E. Smith, H. Z. Bu and D. A. Smith, *Chem. Res. Toxicol.*, 2009, **22**, 357.

93. S. Castellino, M. R. Groseclose and D. Wagner, *Bioanalysis*, 2011, **3**, 2427.

94. M. W. Powley, C. B. Frederick, F. D. Sistare and J. J. DeGeorge, *Chem. Res. Toxicol.*, 2009, **22**, 257.

CHAPTER 10

Integrating Metabolism and Toxicity Properties

MATTHEW SEGALL*[a]

[a]Optibrium Ltd. 7221 Cambridge Research Park, Beach Drive, Cambridge, CB25 9TL, UK
*E-mail: matt.segall@optibrium.com

10.1 Introduction

Identifying a successful, efficacious and safe drug is a delicate balancing act in which many properties must be simultaneously optimised. Achieving potency against a therapeutic target or targets is necessary, but is not sufficient. In order to achieve efficacy, a drug must reach the site of action at a sufficient concentration and for a sufficient duration of time. The drug must ultimately be eliminated, by metabolic or other routes, and both the compound and its metabolites must avoid significant off-target or toxic effects at a therapeutic dose.

For these reasons, it is now common to measure and predict a broad range of absorption, distribution, metabolism, elimination (ADME) and toxicity (ADMET) properties from the early stages of drug discovery, to eliminate unsuitable compounds as early as possible and avoid late-stage, expensive failures in development. These properties and methods for their measurement and prediction are discussed in detail elsewhere in this book. However, the availability of these complex data poses another challenge; how to make effective use of these data to make good decisions regarding the selection

RSC Drug Discovery Series No. 49
New Horizons in Predictive Drug Metabolism and Pharmacokinetics
Edited by Alan G. E. Wilson
© The Royal Society of Chemistry 2016
Published by the Royal Society of Chemistry, www.rsc.org

and design of compounds? The objective is to quickly focus on chemistries with the best chance of success while not missing opportunities by inappropriately rejecting compounds.

It is therefore necessary to integrate all of these early ADMET data in a manner that can be easily interpreted. There are several approaches that may be used to achieve this: where sufficient data on properties governing absorption and distribution are available, they may be used as inputs to physiologically based pharmacokinetic (PBPK) models to predict the concentration–time profile at the site of action and pharmacokinetic (PK) parameters such as clearance and exposure.[1] However, many of the requirements for a successful drug cannot be combined into a single mechanistic model and in some cases the available data may be insufficient to use as inputs to such a model. Therefore, alternative, empirical methods described under the broad term of multi-parameter optimisation (MPO)[2] are also used to guide the broader optimisation challenge.

PBPK modelling is discussed in detail in Chapter 17 of this book, so here I will focus on the application of MPO methods in drug discovery. In this discussion the requirements of an ideal method that will help to guide good decisions in drug discovery should be considered:

- It should be flexible in order to deal with the differing requirements of drug discovery projects that will depend on the therapeutic indication, intended route of administration and other factors. For example, a drug intended for inhaled or topical administration will have quite different requirements for physicochemical properties to a drug intended for oral administration. Similarly, the required safety profile for an oncology drug will differ substantially from that of a cardiovascular therapeutic intended for chronic dosing.
- It is important to remember that the data obtained in early drug discovery have significant uncertainties. These derive from experimental variability or statistical error in predictive methods and mean that the value of compound properties cannot be known with precision; *in vitro* measurements of affinity (K_i or IC_{50}) for the same compound often vary by a factor of 2 to 5 (0.3 to 0.7 log units), while predictive models may have standard errors in prediction in the range of 0.5 to 1 log units, or even more. A further source of uncertainty in the properties measured in early drug discovery is in their relevance to the ultimate behaviour of a compound. There is not a perfect correlation between *in vitro* properties and *in vivo* pharmacokinetics and safety, as illustrated in Figure 10.1. Therefore, the impact of these uncertainties on our ability to confidently distinguish between compounds when making decisions should be considered.[3]
- It is rare to immediately identify an ideal compound and therefore a method for combining multiple properties should provide guidance on the properties with the greatest effect on the quality of a compound. This can guide the optimisation of compounds by identifying the most important factors to address in order to improve a compound's chance of success.

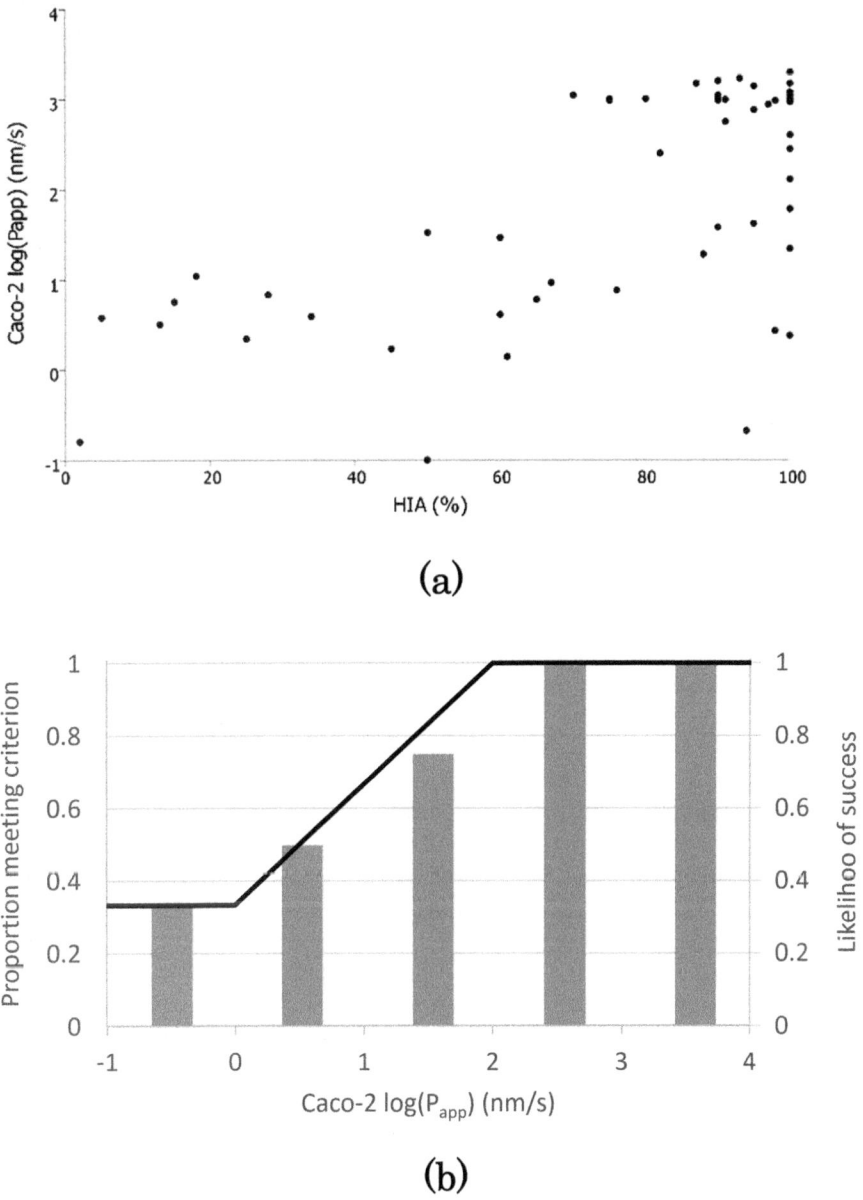

Figure 10.1   (a) Scatter plot of the experimentally measured Caco-2 apparent permeability coefficients (P_{app}) against clinical human intestinal absorption for 52 compounds published by Irvine *et al.*[21] The histogram in
(b) shows the proportion of compounds achieving a human intestinal absorption greater than 50% for Caco-2 P_{app} values binned in one
log-unit ranges. The solid line corresponds to a desirability function
approximately representing the likelihood of success of compounds
for this objective against Caco-2 P_{app}.[3]

The following sections of this chapter will describe a variety of commonly applied MPO methods, provide an example of their application and draw conclusions regarding the state of the art and future directions for the field.

10.2 MPO

The most obvious and widely used approach for MPO is to apply filters to eliminate compounds that do not meet all of the property criteria for a project's objectives. However, the limitations of the available data, as discussed in the introduction to this chapter, mean that this approach is often counterproductive. The limited correlation of early discovery data with the ultimate *in vivo* disposition of a compound means that it is rarely appropriate to impose a hard cut-off with which to reject compounds. Furthermore, the uncertainty in the data implies that, even when a cut-off is used, it is often impossible to say with confidence on which side of the criterion a compound lies. The uncertainties in each filter are compounded when these are applied for multiple property criteria. For example, if we apply 5 filters that are each 80% accurate in distinguishing 'good' from 'bad' compounds, the probability of a perfect compound passing all 5 filters is only 33%, *i.e.* we are twice as likely to reject a perfect compound as to keep it. Moreover, in most drug discovery projects ideal compounds are very rare, and the cost of missing an opportunity is high.

Given the challenge of dealing with multiple, complex properties, there is a tendency to simplify the problem by focussing on a small number of simple, surrogate properties, often described as "drug-like properties". Common examples include the partition coefficient between octanol and water ($\log P$), molecular weight (MW) and counts of simple structural features such as hydrogen bond donors (HDB), hydrogen bond acceptors (HBA), rotatable bonds (ROTB) and aromatic rings (AROM). The most famous example of a rule for combining these properties is Lipinski's Rule of Five (RoF),[4] which defines four simple criteria for $\log P$, MW, HBA and HBD, although numerous other rules have been proposed.[5] These simple 'rules of thumb' have the benefit of being straight-forward and provide guidelines that help medicinal chemists to consider the potential risks associated with the selection of a compound, based on simple, easily understood properties. Furthermore, it is usually easy to recognise the steps needed to modify a compound to comply with these guidelines. However, the simple properties on which they are based typically have a poor correlation with the chance of a compound's success[6] and, all too often, they are applied as hard filters with the risks outlined above.

Another popular trend is to combine target potency with one or more properties to calculate a 'ligand efficiency index' (LEI), which can be used to guide selection or optimisation of compounds. The first example of this was the Ligand Efficiency (LE) equation,[7,8] which relates the free energy of binding to the number of heavy atoms (HAC) in a compound:

$$\text{LE} = \frac{\Delta G}{\text{HAC}} = \frac{RT \ln K}{\text{HAC}} \approx \frac{1.4 \times p\text{IC}_{50}}{\text{HAC}},$$

where $p\mathrm{IC}_{50}$ is the negative logarithm of the IC_{50} in molar concentration. This is motivated by the fact that large compounds tend to exhibit poor physico-chemical and ADME properties. Therefore, of two equipotent compounds, the smaller will typically have a lower risk.

The derivation of LE led to the suggestion of several LEIs, including ligand lipophilicity efficiency (LLE):

$$\mathrm{LLE} = p\mathrm{IC}_{50} - \log P,$$

and several others combining measures of size, lipophilicity and polarity with potency.[9] As with the rules for drug-like properties, LEIs can provide useful guidelines for optimisation of compounds. However, as discussed above, the non-potency properties that contribute to LEIs are imperfect surrogates for the biological properties of a compound and there has been considerable debate regarding the relative merits of different LEIs.[10-12] Of the commonly applied LEIs, it has been suggested that LLE may have the greatest relevance due to its relationship with the thermodynamics of binding[13] and, in particular, the preference for maximising the enthalpic contribution to binding affinity to minimise non-specific or off-target binding. A further note of caution must be sounded because the uncertainties in both the potency and $\log P$ will combine to give a greater uncertainty in LLE, often making it difficult to distinguish between compounds on this basis.

Of course, MPO is not limited to simple compound properties; there are several approaches that can be applied to any data, whether calculated or experimental, and overcome the limitations of simple filters. The most commonly applied methods will be described below and general reviews can be found elsewhere.[2,14,15]

10.2.1 Pareto Optimisation

Pareto optimisation is named after its inventor, an economist who first published the method in the early 20th century.[16] He proposed that, when considering multiple parameters, there may not be a single, optimal solution but a family of solutions that each represent an optimal combination of parameters. Specifically, a Pareto optimal, or 'non-dominated', solution is one for which there is no other solution that is better in all of the parameters. A simple example of this for two parameters is illustrated in Figure 10.2(a).

Pareto optimisation is particularly useful when it is not clear what the 'best' balance of properties may be to achieve a desired outcome. In the example shown in Figure 10.2 for potency and metabolic stability, it would be ideal to find a very stable and highly potent compound. However, in the absence of such a compound, it may be possible to improve efficacy by increasing potency or increasing exposure through greater metabolic stability. Therefore, in this scenario, it would be reasonable to explore a range of compounds that represented different trade-offs between these parameters.

The Pareto-optimal points form a boundary, the 'Pareto front', within the parameter space being explored, as shown in Figure 10.2(a). This concept

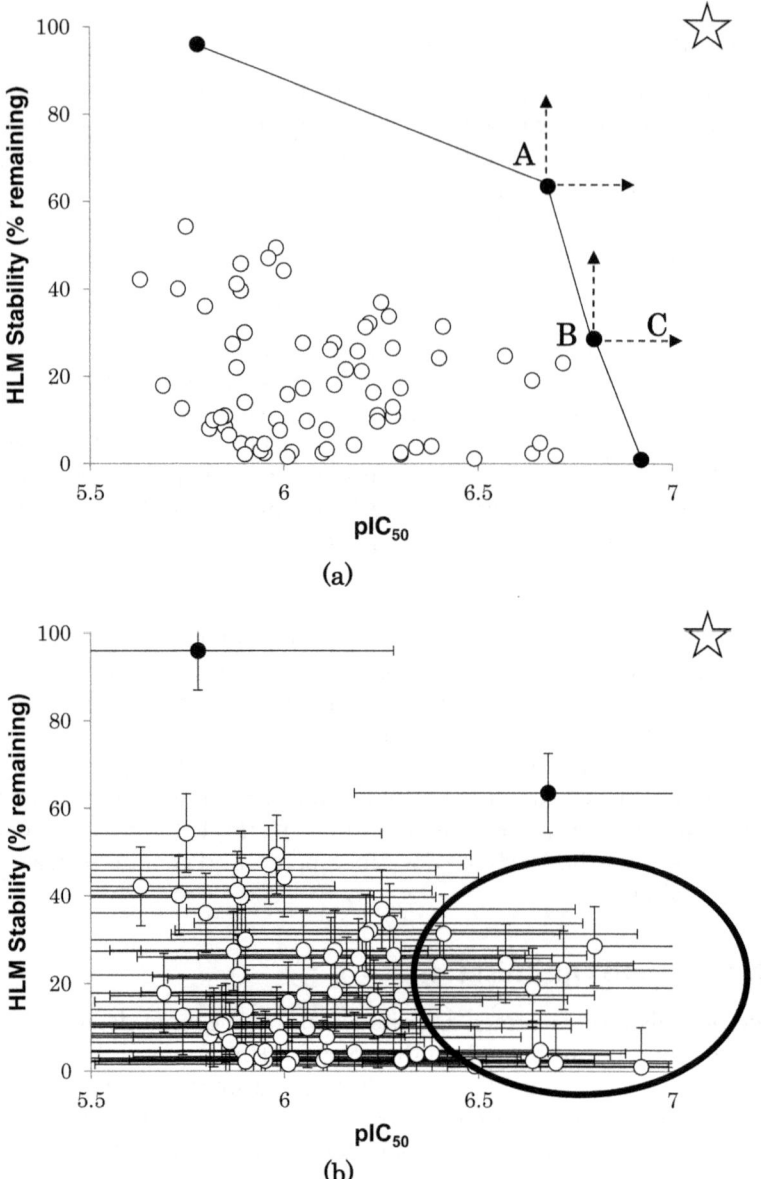

Figure 10.2 Plots illustrating the concept of Pareto optimality in which the ideal outcome corresponds to the top right corner of the plot, as indicated by the star. (a) Shows a scatter plot of data for activity against the therapeutic target and stability in human liver microsomes (HLMs) for a set of 75 compounds. The solid points are Pareto optimal, or 'non-dominated' points; for example, in the case of point A, there are no points with a higher value for both parameters. However, open circles are not Pareto optimal; for example point B is 'dominated' by point C. The solid line joining Pareto optimal compounds is the Pareto front. (b) Shows the same data for which the uncertainty (1 standard deviation) has been illustrated by error bars on each point. From this it is clear that, while two points may be confidently identified as Pareto optimal (solid circles), there are many points in the region indicated by the ellipse that may not be confidently identified as Pareto optimal or otherwise.

may be generalised to a 'Pareto rank' whereby those points on the Pareto front are given a rank of 0, those for which there is only one point better in all parameters are rank 1, *etc.* The Pareto rank can provide a basis for prioritising compounds based on multiple properties.

A limitation of Pareto optimisation is that the number of Pareto optimal solutions can be very large, making it difficult to focus on a small number of high quality compounds. This is particularly the case when simultaneously considering a large number of properties, because the number of Pareto optimal solutions increases exponentially with the number of parameters in the space. Therefore, in practice, Pareto optimisation is typically limited to exploring a maximum of 4–5 parameters. The challenge created by a large number of Pareto optimal solutions is further exacerbated when one considers the impact of uncertainty, whereby it may not be possible to say with confidence which compounds are Pareto optimal, as illustrated in Figure 10.2(b), meaning that it would be necessary to investigate an even larger number of compounds.

One common approach to overcome the limitation on the number of parameters that may be explored simultaneously is to combine multiple properties into a single parameter that can be used as input to Pareto optimisation. For example, multiple ADME-related properties can be combined into a single score and this can be balanced against other factors, such as potency.[17,18] This score could be calculated using one of the methods based on desirability functions, described below.

10.2.2 Desirability Functions

An alternative approach to prioritise compounds based on multiple properties is provided by the use of desirability functions. This was first proposed by Harrington in 1965[19] as a method for combining multiple properties to give a single measure of quality. A desirability function transforms the value of a property onto a scale of 'desirability' from 0 (unacceptable) to 1 (ideal). A desirability function can take any form and some simple examples are shown in Figure 10.3. The use of desirability functions overcomes one of the pitfalls of applying hard filters by allowing more subtle distinctions to be made between similar property values.

Segall and Champness[3] considered the data in Figure 10.1(a), comparing permeability [apparent permeability coefficient (P_{app})] across the human epithelial colorectal adenocarcinoma (Caco-2) cell line[20] with clinically measured human intestinal absorption (HIA), as published by Irvine *et al.*[21] Caco-2 permeation is a commonly used model of absorption across the human intestine and these data indicate that a high Caco-2 permeability would be ideal, because it correlates strongly with good HIA. However, it can be seen that low permeation does not necessarily indicate that the compound will be poorly absorbed. Therefore, it would not be appropriate to apply a hard filter to reject compounds with a low Caco-2 permeability, particularly if other properties of the compound were good. Instead, this can

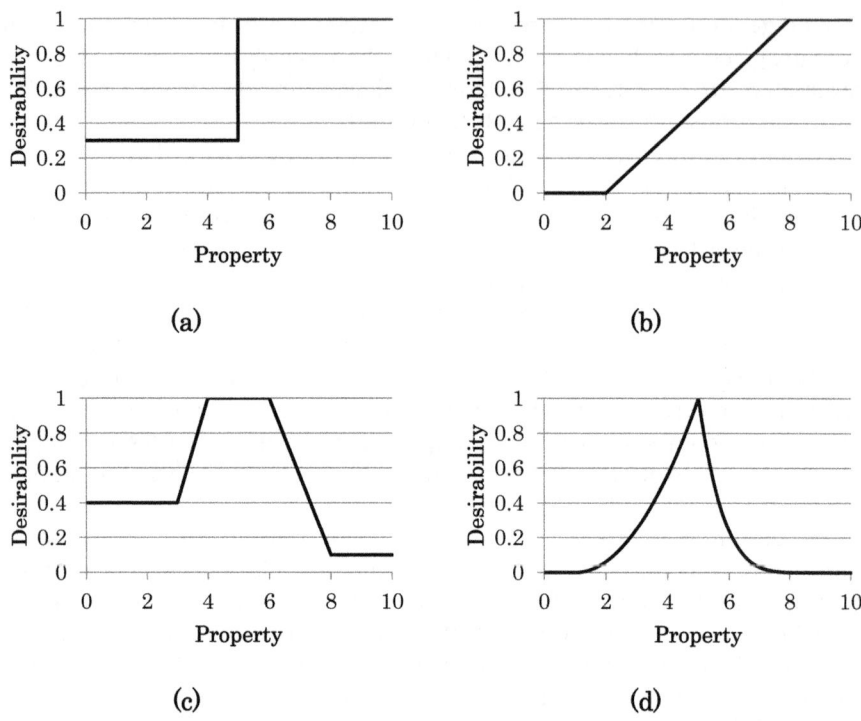

Figure 10.3 Example desirability functions. The functions shown by the bold lines in (a) to (c) are examples of linear desirability functions: (a) is a hard cut-off, but not a filter, because property values that do not achieve the criterion of >5 are less desirable, but will not be rejected outright; (b) defines an ideal property criterion of >8 with linearly increasing desirability above a property value of 2; (c) defines an ideal property range of 4–6 with values exceeding the upper limit being less desirable than those below the lower limit. The boundaries of this range are not hard-cut-offs, but are 'softened' because the desirability above and below the ideal range decreases linearly. The desirability function in (d) is an example of a nonlinear Derringer function[31] with desirability d for property value X defined by: $X < 1$: $d = 0$; $1 < X < 5$: $d = ((X - 1)/4)^2$; $5 < X < 8$: $d = ((9 - X)/4)^5$; $8 < X$: $d = 0$.

be represented as a desirability function for Caco-2 permeation as shown in Figure 10.1(b), which corresponds to the objective of achieving a HIA greater than 50%. The histogram bars indicate the chance of a compound achieving this objective for a measured Caco-2 permeability in one log-unit ranges and the corresponding desirability function is shown, indicating that the ideal outcome would be a Caco-2 permeability above 100 nm s^{-1} [$\log(P_{app}) > 2$]. The worst outcome would be a Caco-2 permeability below 1 nm s^{-1} [$\log(P_{app}) < 0$], where the chance of success is still approximately one third. Between these values, the desirability increases approximately linearly.

A desirability function normalises each property on a scale of desirability between 0 and 1, which makes it convenient to combine the desirabilities of the individual properties into a single score, or 'desirability index', representing the quality of a compound against multiple properties. There are two general approaches to calculating a desirability index from the individual property desirabilities:

$$\text{Additive}: D = \frac{d_1\left(Y_1\right) + d_2\left(Y_2\right) + \cdots + d_n\left(Y_n\right)}{n},$$

$$\text{Multiplicative}: D = (d_1(Y_1) \times d_2(Y_2) \times \ldots \times d_n(Y_n))^{1/n}$$

where D is the overall desirability index, $d_i(Y_i)$ is the desirability score for property Y_i and n is the number of properties. In the two examples above, the score has been normalised by the number of properties by taking the average or geometric mean respectively.

An additive approach has a drawback that the impact of any individual property is limited when a large number of properties are considered; a low desirability for a single property will only have a small effect on the overall score. This may not be appropriate because, in some cases, a single bad result may be enough to 'kill' a compound. For example, a compound with very poor potency (*e.g.* 100 µM) would not be of interest, even if all of its other properties were ideal. The use of a multiplicative approach overcomes this limitation, because a single unacceptable results can be sufficient to 'kill' a compound. However, a multiplicative approach can over-penalise compounds unless the desirability functions are carefully considered, particularly when a poor outcome for one property can be mitigated by a good result for another. In an effort to overcome some of these limitations, an alternative approach was proposed by Nissink and Degorce,[22] whereby the overall score is calculated as a normalised distance between the point $(d_1(Y_1),d_2(Y_2),\ldots, d_n(Y_n))$ and the point corresponding to an ideal compound $(1,1,\ldots,1)$.

Different levels of importance can also be assigned to each property by weighting the contribution of the corresponding desirability in the calculation of the score. Therefore, desirability functions provide a flexible framework with which to tailor the property requirements to the therapeutic objective of a project. Furthermore, it is straightforward to interpret the impact of each property on the overall score of a compound; a low desirability for an individual property highlights an issue that must be addressed to significantly increase the overall quality of a compound.

Of course, in order to define desirability functions for each property of interest it is necessary to know the required property criteria *a priori*. In many cases this can be defined based on the knowledge and experience of a drug discovery project team. Furthermore, if the evidence from downstream experiments, *e.g. in vivo* studies, indicates a different profile may be required, it is straightforward to modify the desirability functions and calculate new scores to ascertain if the priorities of compounds would change. However, with the increasing complexity of the data that are available in early drug discovery, from *in silico* predictions and high-throughput screening, it may not be clear which properties offer the best ability to distinguish between successful and unsuccessful compounds nor what desirability functions should be applied for each of these properties. From this perspective, Pareto optimization can help to explore different property trade-offs. Furthermore, methods such as 'rule induction'[23] can help to explore existing data for compounds for which the outcome is known to identify the most appropriate desirability functions.

10.2.3 Probabilistic Scoring

Desirability functions avoid hard cut-offs that can lead to artificially large distinctions between compounds with similar properties. However, this approach does not explicitly account for the uncertainties in the underlying data and therefore it is not clear when compounds can be confidently distinguished or when the data do not support such a decision. Furthermore, frequently, some data are not available for some compounds and it is not immediately clear how these should be accounted for or what impact the missing data will have on the decisions made.

To address this, the Probabilistic Scoring method[24] builds on desirability functions by explicitly taking the uncertainty of the underlying data into account. The score calculated by this method represents the likelihood of success, *i.e.* the probability of a compound achieving the ideal outcome, as defined by a profile of property criteria, which are each represented by a desirability function (see Figure 10.4 for an example). Furthermore, the uncertainty in the overall score for each compound is calculated, based on the uncertainty in the underlying data, as also illustrated in Figure 10.4. From this it can clearly be seen when the data can separate compounds, but compounds will not be inappropriately rejected based on uncertain data, which could potentially miss valuable opportunities.

This approach can also deal rigorously with missing data, which are equivalent to a very uncertain value. The impact of this uncertainty will be reflected in the overall score. For example, consider a compound that is ideal for all properties except for one important property for which the data are missing. Such a compound will have an intermediate score—an unknown value is better than a value that is known to be poor, but worse than one that is known to be good—and the uncertainty in the overall score will be large. This is because the compound would be perfect if the property were measured and found to be ideal, but if the property value was found to be poor the compound would have a low chance of success. Alternatively, if a different compound had poor values for several properties, but was missing data for one property, both the score and uncertainty would be low; a good value for the missing property will not 'rescue' a compound that 'fails' for several other properties. This makes it clear when measuring missing property values will improve our ability to choose between compounds and help to prioritise experimental effort.

Finally, in a similar manner to simple desirability functions, probabilistic scoring provides feedback on the impact of each property on the overall

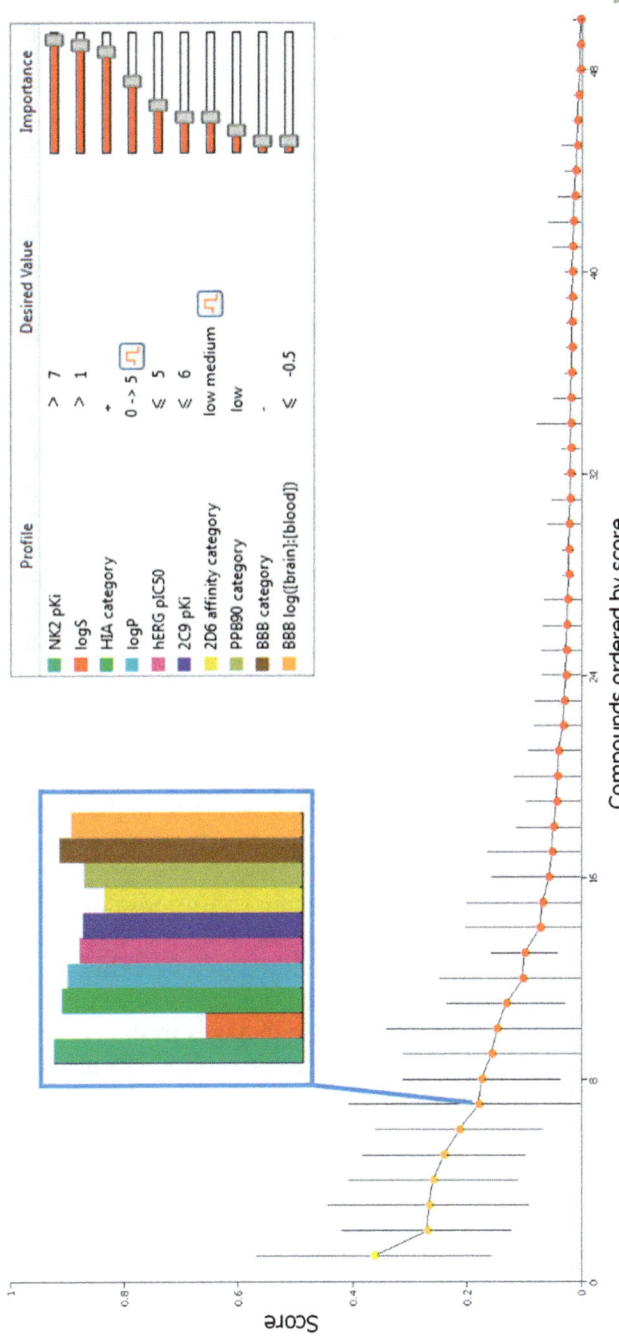

Figure 10.4 This graph shows the compounds in a data set, ordered by their overall scores calculated using the probabilistic scoring method on the axis. The score is calculated against a profile of property criteria (inset), each of which is represented by a desirability function. The score for each compound, representing the likelihood of success against the profile, is plotted on the y axis. Error bars indicate the uncertainty in the overall score for each compound due to the uncertainty in the underlying data. In this case we can see that the error bar for the top-scoring compound overlaps with those for ~15 compounds in the data set, indicating that these compounds cannot be confidently distinguished. The inset histogram shows the contribution of each property to the overall score for a single compound. In the example shown, the most significant issue to address, in order to increase the overall score, is solubility (the colours of the histogram bars correspond to the key in the profile).

quality of a compound. This can be shown as a histogram, as illustrated in Figure 10.4, in which a high bar indicates confidence that a property will meet the ideal requirements with high confidence, while a low bar indicates confidence that the value is very likely be poor for an important property; *i.e.* a critical issue.

10.2.4   Sensitivity to Property Criteria and Importance

When defining a profile of property criteria with which to prioritise compounds, it is not always obvious what the 'right' criteria are and it is important to know if the chosen criteria may be artificially distorting the choice of compounds to pursue. If a small change in a criterion or its importance would lead to a different decision, this can highlight new avenues for exploration and avoid missed opportunities.

Analysing the sensitivity of compound selections to the criteria and their importance by exploring the impact of small changes to these parameters can determine if this is the case. One approach to calculating a 'sensitivity score' is to compare the order in which compounds would be selected, for example using a Spearman's rank correlation coefficient, ρ, between the scores calculated with an original profile and a profile in which a criterion or its importance has been slightly modified. A high correlation (ρ close to 1) would indicate low sensitivity, while a low correlation (ρ close to 0) would mean that there has been a large change in the order of compounds and hence a high sensitivity. Therefore, the sensitivity score can be defined as $1 - \rho$.

However, in calculating the sensitivity, we are most interested in changes to the top-ranked compounds; it does not matter if the order of compounds that we would reject anyway changed. To reflect this, we can restrict the calculation of the rank correlation to the compounds with the highest rank according to the original profile. Also, if we are considering uncertainty, for example with probabilistic scoring, we should neglect changes in rank within the range of uncertainties in the scores because this does not reflect a change in the decision we would make; the changes are in the 'noise'. The calculation of the rank correlation can also be modified to reflect this.

Figure 10.5(a) shows an example of exploring the sensitivity of compound selection from a data set of 191 compounds due to changes in the criterion value for the potency of a compound ($pK_i > 7$) in the profile shown in Figure 10.4. From this it can be seen that the selection of compounds from this data set is highly sensitive to this criterion; an increase of approximately 0.7 log units (to $pK_i > 7.7$) results in a sensitivity of approximately 0.7. The impact of this modification on the scores of the compounds is shown in Figure 10.5(b), indicating a significant change in the top-ranked compounds. Where the prioritisation of compounds is sensitive to one or more parameters of the scoring profile, these parameters should be considered in more detail, because the choice of compounds will depend significantly on the chosen values. If we are confident that the values in the profile are 'correct' we can proceed with the selection of compounds. However, if we are uncertain of the most

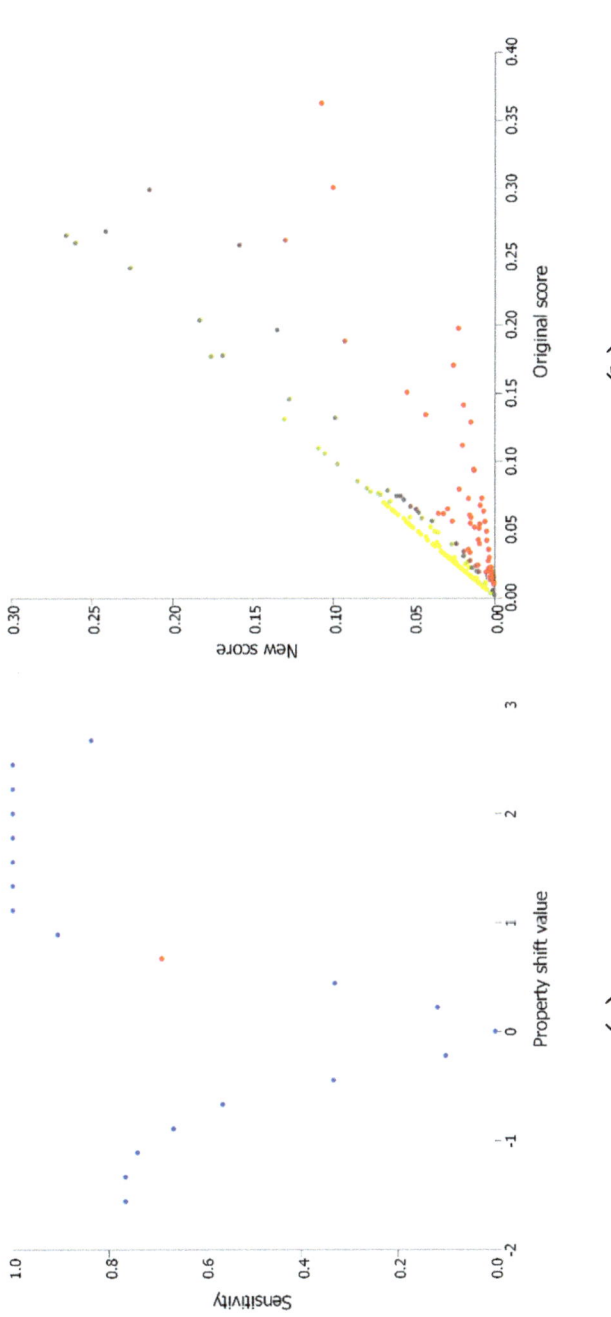

Figure 10.5 Results of a sensitivity analysis for the criterion for pK_i in the profile of property criteria shown in Figure 10.4. (a) Shows a plot of the sensitivity of compound ordering to changes in the criterion around the original criterion of >7. This indicates that small changes in the criterion value results in a high sensitivity, *i.e.* a significant change in the top-ranked compounds. For the point selected in red, corresponding to a criterion of approximately >7.7, the correlation between the original scores and those with the modified criterion (new score) is shown in (b). This helps to identify the compounds for which the ranks change significantly due to the change in the property criterion. Yellow points correspond to compounds for which there is a large increase in rank, red points to those for which there is a large decrease.

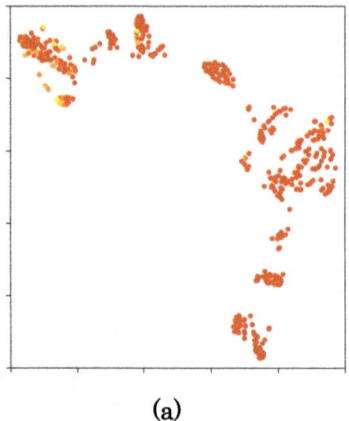

(a)

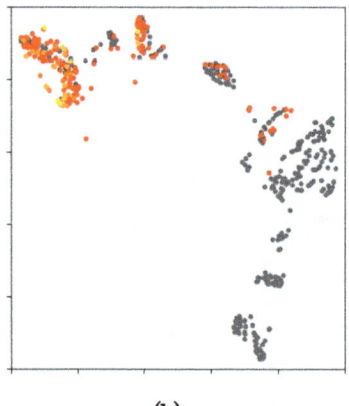

(b)

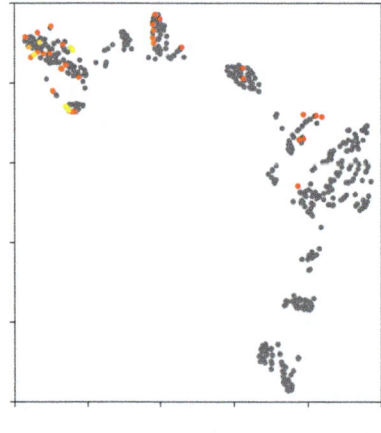

(c)

appropriate values for these parameters, we should consider alternative compounds that would be selected by profiles in which the sensitive parameters have been changed within reasonable ranges. Investigation of these variations may identify alternative compounds that would be valuable to consider, and downstream testing of these would help to determine the most appropriate scoring profile for selecting further high quality compounds.

On the other hand, if the selection of compounds is not sensitive to reasonable changes in the property criteria and their importance, we can proceed with confidence that small uncertainties regarding the most appropriate parameters will not significantly change the direction of the project.

10.3 Example Application: MPO from Hit to Candidate

In this prospective example, the objective of the drug discovery project was to identify a development candidate for a cardiovascular therapeutic. The initial phase of the project involved screening of a focused library of approximately 500 compounds against the primary target. To protect intellectual property rights, the structures of the compounds cannot be revealed here; however the 'chemical space' plots in Figure 10.6 chart the progress of the project as the chemical diversity represented by this library was explored.

The compounds in the library were scored based on the experimentally measured potency (% inhibition) and predictions of a range of ADME properties, including solubility, lipophilicity, human intestinal absorption, inhibition of cytochrome P450 enzymes, blood–brain barrier (BBB) penetration and active efflux by P-glycoprotein (P-gp), using probabilistic scoring and the profile shown in Figure 10.7(a). The distribution of these scores across the

---

Figure 10.6 'Chemical space' plots illustrating the progress of an example project described in Section 10.3. Each point in a chemical space represents a single compound and the proximity of points indicates their structural similarity (2D path-based similarity calculated by a Tanimoto index[32]). The points are coloured by their score against a multi-parameter profile from the highest in yellow to the lowest in red. (a) Shows an initial library of approximately 500 compounds for which target activity had been measured. The points are coloured by the score of the corresponding compound against the profile shown in Figure 10.7(a) for a balance of activity and predicted ADME properties. (b) Shows the compounds chosen for further investigation, including some additional compounds synthesised to expand the most interesting chemotype. The corresponding points are coloured using the same colour scale as (a). (c) Shows 40 compounds that progressed for detailed *in vitro* ADME studies. These focus on the highest scoring compounds from the previous phase, but also include a small number of more diverse compounds to confirm the predictions. The points in (c) are coloured according to the scoring profile shown in Figure 10.7(b) based only on experimentally measured activity and ADME properties.

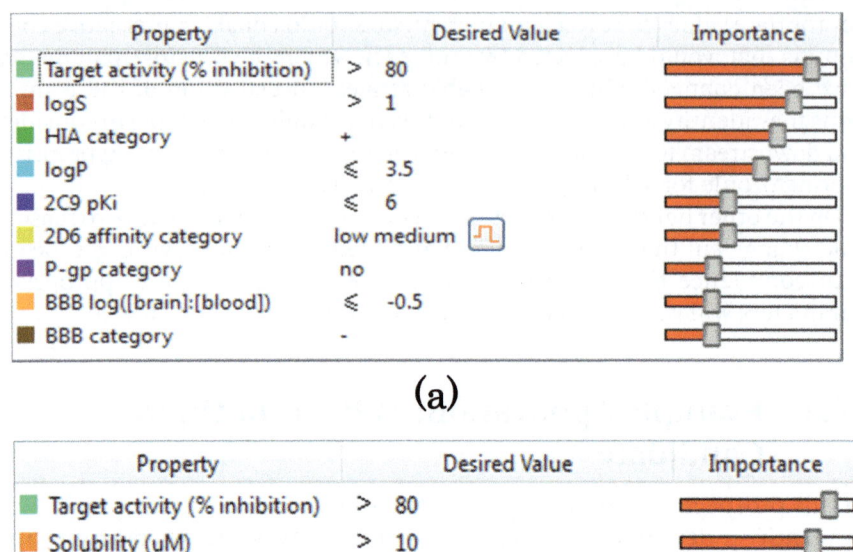

(a)

(b)

Figure 10.7 Property profiles used to prioritise compounds in an example project described in Section 10.3. For each criterion, the desired outcome is shown and the importance of the individual criterion to
the overall objective is illustrated as a red bar. (a) Illustrates a profile of property criteria including experimentally measured target
activity (% inhibition) and predictions of the following properties:
logarithm of aqueous solubility in µM (log S); HIA, based on a cut-
off of 30%; log P; inhibition of the CYP2C9 and CYP2D6 isoforms
of cytochrome P450 (pK_i); categorisation as a P-gp substrate; and
penetration of the BBB. (b) Shows a profile of *in vitro* properties
measured for a subset of the compounds studied in the project:
target activity (% inhibition); solubility (µM); and HLM stability
(% remaining after 40 minutes).

chemical diversity of the library is shown in Figure 10.6(a). This indicates
that the majority of high scoring compounds are concentrated in a small
region of the chemical space (top-left) representing a single chemotype. The
distribution of the scores and their uncertainties are shown in the plot in
Figure 10.8(a), indicating that the highest scoring compounds have a score
of approximately 0.4, representing approximately a 40% chance of success
against the criteria in the profile. However only approximately 10 of these
compounds have a statistically significantly higher score than the remaining
compounds in the library.

Additional compounds were synthesised to expand the highest scoring
chemotype and the potencies of these, along with some of the compounds

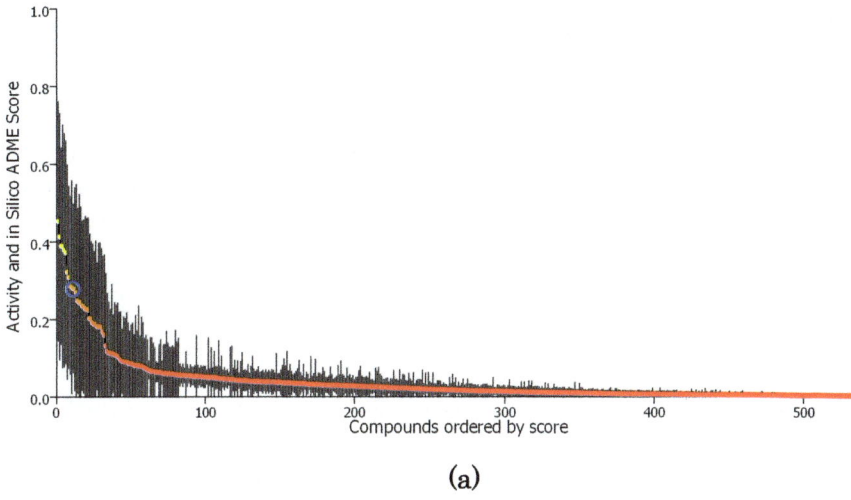

(a)

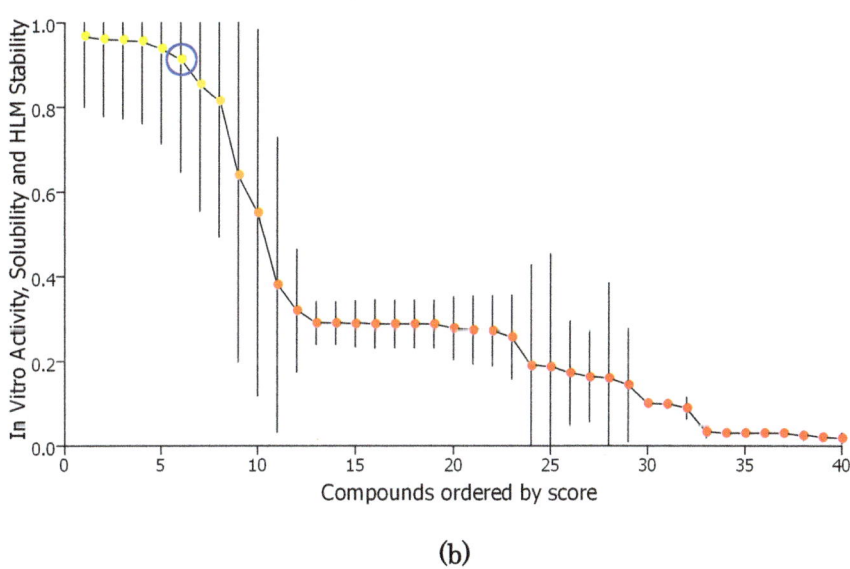

(b)

Figure 10.8 Distribution of scores for compounds in an example project described herein, similar to the plot shown in Figure 10.4. (a) Shows the scores and uncertainties for a library of approximately 500 compounds shown in the chemical space in Figure 10.6(a) and calculated using the profile of property criteria shown in Figure 10.7(a). (b) Shows the scores and uncertainties for a subset of 40 compounds based on experimental data and the profile of property criteria shown in Figure 10.7(b). In each case, the points are coloured by the corresponding score from the highest in yellow to the lowest in red. The compound that was ultimately nominated as a development candidate is highlighted by a blue circle in both plots.

from the initial library, were confirmed. This set comprised approximately 220 compounds and their chemical diversity and scores are illustrated in Figure 10.8(b).

The *in vitro* solubility, and human liver microsomal (HLM) stability were measured for a selected subset of 40 of these compounds, shown in Figure 10.8(c). Here it can be seen that, while the majority of these compounds were selected from the highest scoring clusters, a broader diversity was explored to confirm that the predictions of ADME properties were appropriately selecting high quality compounds. The 40 compounds were scored, based only on the *in vitro* data, using the profile shown in Figure 10.7(b), resulting in the scores shown in Figure 10.8(b). From this set, there are approximately 10 very high scoring compounds, although these cannot be confidently distinguished from one another based on these data.

Further detailed *in vitro* and *in vivo* studies were performed on the highest scoring compounds, to confirm that they exhibited appropriate efficacy, PK and safety profiles, resulting in the nomination of a development candidate, highlighted in Figure 10.8. It is notable that the candidate compound was identified early in the process, saving time and resources that might have been wasted exploring a wider range of chemistries with a low chance of success. However, exploring an appropriate degree of diversity confirmed that opportunities were not missed due to uncertain measurements or predictions.

This example illustrates how MPO, based on a range of experimental and predicted properties, can quickly prioritise high quality compounds and achieve rapid progress from an early hit to an optimised development candidate.

10.4   Conclusion

Psychology research has demonstrated that people are inherently weak at making decisions in the face of complex, uncertain data and drug discovery scientists are, unfortunately, not immune to these effects.[25] With the increasing complexity of ADMET data available from the earliest stages of drug discovery, there is a need for approaches that guide decisions to quickly identify compounds with a high chance of success against the multiple property criteria for a high quality drug.

MPO methods provide frameworks within which to use all of the available data in a consistent and objective way when selecting and optimising compounds. Combined with predictive methods and early ADMET screening these enable high quality compounds and chemical series to be targeted early in the drug discovery process. This facilitates more rapid lead optimisation and results in higher quality candidates for development. The case studies in this chapter and references herein illustrate examples of the application of MPO within drug discovery and the impact that can be achieved.

Further areas of research in MPO, as applied to drug discovery, include the development of methods that help to determine the most appropriate multi-parameter criteria tailored to a specific project's objectives. Methods such as rule induction[23] can explore multi-parameter property spaces to identify scoring profiles that preferentially select compounds with a high chance of success. Furthermore, they can identify the properties that best distinguish between successful and unsuccessful compounds, thereby guiding strategic decisions on allocation of experimental resources in a project to measure the most important properties first.

MPO methods can also be used to guide automatic, or *de novo*, design to develop new strategies for optimisation around a compound or series.[14,26] The first generation of *de novo* design methods were criticised for generating unfeasible structures or compounds with poor properties, but recent developments have focused on generating more relevant chemical structures through the use of medicinal chemistry 'transformation' rules[27] and the use of MPO to guide the optimisation towards high quality compounds. Recent examples, such as that published by Besnard *et al.*,[18] have demonstrated the generation and experimental validation of compounds with a desired profile of activities and properties.

Finally, these computational tools provide an excellent basis for collaboration between project team members from different disciplines: computational and medicinal chemists; drug metabolism/PK scientists; pharmacologists and toxicologists, *etc.* Therefore, it is important that they are accessible and intuitive for scientists in all disciplines. On-going work has led to the design of modern user interfaces that allow scientists to interact with this information in a user-friendly way and quickly identify structure–activity relationships to guide optimisation strategies.[28–30]

References

1. T. Lavé, H. Jones, N. Paquerau, P. Poulin, P. Theil and N. Parrott, *Pharmacokinetic Profiling in Drug Research: Biological, Physicochemical, and Computational Strategies*, ed. B. Testa, S. D. Krämer, H. Wunderli-Allenspach and G. Folkers, Wiley-VCH Verlag GmbH & Co. KGaA, Weinheim, Germany, 2006, pp. 431–439.
2. M. D. Segall, *Curr. Pharm. Des.*, 2012, **18**, 1292.
3. M. D. Segall and E. C. Champness, *J. Comput.–Aided Mol. Des.*, 2015, DOI: 10.1007/s10822-015-9855-2.
4. C. A. Lipinski, F. Lombardo, B. W. Dominy and P. J. Feeney, *Adv. Drug Delivery Rev.*, 1997, **23**, 3.
5. A. T. Garcia-Sosa, U. Maran and C. Hetenyi, *Curr. Med. Chem.*, 2012, **19**, 1646.
6. I. Yusof and M. D. Segall, *Drug Discovery Today*, 2013, **18**, 659.
7. I. D. Kuntz, K. Chen, K. A. Sharp and P. A. Kollman, *Proc. Natl. Acad. Sci. U. S. A.*, 1999, **96**, 9997.
8. A. L. Hopkins, C. R. Groom and A. Alexander, *Drug Discovery Today*, 2004, **9**, 430.
9. C. Abad-Zapatero and J. M. Metz, *Drug Discovery Today*, 2005, **10**, 464.
10. M. D. Shultz, *ACS Med. Chem. Lett.*, 2013, **5**, 2.

11. M. D. Shultz, *Bioorg. Med. Chem. Lett.*, 2013, **23**, 5980.
12. A. L. Hopkins, G. M. Keseru, P. D. Leeson, D. C. Rees and C. H. Reynolds, *Nat. Rev. Drug Discovery*, 2014, **13**, 105.
13. M. D. Shultz, *Bioorg. Med. Chem. Lett.*, 2013, **23**, 5992.
14. M. D. Segall, *Expert Opin. Drug Discovery*, 2014, **9**, 803.
15. C. A. Nicolaou and N. Brown, *Drug Disovery Today: Technol.*, 2013, **10**, e427.
16. W. Jaffe, *J. Econ. Lit.*, 1972, **10**, 1190.
17. J. Kruisselbrink, E. Michael, T. Back, A. Bender, A. Ijzerman, E. van der Horst, M. Ehrgott, C. Fonesca, X. Gandibleux, J.-K. Hao and M. Sevaux, *Lecture Notes in Computer Science: Evolutionary Multi-Criterion Optimization*, Springer, Berlin/Heidelberg, 2009, vol. 5467, pp. 453–467.
18. J. Besnard, G. F. Ruda, V. Setola, K. Abecassis, R. M. Rodriguiz, X. P. Huang, S. Norval, M. F. Sassano, A. I. Shin, L. A. Webste, F. R. Simeons, L. Stojanovski, A. Prat, N. G. Seidah, D. B. Constam, G. R. Bickerton, K. D. Read, W. C. Westel, I. H. Gilbert, B. L. Roth and A. L. Hopkins, *Nature*, 2012, **492**, 215.
19. E. C. Harrington, *Ind. Qual. Control*, 1965, **21**, 494.
20. I. J. Hidalgo, T. J. Raub and R. T. Borchardt, *Gastroenterology*, 1989, **96**, 736.
21. J. D. Irvine, L. Takahashi, K. Lockhart, J. Cheong, J. W. Tolan, H. E. Selick and J. R. Grove, *J. Pharm. Sci.*, 1999, **88**, 28.
22. J. W. M. Nissink and S. Degorce, *Future Med. Chem.*, 2013, **5**, 753.
23. I. Yusof, F. Shah, T. Hashimoto, M. D. Segall and N. Greene, *Drug Discovery Today*, 2014, **19**, 680.
24. M. Segall, A. Beresford, J. Gola, D. Hawksley and M. Tarbit, *Expert Opin. Drug Metab. Toxicol.*, 2006, **2**, 325.
25. A. T. Chadwick and M. D. Segall, *Drug Discovery Today*, 2010, **15**, 561.
26. C. A. Nicolaou, J. Apostolakis and C. S. Pattichis, *J. Chem. Inf. Model.*, 2009, **49**, 295.
27. K. Stewart, M. Shiroda and C. James, *Bioorg. Med. Chem.*, 2006, **14**, 7011.
28. D. K. Agrafiotis and J. M. Wiener, *J. Med. Chem.*, 2010, **53**, 5002.
29. M. D. Segall, E. J. Champness, C. Leeding, J. Chisholm, P. Hunt, A. Elliott, H. Garcia-Martinez, N. Foster and S. Dowling, *Drug Discovery Today*, 2015, **20**, 1093.
30. K. Klein, N. Kriege and P. Mutzel, *Computer Vision, Imaging and Computer Graphics. Theory and Applications*, Springer Berlin, Heidelberg, 2012, vol. 359, pp. 176–192.
31. G. Derringer and R. Suich, *J. Qual. Technol.*, 1980, **12**, 214.
32. D. J. Rogers and T. T. Tanimoto, *Science*, 1960, **132**, 1115.

CHAPTER 11

Metabolomics-Based Approaches to Determine Drug Metabolite Profiles

LISA J. CHRISTOPHER[a], RAMASWAMY IYER[a], JONATHAN L. JOSEPHS[b], AND W. GRIFFITH HUMPHREYS*[a]

[a]Bristol-Myers Squibb Pharmaceutical Co., Department of Biotransformation, Princeton, NJ, 08648, USA; [b]Thermo Fisher Scientific, Bridgewater, NJ, 08873, USA
*E-mail: william.humphreys@bms.com

11.1 Introduction

The availability of robust, accessible high resolution mass spectrometers (HR-MS) has made a huge impact in a number of analytical fields. The application of this instrumentation allows collection of datasets with robust mass accuracy that enable workflows using supervised or unsupervised searches to characterize multiple chemical constituents of a given sample. Examples of these types of application range from metabolomics[1] and biomarker discovery[2] to drug metabolism or forensics. The former studies are typically designed to characterize all chemical species present in a sample and are often looking to characterize changes in signal intensity of high abundance ions. The latter studies, *e.g.*, profiling of drug metabolites, are slightly different in that the ions of interest all arise from a known starting mass, the administered drug, which can be used as a starting point for searches. While

RSC Drug Discovery Series No. 49
New Horizons in Predictive Drug Metabolism and Pharmacokinetics
Edited by Alan G. E. Wilson
© The Royal Society of Chemistry 2016
Published by the Royal Society of Chemistry, www.rsc.org

the design of specific search techniques taking advantage of properties of the drug makes finding drug-related material easier, the fact that these components are typically of low abundance relative to the wide variety of very complex background matrix ions still presents significant challenges. The application of HR-MS technology and the use of metabolomics-related approaches in drug metabolism studies share many similarities to applications in areas such as forensic science and doping control.[3]

Two of the most challenging tasks in metabolite identification by liquid chromatography (LC)/MS are: (1) the rapid assignment of full scan (FS) and MS/MS spectra obtained from *in vitro* samples during optimization; and (2) comprehensive detection and structural elucidation of all metabolites, including those that could be considered trace, and those arising from both predictable and unpredictable biotransformations, in the presence of large amounts of complex interference ions from endogenous components. HR-MS can play a unique role in both of these key activities. Targeted searches for metabolites take advantage of the fact that the majority of drug metabolites can be categorized as predictable, *i.e.*, those formed *via* common biotransformation reactions. Using list searches of exact masses of expected metabolites can lead to rapid assignment of metabolites. Triggered MS/MS spectra can then be used to provide structural assignment. However, there are many examples of important metabolites that arise from uncommon reactions and are thus not easily predicted *a priori*. These metabolites may require additional data mining of HR-MS datasets.

In this chapter, approaches are discussed for drug metabolite identification with HR-MS, including data acquisition and data mining technologies, employed in support of metabolite identification in drug discovery and development.

11.2 Instrumentation

Although high mass accuracy instruments have been available in leading MS laboratories for many years, the first instruments that allowed this technology to be more generally available arrived around 2005. The two technologies that quickly evolved to provide high mass accuracy instruments for general purposes were ion traps and time-of-flight (ToF) instruments. From the early days, both of these instrument classes were capable of providing sufficient accuracy and resolution for the assignment of high probability matches for molecular formulas with the observed molecular weights. Differentiators in the early versions of ion trap and ToF instruments were predominately around mass stability and scan speed, with ion traps having superior mass stability over time but not offering the scan speeds available on ToF instruments. Early ToF instruments needed to be re-calibrated often to retain mass accuracy and did not lend themselves to medium or large sample sets.

The differentiating factors seen with early instruments have in many respects disappeared with the recently introduced HR-MS instruments. These newer mass spectrometers provide high resolution, good scan-to-scan stability and high scan rates. The QEXACTIVE™ provides high resolution [>100 K full width at half maximum (FWHM)] while maintaining high sensitivity, scan speed and very good scan-to-scan stability without use of lock mass, thus enabling extensive quantitative analytical experiments. Coupling this HR-MS technology to ultra high performance LC (UHPLC) or low flow LC technologies offers the opportunity to obtain qualitative and quantitative information on metabolites as well as parents *in vitro* or *in vivo* without sacrificing sensitivity and speed of analysis. UHPLC often allows greater separation capacity and often enables separation of problematic components such as isobaric hydroxylated metabolites and multiple unknown components within an acceptable analysis time. However, the fast separation of UHPLC results in very narrow chromatographic peaks. So the HR-MS used has to scan fast enough to obtain sufficient data points across these narrower peaks for quantitation.

11.3 Identification of Metabolites with HR-MS

Since electrospray instruments were introduced in the 1990s, great efforts were made to develop MS methodologies that enabled fast, sensitive and accurate identification of metabolites. Traditional triple quad methods were conducted using various scanning functions, such as product ion (PI) or neutral loss (NL), to identify metabolite ions. Significant method development was required to generate parent spectra and thus predict fragment ions of metabolites, and the methods often required multiple injections to detect different metabolites. After the introduction of ion trap instrumentation, once metabolite ions were found *via* triple quads, multistage PI scans (MS^n) on an ion trap instrument were carried out to get more detailed fragmentation pathways for structure elucidation. HR-MS instruments were utilized in cases when determination of empirical formulae of metabolites or their fragments was required. This comprehensive approach was effective in identifying unexpected metabolites, but required multiple instruments and several MS experiments. In the past 10 years, new and improved HR-MS instruments and data processing techniques have been developed for metabolite identification. As a result, HR-MS instruments are now capable of accomplishing all requisite metabolite identification tasks with significantly improved productivity and quality. With the use of list search techniques to identify metabolites and to trigger collection of MS/MS spectra, complete metabolite identification and characterization can often be accomplished in one LC run.

The most common method to rapidly identify predictable metabolites is through the use of list searches of the FS-MS data files. The lists can be generated automatically through the use of the HR-MS vendor's software or third party software. All of these software packages come with fairly rigorous methods of generating exact mass *m/z* lists for common metabolites arising from hydroxylation/heteroatom oxidation, heteroatom dealkylation and ester/amide hydrolysis, *etc.* The metabolite peaks can then be visualized by plotting the exact mass chromatograms. This methodology is sufficient for a large proportion of *in vitro* studies where primary metabolites predominate and typically arise from predictable metabolic steps. *In vivo* metabolite identification is often much more challenging with list searches being only the first step in a multistep process that employs MS/MS data analysis and data mining. A detailed discussion of this process can be found in Section 11.6 below.

The most significant bottleneck in the completion of a metabolite identification workflow is the assignment of structure through interpretation of the MS/MS spectra. While there have been some recent developments in software-assisted automated assignment of MS/MS fragments and metabolite structure prediction,[4] this step still requires manual intervention to confirm computer assignments. It is important to note that the high mass accuracy of fragments in MS/MS spectra obtained from HR-MS instruments greatly facilitates the structural work necessary for assignment of metabolite structure and can really drive the automated assignment algorithms.

11.4   Quantitation Strategies

Due to its sensitivity, selectivity and speed of analysis, LC/MS using atmospheric pressure ionization (API) sources has been the method of choice for quantitative analysis of drugs and their metabolites in biological matrices for a number of years. In recent years, there has also been some growth in the number of HR-MS driven quantitation strategies, especially when HR-MS is employed for qualitative analysis. These strategies are usually referred to as "quan/qual". One major drawback of MS is that the MS response of an analyte obtained using an API source depends strongly on the chemical structure of the analyte and the matrix in which the analyte is analyzed, which necessitates the use of a calibration curve prepared from an authentic standard for quantitation. For a drug candidate in the optimization and early development stages, metabolite standards are not routinely available and thus an early estimation of the metabolite concentration measurements must be done by alternative means. In order to obtain quantitative information on metabolites when metabolite standards are not available, the majority of published strategies have revolved around either using the MS response directly or using an orthogonal quantitative technique such as ultraviolet (UV) spectroscopy. There are obvious advantages and disadvantages to both, which impact the quality and throughput of the data, and also how the results can be utilized for decision making.

The use of MS response as a quantitative tool has obvious advantages in throughput, and screening methods built around MS response are by far the best way to achieve relatively high throughput. These screens are well suited for qualitative assays where "yes/no" answers are adequate, but should be considered as quantitative estimates, at best, of metabolite concentration because of the variability in MS response caused by the variability in ionization efficiency based on structure. For this reason other techniques have been explored to correct for the non-universal MS response between parent compounds and metabolites.

UV[5] and nuclear magnetic resonance (NMR)[6] have been used to calibrate the MS response of metabolites relative to parent compounds using biologically generated metabolite standards. Although less sensitive, both detectors have a more universal response than MS. NMR has been found to be more accurate than UV, but it requires the isolation of a few micrograms of metabolites, which can be challenging in the case of minor metabolites from complex biological matrices. On the other hand, UV detection does not require metabolite and UV/photodiode array detectors are readily available in most bioanalytical laboratories.

A radiometric calibration technique has been used to estimate the circulating metabolites in humans by comparing the MS peak areas of the metabolites in plasma with those of a sample spiked with a known amount of radiolabeled metabolites, which are either generated by *in vitro* incubations or isolated from *in vivo* studies.[7] The major limitation of this approach is that it relies on the availability of radiolabeled compounds.

11.5 Utilization of HR-MS in the Discovery/ Optimization Stage

Metabolite detection, identification and quantitation in both *in vitro* and *in vivo* studies play key roles at various stages of drug discovery and development, although the goals of each study place slightly different requirements on instrumentation. Studies during the optimization stage must be able to characterize multiple drug candidates in experimental protocols that have throughput and turnaround times that meet the needs of medicinal chemistry programs. These studies not only reveal biotransformations leading to possible reactive, toxic or human-unique metabolites, but also sometimes result in the discovery of new drug entities in the form of pharmacologically active metabolites. Early studies are typically carried out in *in vitro* systems utilizing subcellular liver fractions or with plasma/serum.

In vitro metabolism screening strategies employing HR-MS technology have been discussed in a number of reports.[8] All of these analytical strategies describe generic systems that can be run with minimal or no optimization prior to running samples from experiments with new drug candidates. The systems usually rely on generic LC systems that provide: (1) adequate separation of parent and metabolites over a broad range of chemotypes; and (2) reasonable run times such that the throughput of the assay is adequate to meet demand from medicinal chemistry efforts. UHPLC is becoming more common as it provides benefits in both separation and run time aspects. Also, the methods all take advantage of the ability of HR-MS instruments to: (1) perform rapid quantitative analysis in order to determine parent disappearance; (2) enable qualitative analysis and assignment of metabolite molecular formulae when run in FS mode; and (3) assign metabolite structures using

MS/MS fragmentation information. The major difference in methods is the strategy to determine estimated metabolite concentrations, which has significant impact on assay design.

Bateman *et al.*[8a] describe a method for analysis of samples from microsome incubations that uses alternate scanning between FS-MS and spectra collected after higher energy collisional dissociation (HCD) fragmentation. The scanning capabilities of the ORBITRAP were deemed sufficient to allow accurate determination of parent concentration and thus parent disappearance values from the incubation samples at various time points. The method then determines metabolites with manual searches of the FS spectra. Finally, the method determines metabolite structures using the fragmentation information contained in the HCD spectra.

The methodology outlined in King *et al.*[8e] takes advantage of the high scanning speeds of the QEXACTIVE instrument to perform rapid quan/qual experiments with *in vitro* metabolism samples. The methods described involve generic ultra performance LC gradient run times of 2 or 10 min depending on the extent of metabolite profiling information required. As above, the parent disappearance rate/extent is determined from FS spectra. Metabolites are determined by matching exact mass lists generated in Thermo Scientific™ LCQUAN™ software to the FS spectra. Quantitative estimates of metabolite concentrations are made based on MS response, although the authors stress that these values are only used to make conclusions based on relative levels in multiple samples not to make absolute determinations.

The method detailed in publications by Grubb and Josephs[8c,8d] involves the combination of UHPLC with an LTQ-ORBITRAP mass spectrometer system for obtaining quantitative and qualitative exposure information on metabolites (Figure 11.1). The method employs incubations at two concentrations, one in a range allowing UV detection of parent and metabolites, and one in a range that is more relevant to typical clinical concentrations and thus more kinetically relevant. The BMS assay is typically run at 0.1–1 and 30 μM as these concentrations were found to best meet the criteria laid out above. Samples from incubations with liver subcellular fractions are analyzed using UHPLC-UV and HR-MS. The UV chromatograms at the highest concentration allow quantitation of the UV response to MS response for each metabolite. The ratio, along with FS-MS detection of a parent and its metabolites, is then used to quantitate the amount of metabolite present in low concentration samples in the range of 0.1–1 μM. The result is a plot of parent disappearance and metabolite formation over time at a concentration more relevant for the determination of *in vitro* clearance and major metabolic pathways. The MS/MS spectra are used to aid in metabolite structure identification. The method is referred to as 'MetPro'.[8c] MetPro is a rapid and efficient means to generate profiles of metabolite concentrations in *in vitro* incubations *versus* time for discovery stage new chemical entities for which metabolite standards may not be available. Absolute amounts can be determined with the key assumption that the UV absorption of parent compounds and metabolites are equivalent.

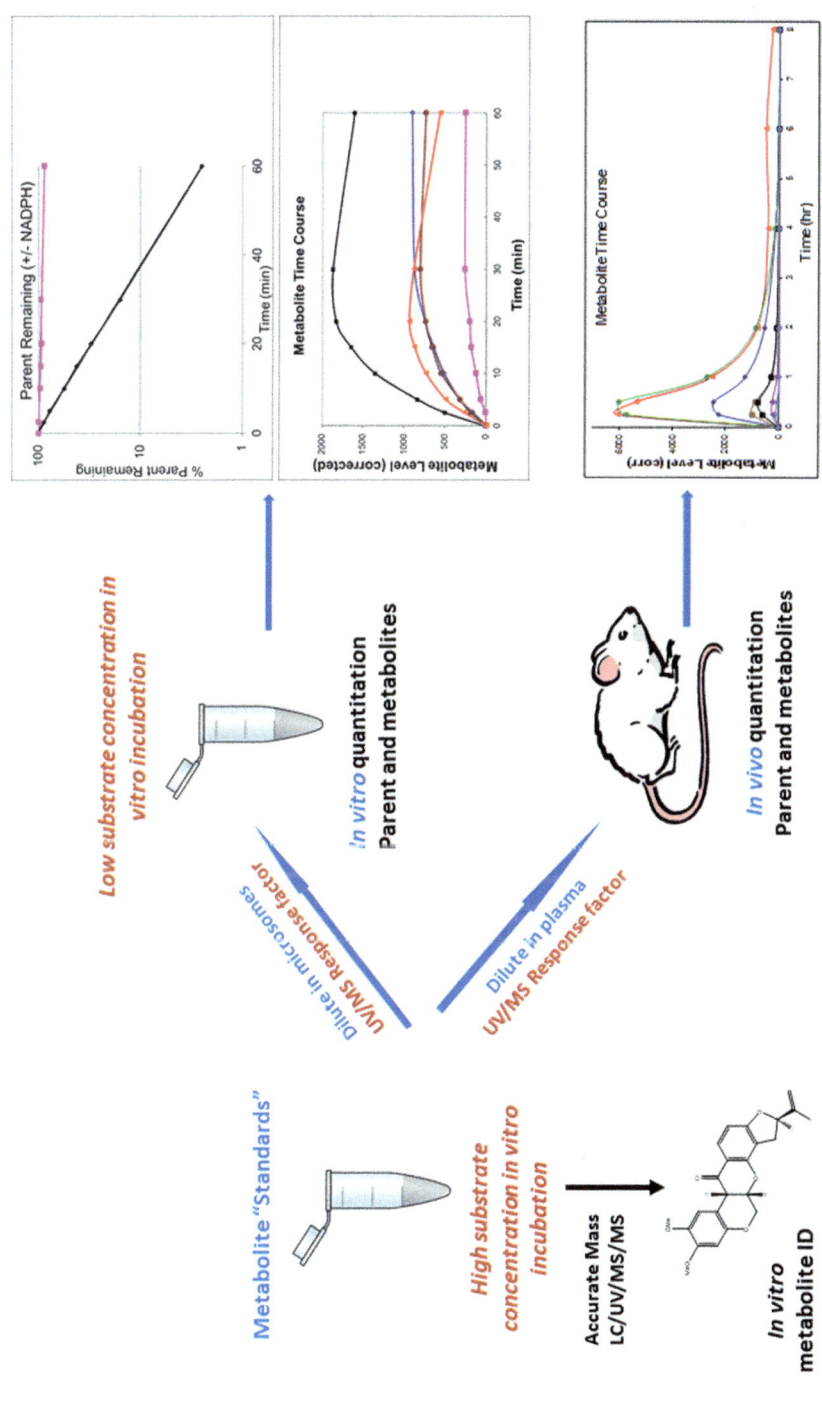

Figure 11.1 Schematic of the workflow used for metabolite identification and UV-based quantitation. Demonstration of the application of MS/UV correction factors for quantitation of metabolites at low substrate concentrations by LC-MS in the absence of authentic standards.

This approach, with use of 'metabolite standards' generated from high concentration *in vitro* incubations,[5,8d] can also be adapted to determine quantitative estimates of plasma metabolites in the absence of chemically synthesized metabolite standards. First, the *in vitro* incubation sample containing all the generated metabolites is diluted in plasma to serve as a single point calibration standard for calculating the metabolite concentrations in plasma samples. The analysis of the plasma samples in question then proceeds utilizing the methodology laid out above for the *in vitro* low concentration samples.

11.6　Utilization of HR-MS in the Development/ Characterization Stage

In early development, metabolite profiling efforts for drug candidates are focused on identifying metabolites in human samples obtained from clinical studies and relating the exposure of metabolites in humans to levels observed in the preclinical toxicology species. Although structural modification often renders a metabolite inactive, some metabolites may retain pharmacological activity or produce off-target toxicity concerns. Since circulating metabolites in particular may contribute to these effects, it is important to identify and fully characterize any abundant plasma metabolites to establish its contribution to the drug's pharmacological effect, and to confirm that its safety has been satisfactorily evaluated through the achievement of adequate exposures in preclinical toxicology species. Furthermore, metabolites present in excreta reflect the overall flux through the various metabolic pathways; quantitative information on drug and metabolite levels in the excreta can be used in conjunction with enzyme phenotyping data to predict variability in pharmacokinetic parameters resulting from genetic polymorphisms of drug metabolizing enzymes or the likelihood and extent of victim drug–drug interactions with co-medications.[7a]

Traditionally, metabolites were identified in samples collected in single-dose radiolabeled absorption, metabolism and excretion (AME) studies after administration of [^{14}C]- or [^{3}H]-labeled drug to animal species and humans. Drug-related components in plasma and excreta samples were chromatographically separated and quantified with online radiometric detection or fraction collection followed by off-line radioactivity analysis. Regions corresponding to prominent radioactive peaks in the resulting radioprofiles were isolated and submitted for analytical assessment (*e.g.*, MS or NMR) or these regions of interest were examined for drug-related products in a parallel LC-MS^n analysis, typically with a low resolution mass spectrometer. Because metabolite identification was reliant on the synthesis of radiolabeled drug, these studies were often conducted later in development. Some of the objectives and processes for conducting human radiolabeled mass balance studies have been summarized.[9]

In 2008 and 2009, respectively, the US Food and Drug Administration (FDA) and the International Conference on Harmonization of Technical Requirements for Registration of Pharmaceuticals for Human Use (ICH) issued guidance documents that outlined requirements for evaluation of safety for drug metabolites.[10a,10b] Identification of the differences in exposure of metabolites between humans and nonclinical species used in toxicology evaluation, particularly those metabolites that were disproportionately high in humans, was encouraged to occur as early as possible in the drug development process. The ICH further focused metabolite safety characterization on abundant metabolites that comprised more than 10% of the total exposure to drug related material in human circulation under steady-state conditions.[11]

The following are necessary components to achieve a metabolite profiling assessment that will satisfy the directives set forth in the guidance documents: (1) a screen to identify circulating human metabolites and elucidate their structures; (2) a steady-state comparison (*e.g.*, after multiple daily drug doses in humans and animals) of whether each metabolite found in human plasma is present in the circulation of at least one of the toxicology species at exposures that are similar to or exceed the human exposure; and (3) if exposure multiples are not obtained for a particular metabolite, an evaluation to determine whether the metabolite comprises more than 10% of the exposure to all drug-related material in human plasma. Several groups have proposed analytical strategies aimed at fulfilling these requirements.[12]

A history of the application of MS in drug metabolism studies was recently reviewed.[13] In recent years, HR-MS has become an increasingly important analytical tool in drug metabolism laboratories. Technological advances in HR-MS such as the Fourier transformation ORBITRAP and ToF instruments have increased their utility for metabolite profiling. In addition to being useful for elucidating structures of drug-related components, the high selectivity of HR-MS instruments combined with advances in software for data acquisition and processing have greatly improved the ability to detect drug metabolites in the presence of endogenous compounds in complex biological samples without needing to rely on the use of a radiolabel.[12a] Significant developments include increased scan and data acquisition rates that enable collection of more comprehensive datasets. In addition, the high resolution information can be exploited using several data mining tools, include background subtraction,[14] mass defect filtering (MDF)[15] and isotope pattern filtering (IPF),[16] or a combination of filtering approaches.[17] Many pharmaceutical companies have started to utilize these timely technological advances in HR-MS to screen and identify metabolites earlier in development (*e.g.*, at the time of the first-in-human or multiple-ascending dose studies) and address requirements outlined in the guidance documents.[18]

The initial screen to identify human metabolites typically involves collection of FS-LC-HR-MS and MS/MS data from select plasma samples collected after administration of a drug candidate to humans. Corresponding samples from subjects dosed with placebo (vehicle control) may be collected and similarly analyzed. With background subtraction, drug-related components can be detected by comparing ions present in the sample data file to those from the control data file. If a particular ion is present in both the sample and control file within an accurate mass- and retention time-tolerance window, it is subtracted from the sample file. Since ions pertaining to the plasma and dosing vehicle are removed during background subtraction, the processed file is enriched for mass data related to drug-related components, thus facilitating metabolite identification.[14] Care must be used in the design of background subtraction algorithms to ensure that background ions are subtracted out while signals of interest are not discarded. Figure 11.2A shows the high resolution total ion chromatogram from an extracted human fecal sample collected 0–96 hours after oral administration of a drug candidate. The chromatogram contains interference peaks from both endogenous materials in the feces as well as numerous polyethylene glycol-related peaks

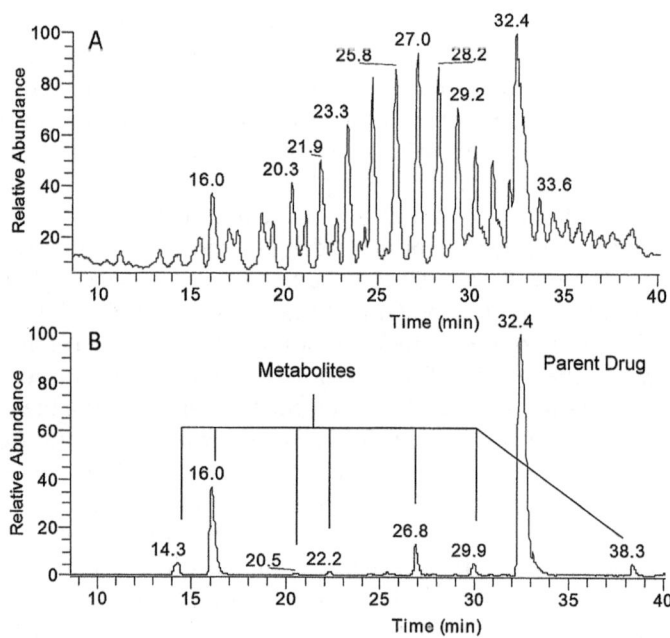

Figure 11.2 Example showing the utility of background subtraction. (A) Full scan total ion chromatogram of extracted pooled fecal sample from healthy subjects treated with a drug candidate. The chromatogram contains many interference peaks, including multiple peaks from polyethylene glycol, which was introduced into the sample during processing. (B) Background subtracted chromatogram of the extracted pooled fecal sample. A full scan total ion chromatogram from an extracted pooled fecal sample from healthy subjects (control sample) was subtracted from the treated subjects, resulting in a simplified chromatogram that is enriched for drug-related peaks. Courtesy of Hong Su, Bristol-Myers Squibb.

that had been introduced into the sample during the preparation/homogenization process. After background subtraction of the data file obtained from a corresponding sample from a placebo-treated subject that was collected, processed and analyzed similarly, the chromatogram was dramatically simplified and drug-related peaks were easily detected (Figure 11.2B). An advantage of background subtraction is that it does not require *a priori* knowledge about the molecular weight or structure of metabolites, and as a result, can identify metabolites that have significant structural changes compared with the structure of the parent molecule.

The mass defect of a compound is defined as the difference between its exact and nominal masses, and is dependent upon its elemental composition and formula weight. Common Phase I and II metabolites typically have mass defects that are within 50 mDa of the parent drug, whereas the mass defects of many of the components in common biological matrices, *e.g.*, plasma, bile and feces, are outside that window.[19] After filtering out data that are more than ±50 mDa outside of the parent drug's mass defect, many of the ions related to endogenous materials are removed, thus simplifying the mass spectra. One disadvantage of MDF is in the detection of metabolites that are formed *via* a substantial structural change to the parent drug, *e.g.*, as a result of an internal cleavage resulting from hydrolysis or dealkylation. The mass defect of the resulting metabolite(s) may be outside of the 50 mDa window, resulting in the mass information for these metabolites being excluded from the dataset. However, if such metabolites can be anticipated, additional mass defect window(s) can be applied.[15]

For drugs that contain a characteristic isotope pattern, such as those containing chlorine or bromine, IPF can be utilized to facilitate the identification of drug-related components that share a similar isotopic pattern as the parent compound. Ions that do not meet predefined tolerance criteria for both the accurate mass difference between characteristic ions (*e.g.*, M, M + 1, M + 2) and the relative abundance of these ions in the pattern are removed, thus enriching the spectrum for drug-related material.[16] This technique does not work well for compounds that do not have a characteristic isotope pattern[17] and it shares a similar liability with MDF in that metabolites arising from a substantial structural change (*e.g.*, loss of a halogen atom that contributes to the isotope pattern for IPF) would be filtered out. However, MDF and IPF do not require analysis of an additional matrix-matched or placebo sample that is needed for the background subtraction technique.[12a]

In practice, researchers have found that applying a combination of filtering techniques to the HR-MS data, including those described above, as well as PI and NL filters, provides the most comprehensive results for extracting and differentiating drug-related peaks from endogenous component peaks in complex *in vivo* samples.[17,20] Once metabolites have been identified through one or more of these techniques, structures of metabolites can be proposed from the accurate mass and MS/MS fragmentation data. Several examples of the application of HR-MS for elucidating metabolite structures were described in a recent review.[21]

If synthetic standards are available for any of the metabolites, plasma concentrations of these metabolites may be determined in individual samples collected at various time points from multiple dose studies in humans and the toxicology species. Metabolite quantification with standards is most often conducted with multiple reaction monitoring (MRM) on triple-quadrupole instruments due to the high sensitivity and specificity it provides. Multiples for human exposure can then be calculated from steady-state exposures determined from the full pharmacokinetic profile of measured metabolites. This proactive approach for metabolite assessment is often employed for metabolites that are known to contribute to pharmacological activity or off-target effects, and are expected to be abundant human circulating metabolites.[12b] While this approach provides the most comprehensive assessment of metabolite exposures, extensive time and resources can be expended synthesizing metabolites and developing and validating LC-MS/MS assays to provide formal quantitative assessment of metabolite concentrations.

More recently, researchers have described several exploratory approaches aimed at evaluating exposure coverage of human metabolites in the toxicology species and/or estimating concentrations of metabolites in human plasma relative to parent drug, without the use of authentic synthetic reference standards or conducting radiolabeled studies. The objectives of these assessments are to identify metabolites that require further evaluation according to the regulatory guidance.[10] In the Hamilton, or time-proportional area under the concentration–time curve (AUC)-pooling approach, appropriate aliquots of pharmacokinetic plasma samples, with the volume of each aliquot defined as a function of its collection time, are combined into one representative sample such that the concentration of each metabolite in the pooled sample is proportional to its AUC exposure.[22] Exposure multiples of human metabolite species are assessed using similarly prepared pooled plasma samples obtained from steady-state multiple-dose studies in humans (at an efficacious dose) and the toxicology species (at dose(s) used for toxicological assessment). To normalize potential matrix differences between species, Gao and co-workers[23] recommended that the pooled sample from each species should be diluted with an equal volume of blank plasma from other species. After extraction, the LC-MS peak area for each metabolite in each sample is determined and the peak area ratios in human *vs.* animal samples are calculated. Either LC-MRM[23] or FS-HR-MS[24] was shown to be suitable for generation of the LC-MS peak areas. Demonstration of a similar or greater peak area for a particular metabolite in the animal species compared with in humans suggests that the metabolite safety would be adequately assessed in the toxicology studies. However, if the human:animal peak area ratio for a particular metabolite is <1, an evaluation to determine whether the metabolite represents >10% of the exposure to drug-related material is needed.

With conventional LC-MS, the MS response can vary greatly between a parent drug and metabolites; therefore, the ability to directly use LC-MS peak areas to estimate metabolite exposure is limited. Consequently, several semi-quantitative approaches to estimate the exposure of metabolites relative to parent in the circulation have been explored. These approaches have utilized isolated metabolites or samples containing mixtures of metabolites from *in vitro* incubations, where the metabolite concentration can be estimated, *e.g.*, by UV response,[25] quantitative ^{1}H[25b] or radioactivity.[7,12b] If enough material is available, these samples can be used as surrogate standards to generate standard curves for the quantification of metabolites in study samples by LC-MS/MS or LC-HR-MS.[7a,12b] Alternatively, LC-MS peak area response factors can be established by relating the estimated concentrations of the metabolite(s) to their LC-MS peak areas. By normalizing the metabolite response factor to that of the parent drug, the concentrations of metabolites in study samples may be estimated.[7b,24] LC-UV responses,[25b] LC-nano-spray ionization-MS[26] and corona charged aerosol detection (CAD)[25a,27] have shown potential to provide more consistent responses between analytes and may also be applied to directly estimate circulating levels of metabolites relative to parent drug. These strategies can be applied to evaluate metabolite concentrations in the same time-proportionally pooled samples described above to evaluate whether any metabolites represent >10% of the exposure to parent drug or drug-related material.[25b] The pooled sample approach has the advantage of being able to estimate metabolite levels with a limited number of samples and reference material. If a metabolite is shown to represent >10% of drug-related material and does not have adequate exposure coverage in the toxicology species, additional bioanalytical and safety assessments may be required, including a more definitive evaluation of exposure coverage using validated LC-MS/MS assays, evaluating metabolite exposures in additional toxicology species, or dosing the metabolite to animals.

Radiolabeled studies are still considered to provide definitive information on absorption, distribution, metabolism and elimination (ADME) of drug candidates.[18] Since the amount of radioactivity that can be administered to human subjects is limited, practically, radiolabeled ADME studies are single dose studies. The radiolabel facilitates determination of mass balance, informs recovery of drug-related material from extracted samples, and permits the quantification of metabolites from plasma and excreta radioprofiles. LC-MS^n analyses performed in conjunction with radioprofiling aid in the identification of radioactive peaks and elucidation of metabolite structures.

In summary, a number of analytical approaches have been described that take advantage of recent advances in MS instrumentation and software to enable identification of drug metabolites and provide semi-quantitative assessments of their exposures at steady-state. The objectives of these assessments are to reveal any human metabolites that do not have adequate exposure coverage in the toxicology species and require further safety assessment. By identifying these metabolites early in clinical development, there is ample time to conduct any additional safety characterization that may be required. Definitive radiolabelled ADME studies, conducted later in development, serve to confirm the metabolite profiling results from studies with unlabeled drug, and provide quantitative information on mass balance and flux through the various metabolic pathways. Ultimately, the data from all studies are integrated to generate a comprehensive account of metabolite safety and drug disposition.

11.7 Summary

The last decade has seen an explosion in the availability of rugged HR-MS instrumentation and these new instruments have quickly taken an indispensable place in laboratories of ADME scientists. The next decade will certainly see improvements in hardware that lead to greater sensitivity, improved accuracy and faster analysis times. However, the more dramatic improvements may well be in the development of software to facilitate tasks such as MS/MS assignment or metabolite ID from complex samples with enhanced data mining. These advances in HR-MS technology will lead to improvements in the speed and quality of ADME characterizations of small molecules and also play a role in how we are able to address ADME related issues for protein therapeutics, millamolecules and other therapeutic modalities.

References

1. (a) D. R. Jones, Z. Wu, D. Chauhan, K. C. Anderson and J. Peng, *Anal. Chem.*, 2014, **86**(7), 3667–3675; (b) X. Liu, Z. Ser and J. W. Locasale, *Anal. Chem.*, 2014, **86**(4), 2175–2184; (c) T. Yu and D. P. Jones, *Bioinformatics*, 2014, **30**(20), 2941–2948.
2. Z. Zeng, X. Liu, W. Dai, P. Yin, L. Zhou, Q. Huang, X. Lin and G. Xu, *Anal. Chem.*, 2014, **86**(8), 3793–3800.
3. (a) T. G. Rosano, S. Na, K. Ihenetu, T. A. Swift and M. Wood, *J. Anal. Toxicol.*, 2014, **38**(8), 495–506; (b) M. Sundstrom, A. Pelander and I. Ojanpera, *Drug Test. Anal.*, 2015, **7**(5), 420–427.
4. (a) I. Zamora, F. Fontaine, B. Serra and G. Plasencia, *Drug Discovery Today: Technol.*, 2013, **10**(1), e199–205; (b) V. Zelesky, R. Schneider, J. Janiszewski, I. Zamora, J. Ferguson and M. Troutman, *Bioanalysis*, 2013, **5**(10), 1165–1179.
5. Y. Yang, M. F. Grubb, C. E. Luk, W. G. Humphreys and J. L. Josephs, *Rapid Commun. Mass Spectrom.*, 2011, **25**(21), 3245–3251.
6. (a) G. J. Dear, A. D. Roberts, C. Beaumont and S. E. North, *J. Chromatogr. B: Anal. Technol. Biomed. Life Sci.*, 2008, **876**(2), 182–190; (b) G. S. Walker, J. N. Bauman, T. F. Ryder, E. B. Smith, D. K. Spracklin and R. S. Obach, *Drug Metab. Dispos.*, 2014, **42**(10), 1627–1639.
7. (a) D. Zhang, N. Raghavan, T. Chando, J. Gambardella, Y. Fu, D. Zhang, S. E. Unger and W. G. Humphreys, *Drug Metab. Lett.*, 2007, **1**(4), 293–298; (b) P. Yi and D. Luffer-Atlas, *Bioanalysis*, 2010, **2**(7), 1195–1210.
8. (a) K. P. Bateman, M. Kellmann, H. Muenster, R. Papp and L. Taylor, *J. Am. Soc. Mass Spectrom.*, 2009, **20**(8), 1441–1450; (b) T. Rousu, J. Hokkanen, O. R. Pelkonen and A. Tolonen, *Front. Pharmacol.*, 2010, **1**, 10;

(c) J. L. Josephs, *Bioanalysis*, 2012, **4**(5), 471–476; (d) M. F. Grubb, W. G. Humphreys and J. L. Josephs, *Bioanalysis*, 2012, **4**(14), 1747–1761; (e) L. King, A. Kotian and M. Jairaj, *Bioanalysis*, 2014, **6**(24), 3337–3348.

9. N. Penner, L. J. Klunk and C. Prakash, *Biopharm. Drug Dispos.*, 2009, **30**(4), 185–203.

10. (a) US Department of Health and Human Services, *F. a. D. A., Center for Drug Evaluation and Research, Guidance for Industry: Safety Testing of Drug Metabolites*, 2008, http://www.fda.gov/cder/guidance/6897fnl.pdf2008; (b) International Conference on Harmonization of Technical Requirements for Registration of Pharmaceuticals for Human Use, *M. R. G., Guidance on Nonclinical Safety Studies for the Conduct of Human Clinical Trials and Marketing Authorization for Pharmaceuticals*, 2009, http://www.ich.org/product/guidelines/multidisciplinary/article/multidisciplinary-guidelines.html.

11. International Conference on Harmonization of Technical Requirements for Registration of Pharmaceuticals for Human Use, *M. R. G., Guidance on Nonclinical Safety Studies for the Conduct of Human Clinical Trials and Marketing Authorization for Pharmaceuticals, Questions and Answers (R2)*, 2012, http://www.ich.org/products/guidelines/multidisciplinary/article/multidisciplinary-guidelines.html.

12. (a) S. Ma and S. K. Chowdhury, *Anal. Chem.*, 2011, **83**(13), 5028–5036; (b) A. F. Aubry, L. J. Christopher, J. Wang, M. Zhu, G. Tirucherai and M. E. Arnold, *Bioanalysis*, 2014, **6**(5), 651–664; (c) H. Gao and R. S. Obach, *Bioanalysis*, 2014, **6**(5), 641–650.

13. B. Wen and M. Zhu, *Drug Metab. Rev.*, 2015, 1–17.

14. (a) H. Zhang and Y. Yang, *J. Mass Spectrom.*, 2008, **43**(9), 1181–1190; (b) P. Zhu, W. Ding, W. Tong, A. Ghosal, K. Alton and S. Chowdhury, *Rapid Commun. Mass Spectrom.*, 2009, **23**(11), 1563–1572.

15. H. Zhang, D. Zhang and K. Ray, *J. Mass Spectrom.*, 2003, **38**(10), 1110–1112.

16. P. Zhu, W. Tong, K. Alton and S. Chowdhury, *Anal. Chem.*, 2009, **81**(14), 5910–5917.

17. F. Cuyckens, R. Hurkmans, J. M. Castro-Perez, L. Leclercq and R. J. Mortishire-Smith, *Rapid Commun. Mass Spectrom.*, 2009, **23**(2), 327–332.

18. J. G. Slatter, N. G. Agrawal and S. K. Chowdhury, *American Society for Clinical Pharmacology and Therapeutics Annual Meeting*, 2014, PII–009.

19. H. Zhang, M. Zhu, K. L. Ray, L. Ma and D. Zhang, *Rapid Commun. Mass Spectrom.*, 2008, **22**(13), 2082–2088.

20. J. Guo, M. Zhang, C. S. Elmore and K. Vishwanathan, *Anal. Chim. Acta*, 2013, **780**, 55–64.

21. D. S. Wagner, J. L. Pirhalla and G. D. Bowers, *Bioanalysis*, 2013, **5**(4), 463–479.

22. (a) R. A. Hamilton, W. R. Garnett and B. J. Kline, *Clin. Pharmacol. Ther.*, 1981, **29**(3), 408–413; (b) C. E. Hop, Z. Wang, Q. Chen and G. Kwei, Plasma-pooling methods to increase throughput for in vivo pharmacokinetic screening, *J. Pharm. Sci.*, 1998, **87**(7), 901–903.

23. H. Gao, S. Deng and R. S. Obach, *Drug Metab. Dispos.*, 2010, **38**(12), 2147–2156.

24. S. Ma, Z. Li, K. J. Lee and S. K. Chowdhury, *Chem. Res. Toxicol.*, 2010, **23**(12), 1871–1873.

25. (a) R. Ramanathan, J. L. Josephs, M. Jemal, M. Arnold and W. G. Humphreys, Novel MS solutions inspired by MIST, *Bioanalysis*, 2010, **2**(7), 1291–1313; (b) K. Vishwanathan, K. Babalola, J. Wang, R. Espina, L. Yu, A. Adedoyin, R. Talaat, A. Mutlib and J. Scatina, *Chem. Res. Toxicol.*, 2009, **22**(2), 311–322.

26. R. Ramanathan, R. Zhong, N. Blumenkrantz, S. K. Chowdhury and K. B. Alton, *J. Am. Soc. Mass Spectrom.*, 2007, **18**(10), 1891–1899.

27. B. Zhang, X. Li and B. Yan, *Anal. Bioanal. Chem.*, 2008, **390**(1), 299–301.

CHAPTER 12

Drug–Drug Interactions: Regulatory and Theoretical Considerations, and an Industry Perspective

CUYUE TANG[a], JEROME HOCHMAN[b], AND
THOMAYANT PRUEKSARITANONT*[b]

[a]Forum Pharmaceuticals Inc., 225 2nd Avenue, Waltham, MA, USA; [b]Merck
Research Laboratories, One Merck Drive, White House Station, NJ, USA
*E-mail: thomayant_prueksaritanont@merck.com

12.1 Introduction

Drug–drug interactions (DDIs) can reduce therapeutic efficacy or enhance toxicity of drugs, and are one of the major causes of drug withdrawal from the market.[1] Regulatory agencies, including the US Food and Drug Administration (FDA) and European Medicines Agency (EMA), have published guidance documents for industry that are designed to help pharmaceutical researchers better characterize and understand DDI potential for a new molecular entity (NME).[1,2] While DDI can result in alterations of either drug pharmacokinetics (PK), pharmacodynamics (PD) or both, it is the PK interactions that have been the main focus for both the US and EU DDI guidelines. Pharmacokinetic drug interactions, typically characterized by alterations

RSC Drug Discovery Series No. 49
New Horizons in Predictive Drug Metabolism and Pharmacokinetics
Edited by Alan G. E. Wilson

in plasma concentration–time profiles, could be mediated *via* mechanistic changes in processes of absorption, distribution, metabolism and/or excretion (ADME) of a drug substance (victim) by another compound (perpetrator) when they are given concomitantly. In both the EU and US, the first DDI guidance was published in 1997,[1,3] and the most recent guidance versions were issued as drafts in 2010 (EMA)[4] and 2012 (US).[5] Compared with earlier editions, both of the new draft guidance documents contain more extensive recommendations on *in vitro* and *in vivo* studies for assessing DDIs mediated *via* drug metabolizing enzymes [cytochrome P450s (CYPs) and non-CYP enzymes] and transporters. The EMA final version was recently issued in July 2012, with an effective date of January 2013.[4] The US guidance has yet to be finalized as of April 2014, the time this chapter was written, and therefore it is possible that some recommendations in the current draft may not be part of the final recommendations.

The primary objectives of this chapter are to (1) outline the similarities and differences in DDI studies and associated approaches recommended by the new draft US and final EU guidance documents, and (2) present an overview of theoretical considerations for DDIs related to absorption and plasma protein binding areas that have received much less attention from regulatory agencies relative to drug metabolizing enzymes and transporters, and (3) offer an industry perspective in applying the regulatory guidance to support drug development.

12.2 Regulatory Guidance on DDI Studies

12.2.1 Overview of Regulatory Guidance with a Focus on Drug Metabolizing Enzymes and Transporters

The latest version of both US and EU guidance documents contain many features that are similar in concept. In particular, both provide more detailed guidance on how to incorporate results from *in vitro* enzyme and transporter studies to inform the nature and extent of clinical DDI studies. Both place an increased emphasis on transporter-based DDI evaluations including recommendation for evaluating many different transporters. However, there are also some major differences between the guidance documents. Key differences include the type of recommended *in vitro* studies, and approaches and criteria used to help determine whether *in vivo* clinical studies are needed. Some specific details are described below.

12.2.1.1 FDA Guidance (Draft 2012)

Compared with the 2006 version, many new studies have been added in the new FDA guidance. With respect to studies on drug metabolizing enzymes, key changes include recommendations on approaches to studying DDIs for substrates of UDP-glucuronosyltransferases (UGTs). However, the draft guidance does not mention DDI evaluations for UGT inhibitors. For *in vitro* evaluations of CYPs, there are no significant changes except explicit inclusion of studies of time-dependent inhibition for all major CYPs. For enzyme induction studies, the recommended end point now is a change of mRNA levels, rather than enzyme activities. Other major changes center around the recommendation of model-based approaches and associated criteria for using *in vitro* CYP inhibition and induction results to determine the need for *in vivo* DDI studies. These approaches are recommended not only for CYP inhibitors or inducers, but also for compounds demonstrating time-dependent inhibition [time-dependent inhibitors (TDIs)], and those with mixed inhibition and induction effects (Figure 4 of the draft guidance). The models included are both basic and mechanistic [static and physiologically based PK (PBPK)] in nature. In particular, mechanistic PBPK models have been emphasized and mentioned numerous times in the guidance. Indeed, while the agency recommends a stepwise, model-based evaluation of interactions due to altered metabolism starting from a basic model for initial assessment, the criteria set for the basic [based on total maximum plasma concentration (C_{max})] and mechanistic static models [with "AUCR" values—fold change in the area under the plasma concentration–time curve (AUC) of a probe substrate in the presence and absence of a perpetrator—of 0.8–1.25] are so conservative that PBPK will ultimately be needed. There are also specific recommendations with respect to testing DDI potential due to metabolites; especially those with circulating levels of $\geq 25\%$ of the parent compound exposure.

On the transporter front, six additional transporters—organic anion transporting polypeptides OATP1B1 (*SLCO1B1*) and OATP1B3 (*SLCO1B3*), organic cation transporter OCT2 (*SLC22A2*), organic anion transporters OAT1 (*SLC22A6*) and OAT3 (*SLC22A8*), and breast cancer resistance protein BCRP (*ABCG2*)—have been included on the list to be studied, in addition to the existing P-glycoprotein (P-gp; *ABCB1*). The guidance on transporters is rather detailed with many decision trees, mirroring what had been proposed by the International Transporter Consortium (ITC) with respect to considerations as to when to conduct *in vitro* and *in vivo* transporter studies, and includes a list of recommended inhibitors and probe substrates.[6] However, the criteria are somewhat more stringent in the guidance. For instance, evaluation of drugs as substrates of OATP1B or OCT/OAT is recommended by the FDA when hepatic elimination or renal secretion accounts for 25% of total clearance, instead of the respective cut-offs of 30% and 50%, as recommended by the ITC. Additionally, the FDA recommends using total C_{max}, as opposed to the unbound C_{max} $(C_{max,u})$ by the ITC, to estimate the value for inhibitor concentration "I_1" for BCRP and P-gp inhibitors, and the cut-off "R" (fold change in exposure of statins, OATP1B substrates) value of 1.25 is calculated based on an absorption rate constant k_a of 0.1 min^{-1} (*versus* an "R" value of 2 calculated based on the k_a value of 0.03 min^{-1} by the ITC) for OATP1B inhibitors. Readers are referred to details described in our earlier publication on this subject.[7]

With respect to *in vivo* DDI studies, one key change involves recommendations to include a third arm in clinical studies to evaluate the time required for activity to return to baseline when evaluating an enzyme inducer or TDI.

For compounds with concurrent inhibition/induction (such as rifampin, which is a known OATP1B inhibitor and CYP3A inducer), additional study arms may be needed to determine the appropriate timing of administration of substrate and the duration of the interaction effect. Additionally, both UGT1A1 and OATP1B1 have now been included on the recommended list for genotyping or phenotyping studies, expanding the original panel of polymorphic enzymes—CYP2C9, 2C19 and 2D6. For the first time, the guidance also includes recommendations to conduct drug interaction studies for therapeutic proteins, with a primary focuses on *in vivo* (much less on *in vitro*) clinical studies for cytokines or cytokine modulators. The changes include recommended tests for these protein-based drug products that will be used in combination therapy with other drug products (small molecule or proteins), or those with the potential for PK or PD related DDIs based on prior experience/known mechanisms. In the absence of clinical studies, general labeling language indicating the potential for interactions with CYPs or transporters is allowed for cytokines/cytokine modulators.

12.2.1.2   *EMA Guidance*

Similarly, there are numerous changes in the latest EMA guidance compared with the 1997 version. While the latest EMA guidance is similar in concept to the 2012 draft FDA guidance, it contains some major differences. Notably, the EMA, and not the FDA, provide guidance on when studies should be performed (*e.g.*, most *in vitro* studies should be before Phase II starts). In addition, the criteria for the level of CYP inhibition, especially for the basic model, to trigger *in vivo* clinical studies are quite different between the two agencies. The EMA favors the use of unbound plasma concentrations to reflect the concentration of the inhibitor at the site where the enzymes reside, whereas the FDA recommends total plasma concentrations are used for the front line predictions, conceivably to force further consideration of the proposed funneling system with mechanistic models as the next in line. Such differences in recommendations can pose a difficult challenge to drug developers especially when the same experimental data may give rise to different predictions and interpretations of DDI potential based upon these different specifications by the authorities. For example, at a given total plasma concentration and based on their respective cut-off criteria, a compound with a very low plasma protein binding value may be viewed of low DDI potential and thus a clinical DDI study would not be required based on the FDA but not the EMA guidance. The opposite would be true for a highly bound drug. Additionally, while the FDA provides specific recommendations on the use of predictive models based on *in vitro* data for compounds with mixed inhibitory and induction effects on CYPs, the EMA specifically states that *in vivo* clinical studies need to be conducted for these compounds, given limited experience in DDI predictions for the mixed inhibitors/inducers. Interestingly, unlike the FDA, the EMA provides no specific guidance on the evaluation of UGT substrates, but instead explicitly recommends testing compounds for inhibition of UGT1A1 and 2B7.

Other major differences are in the area of transporters. The EMA guidance includes human bile salt export pump (BSEP) as another transporter to be studied, primarily for safety reasons, and provides only more general guidance on transporter studies *versus* the prescriptive decision tree approach proposed in the FDA draft guidance. Similar to the criteria used for drug metabolizing enzymes, the EMA uses unbound plasma concentration (*versus* total concentrations recommended by the FDA) for establishing the transporter criteria (see additional details elsewhere[7]). The EMA also provides more clarity on the need to conduct *in vitro* and *in vivo* DDI studies related to metabolites. On the other hand, the EMA guidance focuses only on small molecule drugs; it provides more limited guidance on DDIs related to therapeutic proteins, primarily immunomodulators, in a separate guidance document.[8]

12.2.2 Guidance on DDIs Related to Absorption and Distribution

Unlike the transporters and metabolizing enzymes, the regulatory framework in general does not place emphasis on specific requirements for absorption and altered plasma protein binding due to displacement (dPB). As described below, this is particularly the case for the FDA *versus* EMA guidelines.

12.2.2.1 Absorption Related DDIs

Other than DDIs related to drug transporters at the intestinal level, there is no mention of absorption related DDIs in the FDA 2012 draft drug interaction guidance.[5] Instead, a proposed conceptual framework has recently been published by authors from the FDA outlining a decision tree for assessing DDIs with acid reducing agents for drugs with pH-dependent solubility profiles (primarily weak base drugs).[9] Also included are recommendations on clinical study designs (including selection of acid reducing agents: proton-pump inhibitors or H2-receptor antagonists) to assess pH-dependent DDIs during drug development to inform drug labeling. The EMA guidance[4] covers the potential for interactions that affect both solubility and gastric emptying/intestinal motility, in addition to DDIs related to intestinal transporters. Similar to the FDA proposed framework, the EMA guidance includes some high level recommendations on when to conduct clinical DDI studies with proton-pump inhibitors, H2-receptor antagonists or antacids for compounds with pH-dependent solubility/dissolution profiles.

12.2.2.2 DDIs due to Altered Plasma Protein Binding

Similarly, the FDA guidance provides no specific recommendation with respect to altered dPB. The EMA guidelines specify that the risk should be addressed by *in vitro* displacement studies using therapeutically relevant concentrations. If a clinically relevant interaction is suspected, an *in vivo* study could be performed.[4] The risk factors that are described in the EMA guidance include: (1) being highly bound [arbitrary unbound fraction (f_u) < 1%]; (2) a narrow therapeutic window; and (3) a high hepatic ER if intravenously administered; or (4) a high renal ER. Interestingly, the Japanese guidance also provides similar recommendations, but with some distinctions. The Japanese guidance defines highly bound compounds as those with approximately 90% or higher plasma protein binding, and also adds a requirement for compounds with a small volume of distribution (defined as equal to or less than the extracellular fluid volume; 0.25 L kg^{-1} in humans).[10] As will be discussed below, the cut-off value of 90% binding is conservative based on the theoretical impact on unbound exposure. However, the requirement regarding volume of distribution is considered comprehensive, taking into a consideration the potential dPB impact on half-life ($t_{1/2}$). This aspect could be important for compounds that must maintain minimal concentrations above certain target values to achieve full efficacy, as well as for those whose toxicity is sensitive to $C_{max,u}$.

Interestingly, while DDIs due to dPB appeared to be de-emphasized, both the FDA and EMA [as well as others including the Japanese regulatory agency—Pharmaceuticals Medical Devices Agency (PMDA)] recommend measuring plasma protein binding of compounds exhibiting a high extent of plasma protein binding (the cut-off was not specified) in impaired renal and hepatic models. It is possible that this recommendation may not be related entirely to safety/efficacy considerations, but may be for data interpretation as well. It is known that in these disease conditions, the concentrations of binding proteins vary, thus impacting drug clearance and consequently total drug exposure.

12.3   Theoretical Considerations

12.3.1   Drug Interactions Related to Absorption

12.3.1.1   Introduction

The extent of absorption is determined by the solubility of the drug, the rate of membrane permeation across the intestinal membrane, and the time of exposure (*i.e.*, transit time through the intestine). Each of these variables can be influenced by drug induced changes in physiological or biochemical activities and consequently are potential factors in DDIs. Intestinal absorption is a kinetic process considered to occur under sink conditions in which soluble drug concentrations in the intestinal lumen unidirectionally diffuse across the intestinal epithelium into a relatively large systemic volume (*i.e.*, diffusion from the blood to the intestinal lumen during absorption is insignificant). For most soluble drugs [Biopharmaceutics Classification System (BCS) class 1 and 3], this is a first order process in which the fraction absorbed is an exponential function of the rate of drug permeation across the intestinal epithelium and the time of exposure.[11,12] The rate of permeation is a product of the luminal concentration, the effective permeability coefficient (P_{app}), and the surface area for drug–epithelial interactions. Although some small polar drugs cross the intestinal epithelium by the paracellular route, the majority of drugs undergo transcellular transport in which the drug transits across the cytosol and both the apical and basolateral membranes. For some transcellularly transported drugs, the rate of permeation may potentially be impacted by uptake or efflux transporters expressed in intestinal epithelial cells.[13] The time of interaction is dependent on the intestinal transit time and the window for absorption to occur.[14] For poorly soluble drugs (BSC class 2 and 4), low rates of drug dissolution or drug precipitation in the intestinal tract can further reduce the observed absorption rate and the time of exposure.[12]

12.3.1.2 Drug Interactions Mediated via Changes in Physiological Parameters

The physiology of the gastrointestinal (GI) tract can have a major effect on drug absorption by impacting drug solubility and dissolution, and by altering the time of exposure of a drug to the absorptive intestinal epithelium. The acidic environment of the stomach facilitates dissolution of solid dosage forms and impacts the solubility of some drugs. Acid reducing agents (antacids, H2-receptor antagonists and proton pump inhibitors) can increase gastric pH from normal values of 1.5–3 to values as high as 5–6.[15] Many weakly basic drugs show dramatic changes in solubility over this pH range, resulting in reduced dissolution and bioavailability. Clinical DDIs associated with increased GI pH resulting from acid reducing drugs have been observed with many basic drugs, especially those with pH-dependent solubility. Among 231 new chemical entities (NCEs) approved between 2003 and May 2013, dedicated clinical DDI studies with acid reducing agents were performed on 32 drugs. Half of these drugs showed DDIs resulting in a greater than 25% reduction in drug exposure (AUC) as a consequence of pH associated decreases in solubility.[9] Relatively large reductions (~50–100%) in drug exposure have been reported following co-administration of acid reducing agents with indinavir and atazanavir.[16,17] Consistent with the premise that the effects are due to pH-dependent solubility, lopinavir (a neutral antiretroviral drug) is not subject to acid reducing agent DDIs.[18] Similar to the antiretroviral drugs, many other weak base drugs including triazole antifungal agents (itraconazole, posaconazole and ketoconazole),[19-21] targeted anticancer drugs (dasatinib, gefitinib and erlotinib)[22] and the immunosuppressant prodrug mycophenolate mofetil (but not the active acidic active species mycophenolate)[23] show dramatic reductions in solubility and oral absorption when administered with acid reducing agents. Among 15 drugs that showed clinical pH-dependent DDIs, nearly all were classified as BCS class 2 or 4, suggesting that the anticipated luminal solubility (solubility relative to dose per 250 mL) appears to be the major driver.[9] Thus, more soluble weak bases are not anticipated to be subject to acid associated DDIs,[18,24,25] and the effects of acid reducing agents are highly influenced by the drug formulation.[19,26] For example, itraconazole absorption was inhibited by coadministration with omeprazole when itraconazole was given in a solid dosage form but not as an oral solution, suggesting that dissolution rather than precipitation may be the limiting factor. The magnitude of acid reducing drug interactions can be quite large, and consequently co-dosing of acid reducing drugs with compounds showing decreased solubility at mildly acidic to neutral pHs presents a potential risk of sub-therapeutic exposure.

Drug absorption and PK can also be impacted by GI motility. While GI motility is primarily associated with food effects, some drugs (*e.g.*, metoclopramide, cisapride and erythromycin) increase gastric emptying and intestinal motility, while others (anticholinergic drugs, opioids and anesthetics)[27] can slow these processes. For highly permeable drugs, changes in gastric emptying tend to have little or no impact on the drug AUC, but can change the shape of the absorption curve. Pharmacological acceleration of gastric emptying with metoclopramide in healthy volunteers changed the C_{max} of paracetamol from 12.5 to 20.5 μg mL^{-1}, and time to reach C_{max} (T_{max}) from 120 to 48 min.[28] Conversely, a delay of gastric emptying with propantheline increased the T_{max} from 70 to 160 min and decreased the C_{max} from 26.3 to 17.5 μg mL^{-1}. Under both conditions, the AUC was essentially unchanged relative to controls, suggesting little or no change in the extent of absorption but alterations in the rate of absorption and the shape of the PK profile. In contrast to highly permeable drugs, altered GI motility can affect the extent of absorption measured by AUC for less permeable drugs. In these cases, the time of exposure to the absorptive surface is reduced with accelerated GI transit and therefore could have a greater impact on poorly permeable drugs. Oral absorption of desmopressin (a poorly permeable 9 amino acid peptide) was increased 3-fold in healthy subjects treated with loperamide relative to untreated controls, consistent with enhanced absorption as a consequence of increased intestinal transit time.[29] Similar results correlating increased intestinal transit time and prolonged intestinal exposure with greater absorption have also been reported for the low permeability drugs chlorothiazide, hydrochlorothiazide, cimetidine and ranitidine.[30–32]

12.3.1.3   Interactions Mediated via Drug Transporters

Research into DDIs associated with drug transporters has primarily focused on the impact of efflux transporters. Although DDIs can potentially occur with uptake transporters such as the dipeptide transporter (PEPT1), large neutral amino acid transporter (LNA), monocarboxylate transporter (MCT1) and OATP2B1,[33] drugs with absorption dependent on these transporters are confined to a small structural set of compounds and thus the potential for DDIs is limited to a small subset of drugs. In contrast to the specific structural constraints conferred by nutrient uptake pathways, drugs interacting with efflux transporters tend to be more ubiquitous. The vast majority of studies on intestinal drug interactions are focused on the intestinal efflux transporters P-gp and BCRP.[1–4,6] The impact of efflux transporters is the reduction of intracellular drug concentration through apical drug flux, thereby reducing the effective P_{app} [34] in the absorptive direction (apical to basolateral transport). Models for intestinal absorption show that compounds with a P_{app} exceeding 2×10^{-6} cm s^{-1} in Caco-2 cells[35–37] or exceeding 1.5×10^{-4} cm s^{-1} *in vivo* in perfused human intestine[38,39] tend to be associated with high intestinal absorption irrespective of efflux or uptake transporter activity. Using a single pass perfusion apparatus, Lennernäs and co-workers measured the effective P_{app} over 10 cm long human intestinal segments and confirmed that the relationship between P_{app} and fraction absorbed is indistinguishable between passively absorbed compounds and substrates for uptake and efflux transporters (*i.e.*, all compounds fit the same curve).[14,38–41] Similarly, comparison of P-gp efflux in MDR1-Madin Darby canine kidney (MDCK) cells measured in routine efflux assays (10 or 20 μM) for 136 marketed drugs showed the net P_{app} in the apical to basolateral direction as the primary criterion defining the extent of absorption.[42] Several drugs such as amprenavir, clarithromycin, dipyridamole, domperidone, nelfinavir and ritonavir have high efflux ratios (values of 22–53), but are compatible with high intestinal absorption (human intestinal absorption greater than 60%). Based on this analysis, the authors concluded that compounds with high permeability (BCS class 1) show little impact of P-gp on intestinal absorption, while compounds showing moderate to low P_{app} ($P_{app} \leq 10^{-5}$ cm s^{-1} in *in vitro* transport models) are more susceptible to P-gp attenuation. Consequently, DDIs resulting from inhibition of P-gp efflux are unlikely for compounds with high passive permeability irrespective of their susceptibility to P-gp. Similarly, induction of efflux transporters may introduce further reductions in the effective permeability of P-gp substrates, but the magnitude of these effects is unlikely to be substantial with the exception of compounds with low to moderate permeability.

Pharmacogenetic studies elucidate the potential of transporters to impact drug absorption. In the case of BCRP, the 421C>A single-nucleotide polymorphism (SNP) results in a single glycine to lysine substitution and reduced trafficking of BCRP to the cell surface.[43] This SNP has been associated with increased oral exposure of rosuvastatin and atorvastatin[44] with 72% greater atorvastatin oral exposure observed for healthy subjects homozygous for the 421AA genotype, and 22% and 144% greater rosuvastatin exposure for heterozygous 421AC and homozygous 421AA subjects, respectively. Similarly, the 421C>A SNP is associated with 2.4-fold increase in oral sulfasalazine exposure[44] and a 1.3-fold increase in oral topotecan exposure.[45] However, the impact of the 421C>A SNP on the PK of other BCRP substrates is not as clear cut in as much as imatanib,[46] irinotecan[47] and pitavastatin[48] show little if any impact of this SNP. Similar studies looking at the impact of gene polymorphism on P-gp have been less consistent than for BCRP. While initial studies implicated the MDR1 SNP C3435T with lower P-gp expression and higher absorption of the P-gp substrates digoxin[49] and fexofenadine,[50] other studies failed to show PK changes as a consequence of this SNP.[51–53] It is worth noting that, although polymorphisms suggest the potential for transporter involvement in drug absorption, the magnitude of effects are relatively modest compared with DDIs ascribed to inhibition of metabolism, consistent with the relatively mild impact of efflux transporters on drug absorption. Given that the values presented reflect the impact of the perpetrator on first pass effects as well as absorption, the moderate impact of DDIs on drug exposure suggests that DDIs due to transporter inhibition during absorption are relatively small in comparison with CYP-mediated drug interactions, which are reported to produce over an order of magnitude increase in drug exposure.[54,55] Considering this relatively small magnitude of impact, the pharmacological consequences will likely be clinically important only for drugs with narrow therapeutic margins such as digoxin, where adverse events have been reported with as little as a 2–3-fold increase in systemic exposure.[56,57]

12.3.2 Drug Interactions Related to Altered Plasma Protein Binding

12.3.2.1 Introduction

The majority of drugs bind to certain sites on proteins in plasma at various extents to form drug–protein complexes. It is known that DDIs due to dPB can occur both *in vitro* and *in vivo*, with possible impacts on drug PK, measured as unbound and/or total parameters. According to the free drug hypothesis, only the unbound drug is able to distribute to the target site to elicit desired pharmacological effects, undesired adverse outcomes, and to be metabolized and eliminated.[58–60] At steady-state, the unbound drug concentration is anticipated to be similar on both sides of any biomembrane in the absence of active transport. As a cogent extension, the unbound drug concentration in the plasma at steady-state $(C_{up,ss})$ is considered a reasonable surrogate for the free concentration at target sites, and thus pharmacological activities. Achieving and maintaining desired $C_{up,ss}$ levels is a key consideration for effective drug treatment and thus a focus in the entire process of drug discovery and development. However, the clinical relevance of PK alterations as a result of dPB has been the subject of long-lasting discussions in the past few decades, due partly to the fact that unbound drug concentrations are usually not measured and the measured total drug concentrations are not always reflective of the changes (with respect to direction and/or magnitude) in unbound levels.[61–70] Although theoretical bases and clinical and experimental evidence pointed to the clinical insignificance of dPB for the majority of drugs,[63,65,66,68] interest in this subject remains for scientists in the pharmaceutical industry, academia and regulatory agencies.

12.3.2.2 Impact of dPB on Steady-State Exposure

Using a systematic approach of exposure and equilibration time concepts, and based on the "well-stirred" clearance model, Benet and Hoener provided groundwork in their classic paper entitled "Changes in plasma protein binding have little clinical relevance" in 2002.[68] They concluded that interactions

Table 12.1 Summary of scenarios where dPB may be clinically relevant[a] based on unbound exposure (AUC_u) or $C_{max,u}/C_{min,u}$.

Extent of organ extraction $(ER)^b$	PK parameters	
	AUC_u	$C_{max,u}/C_{min,u}$
Low	No	Yes (only drugs with low V_D)
High	No only for oral drugs eliminated mainly by hepatic clearance; otherwise yes	Yes (effect varies dependent on route of administration and V_D; see text and Schmidt *et al.*[71])

[a]Clinical relevance is usually associated with compounds with a narrow therapeutic index.
[b]ER >0.7 and <0.3 are defined as high and low ER, respectively, based on Wilkinson and Shand.[84]

attributed to dPB are not expected to elicit changes in unbound exposure (measured as unbound AUC or $C_{up,ss}$), a key measure of clinical relevance for oral drugs that are cleared *via* hepatic elimination regardless of their organ extraction ratio (ER; Table 12.1). Most of the drugs available on the market fall under this category. Benet and Hoener arrived at these conclusions by applying the simplest organ clearance model (well-stirred venous equilibration model).[68] In essence, this model suggests that for drugs orally administered and cleared by hepatic elimination, either with a high or low ER, the unbound exposure of the drugs is only determined by the intrinsic clearance (CL_{int}) at a given dose and fraction absorbed. The impact of dPB will be evident only for drugs with parenteral administration or oral drugs eliminated by non-hepatic routes (Table 12.1). In the latter scenario, drugs with a high ER (>0.7) are believed to be affected more significantly than those with a low ER (<0.3), and the net outcome is an increased $C_{up,ss}$ in response to the increased unbound fraction in plasma (f_u). This relationship is also applicable to other situations, including drugs orally administered and eliminated by renal clearance. It is worth noting that marketed oral drugs with a high ER by renal clearance have not been identified to date.[68]

12.3.2.3 Impact of dPB on Temporal Profiles of Plasma Concentrations

The above analyses and conclusions are based on unbound exposure at steady-state, represented by either AUC_u or $C_{up,ss}$. However, for certain classes of compounds, and especially those with a narrow therapeutic index, $C_{max,u}$ and unbound minimum concentration ($C_{min,u}$) could have implications on toxicity and therapeutic failure, respectively. It is known that dPB can impact the time course of C_{up}. In most cases, the impact of dPB is usually transient in nature, with the impact occurring at the initial distribution phase, and affecting the time taken for the increased C_{up} to return to the initial level. The magnitude of the impact is dependent on the PK properties of both the victim drug and the displacer as well as how the displacer is administered. The transient rise in C_{up} for both oral and intravenous drugs will be higher and faster by displacers with more rapid input rates, and the rise in C_{up} will last longer with displaced drugs exhibiting longer $t_{1/2}$.[63]

For this analysis, the impact of dPB on volume of distribution (V_D) needs to be taken into account. It is known that V_D is determined by the extent of drug binding inside and outside the plasma (f_u and fraction of tissue binding, f_{uT}) as well as the actual volume into which the drug distributes (V_T), as described by the following equation:

$$V_D = V_p + \frac{f_u}{f_{uT}} \times V_T$$

By this equation, changes in f_u will have a relatively small impact on low V_D compounds (*i.e.*, $V_D \sim V_p$), while nearly proportional changes in V_D would be observed for high V_D compounds. Using a one-compartmental model, Schmidt *et al.*[71] showed that dPB could impact the $C_{max,u}$ and $C_{min,u}$ (as well as $t_{1/2}$ due to its dependency on V_D and clearance) of low ER drugs (given orally or intravenously) with low V_D, but not high V_D (Table 12.1). However, for high ER compounds, the impact of dPB on these parameters is route dependent. For orally administered high ER drugs, the impact is expected only if the drug also possesses a high V_D, while for intravenous drugs, the impact can be observed for both low and high V_D (Table 12.1). Directionally, an increased f_u will lead to shortened $t_{1/2}$, increased $C_{max,u}$ and decreased $C_{min,u}$ for low ER drugs with low V_D, irrespective of the administration route. The opposite is predicted for compounds with a high ER and high V_D (oral and intravenously administered), or high ER and low V_D (intravenously administered only). Readers are referred to a comprehensive review by Schmidt *et al.*[71] for additional details. Interestingly, this analysis expands the list of possible clinical relevant DDIs due to dPB beyond what has been illustrated based simply on the level of unbound exposure, where changes are anticipated to be minimal for orally administered low ER drugs (the majority of compounds).

Warfarin fits the criteria for potential clinical relevance of dPB on $t_{1/2}$ and thus $C_{max,u}/C_{min,u}$ despite minimal changes in unbound AUC. It is a highly protein bound compound with a narrow therapeutic index, low ER and low V_D properties. Due to its long $t_{1/2}$, the increase in unbound concentrations could remain high for a longer period of time and cause prolonged bleeding times. Not surprisingly, there were many reports of DDIs due to dPB between warfarin and several highly bound drugs, including diflunisal, trichloroacetic acid and phenylbutazone[63] (and references therein). Except with diflunisal, the clinical relevance of these DDIs, although relatively mild, was reported. In the case of diflunisal displacer, the lack of clinical significance was attributed to the slow input of the displacer. For the warfarin–phenylbutazone DDI, Aggeler *et al.*[72] also provided supporting evidence using *in vitro* experiments that showed displacement of warfarin from albumin binding by phenylbutazone. However, the clinical significance of this interaction, which included severe hemorrhagic complications, was shown to be driven primarily by metabolic interactions resulting from the inhibitory effect of phenylbutazone on warfarin metabolic clearance.[73] Reduction in warfarin intrinsic clearance is expected to make the transient rise in its unbound concentrations (as a result of dPB) become more sustained and therefore prolong its pharmacological action. This added metabolic impact is believed to be the key driver for the majority of clinically relevant DDIs observed for several drugs with low ERs, including the reported clinical significance for low ER drugs with narrow therapeutic indices, such as tolbutamide and carbamazepine.[63]

Many anti-infective agents, including ceftriaxone, are characterized by low ER and low V_D. In theory, they may be subject to dPB elicited $t_{1/2}$ shortening and $C_{min,u}$ decrease, and thus potentially result in therapeutic failure. In severe sepsis patients with normal renal function but ~50% decreased albumin concentrations, the clearance and V_D of ceftriaxone increased by 130% and ~50%, respectively. These observations corroborate the notion discussed earlier that altered f_u would elicit differential effects on clearance and V_D for drugs with these PK characteristics. Namely, clearance would vary with f_u proportionally, but V_D less than proportionally. As a result of this differential increase, ceftriaxone displayed a shorter $t_{1/2}$ and its $C_{min,u}$ fell below that required for efficacy when given at normal dosing regimens, necessitating dosage adjustment.[74]

With respect to clinical DDIs of ceftriaxone resulting from dPB, there was a report of decreased total exposure and $t_{1/2}$ (~30%) due to increased total clearance (but not V_D) by probenecid, which is another highly bound compound.[75] This interaction was consistent with the increased f_u of ceftriaxone by probenecid, attributable to a relatively higher affinity binding to albumin by probenecid than ceftriaxone.[76] Interestingly, the interaction was observed in spite of a slight decrease in ceftriaxone renal clearance (~15%) as a result of probenecid inhibiting renal secretion of ceftriaxone *via* renal transporters. Due to the modest impact, the interaction was considered not clinically relevant.

12.3.2.4 Impact of Binding Proteins

Fundamentally, observable DDIs due to dPB should only occur with drugs that bind substantially to binding proteins, simply because changes in free fractions are inconsequential for weakly bound victim drugs. However, for a given binding affinity, the binding magnitude (as reflected by f_u) is also determined by the binding capacity of the protein for the drug. The major binding proteins in the plasma are albumin and α1 acid glycoprotein (AGP). They differ significantly in concentration in the plasma (600–800 μM *versus* 10–20 μM). Albumin is favored by the majority of drugs in the plasma; its high concentration minimizes the impact of a displacer. Therefore, the displacer concentration must be high enough to occupy the majority of the binding sites on the protein to considerably displace the victim drug. It is noteworthy that under some pathological conditions, including burns and sepsis, albumin concentrations could be reduced by as much as half of the normal values,[74] and thus making these patients more amendable to possible DDIs due to protein binding displacement. By contrast, a number of important drugs, typically basic in nature, primarily bind to plasma AGP. In addition to its much lower plasma concentration under physiological conditions (10–20 μM), it is known to fluctuate enormously in some medical conditions, including renal and hepatic impairment.[77] DDIs due to dPB are expected to be more common for drugs that bind primarily to AGP than those that bind mainly to albumin. Drugs that are known to bind primarily to AGP include methadone, propranolol, dipyridamole and vinblastine.[78] It is important to note that many drugs bind to both albumin and AGP.[79] With its high capacity, albumin can "buffer" any change in unbound fraction caused by the displacement of a drug from the low capacity AGP. For these drugs, dPB will have an insignificant impact on their PK.

The important role of AGP in mediating DDIs can be exemplified by recent work regarding PK interactions between telaprevir and methadone.[80] Telaprevir does not significantly bind to human plasma (f_u = 0.24–0.41). It binds mainly to AGP and human serum albumin at concentrations ranging from 0.1 to 20 μM.[81] Methadone, a synthetic narcotic analgesic, binds significantly to human plasma (f_u = 0.15–0.1), primarily to AGP,[82] and is metabolized extensively by CYP3A, 2B6 and 2C19.[83] Based on clearance (3–10 L h^{-1}, label), it is considered to be a low ER compound. As telaprevir has been shown to be a potent inhibitor of CYP3A and some patients treated with telaprevir receive methadone maintenance therapy, a study was conducted to evaluate the potential DDI between telaprevir and methadone.[80] Unexpectedly, it was found that total exposure of R-methadone was reduced by ~30% in the presence of telaprevir, with an increase in the median unbound percentage of R-methadone from 7.9% to 10%, which is roughly a 30% reduction in binding extent in the presence of telaprevir. This is somewhat surprising because the displacer is not highly bound. Telaprevir could even be considered as being weakly bound (with an unbound percentage of approximately 59–76%). However, since telaprevir binds to both AGP and albumin,[81] it can be inferred that this drug has to have a higher affinity to AGP than to albumin, and that the observed extent of dPB is mainly attributable to the low capacity of binding protein and the relatively high exposure of telaprevir of 750 mg every 8 h. This case indicates that significant dPB does not necessarily have to happen to very extensively bound drugs, and underscores the knowledge of the responsible binding protein(s) for both the victim drug and the displacer. Nevertheless, consistent with the above theoretical consideration that dPB has little clinical relevance for oral drugs with low clearance, there was no change in the unbound exposure of R-methadone as a result of dPB.

12.3.2.5 Summary

dPB can cause changes in PK profiles, including the total or unbound AUC or C_{max}/C_{min} of victim drugs possessing high plasma protein binding (typically >90%) and one of the following:

(a) The major binding protein (*e.g.*, AGP) has limited capacity compared with concentrations of displaced drugs and displacers combined. In certain disease states, the binding capacity may be significantly altered; this change needs to be taken into consideration.
(b) Displacers have higher affinities than displaced drugs.

However, dPB's impact can only be considered clinically relevant when it causes appreciable changes in AUC_u or $C_{max,u}/C_{min,u}$. In general, the impact of dPB on the C_{up}–time profile is transient in nature and dependent on the rate of displacer inputs (the faster the input the faster the transient rise) and $t_{1/2}$ of displaced drugs (the longer the $t_{1/2}$ the slower it takes for the rise to return). In addition, the properties (ER, V_D and therapeutic index) and administration route of displaced drugs are critical in determining whether dPB could be of clinical significance:

(a) Changes in AUC_u are least common with oral drugs and most common with intravenous drugs with high ER (Table 12.1).
(b) Increased $C_{max,u}$ and decreased $C_{min,u}$ due to dPB are usually associated with low ER and low V_D drugs regardless of route of administration (Table 12.1). These changes may be of particular importance for drugs whose C_{max} and C_{min} are associated with toxicology and efficacy, respectively.

12.4 Conclusions: An Industry Perspective

Overall, the new guidance documents contain many helpful recommendations for assessing a new drug candidate for its DDI potential mediated *via* drug transporters and drug metabolizing enzymes. However, in contrast to CYP-mediated DDIs where knowledge gained over the past 20–30 years has established a foundation for more quantitative predictions of drug clearance and potential for DDIs, the current understanding of the potential for DDIs arising from interactions with transporters is still in its infancy, and thus it may be premature to provide and apply detailed guidance on transporter studies and associated criteria on a broad basis.[7] Considering that the majority of drug candidates will fail after a first in human trial (>90%) or after a proof of concept (POC) study (>60%), the recommendations and associated criteria proposed in the regulatory guidance should be applied in a stage appropriate manner during drug development. This is particularly true for the transporter related studies, where focus should be primarily on the more established transporters P-gp and OATP1B1. Thus far, the magnitude of DDIs reported in clinical studies with inhibitors or substrates of transporters other than OATP1B, and particularly for the renal transporters OCTs and OATs, is generally <2-fold,[7] and thus clinically manageable. Therefore, for the majority of compounds, routine *in vitro* transporter studies appear unnecessary until after POC studies, apart from for those with a narrow therapeutic index.

Although the major focus on DDIs from the regulatory perspective concerns primarily biochemical evaluation of transporters and metabolism interactions, DDIs due to drug induced changes in GI physiology can be as large as or larger than those ascribed to the biochemical mechanism. At the point that a drug is a candidate for first in man studies, a wealth of knowledge is available on the physical and pharmacological properties of the drug substance. With the exception of BCS 1 drugs, mechanistic studies based on a holistic understanding of the pharmaceutical (including pH-dependent solubility profile) and pharmacological (*e.g.*, impact on GI physiology and therapeutic margin) should provide a more focused and comprehensive understanding of DDI potential in a clinical setting. Applying this directed comprehensive approach would not only provide more relevant information, but could also help resolve/understand interactions between factors (*e.g.*, solubility and transport) that could lead to pharmacologically relevant DDIs.

While a clinically meaningful DDI attributed solely to dPB is not expected to be common, knowledge of the plasma protein binding extent of clinical samples is of important diagnostic value. This is especially true for therapeutic drug monitoring, which is usually performed on the basis of total plasma concentration. Whether total plasma concentration changes or not, information regarding f_u will greatly facilitate data interpretation and diagnosis of hidden culprits. With the advance of methodology for drug measurement and f_u determination, it is desirable to not only determine plasma binding extent but also binding proteins, especially when AGP, due to its low binding capacity and variable levels in various disease states, is suspected to play a major role. Other factors that may have impact on victim intrinsic clearance (*e.g.*, enzyme inhibition/induction) also need to be considered as they may complicate the interpretation of results.

References

1. S. M. Huang, J. M. Strong, L. Zhang, K. S. Reynolds, S. Nallani, R. Temple, *et al.*, *J. Clin. Pharmacol.*, 2008, **48**, 662.
2. European Medicines Agency (EMA), Committee for Human Medicinal Products for Human use (CHMP). Concept paper/recommendation on the need for revision of (CHMP) Note for guidance on the investigation of drug interactions, July 2008.
3. The European Agency for the Evaluation of Medicinal Products (EMEA), Committee for Proprietary Medicinal Products (CPMP). Note for Guidance on the investigation on drug interactions, December 1997.
4. European Medicine Agency (EMA), Committee for Human Medicinal Products (CHMP). Guideline on the Investigation of Drug Interactions, 21 June 2012.

5. U.S. Department of Health and Human Services, Food and Drug Administration, Center for Drug Evaluation and Research (CDER). Guidance for Industry, Drug Interaction Studies—Study Design, Data Analysis, Implications for Dosing, and Labeling Recommendations, February 2012.

6. K. M. Giacomini, S. M. Huang, D. J. Tweedie, L. Z. Benet, K. L. Brouwer, X. Chu, *et al.*, *Nat. Rev. Drug Discovery*, 2010, **9**, 215.

7. T. Prueksaritanont, X. Chu, C. Gibson, D. Cui, K. L. Yee, J. Ballard, T. Cabalu and J. Hochman, *AAPS J.*, 2013, **15**, 629.

8. European Medicines Agency (EMA), Committee for Medicinal Products for Human Use (CHMP). Guideline on the Clinical Investigation of the Pharmacokinetics of Therapeutic proteins, January 2007.

9. L. Zhang, F. Wu, S. C. Lee, H. Zhao and L. Zhang, *Clin. Pharmacol. Ther.*, 2014, **39**, 121.

10. Japanese Ministry of Health, *Labour, and Welfare, Clinical Pharmacokinetic Studies of Pharmaceuticals*, June 1, 2001, www.nihs.go.jp/phar/pdf/ClPkEng011122.pdf.

11. P. J. Sinko, G. D. Leesman and G. L. Amidon, *Pharm. Res.*, 1991, **8**, 979.

12. G. L. Amidon, H. Lennernäs, V. P. Shah and J. R. Crison, *Pharm. Res.*, 1995, **12**, 413.

13. K. Sugano, M. Kansy, P. Artursson, A. Avdeef, S. Bendels, L. Di, G. F. Ecker, B. Faller, H. Fischer, G. Gerebtzoff, H. Lennernaes and F. Senner, *Nat. Rev. Drug Discovery*, 2010, **9**, 597.

14. H. Lennernäs, *Xenobiotica*, 2007, **37**, 1015.

15. A. D. Sutherland, J. R. Maltby, J. P. Sale and C. R. Reid, *Can. J. Anaesth.*, 1987, **34**, 117.

16. H. L. Tappouni, J. C. Rublein, B. J. Donovan, S. B. Hollowell, H. C. Tien, S. S. Min, D. Theodore, N. L. Rezk, P. C. Smith, M. N. Tallman, R. H. Raasch and A. D. Kashuba, *Am. J. Health-Syst. Pharm.*, 2008, **65**, 422.

17. D. L. Tomilo, P. F. Smith, A. B. Ogundele, R. Difrancesco, C. S. Berenson, E. Eberhardt, E. Bednarczyk and G. D. Morse, *Pharmacotherapy*, 2006, **26**, 341.

18. C. E. Klein, Y. L. Chiu, Y. Cai, K. Beck, K. R. King, S. J. Causemaker, T. Doan, H. U. Esslinger, T. J. Podsadecki and G. J. Hanna, *J. Clin. Pharmacol.*, 2008, **48**, 553.

19. S. Jaruratanasirikul and S. Sriwiriyajan, *Eur. J. Clin. Pharmacol.*, 1998, **54**, 155.

20. J. Walravens, J. Brouwers, I. Spriet, J. Tack, P. Annaert and P. Augustijns, *Clin. Pharmacokinet.*, 2011, **50**, 725.

21. E. Lahner, B. Annibale and G. Delle Fave, *Aliment. Pharmacol. Ther.*, 2009, **29**, 1219.

22. G. S. Smelick, T. P. Heffron, L. Chu, B. Dean, D. A. West, S. L. Duvall, B. L. Lum, N. Budha, S. N. Holden, L. Z. Benet, A. Frymoyer, M. J. Dresser and J. A. Ware, *Mol. Pharm.*, 2013, **10**, 4055.

23. M. Miura, S. Satoh, K. Inoue, H. Kagaya, M. Saito, T. Suzuki and T. Habuchi, *Ther. Drug Monit.*, 2008, **30**, 46.

24. J. F. Hilton, D. Tu, L. Seymour, F. A. Shepherd and P. A. Bradbury, *Lung Cancer*, 2013, **82**, 136.

25. M. J. Egorin, D. D. Shah, S. M. Christner, M. A. Yerk, K. A. Komazec, L. R. Appleman, R. L. Redner, B. M. Miller and J. H. Beumer, *Br. J. Clin. Pharmacol.*, 2009, **68**, 370.

26. M. D. Johnson, C. D. Hamilton, R. H. Drew, L. L. Sanders, G. J. Pennick and J. R. Perfect, *J. Antimicrob. Chemother.*, 2003, **51**, 451.

27. J. M. Greiff and D. Rowbotham, *Clin. Pharamcokinetic.*, 1994, **27**, 447.

28. J. Nimmo, R. C. Heading, P. Tothill and L. F. Prescott, *Br. Med. J.*, 1973, **1**, 587.

29. T. Callréus, J. Lundahl, P. Höglund and P. Bengtsson, *Eur. J. Clin. Pharmacol.*, 1999, **55**, 305.

30. S. A. Riley, F. Sutcliffe, M. Kim', M. Kapas, M. Rowland and L. A. Turnberg, *Br. J. Clin. Pharmacol.*, 1992, **34**, 32.

31. H. T. Lee, Y. J. Lee, S. J. Chung and C. K. Shim, *Res. Commun. Mol.*, 2000, **108**, 311.

32. N. Takamatsu, L. S. Welage, Y. Hayashi, R. Yamamoto, J. L. Barnett, V. P. Shah, L. J. Lesko, C. Ramachandran and G. L. Amidon, *Eur. J. Pharm. Biopharm.*, 2002, **53**, 37.

33. M. V. Varma, C. M. Ambler, M. Ullah, C. J. Rotter, H. Sun, J. Litchfield, K. S. Fenner and A. F. El-Kattan, *Curr. Drug Metab.*, 2010, **11**, 730.

34. K. Korzekwa and S. Nagar, *Pharm. Res.*, 2014, **31**, 335.

35. P. Artursson and J. Karlsson, *Biochim. Biophys. Acta*, 1992, **1111**, 204.

36. P. Artursson, K. Palm and K. Luthman, *Adv. Drug Delivery Rev.*, 2001, **46**, 27.

37. D. Sun, H. Lennernäs, L. S. Welage, J. L. Barnett, C. P. Landowski, D. Foster, D. Fleisher, K. D. Lee and G. L. Amidon, *Pharm. Res.*, 2002, **19**, 1400.

38. U. Fagerholm, M. Johansson and H. Lennernäs, *Pharm. Res.*, 1996, **13**, 1336.

39. H. Lennernäs, *J. Pharm. Sci.*, 1998, **87**, 403.

40. A. Lindahl, R. Sandström, A. L. Ungell, B. Abrahamsson, T. W. Knutson, L. Knutson and H. Lennernäs, *Clin. Pharmacol. Ther.*, 1996, **60**, 493.

41. S. Winiwarter, N. M. Bonham, F. Ax, A. Hallberg, H. Lennernäs and A. Karlén, *J. Med. Chem.*, 1998, **41**, 4939.

42. M. V. S. Varma, K. Sateesh and R. Panchagnula, *Mol. Pharm.*, 2005, **2**, 12.

43. B. L. Urquhart, J. A. Ware, R. G. Tirona, R. H. Ho, B. F. Leake, U. I. Schwarz, H. Zaher, J. Palandra, J. C. Gregor, G. K. Dresser and R. B. Kim, *Pharmacogenet. Genomics*, 2008, **18**, 439.

44. J. E. Keskitalo, O. Zolk, M. F. Fromm, K. J. Kurkinen, P. J. Neuvonen and M. Niemi, *Clin. Pharmacol. Ther.*, 2009, **86**, 197.

45. A. Sparreboom, W. J. Loos, H. Burger, T. M. Sissung, J. Verweij, W. D. Figg, K. Nooter and H. Gelderblom, *Cancer Biol. Ther.*, 2005, **4**, 650.

46. E. R. Gardner, H. Burger, R. H. van Schaik, A. T. van Oosterom, E. A. de Bruijn, G. Guetens, H. Prenen, F. A. de Jong, S. D. Baker, S. E. Bates, W. D. Figg, J. Verweij, A. Sparreboom and K. Nooter, *Clin. Pharmacol. Ther.*, 2006, **80**, 192.

47. F. A. de Jong, S. Marsh, R. H. Mathijssen, C. King, J. Verweij, A. Sparreboom and H. L. McLeod, *Clin. Cancer. Res.*, 2004, **10**, 5889.

48. I. Ieiri, S. Suwannakul, K. Maeda, H. Uchimaru, K. Hashimoto, M. Kimura, H. Fujino, M. Hirano, H. Kusuhara, S. Irie, S. Higuchi and Y. Sugiyama, *Clin. Pharmacol. Ther.*, 2007, **82**, 541.

49. C. Verstuyft, M. Schwab, E. Schaeffeler, R. Kerb, U. Brinkmann, P. Jaillon, C. Funck-Brentano and L. Becquemont, *Eur. J. Clin. Pharmacol.*, 2003, **58**, 809.

50. R. B. Kim, B. F. Leake, E. F. Choo, G. K. Dresser, S. V. Kubba, U. I. Schwarz, A. Taylor, H. G. Xie, J. McKinsey, S. Zhou, L. B. Lan, J. D. Schuetz, E. G. Schuetz and G. R. Wilkinson, *Clin. Pharmacol. Ther.*, 2001, **70**, 189.

51. B. Chowbay, H. Li, M. David, Y. B. Cheung and E. J. Lee, *Br. J. Clin. Pharmacol.*, 2005, **60**, 159.

52. S. Drescher, E. Schaeffeler, M. Hitzl, U. Hofmann, M. Schwab, U. Brinkmann, M. Eichelbaum and M. F. Fromm, *Br. J. Clin. Pharmacol.*, 2002, **53**, 526.

53. C. Y. Li, J. Zhang, J. H. Chu, M. J. Xu, W. Z. Ju, F. Liu and J. D. Zou, *Eur. J. Drug Metab. Pharmacokinet.*, 2014, **39**, 121.

54. V. Ancrenaz, J. Déglon, C. Samer, C. Staub, P. Dayer, Y. Daali and J. Desmeules, *Basic Clin. Pharmacol. Toxicol.*, 2013, **112**, 132.

55. C. Schmitt, C. Hofmann, M. Riek, A. Patel and E. Zwanziger, *Pharmacotherapy*, 2009, **29**, 1175.

56. E. B. Leahey Jr, J. A. Reiffel, R. E. Drusin, R. H. Heissenbuttel, W. P. Lovejoy and J. T. Bigger Jr, *JAMA*, 1978, **240**, 533.

57. K. J. DeVores and R. A. Hobbs, *Pharmacotherapy*, 2007, **27**, 472.

58. G. L. Trainor, *Expert Opin. Drug Discovery*, 2007, **2**, 51.

59. D. A. Smith, L. Di and E. H. Kerns, *Nat. Rev. Drug Discovery*, 2010, **9**, 929.

60. S. S. Singh, *Curr. Drug Metab.*, 2006, **7**, 165.

61. E. M. Sellers, *Pharmacology*, 1979, **18**, 225.

62. P. F. D'Arcy and J. C. McElnay, *Pharmacol. Ther.*, 1982, **17**, 211.

63. J. J. MacKichan, *Clin. Pharmacokinet.*, 1989, **16**, 65.

64. P. du Souich, J. Verges and S. Erill, *Clin. Pharmacokinet.*, 1993, **24**, 435.

65. P. E. Rolan, *Br. J. Clin. Pharmacol.*, 1994, **37**, 125.

66. L. N. Sansom and A. M. Evans, *Drug Saf.*, 1995, **12**, 227.

67. A. Sparreboom, K. Nooter, W. J. Loos and J. Verweij, *Neth. J. Med.*, 2001, **59**, 196.

68. L. Z. Benet and B. A. Hoener, *Clin. Pharmacol. Ther.*, 2002, **71**, 115.

69. J. A. Roberts, F. Pea and J. Lipman, *Clin. Pharmacokinet.*, 2013, **52**, 1.

70. J. Heuberger, S. Schmidt and H. Derendorf, *J. Pharm. Sci.*, 2013, **102**, 3458.

71. S. Schmidt, D. Gonzalez and H. Derendorf, *J. Pharm. Sci.*, 2010, **99**, 1107.

72. P. M. Aggeler, R. A. O'Reilly, L. Leong and P. E. Kowitz, *N. Engl. J. Med.*, 1967, **276**, 496.

73. R. A. O'Reilly and D. A. Goulart, *J. Pharmacol. Exp. Ther.*, 1981, **219**, 691.

74. G. M. Joynt, J. Lipman, C. D. Gomersall, R. J. Young, E. L. Wong and T. Gin, *J. Antimicrob. Chemother.*, 2001, **47**, 421.

75. K. Stoeckel, V. Trueb, U. C. Dubach and P. J. McNamara, *Eur. J. Clin. Pharmacol.*, 1988, **34**, 151.

76. P. J. McNamara, V. Trueb and K. Stoeckel, *Biochem. Pharmacol.*, 1990, **40**, 1247.
77. J. M. Kremer, J. Wilting and L. H. Janssen, *Pharmacol. Rev.*, 1988, **40**, 1.
78. Z. Huang and T. Ung, *Curr. Drug Metab.*, 2013, **14**, 226.
79. F. Zsila, I. Fitos, G. Bencze, G. Kéri and L. Orfi, *Curr. Med. Chem.*, 2009, **16**, 1964.
80. R. van Heeswijk, P. Verboven, A. Vandevoorde, P. Vinck, J. Snoeys, G. Boogaerts, E. De Paepe, R. Van Solingen-Ristea, J. Witek and V. Garg, *Antimicrob. Agents Chemother.*, 2013, **57**, 2304.
81. V. Garg, R. S. Kauffman, M. Beaumont and R. P. van Heeswijk, *Antiviral Ther.*, 2012, **17**, 1211.
82. D. C. Lehotay, S. George, M. L. Etter, K. Graybiel, J. C. Eichhorst, B. Fern, W. Wildenboer, P. Selby and B. Kapur, *Clin. Biochem.*, 2005, **38**, 1088.
83. Mallinckrodt Inc., *Methadone FDA label*, 2012, http://www.accessdata.fda.gov/drugsatfda_docs/label/2008/017116s021lbl.pdf, accessed 31 Aug 2013.
84. G. R. Wilkinson and D. G. Shand, *Clin. Pharmacol. Ther.*, 1975, **18**, 377.

CHAPTER 13

Drug–Drug Interactions: Computational Approaches

KAREN ROWLAND-YEO*[a] AND GEOFFREY T. TUCKER[b]

[a]Simcyp Limited, Blades Enterprise Centre, John Street, Sheffield S2 4SU, UK; [b]University of Sheffield, UK
*E-mail: k.r.yeo@simcyp.com

13.1 Introduction

Drug–drug interactions (DDIs) are considered to be responsible for 13% of adverse drug events in elderly patients living in the community[1] and 3% of hospital admissions.[2] However, many of these interactions, which are predominantly due to enzyme inhibition and induction, are likely to be 'silent'[3] in that only the obvious ones are recorded, leading to significant reporting bias.[4]

A responsibility of the pharmaceutical industry and regulatory authorities is to understand the mechanism(s) of DDIs and to provide appropriate warnings through labelling. The need for this vigilance became particularly apparent during the 1990's following the withdrawal of several drugs, notably terfenadine, astemizole, cisapride and mibefradil, as a consequence of unmanageable metabolism-based DDIs that caused severe cardiac toxicity.[5] Up to that time, the selection of DDI studies during drug development was based on two main criteria: the likelihood of co-prescription and therapeutic index. Classically, studies would be done with antipyrine as a model 'victim' and cimetidine as a ubiquitous 'perpetrator', while the list of low therapeutic

RSC Drug Discovery Series No. 49
New Horizons in Predictive Drug Metabolism and Pharmacokinetics
Edited by Alan G. E. Wilson
© The Royal Society of Chemistry 2016
Published by the Royal Society of Chemistry, www.rsc.org

index drugs of concern included warfarin, oral contraceptives, phenytoin, theophylline and cyclosporine. This paradigm underwent significant revision when intelligent use began to be made of the understanding of the substrate selectivity of the enzymes involved in drug metabolism, particularly with respect to the different forms of cytochrome P450 (CYP).[6,7]

Further developments with respect to the prediction of DDIs were based on the coming together of three concepts, namely *in vitro* to *in vivo* extrapolation of metabolic clearance from preclinical data obtained with human tissue, the application of whole body physiologically based pharmacokinetic (PBPK) modelling and the use of correlated Monte Carlo simulation to assess population variability in pharmacokinetics and DDIs.[8,9] This approach, now widely adopted by the pharmaceutical industry[10,11] and drug regulatory authorities,[12–15] allowed the extent of DDIs to be anticipated in preclinical development, with implications for the selection and design of clinical studies, and prediction of their impact in relation to many other patient variables (*e.g.*, demographics, race, genetics, smoking and disease).[16]

13.2 Construction of Models

Both static and dynamic models are used to predict the extent of DDIs resulting from the inhibition and induction of drug metabolising enzymes and transporters. The former models attempt to estimate the fold change in systemic exposure, indicated by the area under the plasma drug concentration–time curve (AUC),[8,17] while the latter are based on full or partial PBPK models that assess changes in the time course of drug concentrations in plasma and tissues.[18–20]

13.2.1 Equations

A number of basic equations expressing the change in systemic exposure of the victim drug in the presence of a perpetrator are used in both static and dynamic models.

In the simplest case, where the clearance of the 'victim' substrate is mediated by a single enzyme that is inhibited competitively by a 'perpetrator' and there is no metabolism in the gut wall, the mean change in AUC after an oral dose (AUC_{po}) is given by eqn (13.1):[17]

$$\frac{AUC_{po}(inh)}{AUC_{po}} = \frac{1}{\left(1 + \dfrac{[I]}{Ku_i}\right)} \tag{13.1}$$

where (inh) refers to the inhibited state, [I] is the inhibitor concentration at the enzyme site and Ku_i is the unbound inhibition constant obtained from *in vitro* studies after accounting for non-specific microsomal binding. For the value of [I], the US Food and Drug Administration (FDA) recommends using the mean maximum total plasma drug concentration of the inhibitor (C_{max})

after the highest clinical dose, to allow a conservative estimate of the extent of inhibition.[21] However, use of the maximum unbound concentration at the inlet to the liver [$Iu_{in,max}$; eqn (13.2)] appears to provide better predictions and a decreased risk of false positives:[22,23]

$$Iu_{in,max} = fu_B \left(I_{max} + \frac{ka \times F_a \times F_G \times Dose}{Q_{H,B}} \right) \tag{13.2}$$

The simplistic approach, based on eqn (13.1), is often used in drug discovery as an initial screen for the assessment of DDI potential. Eqn (13.1) should be expanded to allow for the fact that the inhibited enzyme invariably contributes to a fraction of total metabolic clearance (fm) of the 'victim' drug [eqn (13.3)]:[17]

$$\frac{AUC_{po}(inh)}{AUC_{po}} = \frac{1}{fm \Big/ \left(1 + \dfrac{[I]}{Ku_i}\right) + (1 - fm)} \tag{13.3}$$

When renal clearance (CL$_R$) contributes significantly to the net clearance of the inhibited compound, eqn (13.4) applies:[24]

$$\frac{AUC_{po}(inh)}{AUC_{po}} = \frac{\left(\dfrac{1 + \dfrac{CL_R}{Q_{H,B}}}{\dfrac{fm}{1 + \dfrac{[I]}{Ku_i}} + (1-fm)} + \dfrac{R_B CL_R}{fmCLu_{int,H}} \right)}{1 + CL_R \left(\dfrac{1}{Q_{H,B}} + \dfrac{R_B}{fmCLu_{int,H}} \right)} \tag{13.4}$$

where $Q_{H,B}$ is hepatic blood flow, R_B is the blood:plasma concentration and $CLu_{int,H}$ is the intrinsic unbound hepatic clearance of the victim drug. More complex equations define the cases for multiple enzymes and multiple inhibitors acting through common or independent mechanisms.[8] Thus, for multiple ('p') competitive inhibitors acting *via* the same mechanism to inhibit enzyme 'j' the fold decrease in $CLu_{int,H}$ is given by eqn (13.5):

$$\text{Fold reduction in } CLu_{int,Hj} = 1 + \sum_{k=1}^{p} \frac{[I_k]}{Ku_{i,k}} \tag{13.5}$$

where $[I_k]$ is the concentration of inhibitor 'k' at the enzyme site and $Ku_{i,k}$ is the unbound inhibition constant of inhibitor 'k'. The same equation applies for multiple inhibitors acting at the same enzyme site. However, if the mechanisms of inhibition by multiple inhibitors are different (independent), the fold reduction in clearance would be greater and is given by eqn (13.6):

$$\text{Fold reduction in CLu}_{\text{int,Hj}} = \prod_{k=1}^{p} \frac{[I_k]}{Ku_{i,k}} \tag{13.6}$$

Predictions of time-dependent phenomena require estimates of the turn-over rate constants (k_{deg}) of the affected enzymes.[25] In the case of enzyme induction, values of the maximal level of induced enzyme (E_{max}) and the unbound inducer concentration associated with half maximal induction (ECu_{50}) are also needed [eqn (13.7)]:[26]

$$\text{Fold reduction in CLu}_{\text{int,Hj}} = 1 + \frac{k_{\text{deg}} + \dfrac{[I_k] \times E_{\text{max}}}{[I_k] + ECu_{50}}}{k_{\text{deg}}} \tag{13.7}$$

For time-dependent irreversible (mechanism based) inhibition, values of the rate constant defining the maximal rate of enzyme inactivation (k_{inact}) and the inhibitor concentration associated with half maximal inactivation (K_I) are also required [eqn (13.8)]:[27]

$$\text{Fold reduction in CLu}_{\text{int,Hj}} = \frac{k_{\text{deg}} + \dfrac{[I_k] \times k_{\text{inact}}}{[I_k] + Ku_{I,k}}}{k_{\text{deg}}} \tag{13.8}$$

In view of the presence of drug metabolising enzymes in the gut wall, especially CYP33A4, it is necessary to account for interactions at this site as well as in the liver. Knowing intrinsic clearance per unit of enzyme (from *in vitro* studies) and the overall abundance of the enzyme in the gut, it should be possible to predict net intrinsic clearance by the gut and hence the extent of its inhibition. Exposure to enzymes during transit through the gut wall also depends on the interplay of uptake and efflux transport, passive membrane permeability and enterocytic blood flow. These factors have been accommodated by a model[28] that defines the availability of drug across the gut wall (F_{Gut}) in terms of intrinsic metabolic clearance ($\text{CLu}_{\text{int,Gut}}$), the free fraction of drug at the enzyme site (fu_{Gut}) and nominal blood flow [Q_{Gut}; eqn (13.9)]:

$$F_{\text{Gut}} = \frac{Q_{\text{Gut}}}{Q_{\text{Gut}} + fu_{\text{Gut}} \times \text{CLu}_{\text{int,Gut}}} \tag{13.9}$$

Q_{Gut} can be further decomposed into permeability clearance (CL_{perm}) and villous blood flow (Q_{villi})[28] [eqn (13.10)]:

$$Q_{\text{Gut}} = \frac{CL_{\text{perm}} \times Q_{\text{villi}}}{CL_{\text{perm}} + Q_{\text{villi}}} \tag{13.10}$$

Permeability clearance can be estimated from *in vitro* data (*e.g.*, using Caco-2 cells), enterocellularity and the relative abundance of transporter in the cell system and the gut.

In the presence of an inhibitor that only alters intrinsic gut metabolic clearance, eqn (13.9) can be rewritten to include an estimate of the concentration of inhibitor in the enterocyte ($[I]_{Gut}$), its free fraction in the gut ($fu_{Gut}(I)$) and its inhibitory constant for CYP3A [K_i; eqn (13.11)]:

$$F_{Gut} = \frac{Q_{Gut}}{\left(Q_{Gut} + fu_{Gut} \times CLu_{int,Gut}\right) \Big/ \left(1 + \dfrac{fu_{Gut}(I) \times [I]_{Gut}}{K_i}\right)} \tag{13.11}$$

When the inhibitor is not co-administered with the substrate, the unbound concentration of the inhibitor in the systemic circulation can be used as an estimate of $[I]_{Gut}$. However, when inhibitor and substrate are co-administered the value of $[I]_{Gut}$ may be approximated from the pre-hepatic absorption rate of the inhibitor and an estimate of enterocytic blood flow (Q_{ent}), according to eqn (13.12):[8]

$$[I]_{Gut} = \frac{fa \times ka(I) \times Dose(I)}{Q_{ent}} \tag{13.12}$$

where fa is the fraction of the inhibitor dose that is absorbed into the gut wall and ka(*I*) and Dose(*I*) are the absorption rate constant and dose of inhibitor, respectively. This equation assumes that the inhibitor is not subject to major "first pass" gut metabolism itself.

In the absence of any information on active drug uptake into the enterocyte, fu_{Gut} takes the default value of 1 (which assumes that there is insufficient time for plasma protein binding equilibrium or erythrocyte uptake before the drug is removed from the basolateral side of the enterocyte). However, it may also be set at fu, which assumes that there is sufficient time for plasma protein binding. Although some effort has been made to clarify this issue,[28,29] further research into the value of fu_{Gut} is required.

To predict DDIs at the level of transporters, the 'well-stirred' liver model has been extended to include intrinsic clearances for hepatic uptake (PS_{inf}), sinusoidal efflux (PS_{eff}) and biliary excretion (PS_{ex}), as well as the intrinsic metabolic clearance (CLu_{met}) of unbound drug [eqn (13.13)].[30] The relationship of these parameters can be simplified depending on the relative magnitude of the component clearances. This also leads to different scenarios for the fold change in net intrinsic clearance (by all mechanisms), depending on which transporters are inhibited.[31] The maximum fold change in the net intrinsic clearance due to inhibitory effects on multiple processes is given by eqn (13.14):[32]

$$CL_{int,all} = PS_{inf}\left(\frac{PS_{ex} + CL_{met}}{PS_{eff} + PS_{ex} + CL_{met}}\right) \tag{13.13}$$

$$\text{Fold change in net clearance} \sim \frac{1}{1 + \dfrac{Iu_{in,max}}{K_{i,inf}}} \times \frac{1}{1 + \dfrac{Iu_{in,max}}{K_{i,eff/met}}} \tag{13.14}$$

13.2.2 Static Models

Values of Ku_i, fm and $CLu_{int,H}$, which define the metabolic clearance of the victim in the absence of the perpetrator, can be obtained from *in vitro* studies using human liver microsomes, hepatocytes or recombinant enzymes, with appropriate use of scaling factors (microsomal protein per milligram of liver[33]), hepatocellularity,[33] specific enzyme abundances, and with allowances for non-specific binding in the systems.[8,9] Together with *in vitro* Ku_i values and the appropriate estimate of [I], this generally allows prediction, based on full equations, of the mean extent of DDIs arising purely from competitive enzyme inhibition within 2–3-fold.[11,34,35] Greater precision is obtained with estimates of $CLu_{int,H}$ determined directly from *in vivo* data by parameter estimation, and Ku_i values from *in vivo* studies with other compounds.[36]

Since intestinal first pass metabolism may contribute significantly to low oral drug bioavailability and DDIs, particularly for CYP3A substrates, it is important to know the value of F_{Gut} of victim drugs with some accuracy. In this context, the 'Q_{Gut} model' has been applied with variable success.[28,37] Gertz *et al.* (2010)[37] evaluated drugs with a wide range of physicochemical properties and *in vivo* F_{Gut} values (0.07–0.94). *In vitro* clearance data were obtained from human intestinal and liver microsome pools (n = 105 donors) using the substrate depletion method. Apparent drug permeability (P_{app}) was determined with Caco-2 and Madin–Darby canine kidney cells transfected with the human MDR1 gene (MDCK-MDR1 cells). Good agreement between predicted and *in vivo* F_{Gut} values was observed for drugs with low to medium intestinal extraction ratios (*e.g.*, the predicted value for midazolam of 0.54 was very close to the observed value of 0.51). By contrast, significant under-prediction was demonstrated for drugs with *in vivo* F_{Gut} values of <0.5 (*e.g.*, the predicted value for saquinavir was only 6% of the observed value). Given the current uncertainty in the values of fu_{Gut} and *in vivo* permeability, Mano *et al.* (2015) recommend the determination of control F_{Gut} values from prior *in vivo* data.[36]

The ability to predict the extent of DDIs involving mechanism-based inhibition is particularly dependent on the design and quality of *in vitro* studies. Uncertainties with respect to the values of all three experimental parameters (k_{inact}, K_I and k_{deg}) persist such that any of them may be in error.[38–41] Typically, human liver microsomes or recombinant enzymes are used to determine parameters for mechanism-based inhibition. For mechanism-based inhibition, there is a tendency to over-predict using static models.[34,42,43] However, values based on the use of human hepatocytes appear to be superior, at least with respect to inhibition of CYP3A4, although there is still a trend for over-prediction.[44]

Static approaches have been applied for prediction of the extent of DDIs resulting from enzyme induction.[34,45–50] Einolf *et al.* (2014)[45] evaluated several models for their ability to identify drugs with CYP3A4 induction liability based on *in vitro* mRNA data, namely a correlation approach based on the ratio of the *in vivo* peak plasma drug concentration (C_{max}) to the *in vitro* half-maximal effective concentration (EC_{50}) and a relative induction score, a basic static model that assumed a fixed fm for the victim drug of 1 and no gut wall metabolism, a mechanistic static model (net effect—mechanism-based inhibition and induction) and a mechanistic dynamic (PBPK) model. The correlation approach and the basic static model resulted in no false negatives only when total C_{max} was used, and it was concluded that these models may be sufficient to screen for CYP3A induction liability. Using static models, the mean extent of DDIs as a result of induction were within 1.5- to 3-fold of the observed data depending on the value of [I] used. Others have used mechanistic models to account for simultaneous enzyme inhibition, inactivation and induction with greater success, albeit using an empirical scaling factor for the induction component in the liver and gut wall.[46]

13.2.3 Dynamic Models

Although static models to predict DDIs are used in drug development, and regulators value them as a conservative approach to assess interaction potential, they are increasingly being replaced by dynamic models based on PBPK modelling.[29,51–54] Thus, the advantages of the latter include not only the ability to capture the effect of the change in plasma concentrations of both victim and perpetrator with time as a function of dosage regimens, but also changes in tissue drug exposure, and the ability to assess non-linearity in kinetic processes and inter-subject variability in the extent of DDIs based on Monte Carlo simulation. The classical generic PBPK model assumes passive perfusion-limited uptake into tissues with hepatic clearance defined by the 'well-stirred model',[39] although specific organ sub-models can accommodate permeability-limited drug distribution including the impact of uptake and efflux transporters. Thus, recent extensions of the primary PBPK model include nested gut, brain, liver and kidney sub-models[55,56] that allow more rigorous evaluation of the complex interplay between enzymes and transporters simultaneously at several sites in the body. While bespoke PBPK models can be constructed using software such as Berkeley Madonna and MATLAB, dedicated commercial platforms for PBPK modelling with associated databases have been developed, such as the Simcyp Population-Based Simulator (http://www.simcyp.com), PK-Sim (http://www.systems-biology.com/products/pk-sim.html) and Gastroplus (http://www.simulations-plus.com/). These products are now widely used by the pharmaceutical industry[29,51–54,57] for decisions on candidate selection in drug discovery and for informing the design and selection of Phase I and II studies with respect to first in human dosage, and evaluation of the impact of age (paediatric and geriatric), gender, genetics, disease and formulation on pharmacokinetics, as well as for the heads-up evaluation of DDI potential.

Data necessary for the construction of PBPK models include system parameters (demographics, enzyme and transporter genotypes, organ sizes and blood flows, enzyme and transporter abundances, and gut transit times, *etc.*) and drug parameters (physicochemical properties including aqueous and lipid solubility, permeability, enzyme and transporter kinetics, plasma protein and red cell binding affinities, *etc.*), together with best estimates of variability in relevant individual parameters (Figure 13.1). The equations mentioned previously with respect to the static models are also implemented in the dynamic PBPK models. As with the static models, *in vitro* to *in vivo* extrapolation is necessary if a purely 'bottom-up' approach to predicting DDIs is implemented, although, again the accuracy of predictions is improved when the intrinsic clearance of the victim drug is determined from *in vivo* data by parameter estimation. Similarly, while *in vitro* K_i values may be applied directly, predictions may be improved using values estimated from prior *in vivo* studies with other compounds or using a correlation between $\log P$ (octanol/buffer partition coefficient) and *in vivo* K_i:*in vitro* K_i ratios.[36] Using best estimates of variability in relevant system and drug parameters, the application of Monte Carlo simulation allows the construction of virtual populations to assess the risk extremes of a DDI with respect to age, ethnicity, genotypes and disease, *etc.*[56] When using Monte Carlo simulation it is important to recognise that many of the variables in the system may be correlated in order not to under- or overestimate the extent of DDIs.[58]

The application of PBPK modelling in predicting DDIs involving inhibition of CYP is relatively mature, especially with respect to older drugs.[20,34,59] However, the trend towards the synthesis of highly lipid-soluble compounds, especially those with low metabolic turnover, can be more of a challenge, underlining the need to allow for non-specific binding and to characterise key parameters

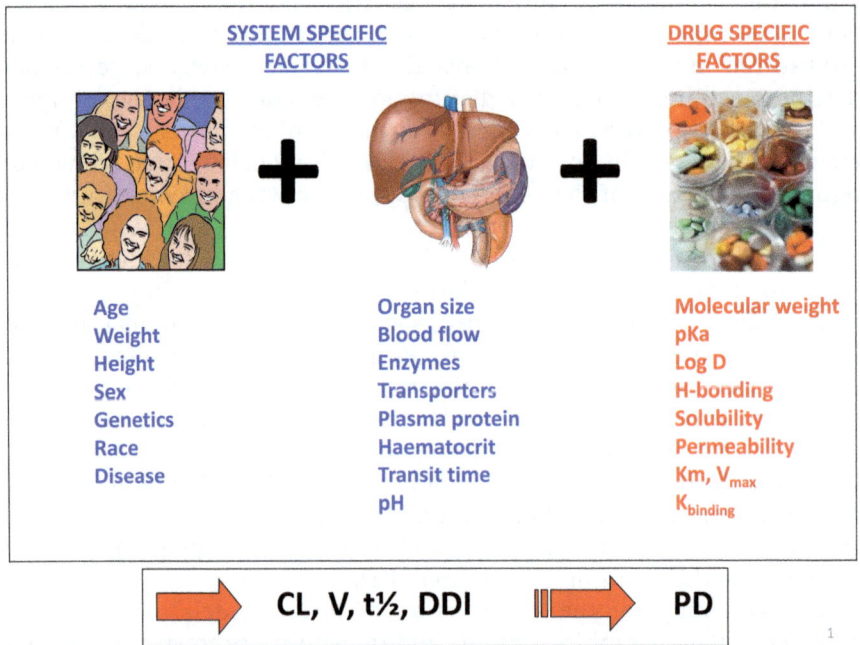

Figure 13.1   Relevant system and drug related parameters required for *in vitro–in vivo* extrapolation and PBPK model development.

from prior *in vivo* data where possible.[36] There is an increasing ability to capture DDIs involving other enzymes such as UDP-glucuronosyltransferases (UGTs),[60,61] while with others (*e.g.*, aldehyde oxidase, esterases and amidases) there remains a need to assess their abundances and to calibrate predictions for new compounds against larger databases.[62] Some success has been achieved with regard to predicting the combined inhibitory effects of parent drug and metabolites, for example for diltiazem and its *N*-desmethyl metabolite, both of which are potent mechanism-based inhibitors of CYP3A4,[20] and for itraconazole and its sequential oxidative products.[59]

Although there are a number of publications indicating that PBPK models have been applied successfully for the quantitative prediction of CYP3A4-mediated induction for drugs in development,[47,63–66] some indicate a tendency for over-prediction.[45] The success of *in vitro* to *in vivo* extrapolation approaches in predicting the extent of enzyme induction depends on a number of factors including the type (induction of mRNA *vs.* enzyme activity) and quality of *in vitro* data, the methods used to analyse the *in vitro* data, the approach used to scale the *in vitro* data to the *in vivo* situation (use of calibrators for *in vitro* and *in vivo* induction data) as well as variability in the data from the clinical studies against which the predictions are compared.

Arguably the greatest contemporary challenge for the prediction of DDIs using PBPK modelling is to incorporate the impact of competition for key transporters. While the equations that extend the well-stirred liver model to include active uptake and efflux (including biliary) clearance are well documented,[30,31] accurate prediction generally requires empirical, compound-dependent scaling factors, especially when multiple transporters are involved.[67–69] Resolution of this issue requires modelling of the prior *in vitro* data obtained using cell systems to determine accurate kinetic parameters, especially for efflux transport where the concentration of drug added to the system cannot be assumed to represent the intracellular concentration,[53,70–73] a better understanding of the fundamental mechanism(s) involved in active transport, and accurate, consensual estimates of the tissue abundances of specific transporters.[73,74] A further consideration is that, while unbound drug concentration is considered to drive metabolic clearance and associated DDIs, in accordance with the 'free-drug hypothesis' and rapid dissociation of drug–plasma protein complexes, the situation may be more complex with regard to transporter processes, requiring consideration of relative on/off rates of plasma binding and the rate of transport.[75]

13.3 Case Studies

To illustrate the contemporary utility of PBPK modelling in anticipating the extent of complex DDIs, four case studies are described involving aripiprazole (metabolised by CYP2D6 and 3A4), repaglinide (metabolised by CYP3A4 and 2C8, and transported in the liver by OATP1B1), clarithromycin (metabolised by CYP3A4) and metformin (transported in the kidney by OCT2, MATE1 and MATE2-K) as victim drugs.

13.3.1 Aripiprazole: Drug Interactions Involving CYP2D6 Poor Metabolisers

Aripiprazole, a partial agonist of dopamine D2 and serotonin 5-HT1A receptors, and an antagonist of serotonin 5-HT2A receptors, is used in the treatment of schizophrenia, bipolar disorder and major depressive disorders. It is metabolised primarily by dehydrogenation, mono-hydroxylation and *N*-dealkylation[76] with major contributions from CYP2D6 and 3A4. CYP2D6 is a polymorphic CYP isozyme, with more than 75 allelic variants currently identified.[77] The polymorphisms can be classified according to one of four levels of activity, namely poor metabolisers (PMs), intermediate metabolisers (IMs), extensive metabolisers (EMs) and ultrarapid metabolisers (UMs). The EM phenotype is expressed by the majority of the population, while the frequency of PMs, who inherit two deficient *CYP2D6* alleles and metabolise substrates at a notably slower rate, is low (8% in Caucasians). The UM phenotype reflects duplication, multiduplication or amplification of active *CYP2D6* genes, including primarily the CYP2D6*2 allele, but also involving CYP2D6*1. Individuals with the UM phenotype are highly likely to encounter loss of therapeutic efficacy at standard doses of major CYP2D6 substrates. IM phenotypes are heterozygous for a defective *CYP2D6* allele, and present with a wide spectrum of metabolic activity ranging from marginally greater than that of the PMs to activity close to that of the EMs.

In CYP2D6 PMs and IMs, plasma aripiprazole concentrations were found to be 1.7- and 1.3-fold higher than those in EMs after oral administration of the drug (10 mg) to steady-state.[78] In addition, co-administration of quinidine (166 mg), a potent CYP2D6 inhibitor, increased the AUC of aripiprazole by 2.1-fold in EMs.[79] After co-administration of ketoconazole (200 mg per day), a potent inhibitor of CYP3A4, with aripiprazole, a 1.6-fold increase in plasma AUC was observed in EMs and IMs.[80]

PBPK modelling (Rowland Yeo, unpublished) has been used to predict the impact of ketoconazole on aripiprazole exposure, with special reference to the risk in CYP2D6 PMs, who were not included in the original *in vivo* study.[80] The initial step in the process was to construct a model for the kinetics of aripiprazole given alone, based on its physicochemical properties and data on its *in vitro* metabolism, and allowing for phenotypic differences in CYP2D6 abundance and activity. The modelling then moved forward to predict the impact of co-administration of ketoconazole based on its exposure and its *in vitro* inhibition constant for CYP3A4. The average predicted and observed increases in the plasma AUC of aripiprazole during co-administration of ketoconazole (200 mg per day) in CYP2D6 EMs were both 1.6-fold (Figure 13.2). A further simulation predicted that co-administration of ketoconazole in CYP2D6 PMs could be expected to result in a 3.3-fold increase in the exposure to aripiprazole, augmenting the already high plasma drug levels in this phenotype (Figure 13.2).

This case study illustrates the value of PBPK modelling in anticipating the extent of DDIs in individuals with different genotypes for drug metabolising enzymes.

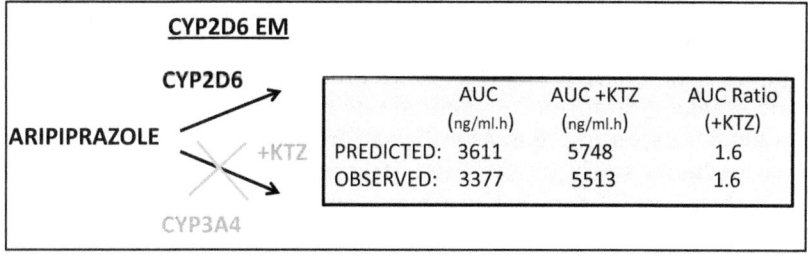

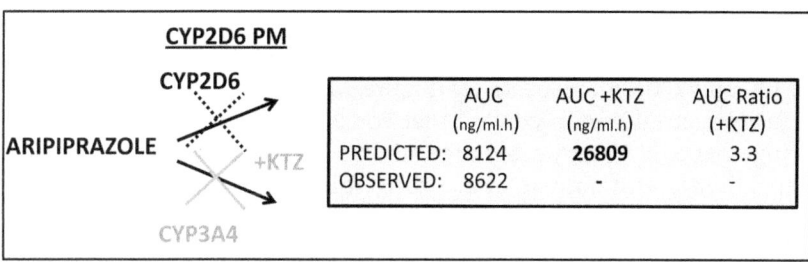

Figure 13.2 Application of PBPK modelling to predict the increase in exposure of aripiprazole in CYP2D6 EMs and PMs following co-administration of ketoconazole (KTZ).

13.3.2 Repaglinide: Drug Interactions Involving Combined Enzyme and Transporter Inhibition

Repaglinide is used to decrease postprandial glucose levels in patients with type 2 diabetes. It has an oral bioavailability of about 60% as a result of considerable first pass metabolism,[81,82] and is metabolised mainly by CYP3A4 and 2C8.[83,84] *In vivo* studies indicate that co-administration of repaglinide (0.25 mg) with trimethoprim (160 mg daily; an inhibitor of CYP2C8) increases its average plasma AUC by 60%, while clarithromycin (250 mg twice daily) and itraconazole (200 mg daily; both inhibitors of CYP3A4) independently raise it by 40%.[85,86] Repaglinide is actively transported into the liver by the organic anion transporting polypeptide OATP1B, as indicated by significantly greater plasma AUC values in carriers relative to non-carriers of a variant of the *SLCO1B1* gene (c.521T_C).[87] An *in vivo* study has shown that co-administration of repaglinide with cyclosporine (100 mg twice daily; an inhibitor of both CYP3A4 and OATP1B1) increases its average plasma exposure by 240%.[84]

PBPK modelling was used to simulate the impact of cyclosporine, trimethoprim and clarithromycin on the systemic exposure of repaglinide when each inhibitor is given separately and when all three compounds are co-administered with repaglinide.[88] The initial step in the modelling process was to construct a model for the kinetics of repaglinide given alone. This required the development of a compound file based on physicochemical properties, plasma binding, red cell/plasma partition and *in vitro* data on the metabolism and transport of the drug. However, using this purely 'bottom-up' approach it was not possible to capture the *in vivo* exposure accurately. Therefore, parameter estimation was used to determine the hepatic uptake clearance of repaglinide by fitting the *in vivo* data of Niemi *et al.* (2003),[85] assuming that, as indicated from prior *in vitro* data, this process is mediated solely by OATP1B1 (Figure 13.3, step 1). The modelling process then moved forward to predict the impact of co-administration of each of the inhibitors, based on the construction of compound files for each one and the input of the relevant *in vitro* constants for enzyme and transporter inhibition. Average predicted increases in the plasma AUC of repaglinide during co-administration of trimethoprim, clarithromycin and cyclosporine of 1.3-, 1.4- and 2.0-fold were consistent with observed values of 1.6-, 1.4- and 2.4-fold, respectively (Figure 13.3, step 2).

A further simulation predicted that co-administration of all three inhibitors together could be expected to result in a 5.6-fold increase in the exposure to repaglinide, with a range of 2.3- to 18-fold within the virtual population. This illustrates the value of asking 'what if' questions with a PBPK model. While the study of the triple combination has not been done, it emphasises the need to evaluate extremes of risk with multi-drug therapy. In this instance, the effects of the inhibitors were essentially additive. In general, the outcome of multiple interactions depends on whether compounds inhibit/induce the

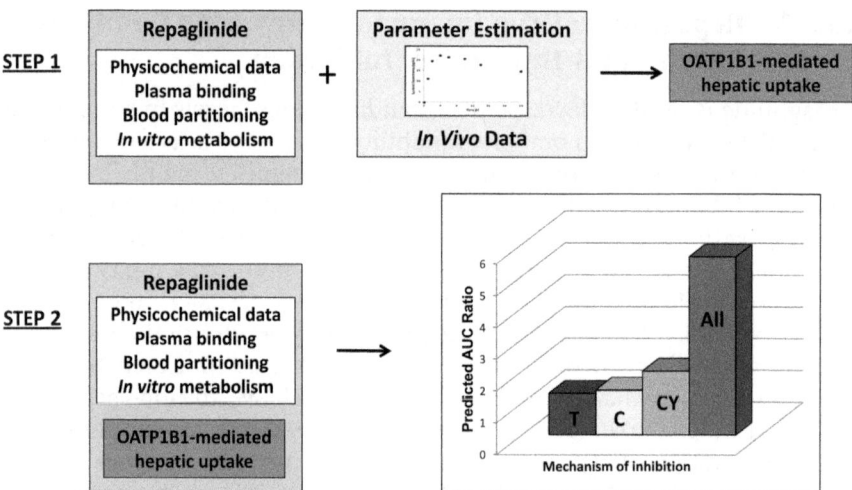

Figure 13.3   Workflow and outcome of PBPK modelling of DDIs with repaglinide. Step 1: use of parameter estimation to describe transporter-mediated hepatic uptake by simulating repaglinide exposure in the absence of interacting drugs. Step 2: use of the optimised model to predict increases in the AUC of repaglinide during co-administration of the CYP2C8 inhibitor trimethoprim (T; 160 mg daily), the CYP3A4 inhibitor clarithromycin (C; 250 mg twice daily) and the CYP3A4 and OATP1B1 inhibitor cyclosporine (CY; 100 mg twice daily).

same or different enzymes and transporters, and whether this is by the same or different mechanisms (*e.g.*, competitive *vs.* irreversible).[8]

13.3.3 Clarithromycin: Drug Interaction in Patients with Renal Impairment

The macrolide antibiotic clarithromycin is extensively metabolised by CYP3A and exhibits nonlinear kinetics as a result of auto-inhibition of the enzyme.[89–91] While renal clearance normally only contributes 20% of the total clearance of clarithromycin,[92] in patients with severe renal impairment the systemic exposure to clarithromycin is significantly increased,[90] indicating the need for a 50% dose reduction. Apart from a decrease in renal clearance this also reflects the down-regulation of CYPs and the accumulation of inhibitory uraemic toxins in renal impairment.[93] Co-administration of ketoconazole (400 mg daily for 5 days) has been shown to increase the mean C_{max} and AUC values for clarithromycin (500 mg twice daily) in healthy subjects by 2.1- and 3.3-fold, respectively.[94]

PBPK modelling was used to predict the impact of ketoconazole on clarithromycin exposure in patients with severe renal impairment, a group that had not been studied previously.[95] Known changes in physiological variables accompanying different degrees of renal impairment (decreases in plasma protein levels and changes in enzyme levels, *etc.*)[39] were incorporated into the model and a compound file for clarithromycin was prepared based on its physicochemical properties and *in vitro* data on its metabolism, with allowance for auto-inhibition of CYP3A4. The model was successful in simulating the plasma concentrations of clarithromycin and in recovering the differences in exposure between healthy subjects and those with severe renal impairment (Figure 13.4A and B). Mean predicted increases in C_{max} and AUC values (1.6- and 2.6-fold, respectively) for clarithromycin after 5 days of co-administration of ketoconazole in healthy subjects were reasonably consistent with the observed data.[94] A lower fold change in AUC was predicted in patients with severe renal failure (1.5 *vs.* 2.6). This reflects the lower baseline abundance of CYP3A4 associated with the disease (Figure 13.4C), *i.e.*, there are fewer enzymes to inhibit (Figure 13.4D).

This case study illustrates the value of PBPK modelling in anticipating the extent of DDIs in patients with severe renal impairment, patients who are difficult to recruit and study.

13.3.4 Metformin: Transporter-Mediated Drug Interaction in the Kidney

As a first-line therapy for type 2 diabetes mellitus, metformin is one of the most widely prescribed drugs. Since it is a hydrophilic base present almost entirely in its cationic form at physiological pH, its pharmacokinetic behaviour is dictated largely by the influence of transporters.[96]

The physicochemical properties of metformin also determine that its elimination is predominantly by renal excretion (80%) with a minor contribution
from metabolism.[97,98] While the magnitudes of documented DDIs affecting
metformin as a victim are not of material clinical significance, the compound
is recommended by the FDA as a probe for OCT2-mediated transport when
investigating possible DDIs with new chemical entities (FDA DDI Guidance,
2012). On this basis, a sound mechanistic understanding of DDIs involving
metformin is important. Such DDIs, involving raised drug exposure in the
kidney, are not necessarily reflected in an equivalent change in systemic
exposure.[99] Within the proximal tubule cells of the kidney, metformin is
actively transported across the basolateral membrane by OCT2 and effluxed
into the tubular fluid at the apical membrane by MATE1 and MATE2-K[100,101]

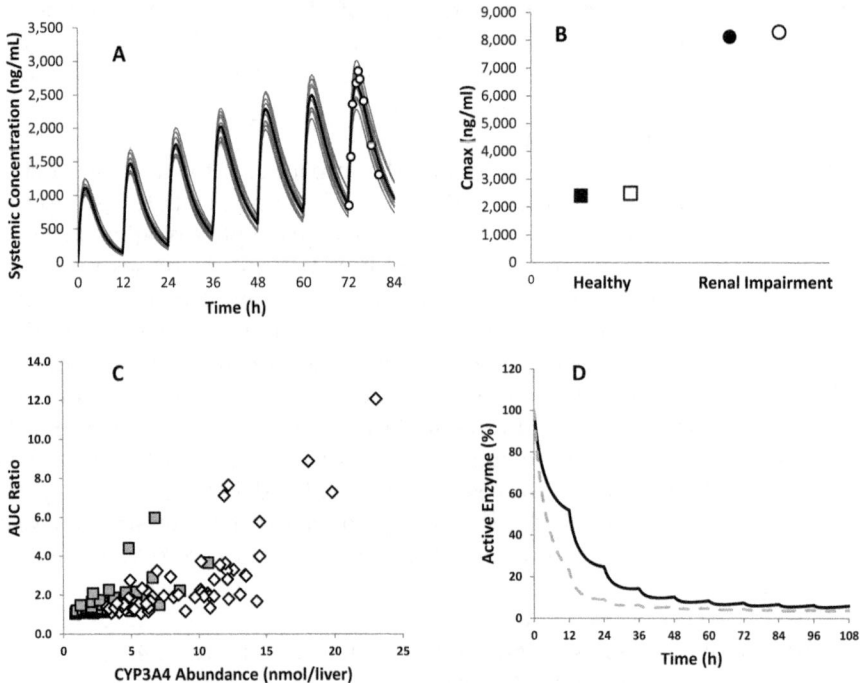

Figure 13.4   (A) Simulated [black line (mean) and grey lines (individual)] and
observed (open circles; Chu *et al.*, 1992) plasma concentrations
of clarithromycin after oral dosing (500 mg twice daily) in healthy
subjects. (B) Predicted (black data points) and observed (open data
points; Davey, 1991)[90] average C_{max} values in healthy subjects and
patients with severe renal impairment. (C) Relationship between
predicted AUC ratio for clarithromycin following co-administration
with ketoconazole and hepatic CYP3A4 abundance at baseline in
healthy subjects (open diamonds) and patients with renal impairment (grey squares). (D) The percentage of active CYP3A4 remaining
in the liver during multiple dose administration of clarithromycin
with ketoconazole in healthy subjects (black line) and subjects with
renal impairment (grey line).

(Figure 13.4). Co-administration of cimetidine, pyrimethamine, trimethoprim, lansoprazole or vandetanib with metformin has been shown to increase its plasma AUC by 1.2–1.7-fold.[102-107] All of these compounds are inhibitors of OCT2, and cimetidine, pyrimethamine and trimethoprim are also inhibitors of MATE transporters.

PBPK modelling incorporating active uptake and efflux of metformin in the kidney and permeability-limited uptake in the liver has been used to predict the effect of co-administration of cimetidine (400 mg twice daily) on the plasma concentrations of metformin (250 mg).[108] A compound file for metformin was constructed based on its physicochemical properties and *in vitro* data on its transport by OCT2 and MATE1 and 2-K in cell systems. This was then used to simulate the plasma drug concentration–time profile after administration of metformin. Input of the *in vitro* inhibition constants for cimetidine with respect to the kidney transporters predicted no effect on plasma metformin concentrations, despite a significant increase in its concentration within the proximal tubule cells. This was clearly inconsistent with the observed 46% increase in systemic exposure.[106,107] In order to render the plasma concentrations of metformin more sensitive to inhibition of MATE1/2-K by cimetidine, the driving force for cellular uptake by OCT2 was augmented with a modulating electrochemical element (Figure 13.5). The OCTs function as electrogenic uniporters, with both membrane potential and the substrate concentration gradient across the membrane providing the driving force for transport.[100,101] This combined electrochemical driving force allows the concentration of cations on one side of a membrane as they move down their electrochemical gradients, to a point that can be defined by their Nernst potentials. The application of functions describing electrochemically mediated OCT2 transport was able to account for a decrease in the driving force for metformin uptake into OCT2 transfected HEK293 cells as its

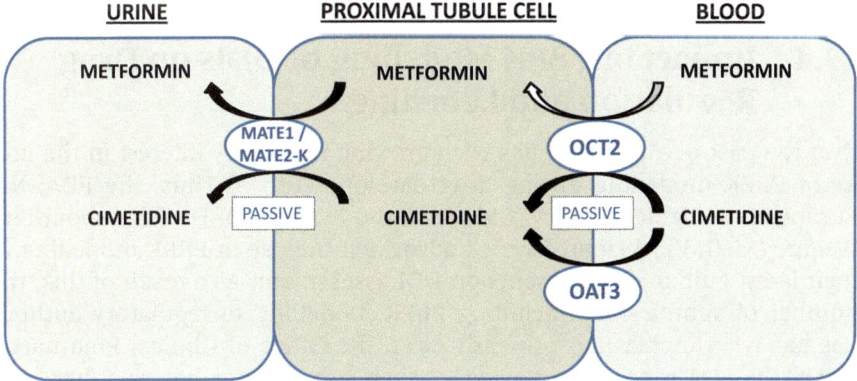

Figure 13.5 A schematic representation of transport processes for metformin and cimetidine and their interaction in renal proximal tubule cells. Black arrows represent active uptake and efflux processes, and the white arrow represents an electrogenic process.

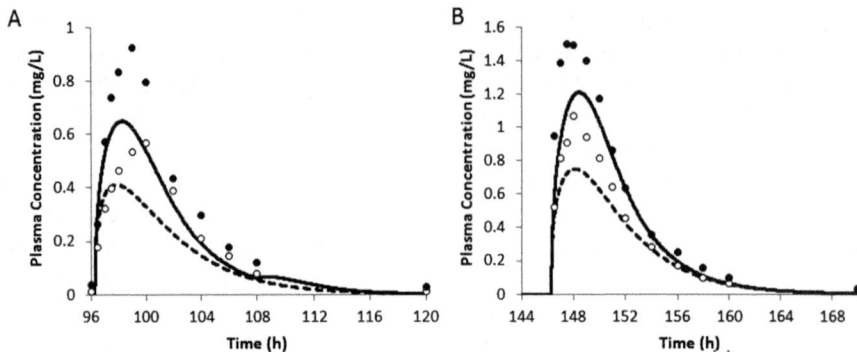

Figure 13.6   Comparison of observed mean plasma metformin concentrations with (filled circles) and without (open circles) co-administration of cimetidine from (A) Somogyi *et al.*, 1987[106] and (B) Wang *et al.*, 2008,[107] and corresponding simulated data with (solid line) and without (dashed line) co-administration of cimetidine. Simulations were performed for a population-representative individual using the electrogenic OCT2 model, and cimetidine K_I's for OCT1, OCT2 and MATE1/2-K decreased by 10- and 20-fold from those determined *in vitro*.

intracellular concentration increased relative to that predicted by a conventional model. Incorporation of this electrogenic model for OCT2 transport within the metformin PBPK model, in association with empirical 10–20-fold scaling factors for the transport of both metformin and cimetidine, allowed resolution of the DDI (Figure 13.6).

This case study reinforces the need to incorporate a better understanding of the mechanisms of drug transport into PBPK models.

13.4   Impact of PBPK Modelling of DDIs on Drug Regulation and Labelling

Over the past decade, there has been growing regulatory interest in the utility of PBPK modelling during drug development.[14,15] Thus, the FDA, the European Medicines Agency (EMA) and the Ministry of Health Labour and Welfare (MHLW) of Japan have all advocated the use of PBPK modelling in their latest guidance documents on DDI assessment. As a result of this, the number of submissions including PBPK modelling to regulatory authorities has been increasing.[12] In early 2011, the Office of Clinical Pharmacology at the FDA reported receiving 13 such submissions between 2008 and July 2010—seven for investigational new drugs (INDs) and six for new drug applications (NDAs). Since then, the FDA has received an additional 20 submissions using PBPK (2 in 2010, 10 in 2011 and 8 in 2012). Of the 33 submissions, 61% were related to the prediction of DDIs.[12] In parallel with the rising number of submissions containing PBPK modelling, it has increasingly utilised *de novo* (*i.e.*, FDA initiated) PBPK in its reviews to help characterise PK in a variety of complex clinical scenarios.

During the past 2 years, there have been more than 15 examples of drug labels informed by PBPK modelling (http://www.accessdata.fda.gov/ drugsatfdadocs). In this context, there is increasing traction with regard to the development of 'virtual labelling' to provide warnings based on PBPK modelling of risk in complex patients with multiple disposing factors influencing drug exposure (DDIs, genetic polymorphisms and specific diseases, *etc.*) that cannot easily be studied in real individuals during drug development. One of the most recent examples, approved by the FDA in November 2013, relates to ibrutinib.[109] This drug is mainly metabolised by CYP3A4 and has an apparent oral clearance of approximately 1000 L h^{-1}, making it highly susceptible to DDIs. Clinical data, including those from studies involving co-administration of ibrutinib with ketoconazole (strong CYP3A inhibitors) and rifampin (strong CYP3A inducer), confirmed this. In the prescribing information for ibrutinib, it was indicated that in a sequential design trial of 18 healthy volunteers, a single dose of 120 mg of ibrutinib was administered alone on day 1 and a single dose of 40 mg was administered on day 7 in combination with 400 mg of ketoconazole (given daily on days 4–9). Dose normalised mean C_{max} and AUC values of ibrutinib on day 7 were increased by 29- and 24-fold, respectively, after co-administration of ketoconazole. Simulations performed using a PBPK model developed for ibrutinib were able to represent the observed data with reasonable accuracy (C_{max} and AUC values were 21- and 30-fold, respectively). Similarly, the predicted 12.5-fold decrease in the AUC of ibrutinib after co-administration of rifampin was consistent with observed data. Prospective application of the 'validated/verified' PBPK model indicated that moderate CYP3A inhibitors (diltiazem and erythromycin) may increase the AUC of ibrutinib 6- to 9-fold in fasted conditions and that a moderate CYP3A inducer (efavirenz) is likely to decrease the AUC of ibrutinib by up to 3-fold. Based on both the observed and simulated interactions with CYP3A perpetrators, ibrutinib dosing recommendations in the presence of CYP3A inhibitors and inducers were made and incorporated into the label.

Another example of the utility of PBPK modelling to inform the drug label is ceritinib.[110] This tyrosine kinase inhibitor is mainly metabolised by CYP3A4 in a time-dependent manner leading to auto-inhibition of its clearance with multiple dosing. Co-administration of a single dose of ceritinib (450 mg) with ketoconazole (200 mg twice daily for 14 days) was found to increase its AUC by 2.9-fold and its C_{max} by 22% in 19 healthy subjects. Co-administration of ceritinib (750 mg) with rifampin (600 mg once daily for 14 days) led to decreases in the C_{max} and AUC of ceritinib of 44% and 70%, respectively. Given that the DDI studies were conducted using single doses of ceritinib the effect of strong perpetrators on steady-state exposure to the drug remained unclear due to the impact of its non-linear time-dependent kinetics. Thus, PBPK modelling was used to simulate a clinically more relevant study design. Predicted changes in the mean steady-state exposure of ceritinib in the presence of ketoconazole and rifampin were 51% (increase) and 6% (decrease), respectively. Therefore, on the basis of the simulations and exposure response data for safety and efficacy, the recommendation was made in the label to avoid concomitant use of strong CYP3A modulators.

A third example of PBPK modelling informing dosage recommendations relates to eliglustat.[111] This drug is highly extracted by the liver on first pass after oral administration. It is mainly metabolised by CYP2D6 with a minor contribution from CYP3A4, and is also a mechanism based inhibitor of CYP2D6. Clinical DDI studies indicated that the systemic exposure of eliglustat (84 mg twice daily) increased by 8.4- and 4.4-fold in CYP2D6 EM subjects in the presence of the strong CYP2D6 inhibitor paroxetine (30 mg once daily) and ketoconazole (400 mg once daily), respectively. Given the complexity of the kinetics of the drug, including the non-linearity due to auto-inhibition of CYP2D6, and the effect of different CYP2D6 genotypes, it was not possible to conduct clinical DDI studies to address all of the issues. Thus, a PBPK model was developed that was able to reflect the prior *in vivo* data accurately, and was then used as a basis for 'virtual' dose recommendations in EMs regarding co-administration of moderate CYP2D6 and CYP3A4 inhibitors (alone and in combination; 3 cases), in IMs for strong and moderate inhibitors of CYP3A4 and CYP2D6 (alone and in combination; 5 cases), and in PMs for strong and moderate CYP3A4 inhibitors (2 cases).

Last year, the FDA held a public workshop entitled "Application of Physiologically based Pharmacokinetic (PBPK) Modelling to Support Dose Selection", focussing on the role of PBPK in drug development and regulation. Representatives from industry, academia and regulatory agencies discussed and debated the acceptance of PBPK modelling during regulatory submission, which culminated in a report providing current perspectives on the application of PBPK in different areas, including its utility, predictive performance and reporting requirements for regulatory submissions.[112,113] Based on regulatory research and review experiences, the FDA's view was that the predictive performance of PBPK models is well established for evaluating the DDI potential of investigational drugs such as those metabolised by CYP3A4 and 2D6.[80,112] However, there was less confidence in the prediction of CYP-mediated DDIs in the gut and those involving time-dependent enzyme inhibition and induction, such that additional research in these areas was recommended. For transporter-mediated interactions, it was felt that data on predictive performance were limited compared with those available for enzyme-based interactions, and that confidence in PBPK modelling varies for different transporters. Research areas such as transporter biology, tissue expression and predicting intracellular drugs were considered to require further investigation.

Another workshop hosted in Europe under the remit of the Ministerial Industry Strategy Group (MISG), the Association of the British Pharmaceutical Industry (ABPI) and Medicines and Healthcare products Regulatory Agency

(MHRA) was held to explore the applications of PBPK modelling and simulation, with a focus on the clinical component of regulatory applications. Topics were selected to be complementary to those discussed at the earlier FDA meeting. A report summarising the meeting outcomes, with a focus on the European regulatory perspective, was published subsequently.[114] One of the key discussion points was drug-related input parameters, particularly with respect to the quality and uncertainty associated with these data. It was indicated that during the drug development process, PBPK modelling should be used to integrate the data and obtain a good quantitative understanding of the various processes contributing to the ADME of a drug. In addition, it was recommended to identify both the 'sensitive' parameters (*e.g.*, k_{deg} for prediction of DDIs involving mechanism based inhibition) and *in vitro* data with uncertainty, and to gauge the effect of these parameters on the predicted outcome of the DDI. It was also acknowledged that system model qualification, especially with continuously emerging data in the literature that require integration into existing databases, is not an area that has been extensively discussed in the PBPK community and that best practices involving computational approaches should be established going forward.

13.5 The Future

While it is encouraging that PBPK models are being used increasingly by the pharmaceutical industry for the prediction of the extent of DDIs, it is apparent that some significant challenges remain that need to be addressed in order to extend the success of this approach. For example, values for many 'system parameters' are lacking, such as the tissue abundances of enzymes other than CYPs and UGTs, and of many transporters. While population files for some ethnic groups (north Europeans, Japanese and Chinese) are reasonably well defined and are being curated, the necessary information for others (*e.g.*, Africans) is still being collated. The quality and reproducibility of *in vitro* data on drug metabolism and transport leaves room for improvement,[53,69,115] and a trend in drug discovery towards the synthesis of relatively large, very lipid-soluble molecules with low metabolic turnover and major impact of transporters also poses a challenge for accurate PBPK modelling. Going forward there is little doubt that *in vitro* transporter kinetics and the factors controlling intracellular drug concentrations will continue to be a major focus for achieving successful prediction. Economic constraints within the pharmaceutical industry leading to growth in pre-competitive research collaborations may help to resolve some of the outstanding issues based on the sharing of information, particularly with respect to system parameters and population and disease data.

Commercial platforms with integrated PBPK models, such as the Simcyp Simulator, GastroPlus™ and PKSIM®, which are used widely in the pharmaceutical industry, are continuously being updated to incorporate scientific developments. Thus, users have to receive sufficient education on the science that is being implemented as well as training on software functionality. This is being provided in the form of workshops and there is increasing interest in teaching these principles in academia. Having said that, experience counts for everything. In the pharmaceutical industry, dedicated users should be assigned in order to develop and retain the skill sets required for application of PBPK models. As a result of the multi-disciplinary aspects of PBPK modelling, users tend to have a wide variety of backgrounds, including drug metabolism, pharmacology, medicine, pharmacy, biophysics, engineering, mathematics, programming and statistics. Thus, it is important to facilitate communication across disciplines.

The extension of PBPK modelling by linking it with mechanistic pharmacodynamic models[116] to assess variability in intrinsic pharmacological response (including that related to receptor genotypes) will continue, as will the amalgamation of bottom-up and top-down approaches in PK to take advantage of the richness of the former with respect to mechanistic understanding and the statistical rigour of the latter with respect to accounting for uncertainty in parameter values.

Currently, PBPK modelling attempts to predict variability in drug exposure in populations and the extremes of risk. A further development would be its direct application in healthcare, concentrating on the individual rather than the population, as an educational tool and for the provision of computerised 'point of care' advice on personalised drug dosage. The safe and effective management of multi-drug treatment of the complex patient with multiple diseases and multiple prescribers requires a truly integrated view of pharmacology and therapeutics. In this context, linking the real patient to his/her 'virtual twin' and a PBPK–pharmacodynamics model in the cloud through a tablet is technically feasible and promises to rapidly predict appropriate individualised/stratified drug dosages, and avoid undesired complex multiple DDIs. Practical issues in making this proposition a reality include the availability of sufficient patient input data (demographics, genotypes, co-medication and biomarkers), adequate confidence in the accuracy of predictions, the availability of a sufficient range of unit dose preparations, the relation of dose prediction (PBPK) to dose adjustment (therapeutic drug monitoring/adaptive feedback) and evidence of cost–benefit for both patients and payers.

References

1. J. H. Gurwitz, T. S. Field, L. R. Harrold, J. Rothschild, K. Debellis, A. C. Seger, C. Cadoret, L. S. Fish, L. Garber, M. Kelleher and D. W. Bates, *JAMA*, 2003, **289**, 1107.
2. C. A. Jankel and L. K. Fitterman, *Drug Saf.*, 1993, **9**, 51.
3. S. Hutson, *Nat. Med.*, 2011, **17**, 6.
4. J. Holm, B. Eiermann, E. Eliasson and B. Mannheimer, *Eur. J. Clin. Pharmacol.*, 2014, **70**, 1375.
5. S. M. Huang, J. M. Strong, L. Zhang, K. S. Reynolds, S. Nallani, R. Temple, S. Abraham, S. A. Habet, R. K. Baweja, G. J. Burckart, S. Chung,

P. Colangelo, D. Frucht, M. D. Green, P. Hepp, E. Karnaukhova, H. S. Ko, J. I. Lee, P. J. Marroum, J. M. Norden, W. Qiu, A. Rahman, S. Sobel, T. Stifano, K. Thummel, X. X. Wei, S. Yasuda, J. H. Zheng, H. Zhao and L. J. Lesko, *J. Clin. Pharmacol.*, 2008, **48**, 662.

6. L. Pichard, I. Fabre, G. Fabre, J. Domergue, B. Saint Aubert, G. Mourad and P. Maurel, *Drug Metab. Dispos.*, 1990, **18**, 595.

7. G. T. Tucker, *Int. J. Clin. Pharmacol., Ther. Toxicol.*, 1992, **30**, 550.

8. A. Rostami-Hodjegan and G. Tucker, *Drug Discovery Today: Technol.*, 2004, **1**, 441.

9. A. Rostami-Hodjegan and G. T. Tucker, *Nat. Rev. Drug Discovery*, 2007, **6**, 140.

10. H. M. Jones, Y. Chen, C. Gibson, T. Heimbach, N. Parrott, S. A. Peters, J. Snoeys, V. V. Upreti, M. Zheng and S. D. Hall, *Clin. Pharmacol. Ther.*, 2015, **97**, 247.

11. C. E. Shardlow, G. T. Generaux, A. H. Patel, G. Tai, T. Tran and J. C. Bloomer, *Drug Metab. Dispos.*, 2013, **41**, 1994.

12. S. M. Huang, D. R. Abernethy, Y. Wang, P. Zhao and I. Zineh, *J. Pharm. Sci.*, 2013, **102**, 2912.

13. S. M. Huang and M. Rowland, *Clin. Pharmacol. Ther.*, 2012, **91**, 542.

14. P. Zhao, M. Rowland and S. M. Huang, *Clin. Pharmacol. Ther.*, 2012, **92**, 17.

15. P. Zhao, L. Zhang, J. A. Grillo, Q. Liu, J. M. Bullock, Y. J. Moon, P. Song, S. S. Brar, R. Madabushi, T. C. Wu, B. P. Booth, N. A. Rahman, K. S. Reynolds, E. Gil Berglund, L. J. Lesko and S. M. Huang, *Clin. Pharmacol. Ther.*, 2011, **89**, 259.

16. M. Rowland, C. Peck and G. Tucker, *Annu. Rev. Pharmacol. Toxicol.*, 2011, **51**, 45.

17. M. Rowland and S. Matin, *J. Pharmacokinet. Biopharm.*, 1973, **1**, 553.

18. H. Jones and K. Rowland-Yeo, *CPT: Pharmacometrics Syst. Pharmacol.*, 2013, **2**, e63.

19. M. Kato, T. Tachibana, K. Ito and Y. Sugiyama, *Drug Metab. Pharmacokinet.*, 2003, **18**, 121.

20. K. Rowland Yeo, M. Jamei, J. Yang, G. T. Tucker and A. Rostami-Hodjegan, *Eur. J. Pharm. Sci.*, 2010, **39**, 298.

21. US Food and Drug Administration, *HSS and CDER. Guidance for Industry: Drug Interactions Studies – Study Design, Data Analysis, Implications for Dosing, and Labeling Recommendations*, FDA, Silver Spring, 2012.

22. K. Ito, H. S. Brown and J. B. Houston, *Br. J. Clin. Pharmacol.*, 2004, **57**, 473.

23. K. Ito, K. Chiba, M. Horikawa, M. Ishigami, N. Mizuno, J. Aoki, Y. Gotoh, T. Iwatsubo, S. Kanamitsu, M. Kato, I. Kawahara, K. Niinuma, A. Nishino, N. Sato, Y. Tsukamoto, K. Ueda, T. Itoh and Y. Sugiyama, *AAPS J.*, 2002, **4**, E25.

24. A. Hisaka, Y. Ohno, T. Yamamoto and H. Suzuki, *Drug Metab. Pharmacokinet.*, 2010, **25**, 48.

25. J. Yang, M. Liao, M. Shou, M. Jamei, K. R. Yeo, G. T. Tucker and A. Rostami-Hodjegan, *Curr. Drug Metab.*, 2008, **9**, 384.
26. L. M. Almond, J. Yang, M. Jamei, G. T. Tucker and A. Rostami-Hodjegan, *Curr. Drug Metab.*, 2009, **10**, 420.
27. Y. H. Wang, D. R. Jones and S. D. Hall, *Drug Metab. Dispos.*, 2004, **32**, 259.
28. J. Yang, M. Jamei, K. R. Yeo, G. T. Tucker and A. Rostami-Hodjegan, *Curr. Drug Metab.*, 2007, **8**, 676.
29. V. K. Sinha, J. Snoeys, N. V. Osselaer, A. V. Peer, C. Mackie and D. Heald, *Biopharm. Drug Dispos.*, 2012, **33**, 111.
30. Y. Shitara, T. Horie and Y. Sugiyama, *Eur. J. Pharm. Sci.*, 2006, **27**, 425.
31. K. Maeda and Y. Sugiyama, Prediction of Hepatic Transporter-Mediated Drug–Drug Interaction from In Vitro Data, in *Transporters in Drug Development*, ed. Sugiyama Y and Steffansen B, Springer, New York, 2013, ch. 6, p. 121.
32. K. Ueda, Y. Kato, K. Komatsu and Y. Sugiyama, *J. Pharmacol. Exp. Ther.*, 2001, **297**, 1036.
33. Z. E. Barter, M. K. Bayliss, P. H. Beaune, A. R. Boobis, D. J. Carlile, R. J. Edwards, J. B. Houston, B. G. Lake, J. C. Lipscomb, O. R. Pelkonen, G. T. Tucker and A. Rostami-Hodjegan, *Curr. Drug Metab.*, 2007, **8**, 33.
34. H. J. Einolf, *Xenobiotica*, 2007, **37**, 1257.
35. E. J. Guest, K. Rowland-Yeo, A. Rostami-Hodjegan, G. T. Tucker, J. B. Houston and A. Galetin, *Br. J. Clin. Pharmacol.*, 2011, **71**, 72.
36. Y. Mano, Y. Sugiyama and K. Ito, *J. Pharm. Sci.*, 2015, **104**, 3183.
37. M. Gertz, A. Harrison, J. B. Houston and A. Galetin, *Drug Metab. Dispos.*, 2010, **38**, 1147.
38. F. Ghanbari, K. Rowland-Yeo, J. C. Bloomer, S. E. Clarke, M. S. Lennard, G. T. Tucker and A. Rostami-Hodjegan, *Curr. Drug Metab.*, 2006, **7**, 315.
39. K. Rowland Yeo, R. L. Walsky, M. Jamei, A. Rostami-Hodjegan and G. T. Tucker, *Eur. J. Pharm. Sci.*, 2011, **43**, 160.
40. J. Yang, M. Jamei, K. R. Yeo, G. T. Tucker and A. Rostami-Hodjegan, *Eur. J. Pharm. Sci.*, 2005, **26**, 334.
41. J. Yang, M. Jamei, K. R. Yeo, G. T. Tucker and A. Rostami-Hodjegan, *Eur. J. Pharm. Sci.*, 2007, **31**, 232.
42. J. R. Kenny, S. Mukadam, C. Zhang, S. Tay, C. Collins, A. Galetin and S. C. Khojasteh, *Pharm. Res.*, 2012, **29**, 1960.
43. Y. H. Wang, *Drug Metab. Dispos.*, 2010, **38**, 1094.
44. Y. Chen, L. Liu, M. Monshouwer and A. J. Fretland, *Drug Metab. Dispos.*, 2011, **39**, 2085.
45. H. J. Einolf, L. Chen, O. A. Fahmi, C. R. Gibson, R. S. Obach, M. Shebley, J. Silva, M. W. Sinz, J. D. Unadkat, L. Zhang and P. Zhao, *Clin. Pharmacol. Ther.*, 2014, **95**, 179.
46. O. A. Fahmi, T. S. Maurer, M. Kish, E. Cardenas, S. Boldt and D. Nettleton, *Drug Metab. Dispos.*, 2008, **36**, 1698.
47. K. Grime, D. D. Ferguson and R. J. Riley, *Curr. Drug Metab.*, 2010, **11**, 870.

48. S. L. Ripp, J. B. Mills, O. A. Fahmi, K. A. Trevena, J. L. Liras, T. S. Maurer and S. M. de Morais, *Drug Metab. Dispos.*, 2006, **34**, 1742.

49. M. Shou, M. Hayashi, Y. Pan, Y. Xu, K. Morrissey, L. Xu and G. L. Skiles, *Drug Metab. Dispos.*, 2008, **36**, 2355.

50. M. L. Vieira, B. Kirby, I. Ragueneau-Majlessi, A. Galetin, J. Y. Chien, H. J. Einolf, O. A. Fahmi, V. Fischer, A. Fretland, K. Grime, S. D. Hall, R. Higgs, D. Plowchalk, R. Riley, E. Seibert, K. Skordos, J. Snoeys, K. Venkatakrishnan, T. Waterhouse, R. S. Obach, E. G. Berglund, L. Zhang, P. Zhao, K. S. Reynolds and S. M. Huang, *Clin. Pharmacol. Ther.*, 2014, **95**, 189.

51. Y. Chen, J. Y. Jin, S. Mukadam, V. Malhi and J. R. Kenny, *Biopharm. Drug Dispos.*, 2012, **33**, 85.

52. S. S. De Buck, V. K. Sinha, L. A. Fenu, M. J. Nijsen, C. E. Mackie and R. A. Gilissen, *Drug Metab. Dispos.*, 2007, **35**, 1766.

53. H. M. Jones, H. A. Barton, Y. Lai, Y. A. Bi, E. Kimoto, S. Kempshall, S. C. Tate, A. El-Kattan, J. B. Houston, A. Galetin and K. S. Fenner, *Drug Metab. Dispos.*, 2012, **40**, 1007.

54. H. M. Jones, I. B. Gardner, W. T. Collard, P. J. Stanley, P. Oxley, N. A. Hosea, D. Plowchalk, S. Gernhardt, J. Lin, M. Dickins, S. R. Rahavendran, B. C. Jones, K. J. Watson, H. Pertinez, V. Kumar and S. Cole, *Clin. Pharmacokinet.*, 2011, **50**, 331.

55. M. Jamei, F. Bajot, S. Neuhoff, Z. Barter, J. Yang, A. Rostami-Hodjegan and K. Rowland-Yeo, *Clin. Pharmacokinet.*, 2014, **53**, 73.

56. M. Jamei, G. L. Dickinson and A. Rostami-Hodjegan, *Drug Metab. Pharmacokinet.*, 2009, **24**, 53.

57. F. Bouzom, K. Ball, N. Perdaems and B. Walther, *Biopharm. Drug Dispos.*, 2012, **33**, 55.

58. B. Achour, J. Barber and A. Rostami-Hodjegan, *Drug Metab. Dispos.*, 2014, **42**, 1349.

59. I. Templeton, C. C. Peng, K. E. Thummel, C. Davis, K. L. Kunze and N. Isoherranen, *Clin. Pharmacol. Ther.*, 2010, **88**, 499.

60. J. O. Miners, P. I. Mackenzie and K. M. Knights, *Drug Metab. Rev.*, 2010, **42**, 196.

61. J. Zhou and J. O. Miners, *Methods Mol. Biol.*, 2014, **1113**, 203.

62. J. M. Hutzler, R. S. Obach, D. Dalvie and M. A. Zientek, *Expert Opin. Drug Metab. Toxicol.*, 2013, **9**, 153.

63. S. Dhuria, H. Einolf, J. Mangold, S. Sen, H. Gu, L. Wang and S. Cameron, *J. Clin. Pharmacol.*, 2013, **53**, 642.

64. K. Gandelman, T. Zhu, O. A. Fahmi, P. Glue, K. Lian, R. S. Obach and B. Damle, *J. Clin. Pharmacol.*, 2011, **51**, 229.

65. R. Greupink, M. Schreurs, M. S. Benne, M. T. Huisman and F. G. Russel, *Eur. J. Pharm. Sci.*, 2013, **49**, 819.

66. Y. Xu, Y. Zhou, M. Hayashi, M. Shou and G. L. Skiles, *Drug Metab. Dispos.*, 2011, **39**, 1139.

67. H. A. Barton, Y. Lai, T. C. Goosen, H. M. Jones, A. F. El-Kattan, J. R. Gosset, J. Lin and M. V. Varma, *Expert Opin. Drug Metab. Toxicol.*, 2013, **9**, 459.

68. J. B. Houston, K. Rowland-Yeo and U. Zanelli, *Toxicol. In Vitro*, 2012, **26**, 1265.

69. M. J. Zamek-Gliszczynski, C. A. Lee, A. Poirier, J. Bentz, X. Chu, H. Ellens, T. Ishikawa, M. Jamei, J. C. Kalvass, S. Nagar, K. S. Pang, K. Korzekwa, P. W. Swaan, M. E. Taub, P. Zhao and A. Galetin, *Clin. Pharmacol. Ther.*, 2013, **94**, 64.

70. X. Chu, K. Korzekwa, R. Elsby, K. Fenner, A. Galetin, Y. Lai, P. Matsson, A. Moss, S. Nagar, G. R. Rosania, J. P. Bai, J. W. Polli, Y. Sugiyama and K. L. Brouwer, *Clin. Pharmacol. Ther.*, 2013, **94**, 126.

71. R. Li, H. A. Barton and M. V. Varma, *Clin. Pharmacokinet.*, 2014, **53**, 659.

72. S. Nagar, J. Tucker, E. A. Weiskircher, S. Bhoopathy, I. J. Hidalgo and K. Korzekwa, *Pharm. Res.*, 2014, **31**, 347.

73. N. D. Pfeifer, R. N. Hardwick and K. L. Brouwer, *Annu. Rev. Pharmacol. Toxicol.*, 2014, **54**, 509.

74. J. Badee, B. Achour, A. Rostami-Hodjegan and A. Galetin, *Drug Metab. Dispos.*, 2015, **43**, 424.

75. M. Baker and T. Parton, *Xenobiotica*, 2007, **37**, 1110.

76. J. N. Bauman, K. S. Frederick, A. Sawant, R. L. Walsky, L. M. Cox, R. S. Obach and A. S. Kalgutkar, *Drug Metab. Dispos.*, 2008, **36**, 1016.

77. S. Bernard, K. A. Neville, A. T. Nguyen and D. A. Flockhart, *Oncologist*, 2006, **11**, 126.

78. M. Hendset, M. Hermann, H. Lunde, H. Refsum and E. Molden, *Eur. J. Clin. Pharmacol.*, 2007, **63**, 1147.

79. US Food and Drug Administration, *Medical Review(s) Part 1-4: Review and Evaluation of Clinical Data NDA #021-436: US FDA Center for Drug Evaluation and Research*, 2002.

80. M. D. Vieira, M. J. Kim, S. Apparaju, V. Sinha, I. Zineh, S. M. Huang and P. Zhao, *Clin. Pharmacol. Ther.*, 2014, **95**, 550.

81. V. Hatorp, S. Oliver and C. A. Su, *Int. J. Clin. Pharmacol. Ther.*, 1998, **36**, 636.

82. P. N. van Heiningen, V. Hatorp, K. Kramer Nielsen, K. T. Hansen, J. J. van Lier, N. C. De Merbel, B. Oosterhuis and J. H. Jonkman, *Eur. J. Clin. Pharmacol.*, 1999, **55**, 521.

83. T. B. Bidstrup, I. Bjornsdottir, U. G. Sidelmann, M. S. Thomsen and K. T. Hansen, *Br. J. Clin. Pharmacol.*, 2003, **56**, 305.

84. L. I. Kajosaari, J. Laitila, P. J. Neuvonen and J. T. Backman, *Basic Clin. Pharmacol. Toxicol.*, 2005, **97**, 249.

85. M. Niemi, J. T. Backman, M. Neuvonen and P. J. Neuvonen, *Diabetologia*, 2003, **46**, 347.

86. M. Niemi, P. J. Neuvonen and K. T. Kivisto, *Clin. Pharmacol. Ther.*, 2001, **70**, 58.

87. A. Kalliokoski and M. Niemi, *Br. J. Pharmacol.*, 2009, **158**, 693.

88. K. Rowland-Yeo, M. Jamei, M. Aarabi and A. Rostami-Hodjegan, Application of Physiologically based pharmacokinetic (PBPK) modelling for prediction of complex drug-drug interactions (DDIs) involving OAT-P1B1-mediated uptake and cytochrome P450 (CYP) metabolism and

multiple inhibitors. Presidential Trainee Awards: Gaylord National Hotel and Convention Center, 2012, National Harbor, Maryland: Clinical Pharmacology & Therapeutics.

89. S. Y. Chu, L. T. Sennello, S. T. Bunnell, L. L. Varga, D. S. Wilson and R. C. Sonders, *Antimicrob. Agents Chemother.*, 1992, **36**, 2447.
90. P. G. Davey, *J. Hosp. Infect.*, 1991, **19**(Suppl A), 29.
91. A. D. Rodrigues, E. M. Roberts, D. J. Mulford, Y. Yao and D. Ouellet, *Drug Metab. Dispos.*, 1997, **25**, 623.
92. K. A. Rodvold, *Clin. Pharmacokinet.*, 1999, **37**, 385.
93. V. Pichette and F. A. Leblond, *Curr. Drug Metab.*, 2003, **4**, 91.
94. J. Shi, S. Chapel, G. Montay, P. Hardy, J. S. Barrett, D. Sica, S. K. Swan, R. Noveck, B. Leroy and V. O. Bhargava, *Int. J. Clin. Pharmacol. Ther.*, 2005, **43**, 123.
95. M. A. Tortorici, D. L. Cutler, A. Hazra, T. D. Nolin, K. Rowland-Yeo and K. Venkatakrishnan, *J. Clin. Pharmacol.*, 2014, **55**, 241.
96. G. G. Graham, J. Punt, M. Arora, R. O. Day, M. P. Doogue, J. K. Duong, T. J. Furlong, J. R. Greenfield, L. C. Greenup, C. M. Kirkpatrick, J. E. Ray, P. Timmins and K. M. Williams, *Clin. Pharmacokinet.*, 2011, **50**, 81.
97. C. R. Sirtori, G. Franceschini, M. Galli-Kienle, G. Cighetti, G. Galli, A. Bondioli and F. Conti, *Clin. Pharmacol. Ther.*, 1978, **24**, 683.
98. G. T. Tucker, C. Casey, P. J. Phillips, H. Connor, J. D. Ward and H. F. Woods, *Br. J. Clin. Pharmacol.*, 1981, **12**, 235.
99. J. A. Sprowl and A. Sparreboom, *Drug Metab. Dispos.*, 2014, **42**, 611.
100. H. Koepsell, K. Lips and C. Volk, *Pharm. Res.*, 2007, **24**, 1227.
101. R. M. Pelis and S. H. Wright, *Compr. Physiol.*, 2011, **1**, 1795.
102. Y. Ding, Y. Jia, Y. Song, C. Lu, Y. Li, M. Chen, M. Wang and A. Wen, *Eur. J. Clin. Pharmacol.*, 2014, **70**, 141.
103. B. Grun, M. K. Kiessling, J. Burhenne, K. D. Riedel, J. Weiss, G. Rauch, W. E. Haefeli and D. Czock, *Br. J. Clin. Pharmacol.*, 2013, **76**, 787.
104. S. Johansson, J. Read, S. Oliver, M. Steinberg, Y. Li, E. Lisbon, D. Mathews, P. T. Leese and P. Martin, *Clin. Pharmacokinet.*, 2014, **53**, 837.
105. H. Kusuhara, S. Ito, Y. Kumagai, M. Jiang, T. Shiroshita, Y. Moriyama, K. Inoue, H. Yuasa and Y. Sugiyama, *Clin. Pharmacol. Ther.*, 2011, **89**, 837.
106. A. Somogyi, C. Stockley, J. Keal, P. Rolan and F. Bochner, *Br. J. Clin. Pharmacol.*, 1987, **23**, 545.
107. Z. J. Wang, O. Q. Yin, B. Tomlinson and M. S. Chow, *Pharmacogenet. Genomics*, 2008, **18**, 637.
108. H. Burt, S. Neuhoff, M. Jamei, A. Rostami-Hodjegan, G. Tucker and K. Rowland-Yeo, *The Application of PBPK modelling to investigate the OCT/MATE transporter DDI between metformin and cimetidine. HGMP/DMDG Open Meeting*, 2014, Paris.
109. US Food and Drug Administration. *Imbruvica (Ibrutinib): US Food and Drug Administration*, 2013, contract no.: 10th June.
110. US Food and Drug Administration. *Zykadia (Ceritinib): US Food and Drug Administration*, 2014, contract no.: 10th June.

111. US Food and Drug Administration. *Cerdelga (Eliglustat): US Food and Drug Administration*, 2014, contract no.: 10th June.

112. C. Wagner, Y. Pan, V. Hsu, J. A. Grillo, L. Zhang, K. S. Reynolds, V. Sinha and P. Zhao, *Clin. Pharmacokinet.*, 2015, **54**, 117.

113. C. Wagner, P. Zhao, Y. Pan, V. Hsu, J. Grillo, S. M. Huang and V. Sinha, *CPT: Pharmacometrics Syst. Pharmacol.*, 2015, **4**, 226.

114. T. Shepard, G. Scott, S. Cole, A. Nordmark and F. Bouzom, *CPT: Pharmacometrics Syst. Pharmacol.*, 2015, **4**, 221.

115. K. L. Brouwer, D. Keppler, K. A. Hoffmaster, D. A. Bow, Y. Cheng, Y. Lai, J. E. Palm, B. Stieger and R. Evers, *Clin. Pharmacol. Ther.*, 2013, **94**, 95.

116. P. Vicini and P. H. van der Graaf, *Clin. Pharmacol. Ther.*, 2013, **93**, 379.

CHAPTER 14

Induction of Hepatic Cytochrome P450 Enzymes: Importance in Drug Development and Toxicity

BRIAN G. LAKE*[a] AND ROGER J. PRICE[a]

[a]Centre for Toxicology, Faculty of Health and Medical Sciences, University of Surrey, Guildford, Surrey, GU2 7XH, UK
*E-mail: blake@lfrmolecular.com

14.1 Introduction

Man is surrounded in his environment by a multitude of chemicals that cannot be used for either the production of energy (*i.e.* as nutrients) or for the elaboration of tissue components. Such chemicals are thus consequently foreign to the normal metabolic pathways of humans and hence have been termed as foreign compounds or xenobiotics. Xenobiotics to which man is exposed include pharmaceutical agents, pesticides, food chemicals, industrial chemicals, natural products and environmental contaminants. Throughout evolution, mammals have developed a series of enzyme systems to detoxify xenobiotics and promote their excretion from the body.[1,2] While the liver is the major site of xenobiotic metabolism in mammals, xenobiotic metabolising enzymes are also found in other tissues, including the

RSC Drug Discovery Series No. 49
New Horizons in Predictive Drug Metabolism and Pharmacokinetics
Edited by Alan G. E. Wilson
© The Royal Society of Chemistry 2016
Published by the Royal Society of Chemistry, www.rsc.org

intestine, lung and skin, which can be the first sites of entry of a xenobiotic into the organism.

Enzymatic pathways of xenobiotic metabolism have been divided into phase I and II, with phase I enzymes introducing or unmasking a functional group in the xenobiotic, while phase II enzymes conjugate functional groups to make the product more polar and hence favour excretion from the body.[1-3] The most important phase I enzymes comprise the cytochrome P450 (CYP) superfamily, which catalyse the oxygenation of a multitude of xenobiotics.[3-7] Other phase I enzymes include carboxylesterase, flavin monooxygenase and aldehyde dehydrogenase enzymes. Phase II enzymes include epoxide hydrolase, N-acetyltransferase, UDP-glucuronosyltransferase (UGT), sulphotransferase and glutathione S-transferase enzymes. This chapter will focus on human and rodent (namely the rat and mouse) hepatic CYP enzymes, and the importance of induction of CYP enzymes in drug–drug interactions in humans and in nongenotoxic tumour formation in chronic rodent toxicity studies.

14.2   Hepatic CYP Enzymes

Hepatic CYP enzymes involved in the metabolism of therapeutic agents and other xenobiotics are primarily located in the endoplasmic reticulum, with other CYP enzymes involved in steroid hormone biosynthesis and vitamin D metabolism being located in mitochondria. In both rodent and human liver, the microsomal fraction contains a range of CYP enzymes including members of the CYP1A, CYP2A, CYP2B, CYP2C, CYP2D, CYP2E, CYP3A and CYP4A subfamilies.[4-9] Table 14.1 lists some CYP enzymes present in rat, mouse and human liver. Important human hepatic CYP enzymes involved in the metabolism of therapeutic agents include CYP1A2, CYP2B6, CYP2C8, CYP2C9, CYP2C19, CYP2D6, CYP3A4 and CYP3A5, with some drugs and other xenobiotics also being metabolised by other CYP enzymes including

Table 14.1   Some human, rat and mouse hepatic CYP enzymes.

CYP subfamily	Species[a]		
	Human	Rat	Mouse
CYP1A	CYP1A2	CYP1A2	Cyp1a2
CYP2A	CYP2A6	CYP2A1, CYP2A2	Cyp2a4, Cyp2a5
CYP2B	CYP2B6	CYP2B1, CYP2B2	Cyp2b9, Cyp2b10
CYP2C	CYP2C8, CYP2C9, CYP2C19	CYP2C6, CYP2C7, CYP2C11, CYP2C12	Cyp2c29, Cyp2c37, Cyp2c38, Cyp2c40
CYP2D	CYP2D6	CYP2D1, CYP2D2, CYP2D3	Cyp2d22
CYP2E	CYP2E1	CYP2E1	Cyp2e1
CYP3A	CYP3A4, CYP3A5	CYP3A1, CYP3A2	Cyp3a11
CYP4A	CYP4A11	CYP4A1, CYP4A2, CYP4A3	Cyp4a10, Cyp4a12, Cyp4a14

[a]For further details see Pelkonen *et al.* (2008),[6] Martignoni *et al.* (2006)[7] and Lake (2009).[8]

CYP2A6 and CYP2E1. Unlike other hepatic CYP enzymes, CYP4A11 is primarily involved in the metabolism of endogenous substrates such as fatty acids, prostaglandins and leukotricnes.[8,9] Levels of CYP1A2, CYP2A6, CYP2B6, CYP2C8, CYP2C9, CYP2C19, CYP2D6, CYP2E1 and CYP3A4/CYP3A5 enzymes in human liver have been reported to account for >10, ~10, <5, ~5, >15, <5, <5, ~15 and >35%, respectively, of the total CYP enzyme content.[6] In terms of drug metabolism, it has been estimated that CYP2B6, CYP2C, CYP2D6 and CYP3A4 metabolise around 25, 16, 30 and 50%, respectively, of marketed therapeutic agents.[7]

As in human liver, both rat and mouse liver contain members of the CYP1A, CYP2A, CYP2B, CYP2C, CYP2D, CYP2E, CYP3A and CYP4A subfamilies (Table 14.1). While some xenobiotics are metabolised by the same CYP subfamily enzymes in human, rat and mouse liver, species differences in substrate specificity are known to exist. For example, testosterone is metabolised to 6β-hydroxytestosterone by human, rat and mouse CYP3A subfamily enzymes.[3] However, while coumarin is a substrate for human CYP2A6 and mouse Cyp2a5, these two CYP enzymes exhibit poor steroid metabolising activity.[10] By contrast, mouse Cyp2a4 and rat CYP3A1 and CYP3A2 all metabolise testosterone to 7α- and/or 15-α-hydroxytestosterone, but do not catalyse the 7-hydroxylation of coumarin.

14.3 Induction of Hepatic CYP Enzymes

Enzyme induction is a process by which a chemical induces the expression of an enzyme. Classically, induction is due to the *de novo* synthesis of new enzyme molecules as a result of increased transcription of the respective gene following treatment with the inducing agent. However, this is not the only mechanism of induction of hepatic CYP enzymes.

The ability of chemicals to induce hepatic CYP and other xenobiotic metabolising enzymes has been known for many years.[2,4] Early examples of inducers of hepatic CYP enzymes include phenobarbitone [phenobarbital (PB)] and its sodium salt (NaPB), together with polycyclic hydrocarbons, such as benzo(a)pyrene and 20-methylcholanthrene (20MC). It is now well established that hepatic microsomal CYP enzymes in both humans and rodents can be induced by many chemicals, including therapeutic agents, pesticides, food additives, industrial chemicals, natural products and environmental contaminants.[4-7] Some known inducers of human and rodent hepatic CYP enzymes are shown in Table 14.2. Human hepatic CYP enzymes can also be induced by polycyclic hydrocarbons present in cigarette smoke and barbecued meat, by consumption of a high protein/low carbohydrate diet, by intake of cruciferous vegetables (*e.g.* broccoli, Brussels sprouts and cabbage) and by certain herbal preparations.[3,5,6,11,12]

The induction of CYP enzymes normally occurs by receptor mediated mechanisms leading to an increase in gene transcription.[4,6,13,14] For example, important receptors involved in the induction of CYP1A, CYP2B, CYP3A

Table 14.2   Some examples of compounds that can induce human or rodent hepatic CYP enzymes.

CYP subfamily	Inducer[a]	
	Human	Rat and/or mouse
CYP1A	BNF, 20MC, omeprazole, TCDD	BNF, 20MC, TCDD
CYP2A	DEX, PB, RIF	PB, pyrazole, TCPOBOP
CYP2B	CARB, CITCO, PB, PHEN, RIF	Chlordane, DDT, DEX, dieldrin, oxazepam, PB, TCPOBOP
CYP2C	CARB, DEX, PB, RIF	PB, TCPOBOP
CYP2E	Ethanol, isoniazid	Ethanol, isoniazid
CYP3A	CARB, DEX, PB, PHEN, RIF	DEX, PB, PCN, TAO
CYP4A	Some evidence for a small effect of rodent CYP4A inducers	Clofibric acid, ciprofibrate, DEHP, methylclofenapate, nafenopin, Wy-14,643

[a]CARB: carbamazepine; DDT: 1,1,1-trichloro-2,2-bis(4-chlorophenyl)ethane; PHEN: phenytoin; TCDD: 2,3,7,8-tetrachlorodibenzo-*p*-dioxin. For further details see Parkinson (2001),[3] Pelkonen *et al.* (1998),[5] Pelkonen *et al.* (2008),[6] Martignoni *et al.* (2006)[7] and Lake (2009).[8]

and CYP4A subfamily enzymes comprise, respectively, the aryl hydrocarbon receptor (AhR), the constitutive androstane receptor (CAR), the pregnane X receptor (PXR) and the peroxisome proliferator-activated receptor alpha (PPARα).[4,6,13,14] Other receptors involved in the regulation of hepatic CYP enzymes include the glucocorticoid receptor, vitamin D receptor, farnesoid X receptor, liver X receptor and hepatocyte nuclear factor-4.[15,16]

While AhR is a member of the Per-Arnt-Sim (PAS) family of transcription factors, CAR, PXR and PPARα are members of the nuclear receptor superfamily.[4,13,14] The AhR is activated by binding to the inducing agent, which then binds to the AhR nuclear translocator (Arnt) forming a heterodimer that can bind to response elements in DNA. Human CYP1A subfamily members comprise CYP1A1 and CYP1A2, the former being essentially an extrahepatic enzyme and hence only CYP1A2 will be considered in this chapter. The induction of hepatic CYP1A2 can also occur by an AhR-independent pathway through activation of CAR.[17]

After activation by the inducing agent, the nuclear receptors CAR, PXR and PPARα all heterodimerise with the retinoid X receptor (RXR), and bind to response elements in DNA. Although CYP inducing agents are normally considered to bind as ligands to the receptors, CAR in particular can be activated without direct ligand binding by an indirect or ligand-independent mechanism.[4,6,15] For example, the activation of CAR by PB is indirect and involves a dephosphorylation reaction at threonine 38 (human) or serine 202 (mouse), apparently signalling through the epidermal growth factor receptor, leading to the nuclear translocation of CAR.[15,18–21] In addition, while most compounds are considered to be agonists of PPARα, receptor binding has only been demonstrated for a few compounds.[22] Thus, for the purposes of this chapter, inducing agents will be referred to as activators of CAR, PPARα or other receptors, without any consideration of the precise mechanism of receptor activation.

The activation of receptors such as CAR and PPARα results in effects on a wide range of genes, including those involved in phase I and II xenobiotic metabolism, phase III transporters, and in genes involved in physiological processes including energy metabolism, cell proliferation and apoptosis.[4,6,15,23] Thus hepatic CYP enzyme induction is just one facet of a pleiotropic response to receptor activation by the inducing agent.

Many studies have demonstrated that there can be considerable cross-talk between receptors involved in the regulation of hepatic CYP enzymes.[6,13–16,24] For example, there is a high degree of similarity between CAR and PXR, with compounds such as PB being activators of both nuclear receptors.[25–27] Several investigations have shown that CAR and PXR can regulate overlapping but distinct sets of genes, including genes involved in hepatic xenobiotic metabolism.[26,28,29] Studies in human hepatocytes with PB have demonstrated that the induction of CYP2B and CYP3A enzymes is mediated through CAR, PXR and the glucocorticoid receptor.[30,31] Similarly, investigations in rodents have shown that due to cross-talk between receptors CYP2B inducers often also induce CYP2A, CYP2C and CYP3A enzymes, whereas CYP3A inducers often also induce CYP2B enzymes.[5,15,32–34] In addition, some PPARα activators, which induce CYP4A enzymes, have also been shown to induce CYP2B and other CYP enzymes in rodent liver.[15,22,35]

In contrast to the induction of CYP2B and some other hepatic CYP enzymes, the induction of CYP2E1 does not occur by a receptor mediated mechanism.[6,11,14] CYP2E1 induction by agents such as isoniazid and ethanol involves a post-translational mechanism *via* stabilisation of the enzyme mRNA and protein. While many CYP enzymes are inducible by drugs and other chemicals in both human and rodent liver, CYP2D subfamily enzymes are usually considered to be refractory to such agents.[3,5,6]

Various studies have demonstrated that there are marked interindividual differences between humans in both the levels of hepatic CYP enzymes and in the inducibility of these enzymes. Such interindividual differences can be due to various environmental factors (*e.g.* diet, cigarette smoking or exposure to enzyme inducing agents), as well as to polymorphisms in CYP genes, nuclear receptors, regulatory proteins and transporters.[36]

14.4 Species Differences in Induction of Hepatic CYP Enzymes

The ability of a compound to induce hepatic CYP enzymes in either rats or mice may indicate a potential to induce hepatic CYP enzymes in humans. However, apart from metabolism and pharmacokinetic considerations, there are now many examples of marked species differences between rodents and humans in hepatic CYP enzyme induction.[6,7,11,14] Thus some compounds that induce hepatic CYP enzymes in rodents are either ineffective or much less potent in humans or *vice versa*. Moreover, species differences also exist between the rat and mouse in their response to inducers of hepatic CYP enzymes.

Omeprazole is known to induce hepatic CYP1A2 in humans, but has little effect on hepatic CYP1A enzymes in the rat and mouse.[11,13] The compound 1,4-bis[2-(3,5-dichloropyridyloxy)]benzene (TCPOBOP) is a potent activator of mouse CAR, but not of human CAR.[6,11,13,37] In contrast to TCPOBOP, the compound 6-(4-chlorophenyl)imidazo[2,1-*b*][1,3]thiazole-5-carbaldehyde *O*-(3,4-dichlorbenzyl)oxime (CITCO) is a potent activator of human CAR.[6,38] While in a short term study PB was shown to induce CYP2B enzymes in both rats and mice, TCPOBOP only induced CYP2B enzymes in mice.[39] However, in other studies high doses of TCPOBOP have been shown to induce CYP2B enzymes in rats.[40] Tamoxifen has been shown to induce hepatic CYP2B and CYP3A enzymes in the rat, but had little effect on CYP enzyme activities in two strains of mice; whereas 4-vinylcyclohexene induced hepatic CYP2A and CYP2B enzymes in the mouse but not in the rat.[41,42]

Rifampicin (RIF) is a known inducer of hepatic CYP3A and other CYP enzymes in humans *in vivo* and *in vitro* in cultured human hepatocytes, but produces only small effects in the rat and mouse.[6,11,43] By contrast, pregnenolone-16α-carbonitrile (PCN) is a good inducer of CYP3A enzymes in the rat and mouse, but has little effect in human hepatocytes.[11]

A number of PPARα activators have been shown to induce hepatic CYP4A enzymes in the rat and mouse, both after *in vivo* administration and in cultured hepatocytes. However, rodent PPARα activators appear to produce only relatively small effects on CYP4A11 mRNA and protein levels in human hepatocytes.[8,44]

Species differences in hepatic CYP enzyme induction are attributable to differences in the receptors involved.[13,14] The species differences observed with both CAR and PXR activators are due to differences in the ligand binding domains of these two nuclear receptors. For example, while both PCN and dexamethasone (DEX) induced Cyp3a11 in wild type mice, in humanised mice (where mouse PXR was replaced by its human counterpart) hepatic Cyp3a11 was induced by RIF and not by PCN.[45]

14.5   Methods to Assess Hepatic CYP Enzyme Induction in Humans and Rodents

If a new chemical entity produces an induction of hepatic CYP enzymes in either rat or mouse, the compound may also be an inducer of hepatic CYP enzymes in humans if administered at a sufficient dosage. However, as described in Section 14.4, there are many examples of species differences in the induction of hepatic CYP enzymes. It is therefore necessary to confirm the potential of a compound to induce human hepatic CYP enzymes in studies using human material. As described in Section 14.5.1, cultured human hepatocytes are a well established *in vitro* test system to screen chemicals for their ability to induce human hepatic CYP enzymes.

14.5.1 Studies in Humans

The induction of hepatic CYP enzymes in humans can be assessed by either *in vivo* studies or *in vitro* investigations such as the use of cultured human hepatocytes. In addition, reporter gene constructs and endogenous metabolite ratios can also provide useful information on the potential of a test compound to stimulate human hepatic CYP enzymes.[6,11,13,14] For *in vivo* studies, following administration of the test compound to human volunteers, the induction of hepatic CYP enzymes can be evaluated by the effects on the kinetics of CYP probe substrates determined in blood and urine, and in some instances in saliva or expired air. Thus, for example, the kinetics of caffeine elimination determined in saliva can be employed as a marker of CYP1A2 induction in humans.[6] For other human CYP enzymes suitable probe substrates include coumarin, diclofenac, dextromethorphan and midazolam for CYP2A6, CYP2C9, CYP2D6 and CYP3A4, respectively.[5,6] It is also possible to administer a cocktail of CYP substrates in order to determine their effects on a number of hepatic CYP enzymes.[46] The induction of human hepatic CYP enzymes can also be assessed by determining levels of some endogenous compounds in urine, including D-glucaric acid and 6β-hydroxycortisol. Indeed, the urinary ratios of both 6β-hydroxycortisol:cortisol and 4β-hydroxycholesterol:cholesterol have been employed as non-invasive markers for CYP3A induction in humans.[6,13,46]

It is also possible to assess the potential for a test compound to induce human hepatic CYP enzymes by employing *in vitro* systems such as cultured hepatocytes, precision-cut liver slices, some cell lines and reporter gene constructs. Of these various *in vitro* systems, cultured human hepatocytes may be considered the "gold standard". The improvement of cell isolation and culture techniques has established human hepatocytes as a reliable *in vitro* system to screen chemicals for induction of hepatic CYP enzymes.[11,47] Another significant advantage of the use of human hepatocytes has been the successful development of cryopreservation procedures, with cryopreserved induction-qualified human hepatocytes now commercially available from a number of suppliers. The availability of good quality plateable cryopreserved human hepatocytes permits experiments to be conducted when required (*i.e.* no waiting for suitable donor tissue to become available) and also allows repeat experiments to be performed with hepatocyte preparations from the same donor.[47,48] The induction of CYP enzymes in cultured human hepatocytes can be assessed by the measurement of mRNA levels, CYP-dependent enzyme activities and CYP protein levels. Only small numbers of cells are required for CYP mRNA studies, with incubations being performed in a 96-well plate format, which permits the use of robotic systems to extract total RNA and subsequently to determine CYP mRNA levels by a real-time quantitative reverse transcription-polymerase chain reaction procedure (*e.g.* TaqMan®). CYP-dependent enzyme activities can either be determined in intact hepatocytes by adding the CYP substrates to the medium or by treating the cells with the test chemical and then removing the cells for subsequent preparation of subcellular fractions (*e.g.* microsomes). In terms of intact cells, a number of fluorescent substrates (*e.g.* 7-ethoxyresorufin and 7-benzyloxy-4-trifluoromethylcoumarin) are available for use in a 96-well plate format.[49,50] CYP substrate metabolism can also be determined in intact hepatocyte monolayers utilising liquid chromatography-tandem mass spectrometry analysis of metabolites.[48,51,52] When performing CYP substrate metabolism studies with intact hepatocytes, it may be necessary to enzymatically hydrolyse metabolites conjugated with D-glucuronic acid and/or sulphate prior to analysis in order to determine the total rate of metabolism of the substrate. Suitable substrates for assessing the effects on CYPs in cultured human hepatocytes comprise either phenacetin or 7-ethoxyresorufin for CYP1A2, bupropion for CYP2B6, either diclofenac or tolbutamide for CYP2C9, and either midazolam or testosterone for CYP3A4.[6] As with human *in vivo* studies, it is possible to use a cocktail of CYP substrates in studies with cultured hepatocytes or cell lines to determine effects on a number of CYP enzymes.[48,51,52] Levels of CYP enzyme proteins can be determined in subcellular fractions prepared from cultured hepatocytes using either Western immunoblotting or the more quantitative technique of enzyme-linked immunoassay (ELISA). For both Western immunoblotting and ELISA studies suitable CYP subfamily-specific antibodies are required. While CYP enzyme activities have been utilised as an endpoint in many studies, some CYP inducers, such as ritonavir and troleandomycin (TAO), can also result in enzyme inhibition.[6,11] Thus for such compounds the determination of CYP mRNA levels and/or CYP protein levels will also be useful endpoints to detect induction. For all endpoints, it is important to include positive controls in each experiment in order to confirm the functional viability of the hepatocyte preparations used. Suitable positive controls for studies in human hepatocytes include β-naphthoflavone (BNF), PB and RIF for CYP1A2, CYP2B6 and CYP3A4, respectively, with PB and RIF normally inducing both CYP2B6 and CYP3A4.[11,48,53]

A number of CYP enzymes, including CYP1A2, CYP2A6, CYP2B6, CYP2C8, CYP2C9, CYP2C19 and CYP3A4, are known to be inducible in cultured human hepatocytes.[6,11,30,31,53,54] For general screening with cultured human hepatocytes it may be necessary to just evaluate effects on CYP1A2 and CYP3A4, because there is co-regulation of CYP3A, CYP2B and CYP2C induction.[30,31,53] However, it is also useful to evaluate the effect of a test chemical on CYP2B6, as some CAR activators do not produce a marked induction of CYP3A4.[11]

Studies with cultured human hepatocytes can thus identify the potential of a compound to induce human hepatic CYP enzymes. However, attention needs to be paid to the concentrations that are effective at inducing CYP enzymes in cultured hepatocytes *in vitro*, compared with the likely *in vivo* exposure after treatment with the chemical. For example, while eletriptan can induce CYP3A enzymes in cultured human hepatocytes, such induction is only observed at high concentrations in the culture medium, which are unlikely to be achieved in human liver *in vivo* after treatment with therapeutic doses of eletriptan.[55]

Apart from cultured human hepatocytes, other available *in vitro* systems include precision-cut liver slices, cell lines and reporter gene constructs.[6] Most studies with precision-cut liver slices have employed freshly cut slices, which means that studies can only be undertaken when suitable tissue is available from human donors. Precision-cut liver slices maintain tissue architecture, making it is possible to utilise immunocytochemical methods to study effects on CYP enzymes in different parts of the liver lobule. Like hepatocytes, CYP enzyme measurements can be made using either intact slices or subcellular fractions prepared from the slices.[56,57]

Generally, cell lines are inferior to human hepatocytes for CYP induction studies.[11,47] For example, the human hepatoma HepG2 cell line contains only low levels of CAR, PXR, CYP1A2, CYP2C9 and CYP3A4 compared with primary human hepatocytes. Fa2N-4 cells are derived from primary human hepatocytes by transfection with the SV40 large T-antigen. The expression of AhR and PXR in these cells is similar to human hepatocytes and the induction of CYP1A2, CYP2C9 and CYP3A4 has been demonstrated. However, CAR expression is deficient in Fa2N-4 cells and hence such cells are not representative of cultured human hepatocytes. HepaRG cells are derived from a hepatocellular carcinoma and consist of two cell types. In order to obtain a liver-like function the cells must be cultured in medium containing dimethyl sulphoxide. Such cells do contain AhR, CAR and PXR, and the induction of CYP1A2, CYP2B6, CYP2C9, CYP2C19 and CYP3A4 has been demonstrated in this cell line.[51,52,58] HepaRG cells are thus a potentially useful alternative to cultured human hepatocytes for some applications.

A number of reporter gene assays have been developed to screen chemicals for effects on either nuclear receptors or on CYP enzymes. Available systems include assays for human CAR and PXR activation and for CYP2B6 and CYP3A4.[6,25,27,59] Such systems are valuable for initial high throughput screening studies at the early stages of compound selection and development, but should not be considered as a substitute for studies with human hepatocytes.

14.5.2 Studies in Rodents

The induction of hepatic CYP enzymes in rodents can be assessed by *in vitro*, *ex vivo* and *in vivo* methods. In the early stages of compound development, where only small amounts of compounds are available, use can be made of primary hepatocyte cultures. Many studies have demonstrated that the induction of CYP enzymes in various subfamilies can be readily demonstrated in cultured rat and mouse hepatocytes. As with human hepatocytes, CYP enzyme induction can be assessed by measuring CYP mRNA levels, CYP enzyme activities and CYP protein levels. Overall, *in vitro* studies with cultured hepatocytes can be useful for initial compound screening and for subsequent candidate selection from a series of compounds.

The induction of hepatic CYP enzymes in rodents can be readily assessed by the *ex vivo* analysis of liver samples from toxicology studies (*e.g.* 7, 14, 28 and 90 day studies). The focus of such studies is normally to assess CYP1A, CYP2B,

CYP3A and CYP4A enzyme induction. If required, screening for induction of other CYP enzymes (*e.g.* CYP2E1) can be added to such studies. To gain an initial assessment of potential CYP enzyme induction, it is useful to determine both hepatic microsomal CYP and protein content. With respect to hepatic microsomal total CYP content, many CYP enzyme inducers increase total CYP content and hence, while not providing any information on which CYP subfamily/subfamilies are induced, this simple measurement clearly identifies the test compound as a CYP enzyme inducer.[34,60] Similarly, treatment with many rodent hepatic CYP enzyme inducers results in a proliferation of the smooth endoplasmic reticulum.[33,34,60] When preparing microsomal fractions from liver samples by normal differential centrifugation procedures, losses will occur and hence observed microsomal protein yield will be lower than the theoretical yield of microsomal content. However, the determination of hepatic microsomal protein content provides a simple measurement of whether treatment with a compound has resulted in an increase in the endoplasmic reticulum of hepatocytes, and hence can provide some information on whether the compound may be an inducer of hepatic CYP enzymes.

To gain information on whether a compound is an inducer of hepatic microsomal CYP enzymes in a specific subfamily/subfamilies, available experimental procedures include determination of the effects on CYP mRNA levels, marker enzyme activities and CYP protein levels. Table 14.3 shows some recommended mRNA and CYP-dependent enzyme activity markers to assess the induction of CYP1A, CYP2B, CYP3A and CYP4A enzymes in rat and mouse liver.

With respect to the measurement of CYP-dependent enzyme activities, some care is required in the interpretation of the data obtained. For example, while 7-ethoxyresorufin *O*-deethylase is a good marker for determination

Table 14.3 Some mRNA and enzyme activity markers for the induction of CYP enzymes in rat and mouse liver.

	mRNA		CYP enzyme activity	
CYP subfamily	Rat	Mouse	Preferred	Alternative
CYP1A	CYP1A2	Cyp1a2	7-Ethoxyresorufin *O*-deethylase	7-Methoxyresorufin *O*-demethylase
CYP2B	CYP2B1	Cyp2b10	7-Pentoxyresorufin *O* depentylase	7-Benzyloxyresorufin *O*-debenzylase Testosterone 16β-hydroxylase
CYP3A	CYP3A1	Cyp3a11	Testosterone 6β-hydroxylase	7-Benzyloxyquinoline *O*-debenzylase
CYP4A	CYP4A1	Cyp4a10	Lauric acid 12-hydroxylase	[Palmitoyl-CoA oxidation[a]]

[a]Rodent PPARα agonists induce both peroxisomal and microsomal (CYP4A-dependent) and fatty acid oxidising enzymes. Cyanide-insensitive palmitoyl-CoA oxidation is a specific measure of the peroxisomal fatty acid β-oxidation cycle and hence may be employed as an alternative endpoint to microsomal lauric acid 12-hydroxylase activity when screening for effects on CYP4A enzymes.[8]

of the effects of a compound on hepatic microsomal CYP1A enzymes, this enzyme activity will be increased to a small extent by other CYP subfamily enzyme inducers, such as PB.[60-62] In the case of PB and other CYP2B subfamily enzyme inducers, the effect on the CYP1A marker 7-ethoxyresorufin *O*-deethylase will be much less than the effect on the CYP2B marker 7-pentoxyresorufin *O*-depentylase. If the assessment of effects on CYP2E1 is required, a commonly employed enzyme activity marker is 4-nitrophenol hydroxylase.[3] However, while this enzyme's activity is increased by CYP2E inducers, such as isoniazid, it is not a specific marker for hepatic CYP2E1.

Hepatic microsomal CYP enzyme induction in rodent liver can also be assessed by the measurement of CYP protein levels by employing suitable CYP subfamily-specific antibodies with either Western immunoblotting or ELISA assays. The determination of CYP protein levels may be useful when administration of a test compound results in the inhibition of CYP enzyme activities due to the presence of tight binding metabolites. For example, treatment with the CYP3A inducers TAO and clotrimazole can result in an apparent inhibition rather than induction of CYP enzyme activities, with TAO also interfering with the spectral determination of total CYP content in rat liver microsomes.[34]

The induction of CYP enzymes in rodent liver *in vivo* may be indicated by changes in the pharmacokinetics of the test compound due to autoinduction. This may result in reduced test compound exposure in rodent toxicity studies and hence in the inadequate safety assessment of the test compound.

If studies with normal (*i.e.* wild type) animals indicate that the compound is an inducer of one or more CYP enzyme subfamilies, this conclusion can be confirmed by the use of transgenic animals that lack nuclear and other receptors for hepatic CYP enzyme induction. For mice, animals lacking the nuclear receptors CAR, PXR and PPARα are commercially available, with CAR knockout rats also now available. Thus the CAR activator PB will not induce CYP2B enzymes in CAR knockout mice and the PPARα activator Wy-14,643 will not induce CYP4A enzymes in PPARα knockout mice.[63-66]

14.6 Importance of Hepatic CYP Enzyme Induction

Drug therapy in humans often involves the administration of multiple therapeutic agents, which can lead to drug–drug interactions.[6,13,14] Such drug–drug interactions may be due to one drug either inhibiting or inducing the metabolism of another drug with resultant alterations in the pharmacological effects of the co-administered therapeutic agent. Only drug–drug interactions due to enzyme induction will be considered in this chapter. In contrast to humans, due to receptor activation, hepatic CYP enzyme induction by nongenotoxic agents in rodents may be associated with the formation of tumours in the liver and other tissues such as the thyroid gland. For example, liver tumour formation in rodents can be associated with the activation of either CAR or PPARα. The modes of action (MOAs) for rodent liver tumour formation by nongenotoxic CAR and PPARα activators, together with a MOA for rodent thyroid gland tumour formation also involving hepatic enzyme induction, are considered below.

14.6.1 Adverse Effects of Hepatic CYP Enzyme Induction in Humans

Hepatic CYP enzyme induction in humans can occur following the administration of therapeutic agents and by other factors such as the consumption of herbal remedies, certain foodstuffs, industrial chemicals and environmental pollutants.[6,11,13,14] The induction of hepatic CYP enzymes can affect the metabolism and pharmacological effects of therapeutic agents in two ways. For compounds where the parent form is the active therapeutic agent, CYP induction can result in increased metabolism and elimination resulting in a reduction in the desired pharmacological effect of the parent drug. Conversely, for prodrugs where the desired pharmacological effect is due to one or more metabolite(s), CYP induction can result in an increased or prolonged pharmacological effect.

One much studied therapeutic agent is RIF, which is a potent inducer of a number of human hepatic CYP enzymes including CYP2B6, CYP2C9, CYP2C19 and CYP3A4.[5-7] The administration of RIF to human subjects has been shown to increase the clearance of many therapeutic agents that are metabolised by CYP2C and CYP3A enzymes. For example, the treatment of human subjects with RIF has been shown to enhance the metabolism of rosiglitazone, (*S*)-warfarin and (*R*)-warfarin, which are predominantly metabolised by CYP2C enzymes, resulting in reduced area under the plasma concentration–time curve profiles.[14] Similarly, RIF treatment has been shown to result in reduced area under the plasma concentration–time curve profiles in human subjects given cyclosporin, diazepam, indinavir, midazolam, nifedipine, triazolam and zolpidem, which are predominantly metabolised by CY3A enzymes.[14] Such effects can result in clinically important drug–drug interactions due to the induction of hepatic CYP enzymes. Examples of such drug–drug interactions include cyclosporin (reduction in blood levels of the immunosuppressive agent leading to organ transplant rejection), the human immunodeficiency virus (HIV) protease inhibitors indinavir, ritonavir and saquinavir (reduced systemic exposure leading to a diminished antiretroviral effect), oral contraceptives (unplanned pregnancies), and warfarin (reduced anticoagulant effect).[6,13,14]

The induction of human hepatic CYP enzymes may result in enhanced toxicity of drugs and other chemicals. For example, paracetamol (acetaminophen) is metabolised by CYP2E1 to a reactive metabolite, namely *N*-acetyl-*p*-benzoquinone imine. As CYP2E1 is induced in subjects who consume large quantities of alcohol, such subjects can be more susceptible to paracetamol-induced hepatotoxicity.[5,14]

As well as drugs and other xenobiotics, human hepatic CYP enzymes can also metabolise endogenous compounds such as folic acid, steroids and vitamin D. The chronic administration of CYP enzyme inducing anticonvulsant drugs has been shown to be associated with disorders of bone metabolism in epileptic subjects.[67,68]

A number of herbal remedies have also been shown to induce human hepatic CYP enzymes.[6,11,69] One much studied example is that of St John's wort, which is prepared from the flowers and leaves of the plant *Hypericum perforatum* and is used as an antidepressant. One component of St John's wort is hyperforin, a lipophilic acylphloroglucinol that is a known PXR activator and inducer of CYP3A4 mRNA in cultured human hepatocytes. In addition, while extracts of St John's wort can inhibit human hepatic CYP enzymes *in vitro*, studies in human subjects have demonstrated increased levels of hepatic CYP3A4 and intestinal CYP3A4 and P-glycoprotein. Such effects have resulted in several reports of a reduction in the therapeutic effect of the immunosuppressive agent cyclosporin, resulting in tissue rejection. Other reported drug–drug interactions with St John's wort include interactions with the HIV protease inhibitor indinavir, the anticoagulant warfarin and oral contraceptives. All of these St John's wort–drug interactions appear to be attributable to enzyme induction, in particular to the stimulation of the hepatic CYP3A4 enzyme. Several other herbal preparations have also been shown to either induce or inhibit hepatic CYP enzymes in humans and rodents.[69]

14.6.2 Adverse Effects of Hepatic CYP Enzyme Induction in Rodents

The induction of hepatic CYP enzymes in rodents can be associated with tumour formation in both the liver and other tissues. Indeed, in the liver the activation of receptors for CYP enzyme induction, such as CAR and PPARα, results not only in the induction of CYP and other xenobiotic metabolising enzymes, but also genes associated with a number of physiological processes, including cell proliferation and apoptosis. Hepatic CYP enzyme induction is thus part of a pleotropic response to the chemical inducer that is not restricted solely to effects on xenobiotic metabolising enzyme activities.

In recent years frameworks have been established for analysing the MOAs by which chemicals can produce tumours in the liver and other organs of rodents, and the relevance of such tumours for human risk assessment have been developed by both the International Programme on Chemical Safety (IPCS) and by the International Life Sciences Institute's Risk Sciences Institute.[70–72] In order to assess the human relevance of a proposed rodent MOA for tumour formation, the IPCS Human Relevance Framework requires answers to the three questions listed below:

1. Is the weight of evidence sufficient to establish a MOA in animals?
2. Can human relevance of the MOA be reasonably excluded on the basis of fundamental qualitative differences in key events between experimental animals and humans?
3. Can the human relevance of the MOA be reasonably excluded on the basis of quantitative differences in either kinetic or dynamic factors between animals and humans?[71]

The liver is a common site of tumour formation in rat and mouse carcinogenicity studies.[73] For nongenotoxic agents, established MOAs for rodent liver tumour formation include activation of AhR, activation of CAR, activation of PPARα, cytotoxicity, hormonal perturbation, immunosuppression and porphyria.[8,21,22,70,74–77] In addition, a number of nongenotoxic chemicals have been shown to produce thyroid tumours in rodents.[78–80] The MOAs by which nongenotoxic chemicals may disrupt thyroid gland function include interference with thyroid hormone synthesis or secretion, increased thyroid hormone catabolism and excretion, and disruption of the conversion of thyroxine (T_4) to triiodothyronine (T_3).[80] This chapter will focus on rodent liver tumour formation by MOAs involving activation of CAR and PPARα, together with thyroid gland tumour formation due to induction of hepatic xenobiotic metabolising enzymes.

14.6.2.1   Rodent Liver Tumour Formation Due to CAR or PPARα Activation

With respect to the relevance of the hepatocarcinogenic hazard of nongenotoxic rodent CYP inducers for humans, two well established MOAs for rodent liver tumour formation by nongenotoxic CYP enzyme inducers comprise compounds that activate either CAR or PPARα. MOA analysis for both CAR activators and PPARα activators have been described in a number of publications.[8,21,22,74–76] More recently, MOA evaluations for these two classes of nongenotoxic rodent hepatocarcinogen were developed in two published papers from a Nuclear Receptors Workshop held in September 2010 and will be described below. At this meeting, to derive MOAs for these two classes of nongenotoxic CYP inducers, the IPCS Human Relevance Framework described above was modified to consider agreed definitions for key events, and also for associative events and modulating factors.[21,22] While key events are required events for the MOA, associative events are not causal necessary key events, but can be reliable indicators of key events. Although modulating factors are not necessary to induce tumour formation, such factors may modulate the dose response or the probability of inducing tumour formation.

The key events, together with some associative events and modulating factors for the MOAs for rodent liver tumour formation by CAR and PPARα activators are shown in Table 14.4. For CAR, the model compound was PB, whereas for PPARα data for a number of PPARα activators including di-(2-ethylhexyl)phthalate (DEHP) and gemfibrozil were used.[21,22] In terms of key events for both MOAs, the first step is receptor activation, which leads to increased cell proliferation, the formation of altered foci and subsequently liver tumour formation. The mitogenic effects of both CAR and PPARα activators in rodent liver are thus pivotal to subsequent liver tumour formation. The associative events and modulating factors for

Table 14.4   Key and associative events and modulating factors for the MOAs for rodent liver tumour formation by CAR and PPARα activators.[a]

Parameter	CAR activators	PPARα activators
Key events	CAR activation	PPARα activation
	Altered gene expression specific to CAR activation	Alteration in cell growth pathways
	Increased cell proliferation	Perturbation of cell growth and survival
	Clonal expansion leading to altered foci	Selective clonal expansion of preneoplastic foci cells
	Liver adenomas/carcinomas	Liver tumours
Associative events and modulating factors	Altered epigenetic changes specific to CAR activation	Alterations in lipid metabolising and lipid transport enzymes
	CYP2B induction	Hypolipidaemic effect
	Liver hypertrophy	Increases in oxidative stress
	Inhibition of apoptosis	NF-κB activation
	Inhibition of gap junctional intercellular communication	Inhibition of gap junctional intercellular communication

[a]For further details see Elcombe *et al.* (2014)[21] and Corton *et al.* (2014).[22]

both MOAs include induction of CYP2B enzymes and liver hypertrophy for CAR activators, and effects on lipid metabolising and lipid transport enzymes, and a hypolipidaemic effect for PPARα activators. Both CAR and PPARα activators can inhibit gap junctional intercellular communication in rodent liver.

Thus in agreement with previous evaluations, robust MOAs for rodent liver tumour formation by both CAR and PPARα activators were established.[21,22] In terms of the human relevance of these rodent liver tumour MOAs, the key species difference is that while CAR and PPARα activators are mitogenic agents in rodent hepatocytes, they do not appear to stimulate replicative DNA synthesis in human hepatocytes. However, some of the other effects of CAR and PPARα activators observed in rodents can also be observed in humans. For example, for CAR activators CYP enzymes (*e.g.* CYP2B6 and CYP3A4) can be induced in human liver, and PPARα activators can produce a hypolipidaemic effect in humans.[21,22]

The key role of increased cell proliferation in these two MOAs for rodent liver tumour formation has been demonstrated in studies performed in mice lacking either CAR or PPARα. Thus in CAR knockout mice, PB does not stimulate replicative DNA synthesis in hepatocytes and does not promote liver tumour formation after treatment with a genotoxic carcinogen.[63–65] Similarly, the potent PPARα activator Wy-14,643 does not stimulate replicative DNA synthesis in hepatocytes and does not produce liver tumours in PPARα knockout mice.[81]

The observation that both CAR and PPARα activators do not stimulate replicative DNA synthesis in human liver comes from *in vitro* studies with cultured human hepatocytes and *in vivo* studies with humanised mice. The effects of a number of CAR and PPARα activators on replicative DNA synthesis in cultured rat and human hepatocytes is shown in Table 14.5. In keeping with *in vivo* studies, the CYP2B and CYP4A inducers listed all stimulate replicative DNA synthesis in cultured rat hepatocytes.[82–89] On the other hand, such compounds do not appear to stimulate replicative DNA synthesis in cultured human hepatocytes. However, while human hepatocytes are refractory to the effects of rodent CAR and PPARα activators, replicative DNA synthesis could be stimulated in cultured human hepatocytes with either epidermal growth factor or hepatocyte growth factor, thus confirming the functional viability of the human hepatocyte preparations used. In a recent *in vivo* study, the effect of NaPB was studied in chimeric mice with humanised livers and in CD-1 mice and Wistar rats.[90] The chimeric mice were obtained by transplanting human heptatocytes into albumin enhancer/promoter driven urokinase-type plasminogen activator-transgenic severe combined immunodeficiency (uPA/SCID) mice. While NaPB could produce liver hypertrophy and induction of CYP enzymes in CD-1 mice, Wistar rats and humanised mice, stimulation of replicative DNA synthesis was only observed in CD-1 mice and Wistar rats. It should be noted

Table 14.5 Examples of species differences in the effects of CYP2B and CYP4A enzyme inducers on replicative DNA synthesis in cultured rat and human hepatocytes.

CYP enzyme inducer	Compound	Replicative DNA synthesis[a] Rat	Human	References
CYP2B	α-Hexachlorocyclohexane	Yes	No	82
	Metofluthrin	Yes	No	83 and 84
	PB	Yes	No	82–84
	Pyrethrins	Yes	No	85
CYP4A	Bezafibrate	Yes	No	86
	Ciprofibrate	Yes	No	86 and 87
	Clofibric acid	Yes	No	86
	DEHP	Yes	No	86
	Diisononyl phthalate	Yes	No	88
	2-Ethylhexanoic acid	Yes	No	89
	Fomesafen	Yes	No	89
	Methylclofenapate	Yes	No	89
	Mono-(2-ethylhexyl) phthalate	Yes	No	88
	Nafenopin	Yes	No	82 and 86

[a]Hepatocyte replicative DNA synthesis was determined as the hepatocyte labelling index or by incorporation of either BrdU or [³H]thymidine into DNA. Response is defined as: Yes: increase in replicative DNA synthesis; or No: no or little increase in replicative DNA synthesis.

that the humanised mice were given doses of NaPB up to the maximum tolerated dose, which resulted in PB blood levels 3–5-fold higher than those observed in human subjects given therapeutic doses of PB. For PPARα activators, studies have been conducted with transgenic mice in which mouse PPARα has been replaced with human PPARα. While treatment of the PPARα-humanised mice with Wy-14,643 resulted in an induction of fatty acid oxidation genes and a reduction in serum triglyceride levels, there was no induction of cell cycle genes and no increase in replicative DNA synthesis.[91,92] Although Wy-14,643 produced adenomas and carcinomas in wild type mice, only a single adenoma was observed in 1 out of 20 PPARα-humanised mice.[93] This single adenoma was morphologically similar to a spontaneous mouse liver tumour and hence may not have arisen as a consequence of Wy-14,643 treatment. The hepatic effects of the PPARα activator fenofibrate have also been studied in wild type and chimeric mice with humanised livers employing the same chimeric mouse model described above. While fenofibrate increased replicative DNA synthesis in hepatocytes of wild type mice, there was no stimulation of replicative DNA synthesis in the human hepatocytes of the chimeric mice.[94] Overall, the available studies with both cultured human hepatocytes *in vitro* and with humanised mice *in vivo* provide convincing evidence that human hepatocytes are refractory to the mitogenic effects of rodent CAR and PPARα activators.

For CAR activators, based on the marked species difference in effects on replicative DNA synthesis, the Workshop panel concluded that the MOA for PB-induced rodent liver tumour formation was qualitatively not plausible for humans.[21] The PPARα Workshop panel concluded that there were significant quantitative differences in PPARα activator-induced effects between rodents and humans and hence the majority of the panel felt that the rodent MOA was not relevant to humans.[22]

The conclusion that the MOAs for rodent liver tumour formation by CAR and PPARα activators are not relevant for humans is supported by available epidemiological data.[21,22] For example, a recent evaluation of the available literature for PB concluded that there was no evidence of a specific role of PB in human liver cancer risk.[95] Moreover, in such studies showing no evidence of increased cancer risk, the subjects received PB for many years at doses that produced similar plasma concentrations to those that are carcinogenic in mice. In addition, epidemiological studies in humans given the hypolipidaemic drugs clofibrate and gemfibrozil have not demonstrated any increase in cancer mortality.[22]

The literature does contain some examples of the application of the IPCS MOA framework to rodent liver tumours induced by some pesticides. For example, CAR activation MOAs have been established for cyproconazole, metofluthrin, propiconazole, pyrethrins and sulfoxaflor, which all produce liver tumours in rats and/or mice.[85,96–101] In addition, the mouse liver tumours produced by the herbicide pronamide have been shown to be due to activation of both CAR and PPARα.[102]

14.6.2.2 Rodent Thyroid Gland Tumour Formation Due to Hepatic Enzyme Induction

A number of nongenotoxic chemicals have been shown to produce thyroid tumours in rodents by a MOA in which circulating thyroid hormone levels are decreased as a result of increased hepatic metabolism and clearance.[70,78,80] For example, PB is known to promote rodent thyroid gland follicular cell tumours and a MOA involving induction of hepatic xenobiotic metabolising enzymes has been established.[70] Generally, for this MOA rats are more susceptible than mice, with male rats being more susceptible than female rats.[78,79] The MOA for PB-induced rodent thyroid gland follicular cell tumour formation involves hormonal dysfunction due to induction of hepatic phase II conjugative enzymes.[70,80,103–107] In this MOA, thyroxine T_4 conjugation is enhanced due to the stimulation of hepatic microsomal UGT activities toward T_4 as substrate. Such hepatic enzyme induction results in increased biliary excretion of T_4 and a decrease in serum T_3 and/or T_4 levels, which results in a compensatory increase in serum thyroid stimulating hormone (TSH) levels. In the rodent thyroid gland the increase in TSH levels results in thyroid gland follicular cell growth and hyperplasia. The chronic stimulation of the rodent thyroid gland by TSH is known to result in thyroid follicular cell hyperplasia and subsequently in the formation of thyroid follicular cell adenomas and carcinomas.[78,80,104]

The IPCS framework was applied to evaluate a MOA for rat thyroid gland follicular cell tumours produced by the herbicide thiazopyr.[108] MOA studies in the rat demonstrated that treatment with thiazopyr resulted in increased thyroid gland weight, thyroid gland follicular cell hypertrophy, increased biliary excretion of T_4, decreased serum T_4 levels, increased serum TSH levels and an induction of hepatic microsomal UGT activity towards T_4 as substrate.[108,109] Table 14.6 shows the key events identified for thiazopyr-induced rat thyroid gland follicular cell tumour formation. Another example of the application of this MOA was in studies with pyrethrins (the insecticide components of pyrethrum extract), which have also been shown to produce thyroid gland follicular cell tumours in rats.[110] MOA studies demonstrated that the treatment of rats with pyrethrins resulted in increased thyroid gland weight, thyroid gland follicular cell hypertrophy, increased thyroid gland follicular cell replicative DNA synthesis, decreased serum T_3 and T_4 levels, increased serum TSH levels,

Table 14.6 Key events for the MOA of thiazopyr-induced rat thyroid gland tumour formation.

Key event[a]
Induction of hepatic UGT activity
Increase in hepatic metabolism and biliary excretion of T_4
Decrease in serum T_4 half-life and concentration
Increase in circulating TSH concentration
Cellular thyroid hypertrophy and follicular cell hyperplasia

[a]Key events taken from Dellarco *et al.* (2006).[108]

and an induction of hepatic microsomal UGT activity towards T_4 as substrate. In addition to PB and pyrethrins, which are CYP2B inducers and hence CAR activators, the CYP3A inducer PCN has also been shown to increase thyroid gland weight, increase thyroid gland follicular cell replicative DNA synthesis, increase biliary excretion of T_4, decrease serum T_4 levels, increase serum TSH levels and increase hepatic microsomal UGT activity towards T_4 as substrate in the rat.[105–107,111] Thus, this MOA for rodent thyroid gland follicular cell tumour formation is not restricted to CAR activators, but could also apply to activators of PXR and other receptors, where receptor activation results in an induction of hepatic microsomal UGT activity towards T_4 as substrate.

While this MOA is well established in rodents, it is not applicable to humans because of quantitative species differences.[70,78,80,104] Compared with humans, rats have higher constitutive serum TSH levels and shorter half-lives of both T_3 and T_4. The much greater half-lives of serum T_3 and T_4 in humans are due to the presence of a high-affinity serum T_4-binding globulin, which is absent in the rat. While T_4 can be bound to serum transthyretin and albumin in rats, these proteins have a much lower affinity for T_4 than human thyroxine-binding globulin. Hence, in the rat, unlike humans, a substantial portion of serum T_4 will be unbound. In rodents a number of hepatic CYP enzyme inducers have been shown to increase serum TSH levels, whereas in humans, studies with enzyme inducers such as PB and RIF have demonstrated that, while serum T_4 levels may be affected, no increase is observed in TSH levels.[104] In addition, there is no epidemiological evidence in humans associating prolonged administration of PB with an increased incidence of thyroid gland cancer.[70,104] Overall, this MOA for rodent liver tumour formation is quantitatively not plausible for humans.

14.7 Conclusions

A wide variety of chemicals can induce hepatic CYP enzymes in humans and in rodents. The induction of CYP enzymes normally occurs by receptor mediated mechanisms leading to an increase in gene transcription. While some compounds induce CYP enzymes in both humans and rodents, marked species differences can exist. Hepatic CYP enzyme induction can produce adverse effects in humans due to enhanced metabolism of therapeutic agents. In some instances, the induction of hepatic CYP and other xenobiotic metabolising enzymes in rodents can be associated with tumour formation in the liver and other tissues.

References

1. R. T. Williams, *Detoxication Mechanisms: The Metabolism and Detoxication of Drugs, Toxic Substances and Other Organic Compounds*, Chapman and Hall, London, 2nd edn, 1959.
2. D. V. Parke, *The Biochemistry of Foreign Compounds*, Pergamon, Oxford, 1968.

3. A. Parkinson, in *Casarett and Doull's Toxicology: the Basic Science of Poisons*, ed. C. D. Klaassen, McGraw Hill, New York, 6th edn, 2001, p. 133.

4. C. J. Omiecinski, J. P. Vanden Heuvel, G. H. Perdew and J. M. Peters, *Toxicol. Sci.*, 2011, **120**(1), S49.

5. O. Pelkonen, J. Mäenpää, P. Taavitsainen, A. Rautio and H. Raunio, *Xenobiotica*, 1998, **28**, 1203.

6. O. Pelkonen, M. Turpeinen, J. Hakkola, P. Honkakoski, J. Hukkanen and H. Raunio, *Arch. Toxicol.*, 2008, **82**, 667.

7. M. Martignoni, G. M. M. Groothuis and R. de Kanter, *Expert Opin. Drug Metab. Toxicol.*, 2006, **2**, 875.

8. B. G. Lake, *Xenobiotica*, 2009, **39**, 582.

9. A. E. Rettie and E. J. Kelly, in *Cytochromes P450: Role in the Metabolism and Toxicity of Drugs and Other Xenobiotics*, ed. C. Ioannides, RSC Publishing, Cambridge, 2008, p. 384.

10. H. Raunio, J. Hakkola and O. Pelkonen, in *Cytochromes P450: Role in the Metabolism and Toxicity of Drugs and Other Xenobiotics*, ed. C. Ioannides, RSC Publishing, Cambridge, 2008, p. 150.

11. N. J. Hewitt, E. L. LeCluyse and S. S. Ferguson, *Xenobiotica*, 2007, **37**, 1196.

12. D. T. Verhoeven, H. Verhagen, R. A. Goldbohm, P. A. van den Brandt and G. van Poppel, *Chem.-Biol. Interact.*, 1997, **103**, 79.

13. M. Dickins, *Curr. Top. Med. Chem.*, 2004, **4**, 1745.

14. J. H. Lin, *Pharm. Res.*, 2006, **23**, 1089.

15. K. Yoshinari, E. Tien, M. Negishi and P. Honkakoski, in *Cytochromes P450: Role in the Metabolism and Toxicity of Drugs and Other Xenobiotics*, ed. C. Ioannides, RSC Publishing, Cambridge, 2008, p. 417.

16. J.-M. Pascussi, S. Gebal-Chaloin, L. Drocourt, E. Assénat, D. Larrey, L. Pichard-Garcia, M.-J. Vilarem and P. Maurel, *Xenobiotica*, 2004, **34**, 633.

17. K. Yoshinari, N. Yoda, T. Toriyabe and Y. Yamazoe, *Biochem. Pharmacol.*, 2010, **79**, 261.

18. F. Hosseinpour, R. Moore, M. Negishi and T. Sueyoshi, *Mol. Pharmacol.*, 2006, **69**, 1095.

19. S. Mutoh, M. Osabe, K. Inoue, R. Moore, L. Pedersen, L. Perera, Y. Rebolloso, T. Sueyoshi and M. Negishi, *J. Biol. Chem.*, 2009, **284**, 34785.

20. S. Mutoh, M. Sobhany, R. Moore, L. Perera, L. Pedersen, T. Sueyoshi and M. Negishi, *Sci. Signal.*, 2013, **6**, ra31.

21. C. R. Elcombe, R. C. Peffer, D. C. Wolf, J. Bailey, R. Bars, D. Bell, R. C. Cattley, S. S. Ferguson, D. Geter, A. Goetz, J. I. Goodman, S. Hester, A. Jacobs, C. J. Omiecinski, R. Schoeny, W. Xie and B. G. Lake, *Crit. Rev. Toxicol.*, 2014, **44**, 64.

22. J. C. Corton, M. L. Cunningham, B. T. Hummer, C. Lau, B. Meek, J. M. Peters, J. A. Popp, L. Rhomberg, J. Seed and J. E. Klaunig, *Crit. Rev. Toxicol.*, 2014, **44**, 1.

23. E. S. Tien and M. Negishi, *Xenobiotica*, 2006, **36**, 1152.

24. W. Xie, J. L. Barwick, C. M. Simon, A. M. Pierce, S. Safe, B. Blumberg, P. S. Guzelian and R. M. Evans, *Genes Dev.*, 2000, **14**, 3014.

25. L. B. Moore, D. J. Parks, S. A. Jones, R. K. Bledsoe, T. G. Consler, J. B. Stimmel, B. Goodwin, C. Liddle, S. G. Blanchard, T. M. Willson, J. L. Collins and S. A. Kliewer, *J. Biol. Chem.*, 2000, **275**, 15112.

26. J. T. Moore, L. B. Moore, J. M. Maglich and S. A. Kliewer, *Biochim. Biophys. Acta*, 2003, **1619**, 235.

27. S. R. Faucette, T.-C. Zhang, R. Moore, T. Sueyoshi, C. J. Omiecinski, E. L. LeCluyse, M. Negishi and H. Wang, *J. Pharmacol. Exp. Ther.*, 2007, **320**, 72.

28. P. Wei, J. Zhang, D. H. Dowhan, Y. Han and D. D. Moore, *Pharmacogenomics J.*, 2002, **2**, 117.

29. J. M. Maglich, C. M. Stoltz, B. Goodwin, D. Hawkins-Brown, J. T. Moore and S. A. Kliewer, *Mol. Pharmacol.*, 2002, **62**, 638.

30. S. Gerbal-Chaloin, J.-M. Pascussi, L. Pichard-Garcia, M. Daujat, F. Waechter, J.-M. Fabre, N. Carrère and P. Maurel, *Drug Metab. Dispos.*, 2001, **29**, 242.

31. H. Wang, S. R. Faucette, D. Gilbert, S. L. Jolley, T. Sueyoshi, M. Negishi and E. L. LeCluyse, *Drug Metab. Dispos.*, 2003, **31**, 620.

32. D. J. Waxman and L. Azaroff, *Biochem. J.*, 1992, **281**, 577.

33. R. W. Nims and R. A. Lubet, in *Cytochromes P450: Metabolic and Toxicological Aspects*, ed. C. Ioannides, CRC Press, Boca Raton, 1996, p. 135.

34. B. G. Lake, A. B. Renwick, M. E. Cunninghame, R. J. Price, D. Surry and D. C. Evans, *Toxicology*, 1998, **131**, 9.

35. R. G. Bars, A. M. Mitchell, C. R. Wolf and C. R. Elcombe, *Biochem. J.*, 1989, **262**, 151.

36. C. Tang, J. H. Lin and A. Y. H. Lu, *Drug Metab. Dispos.*, 2005, **33**, 603.

37. I. Tzameli, P. Pissios, E. G. Schuetz and D. D. Moore, *Mol. Cell. Biol.*, 2000, **20**, 2951.

38. J. M. Maglich, D. J. Parks, L. B. Moore, J. L. Collins, B. Goodwin, A. N. Billin, C. A. Stoltz, S. A. Kliewer, M. H. Lambert, T. M. Willson and J. T. Moore, *J. Biol. Chem.*, 2003, **278**, 17277.

39. V. O. Pustylnyak, A. N. Lebedev, L. F. Gulyaeva, V. V. Lyakhovich and N. M. Slynko, *Life Sci.*, 2007, **80**, 324.

40. B. A. Diwan, J. R. Henneman, J. M. Rice and R. W. Nims, *Carcinogenesis*, 1996, **17**, 37.

41. I. N. White, A. Davies, L. L. Smith, S. Dawson and F. De Matteis, *Biochem. Pharmacol.*, 1993, **45**, 21.

42. S. M. Fontaine, P. B. Hoyer, J. R. Halpert and I. G. Sipes, *Drug Metab. Dispos.*, 2001, **29**, 1236.

43. S. A. Jones, L. B. Moore, J. L. Shenk, G. B. Wisely, G. A. Hamilton, D. D. McKee, N. C. Tomkinson, E. L. LeCluyse, M. H. Lambert, T. M. Willson, S. A. Kliewer and J. T. Moore, *Mol. Endocrinol.*, 2000, **14**, 27.

44. L. Richert, C. Lamboley, C. Viollon-Abadie, P. Grass, N. Hartmann, S. Laurent, B. Heyd, G. Mantion, S.-D. Chibout and F. Staedtler, *Toxicol. Appl. Pharmacol.*, 2003, **191**, 130.

45. W. Xie, J. L. Barwick, M. Downes, B. Blumberg, C. M. Simon, M. C. Nelson, B. A. Neuschwander-Tetri, E. M. Brunt, P. S. Guzelian and R. M. Evans, *Nature*, 2000, **406**, 435.

46. K. P. Kanebratt, U. Diczfalusy, T. Bäckström, E. Sparve, E. Bredberg, Y. Böttiger, T. B. Andersson and L. Bertilsson, *Clin. Pharmacol. Ther.*, 2008, **84**, 589.

47. E. L. LeCluyse, R. P. Witek, M. E. Andersen and M. J. Powers, *Crit. Rev. Toxicol.*, 2012, **42**, 501.

48. E. Alexandre, A. Baze, C. Parmentier, C. Desbans, D. Pekthong, B. Gerin, C. Wack, P. Bachellier, B. Heyd, J.-C. Weber and L. Richert, *Xenobiotica*, 2012, **42**, 968.

49. R. J. Price, D. Surry, A. B. Renwick, G. Meneses-Lorente, B. G. Lake and D. C. Evans, *Xenobiotica*, 2000, **30**, 781.

50. M. T. Donato, N. Jiménez, J. V. Castell and M. J. Gómez-Lechón, *Drug Metab. Dispos.*, 2004, **32**, 699.

51. K. P. Kanebratt and T. B. Andersson, *Drug Metab. Dispos.*, 2008, **36**, 137.

52. M. Turpeinen, A. Tolonen, C. Chesne, A. Guillouzo, J. Uusitalo and O. Pelkonen, *Toxicol. In Vitro*, 2009, **23**, 748.

53. S. R. Faucette, H. Wang, G. A. Hamilton, S. L. Jolley, D. Gilbert, C. Lindley, B. Yan, M. Negishi and E. L. LeCluyse, *Drug Metab. Dispos.*, 2004, **32**, 348.

54. A. Madan, R. A. Graham, K. M. Carroll, D. R. Mudra, L. A. Burton, L. A. Krueger, A. D. Downey, M. Czerwinski, J. Forster, M. D. Ribadeneira, L.-S. Gan, E. L. LeCluyse, K. Zech, P. Robertson, Jr., P. Koch, L. Antonian, G. Wagner, L. Yu and A. Parkinson, *Drug Metab. Dispos.*, 2003, **31**, 421.

55. L. Pichard-Garcia, R. Hyland, J. Baulieu, J.-M. Fabre, A. Milton and P. Maurel, *Drug Metab. Dispos.*, 2000, **28**, 51.

56. B. G. Lake and R. J. Price, *Xenobiotica*, 2013, **43**, 41.

57. C. Ioannides, *Xenobiotica*, 2013, **43**, 15.

58. D. F. McGinnity, G. Zhang, J. R. Kenny, G. A. Hamilton, S. Otmani, K. R. Stams, S. Haney, P. Brassil, D. M. Stresser and R. J. Riley, *Drug Metab. Dispos.*, 2009, **37**, 1259.

59. S. R. Faucette, T. Sueyoshi, C. M. Smith, M. Negishi, E. L. LeCluyse and H. Wang, *J. Pharmacol. Exp. Ther.*, 2006, **317**, 1200.

60. A. B. Renwick, G. Lavignette, P. D. Worboys, B. Williams, D. Surry, D. F. V. Lewis, R. J. Price, B. G. Lake and D. C. Evans, *Xenobiotica*, 2001, **31**, 861.

61. M. D. Burke, S. Thompson, C. R. Elcombe, J. Halpert, T. Haaparanta and R. T. Mayer, *Biochem. Pharmacol.*, 1985, **34**, 3337.

62. P. V. Nerurkar, S. S. Park, P. E. Thomas, R. W. Nims and R. A. Lubet, *Biochem. Pharmacol.*, 1993, **46**, 933.

63. P. Wie, J. Zhang, M. Egan-Hafley, S. Liang and D. D. Moore, *Nature*, 2000, **407**, 920.

64. W. Huang, J. Zhang, M. Washington, J. Liu, J. M. Parant, G. Lozano and D. D. Moore, *Mol. Endocrinol.*, 2005, **19**, 1646.

65. Y. Yamamoto, R. Moore, T. L. Goldsworthy, M. Negishi and R. R. Maronpot, *Cancer Res.*, 2004, **64**, 7197.

66. S. S.-T. Lee, T. Pineau, J. Drago, E. J. Lee, J. W. Owens, D. L. Kroetz, P. M. Fernandez-Salguero, H. Westphal and F. J. Gonzalez, *Mol. Cell. Biol.*, 1995, **15**, 3012.

67. D. L. Andress, J. Ozuna, D. Tirschwell, L. Grande, M. Johnson, A. F. Jacobson and W. Spain, *Arch. Neurol.*, 2002, **59**, 781.
68. A. M. Pack, M. J. Morrell, R. Marcus, L. Holloway, E. Flaster, S. Dŏne, A. Randall, C. Searle and E. Shane, *Ann. Neurol.*, 2005, **57**, 252.
69. C. Ioannides, *Xenobiotica*, 2002, **32**, 451.
70. M. E. Meek, J. R. Bucher, S. M. Cohen, V. Dellarco, R. N. Hill, L. D. Lehman-McKeeman, D. G. Longfellow, T. Pastoor, J. Seed and D. E. Patton, *Crit. Rev. Toxicol.*, 2003, **33**, 591.
71. A. R. Boobis, S. M. Cohen, V. Dellarco, D. McGregor, M. E. Meek, C. Vickers, D. Willcocks and W. Farland, *Crit. Rev. Toxicol.*, 2006, **36**, 781.
72. M. E. Meek, A. Boobis, I. Cote, V. Dellarco, G. Fotakis, S. Munn, J. Seed and C. Vickers, *J. Appl. Toxicol.*, 2014, **34**, 1.
73. L. S. Gold, N. B. Manley, T. H. Slone and J. M. Ward, *Toxicol. Pathol.*, 2001, **29**, 639.
74. M. P. Holsapple, H. C. Pitot, S. M. Cohen, A. R. Boobis, J. E. Klaunig, T. Pastoor, V. L. Dellarco and Y. P. Dragan, *Toxicol. Sci.*, 2006, **89**, 51.
75. S. M. Cohen, *Toxicol. Pathol.*, 2010, **38**, 487.
76. J. E. Klaunig, M. A. Babich, K. P. Baetcke, J. C. Cook, J. C. Corton, R. M. David, J. G. DeLuca, D. Y. Lai, R. H. McKee, J. M. Peters, R. A. Roberts and P. A. Fenner-Crisp, *Crit. Rev. Toxicol.*, 2003, **33**, 655.
77. R. A. Budinsky, D. Schrenk, T. Simon, M. Van den Berg, J. F. Reichard, J. B. Silkworth, L. L. Aylward, A. Brix, T. Gasiewicz, N. Kaminski, G. Perdew, T. B. Starr, N. J. Walker and J. C. Rowlands, *Crit. Rev. Toxicol.*, 2014, **44**, 83.
78. R. N. Hill, T. M. Crisp, P. M. Hurley, S. L. Rosenthal and D. V. Singh, *Environ. Health Perspect.*, 1998, **106**, 447.
79. P. M. Hurley, R. N. Hill and R. J. Whiting, *Environ. Health Perspect.*, 1998, **106**, 437.
80. C. C. Capen, in *Casarett and Doull's Toxicology: the Basic Science of Poisons*, ed. C. D. Klaassen, McGraw Hill, New York, 6th edn, 2001, p. 711.
81. J. M. Peters, R. C. Cattley and F. J. Gonzalez, *Carcinogeneis*, 1997, **18**, 2029.
82. W. Parzefall, E. Erber, R. Sedivy and R. Schulte-Hermann, *Cancer Res.*, 1991, **51**, 1143.
83. Y. Hirose, H. Nagahori, T. Yamada, Y. Deguchi, Y. Tomigahara, K. Nishioka, S. Uwagawa, S. Kawamura, N. Isobe, B. G. Lake and Y. Okuno, *Toxicology*, 2009, **258**, 64.
84. T. Yamada, H. Kikumoto, B. G. Lake and S. Kawamura, *Toxicol. Res.*, 2015, **4**, 901.
85. T. G. Osimitz and B. G. Lake, *Crit. Rev. Toxicol.*, 2009, **39**, 501.
86. V. Goll, E. Alexandre, C. Viollin-Abadie, L. Nicod, D. Jaeck and L. Richert, *Toxicol. Appl. Pharmacol.*, 1999, **160**, 21.
87. C. E. Perrone, L. Shao and G. M. Williams, *Toxicol. Appl. Pharmacol.*, 1998, **150**, 277.
88. S. C. Hasmall, N. H. James, N. Macdonald, D. West, S. Chevalier, S. C. Cosulich and R. A. Roberts, *Arch. Toxicol.*, 1999, **73**, 451.

89. C. R. Elcombe, D. R. Bell, E. Elias, S. C. Hasmall and N. J. Plant, *Ann. N. Y. Acad. Sci.*, 1996, **804**, 628.

90. T. Yamada, Y. Okuda, M. Kushida, T. Sumida, H. Takeuchi, H. Nagahori, T. Fukuda, B. G. Lake, S. M. Cohen and S. Kawamura, *Toxicol. Sci.*, 2014, **142**, 137.

91. C. Cheung, T. E. Akiyama, J. M. Ward, C. J. Nicol, L. Feigenbaum, C. Vinson and F. J. Gonzalez, *Cancer Res.*, 2004, **64**, 3849.

92. Q. Yang, T. Nagano, Y. Shah, C. Cheung, S. Ito and F. J. Gonzalez, *Toxicol. Sci.*, 2008, **101**, 132.

93. K. Morimura, C. Cheung, J. M. Ward, J. K. Reddy and F. J. Gonzalez, *Carcinogenesis*, 2006, **27**, 1074.

94. C. Tateno, T. Yamamoto, R. Utoh, C. Yamasaki, Y. Ishida, Y. Myoken, K. Oofusa, M. Okada, N. Tsutsui and K. Yoshizato, *Toxicol. Pathol.*, 2015, **43**, 233.

95. C. La Vecchia and E. Negri, *Eur. J. Cancer Prev.*, 2014, **23**, 1.

96. R. C. Peffer, J. G. Moggs, T. Pastoor, R. A. Currie, J. Wright, G. Milburn, F. Waechter and I. Rusyn, *Toxicol. Sci.*, 2007, **99**, 315.

97. T. Yamada, S. Uwagawa, Y. Ukono, S. M. Cohen and H. Kaneko, *Toxicol. Sci.*, 2009, **108**, 59.

98. Y. Deguchi, T. Yamada, Y. Hirose, H. Nagahori, M. Kushida, K. Sumida, T. Sukata, Y. Tomigahara, K. Nishioka, S. Uwagawa, S. Kawamura and Y. Okuno, *Toxicol. Sci.*, 2009, **108**, 69.

99. R. A. Currie, R. C. Peffer, A. K. Goetz, C. J. Omiecinski and J. Goodman, *Toxicology*, 2014, **321**, 80.

100. R. J. Price, D. G. Walters, J. M. Finch, K. L. Gabriel, C. C. Capen, T. G. Osimitz and B. G. Lake, *Toxicol. Appl. Pharmacol.*, 2007, **218**, 186.

101. M. J. LeBaron, D. R. Geter, R. J. Rasoulpour, B. B. Gollapudi, J. Thomas, J. Murray, H. L. Kan, A. J. Wood, C. Elcombe, A. Vardy, J. McEwan, C. Terry and R. Billington, *Toxicol. Appl. Pharmacol.*, 2013, **270**, 164.

102. M. J. LeBaron, R. J. Rasoulpour, B. B. Gollapudi, R. Sura, H. L. Kan, M. R. Schisler, L. H. Pottenger, S. Papineni and D. L. Eisenbrandt, *Toxicol. Sci.*, 2014, **142**, 74.

103. R. M. McClain, A. A. Levin, R. Posch and J. C. Downing, *Toxicol. Appl. Pharmacol.*, 1989, **99**, 216.

104. P. G. Curran and L. J. DeGroot, *Endocr. Rev.*, 1991, **12**, 135.

105. R. A. Barter and C. D. Klaassen, *Toxicol. Appl. Pharmacol.*, 1994, **128**, 9.

106. A. Hood, R. Hashmi and C. D. Klaassen, *Toxicol. Appl. Pharmacol.*, 1999, **160**, 163.

107. A. Hood, J. Liu and C. D. Klaassen, *Toxicol. Sci.*, 1999, **50**, 45.

108. V. L. Dellarco, D. McGregor, C. Berry, S. M. Cohen and A. R. Boobis, *Crit. Rev. Toxicol.*, 2006, **36**, 793.

109. K. J. Hotz, A. G. E. Wilson, D. C. Thake, M. V. Roloff, C. C. Capen, J. M. Kronenberg and D. W. Brewster, *Toxicol. Appl. Pharmacol.*, 1997, **142**, 133.

110. J. M. Finch, T. G. Osimitz, K. L. Gabriel, T. Martin, W. J. Henderson, C. C. Capen, W. H. Butler and B. G. Lake, *Toxicol. Appl. Pharmacol.*, 2006, **214**, 253.

111. N. R. Vansell and C. D. Klaassen, *Toxicol. Appl. Pharmacol.*, 2001, **176**, 187.

CHAPTER 15

Current Status and Implications of Transporters: QSAR Analysis Method to Evaluate Drug–Drug Interactions of Human Bile Salt Export Pump (ABCB11/BSEP) and Prediction of Intrahepatic Cholestasis Risk

TOSHIHISA ISHIKAWA*[a,b], TAKEAKI FUKAMI[c],
MAKOTO NAGAKURA[c], AND HIROYUKI HIRANO[†b]

[a]NGO Personalized Medicine & Healthcare, 4-17-30 Kiriga-oka, Midori-ku, Yokohama 226-0016, Japan; [b]Graduate School of Bioscience and Biotechnology, Tokyo Institute of Technology, Nagatsuta, Yokohama 226-8501, Japan; [c]BioTec Co., Ltd, 2-29-4 Yushima, Bunkyo-ku, Tokyo 113-0034, Japan
*E-mail: toshihisa.ishikawa.r@gmail.com

[†]Present address: Center for Sustainable Resource Science, RIKEN, 2-1 Hirosawa, Wako 351-0198, Japan.

RSC Drug Discovery Series No. 49
New Horizons in Predictive Drug Metabolism and Pharmacokinetics
Edited by Alan G. E. Wilson
© The Royal Society of Chemistry 2016
Published by the Royal Society of Chemistry, www.rsc.org

15.1 Introduction

In the final decade of the 20th century, the development of high-throughput screening and combinatorial chemistry technologies helped to accelerate the process of drug discovery. In the 21st century, emerging genomic technologies (*i.e.* human genome analysis by next-generation sequencing, bioinformatics, systems biology, functional genomics, and pharmacogenomics) have been shifting the paradigm for drug discovery and development. However, drug discovery and development are high-risk and high-stakes ventures with long and costly timelines.[1,2] Indeed, drug-induced hepatotoxicity remains one of the major problems in drug discovery and development.[3] Over 90% of market withdrawals are caused by drug toxicity. As exemplified by troglitazone, hepatotoxicity and cardiovascular toxicity have been shown to be the major causes of market withdrawals in recent years.[4]

In clinical Phases I–III, 43% of drug development project terminations were due to insufficient efficacy of the investigated compound.[4] Selection of candidate compounds for preclinical studies in the drug discovery process is a critical step that can determine the speed and cost of clinical development. The attrition of drug candidates in preclinical and clinical development stages is a major issue in drug design. In at least 30% of cases, this attrition is due to poor pharmacokinetics and toxicity. Since drug development costs have exponentially increased during the past 20 years, pharmaceutical companies have begun to seriously re-evaluate their current strategies of drug discovery and development.[1,2]

Accumulating evidence strongly suggests that, besides drug metabolizing enzymes, drug transporters, including ATP-binding cassette (ABC) transporters and solute carriers (SLC), play pivotal roles in determining the pharmacokinetics profile of drugs, as well as the overall pharmacological effect and drug concentration at the target site. In light of this, the International Transporter Consortium (ITC) was founded to discuss and evaluate the contribution of drug transporters to pharmacokinetics and pharmacodynamics in drug discovery and development stages.[5] As part of the activities of the ITC, the authors have proposed that transport mechanism-based designs might help to create new, pharmacokinetically advantageous drugs, and as such this should be considered an important component of drug design strategy.

In general, both ABC and SLC transporters exhibit broad substrate specificity toward structurally diverse compounds. It is important to gain insight into the relationship between the molecular structures of compounds (drug or candidates) and the interaction with drug transporters of interest. Since quantitative structure–activity relationship (QSAR) analysis is a practical approach by which chemical structures are quantitatively correlated with biological activity or chemical reactivity, we developed a new QSAR algorithm to evaluate drug–ABC transporter interactions. In addition, to support the QSAR analysis approach, we established a high-speed screening method to increase the throughput for analyzing the interactions of ABC transporters with drugs. Based on both experimental results and computational QSAR analysis data, it has become easier to gain insight into the molecular mechanism underlying ABC transporter-mediated drug–drug interactions.

15.2 QSAR Analysis

15.2.1 Historical Background of QSAR Analysis

In principle, biological activity can be expressed quantitatively as a function of the structure described by electronic attributes, hydrophobicity, and steric properties.[6] Additionally, when physicochemical properties or structures are expressed by numbers, we can calculate a mathematical relationship, or quantitative structure–activity relationship, between the two. The mathematical expression can be used to predict the biological response of other chemical structures. Recent computational techniques have allowed us to delineate and refine the many variables and approaches that define the QSAR paradigm.

It was more than a century ago that the QSAR paradigm first found its way into the practice of pharmaceutical chemistry and toxicology. Crum-Brown and Fraser expressed the idea that physiological action of a substrate or ligand could be expressed as a function of its chemical composition and constitution.[7] In 1893, Richert demonstrated that the cytotoxicity of a diverse set of simple organic molecules was inversely related to their corresponding water solubilities.[7] In the 20th century, Meyer and Overton independently suggested that the narcotic (depressant) action of a group of organic compounds was correlated with their olive oil/water partition coefficients in a parallel manner.[7] In 1939, Ferguson introduced a thermodynamic generalization to the correlation of depressant action with relative saturation of volatile compounds.[7] Bell and Robin, on the other hand, established the importance of ionization of bases and weak acids in bacteriostatic activity.[8] The modern QSAR paradigm with the molecular mechanistic basis was implemented by Hansch and Fujita. Using the octanol/water system, a whole series of partition coefficients were measured, and thus a new hydrophobic scale was introduced.[7]

In the QSAR paradigm, the basic assumption for all molecule-based hypotheses is that similar molecules have similar activities. The underlying problem is, therefore, how to define a small difference at the molecular level, since each kind of activity, *e.g.* reaction ability, biotransformation ability, solubility, target activity, and so on, might depend on another difference.

15.2.2 Application of New QSAR Analysis to Human ABC Transporters

In the human body, drugs are not only enzymatically metabolized but also transported by various carriers, including members of the SLC superfamily and the ABC superfamily. Transporter proteins mediating the uptake and efflux of small molecules into and out of cells are key determinants of the *in vivo* distribution and elimination of many drugs and endogenous substances.[5] Those drug transporter proteins have broad substrate specificity. Therefore, based on the physicochemical properties of drugs, it is important to predict which drug is transported by which transporter(s). To gain systematic insight into the relationship between the chemical structure of drugs and the substrate specificity of drug transporters, we therefore developed a new QSAR analysis method by introducing chemical fragmentation codes (CFCs), as described below.

15.3 High-Speed Screening

15.3.1 Expression of Human ABCB11 in Sf9 Insect Cells and Preparation of Plasma Membrane Vesicles

Before implementing QSAR analysis for transporters, we developed a high-speed screening system where membrane vesicles expressing human ABC transporters were used as biological material. Today, the isolated membrane vesicles from insect cells provide a practical tool for low-cost and high-throughput analysis of ABC transporters.[8,9] Baculovirus-infected insect cells have successfully been employed to give relatively high protein expression yields; for example, *Spodoptera frugiperda* (Sf9) cells are widely used to obtain membranes overexpressing various ABC transporters.

In order to investigate the inhibition of bile acid transport by different drugs, we first cloned the cDNA of human *ABCB11* (wild type) from a human liver cDNA library.[9] Human ABCB11 is the ABC transporter responsible for hepatobiliary elimination of bile acids (Figure 15.1). The cDNA of human *ABCB11* was inserted into the pFastBac1 vector between the restriction enzyme sites of *Not*I and *Hin*dIII.[9] To express ABCB11 in insect cells, we generated recombinant baculoviruses with the Bac-to-Bac baculovirus expression system.[9] Insect *S. frugiperda* Sf9 cells (1×10^6 cells mL^{-1}) were infected with the recombinant baculoviruses and cultured in EX-CELL™ 420 insect serum-free medium (JRH Biosciences, Inc., Lenexa, KZ, USA) at 27 °C with gentle shaking. The expression of ABCB11 in Sf9 cells increased during the incubation. The cell size and morphology of the infected cells changed dramatically. The cell viability started to decrease after day 4.[9] The membrane morphology of infected Sf9 cells changed greatly; in particular, numerous pores were observed in the cell membrane on day 5. Membrane vesicles prepared from those cells (day 5) are useless for transport experiments. It is important to maintain high integrity of the plasma membrane vesicles used in transport assays. In other words, the membrane vesicles have to be completely sealed. Therefore, we harvested Sf9 cells on day 3, when cell viability was maintained at high levels (>90%).[9]

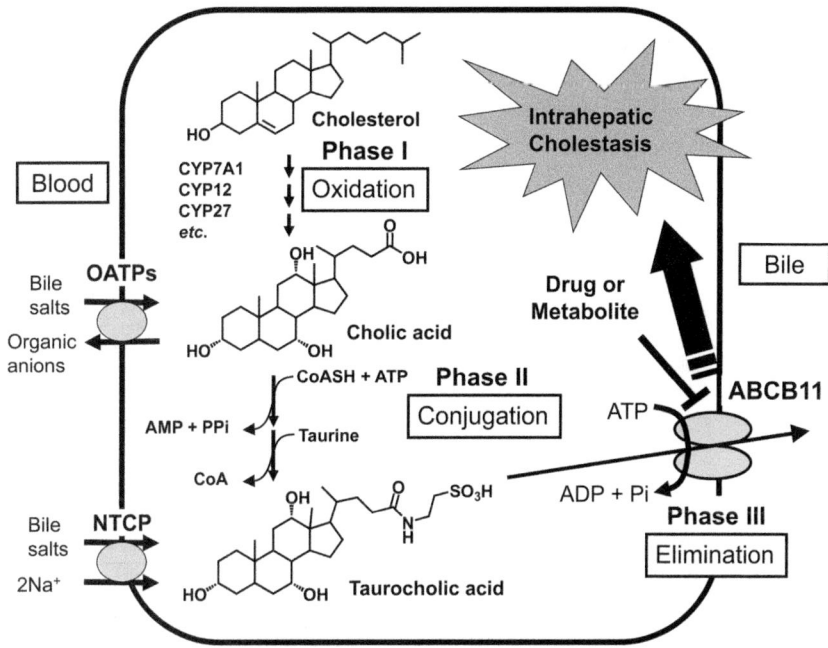

Figure 15.1 Schematic illustration of cholesterol metabolism in the liver, uptake of bile acids, and ABCB11-mediated hepatobiliary excretion of taurocholic acid. Cholesterol is metabolized to cholic acid *via* oxidative reactions catalyzed by CYP7A1, 12, and 27, *etc.* (Phase I oxidation step). Cholic acid, thus formed, undergoes conjugation with taurine to form taurocholic acid (Phase II conjugation step). Bile acids, including taurocholic acid, are actively transported from the blood circulation system to the liver by the action of OATPs and NTCP expressed in the basolateral membrane of hepatocytes. Taurocholic acid and other bile acids are subsequently transported by ABCB11 from liver cells to the bile canaliculi across the apical membrane of hepatocytes (Phase III elimination step).

The harvested cells were washed with phosphate-buffered saline (PBS) at 4 °C and collected by centrifugation. The resulting cell pellet was subsequently diluted 40-fold with a hypotonic buffer (0.5 mM Tris/HEPES, pH 7.4, 0.1 mM EGTA, and 1 μM leupeptin), and then homogenized with a Potter-Elvehjem homogenizer, as shown in Figure 15.2. Addition of leupeptin at this step is important to inhibit the cysteine protease of baculoviruses. Leupeptin (10 μg mL^{-1}) is a potent inhibitor of the degradation of the ABCB11 protein in membrane vesicles prepared from baculovirus-infected Sf9 cells. The plasma membrane fraction was collected by discontinuous sucrose-density gradient centrifugation (100 000 × *g*, 30 min).[9] The membrane vesicles were prepared as shown in Figure 15.2 and then stored at −80 °C. Repeated freeze–thaw of the membrane vesicle preparation should be avoided.

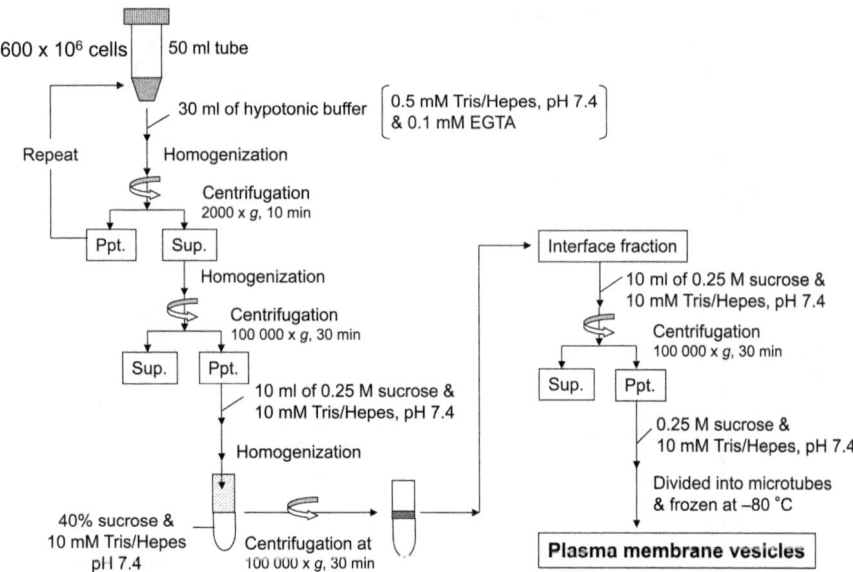

Figure 15.2 Procedure to prepare plasma membrane vesicles from Sf9 insect cell expressing human ABCB11. *S. frugiperda* Sf9 insect cells were grown in EX-CELL™ 420 insect serum-free medium supplemented with 1% (v/v) heat-inactivated fetal calf serum (FCS), penicillin (100 U mL⁻¹), and streptomycin (100 μg mL⁻¹; Invitrogen Co., Carlsbad, CA, USA) with gentle shaking at 27 °C. Sf9 cells (1×10^6 cells mL⁻¹) were then infected with human ABCB11-recombinant baculoviruses and cultured in EX-CELL 420 insect serum-free medium at 27 °C with gentle shaking. Three days after infection, Sf9 cells were harvested by centrifugation. The resulting cell pellet was diluted 40-fold with a hypotonic buffer (0.5 mM Tris/HEPES, pH 7.4, 0.1 mM EGTA) containing leupeptin (10 μg mL⁻¹), and then homogenized with a Potter-Elvehjem homogenizer. After centrifugation at $2000 \times g$, the supernatant (Sup.) was further centrifuged at $100\,000 \times g$ for 30 min. The resulting pellet was suspended in 0.25 M sucrose containing 10 mM Tris/HEPES, pH 7.4 and leupeptin (10 μg mL⁻¹). The crude membrane fraction was layered over 40% (w/v) sucrose solution and centrifuged at $100\,000 \times g$ for 30 min. The turbid layer at the interface was collected, suspended in 0.25 M sucrose containing 10 mM Tris/HEPES, pH 7.4, and centrifuged at $100\,000 \times g$ for 30 min. The membrane fraction was collected and re-suspended in a small volume (150–250 μL) of 0.25 M sucrose containing 10 mM Tris/HEPES, pH 7.4. After the protein concentration was measured by the BCA Protein Assay Kit (PIERCE, Rockford, IL, USA), the membrane solution was stored at −80 °C until it was used. Ppt.: precipitate.

15.3.2 High-Speed Screening of ATP-Dependent [¹⁴C]taurocholate Transport Mediated by Human ABCB11

To discern the contribution of ABCB11 to drug interactions, it is critical to explore and demonstrate methods for systematically characterizing and quantifying the inhibition of ABCB11-mediated transport. However, a new

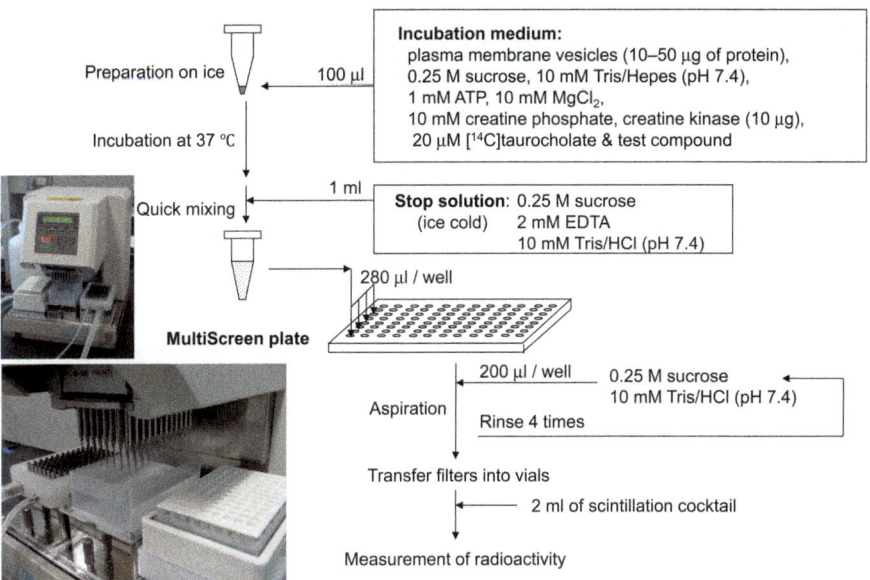

Figure 15.3   Procedure to measure ATP-dependent taurocholate transport mediated by ABCB11 and the inhibition of ABCB11-mediated taurocholate transport by test compounds. The standard incubation medium contained the plasma membrane vesicles (50 μg of protein), 20 μM [^{14}C]taurocholate, 0.25 M sucrose, 10 mM Tris/HEPES, pH 7.4, 10 mM MgCl$_2$, 1 mM ATP, 10 mM creatine phosphate, and 100 μg mL^{-1} creatine kinase in a final volume of 100 μL, and the incubation was carried out at 37 °C. After a specified time (15 min for the standard condition), the reaction medium was mixed with 1 mL of ice cold stop solution (0.25 M sucrose, 10 mM Tris/HEPES, pH 7.4, and 2 mM EDTA) to terminate the transport reaction. The chelating agent EDTA traps Mg^{2+}, which is a prerequisite for the ATP-dependent transport function of ABCB11. Subsequently, aliquots (280 μL per well) of the resulting mixture were transferred to MultiScreen™ plates. Under aspiration, each well of the plate was rinsed four times with the 0.25 M sucrose solution containing 10 mM Tris/HCl, pH 7.4 (4 × 200 μL for each well) in an EDR384S system (BioTec, Tokyo, Japan). The [^{14}C]taurocholate incorporated into the vesicles was measured by counting the radioactivity remaining on the filter of the MultiScreen plates.

automated system was urgently needed to enhance the throughput of transport experiments. In this context, we developed a high-speed screening system by introducing 96-well MultiScreen™ plates (Millipore Corp., Billerica, MA) and an automated multi-dispenser system.[9,10] Figure 15.3 depicts the procedure for high-speed screening of ATP-dependent [^{14}C]taurocholate transport mediated by ABCB11. Figure 15.4A shows the time courses of [^{14}C]taurocholate transport into membrane vesicles in the presence and absence of ATP. ATP-dependent [^{14}C]taurocholate transport exhibited saturation kinetics with an apparent Km value of about 10 μM for taurocholate (Figure 15.4B).[9]

We have used this new screening system to investigate the interaction of ABCB11 with a variety of test compounds. We selected structurally diverse

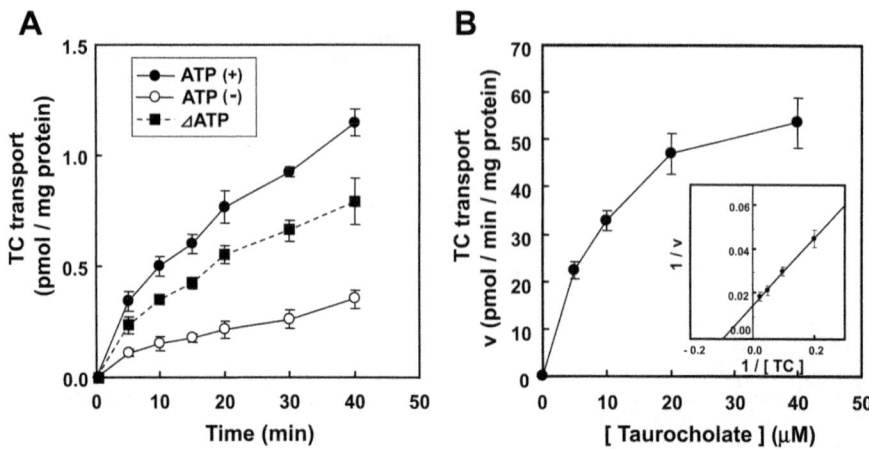

Figure 15.4   Time courses of taurocholate transport into membrane vesicles in the presence or absence of ATP (A) and the effect of taurocholate concentration on the rate of ATP-dependent taurocholate transport (B). [^{14}C]taurocholate (TC) transport was measured in the standard incubation medium (0.25 M sucrose and 10 mM Tris/HEPES, pH 7.4, 10 mM creatine phosphate, 100 μg mL^{-1} creatine kinase, 10 mM MgCl$_2$), as described in Figure 15.3. The Lineweaver–Burk plot of TC concentration *vs.* transport rate is depicted in the inset. Reprinted with permission from Hirano *et al.*, *Mol. Pharm.*, 2006, **3**, 252–265. Copyright 2006 American Chemical Society.

test compounds to examine our hypothesis that common chemical components may be involved in the inhibition of ABCB11-mediated taurocholate transport.[9] The selected test compounds were classified into seven groups: A, neurotransmitters; B, vasodilators; C, potassium channel modulators; D, steroids; E, non-steroidal anti-inflammatory drugs (NSAIDs); F, anti-cancer drugs; and G, miscellaneous. Figure 15.5 summarizes the inhibitory effects of the test compounds on ABCB11-mediated taurocholate transport. It is important to note that the inhibition profile for ABCB11 is very similar to the ATPase profile for ABCB1. Vasodilators, *e.g.* fendiline (B-5), prenylamine (B-6), and nicardipine (B-7) strongly inhibited ABCB11-mediated taurocholate transport. On the other hand, steroids, such as dexamethasone (C-1), betamethasone (C-2), prednisolone (C-3), and cortisone (C-4) did not significantly inhibit ABCB11-mediated taurocholate transport.

15.4   QSAR Analysis of Inhibition of Human ABCB11

15.4.1   New QSAR Analysis Using CFCs

To gain insight into the relationship between the chemical structures of the test compounds and the inhibition of ABCB11-mediated taurocholate transport activity, we developed a new QSAR analysis method by introducing the use of "chemical fragmentation codes" to describe the chemical structures of a variety of drugs and natural compounds.[9]

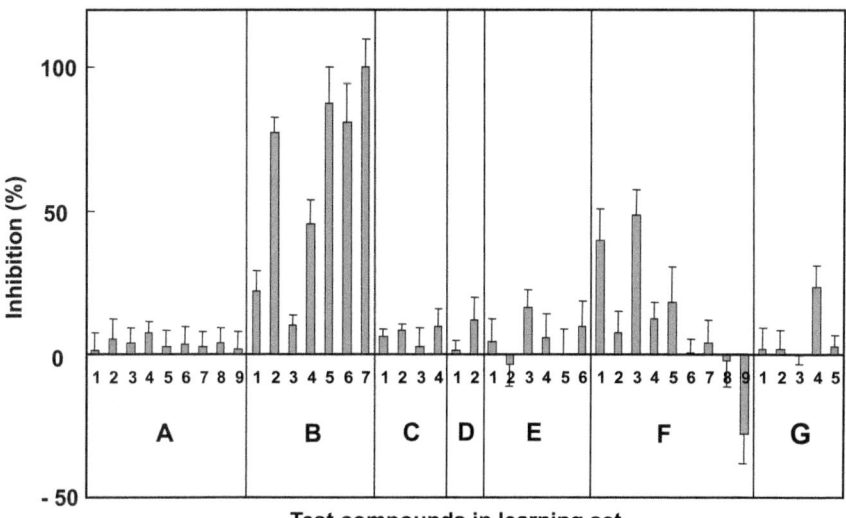

Figure 15.5 Inhibition of ABCB11-mediated taurocholate transport by different test compounds. Inhibition (%) of ABCB11-mediated taurocholate transport by different test compounds is expressed as the relative values compared with the transport activity measured without test compounds (0% inhibition). The test compounds used are classified into seven groups: A, neurotransmitters; B, vasodilators; C, steroids; D, potassium channel modulators; E, NSAIDs; F, anti-cancer drugs; and G, miscellaneous. These groups represent: glycine (A-1), glutamic acid (A-2), dopamine (A-3), norepinephrine (A-4), epinephrine (A-5), GABA (A-6), histamine (A-7), serotonin (A-8), melatonin (A-9), verapamil (B-1), nifedipine (B-2), diltiazem (B-3), bepridil (B-4), fendiline (B-5), prenylamine (B-6), nicardipine (B-7), dexamethasone (C-1), betamethasone (C-2), prednisolone (C-3), cortisone (C-4), nicorandil (D-1), pinacidil (D-2), acetylsalicylic acid (E-1), indomethacin (E-2), acemetacin (E-3), ibuprofen (E-4), naproxen (E-5), mepirizole (E-6), vinblastine (F-1), etoposide (F-2), actinomycin D (F-3), daunorubicin (F-4), paclitaxel (F-5), methotrexate (F-6), doxorubicin (F-7), 5-fluorouracil (F-8), mitoxantrone (F-9), quinidine (G-1), *p*-aminohippuric acid (G-2), penicillin G (G-3), novobiocin (G-4), and prazosin (G-5). Reprinted with permission from Hirano *et al., Mol. Pharm.,* 2006, **3**, 252–265. Copyright 2006 American Chemical Society.

The CFCs were originally created to answer the need to access information on the increasing number of chemical patents. These CFCs are a set of alpha-numeric symbols, each representing a fragment of a chemical structure, that were developed by Derwent Information, Ltd, as an indexing language suitable for describing chemical structures. The Markush TOPFRAG program is a tool for searching the chemical structures and structural information in Derwent's online databases.[11,12]

We applied these CFCs to the QSAR analysis of ABCB11–drug interactions.[9] Our approach is unique in that the extent of ABCB11-mediated taurocholate transport inhibition is described as a linear combination of CFCs, and that the coefficient "$C(i)$" for each CFC reflects the extent of the contribution of a specific chemical moiety to interactions with the ABCB11 protein. Namely, the chemical fragmentation coefficient is defined as the contribution to the activity (here the ability to inhibit taurocholate transport) that is attributable to the presence of a particular chemical moiety in the test compound. We formulated the extent of inhibition of ABCB11-mediated taurocholate transport as a linear combination of CFCs, each of which is weighted by the corresponding coefficient as follows:

$$\text{ABCB11 inhibition (\%)} = \sum C(i) \times \text{Score (i)} + \text{Constant}$$

where the symbol (i) designates a specific chemical fragmentation[9] and the "score" is the presence [≥1] or absence [0] of the corresponding CFC(i) in the chemical structure of a test compound (see Table 15.1). Based on the CFCs thus obtained, and comparison with the observed inhibition of transport activity for each test compound, we have calculated chemical fragmentation coefficients, $C(i)$, by multiple linear regression analysis, to delineate the relationship between the structural components and the extent of ABCB11 inhibition. In this way, we could identify one set of CFCs that are closely related to the inhibition of ABCB11 transporter activity. Explanations for these CFCs are also given in Table 15.1. We use the descriptors of M132, ESTR, R-CC, H181, MN-HC, and OH-ALP to represent multiple CFCs. Based on the results of the multiple linear regression analysis, we calculated the values of predicted inhibition and compared them with the observed values. As demonstrated in Table 15.1 and Figure 15.6, the prediction of transport inhibition correlated well with the observed values of inhibition. The R^2 value was estimated to be 0.952.[9]

The structural components represented by the CFCs of M132 and H181, as well as by the descriptors of ESTR, R-CC, and MN-HC positively contribute to the inhibition, whereas the descriptor of OH-ALP (–OH groups bonded to aliphatic carbon) had a negative contribution. As summarized in Table 15.1, the descriptor ESTR, including CFCs J211 and J212, had a relatively large positive coefficient, $C(\text{ESTR}) = 31.47$, suggesting that an ester (thioester) group bonded to the carbon of a heterocyclic ring is an important component for the interaction with the ABCB11 protein. In addition, the data for R-CC (Table 15.1) suggest that carbocyclic systems with at least one aromatic ring are also important chemical moieties for the interaction with ABCB11. These QSAR profiles for ABCB11 are distinct from those for ABCG2, another human ABC transporter.[8]

15.4.2 Application of QSAR to Predict Inhibition of ABCB11 by Troglitazone

In the case of troglitazone, the CFCs M132, J211, M531, and M521 are involved in its chemical structure.[9] Structural components corresponding to those CFCs are indicated in Figure 15.7. Based on the QSAR calculation [ABCB11 inhibition (%) = $C(\text{M132}) + C(\text{J211}) + C(\text{M531}) + C(\text{M521}) +$ constant], the inhibition of taurocholate transport by troglitazone is estimated to be 81.11%, which is in accordance with the observed value of 90.06% (Figure 15.6).

It has been reported that troglitazone sulfate efficiently forms and accumulates in liver tissue and that it strongly inhibits rat Abcb11 (IC$_{50}$ value of

Table 15.1 Definition of descriptors and CFCs contributing to the inhibition of ABCB11-mediated taurocholate transport.[a] Reprinted with permission from Hirano *et al.*, *Mol. Pharm.*, 2006, **3**, 252–265. Copyright 2006 American Chemical Society.

Descriptor	Coefficient	(95% reliability)	CFC	Definition	Score
M132	35.07	(±8.99)	M132	Ring-linking group containing one C atom (except for M131 >C=W, W: heteroatom)	1
ESTR	31.47	(±4.97)	J211	One ester (thioester) group bonded to heterocyclic C *via* >C=O (>C=S)	1
			J212	Two or more ester (thioester) groups bonded to heterocyclic C *via* >C=O (>C=S)	2
R-CC	14.41	(±2.91)	M530	No carbocyclic system with at least one aromatic ring	0
			M531	One carbocyclic system with at least one aromatic ring	1
			M532	Two carbocyclic systems with at least one aromatic ring	2
			M533	Three or more carbocyclic systems with at least one aromatic ring	3
H181	10.95	(±4.86)	H181	One amine bonded to aliphatic C	1
MN-HC	9.66	(±4.22)	M520	No mononuclear heterocycle	0
			M521	One mononuclear heterocycle	1
			M522	Two mononuclear heterocycles	2
			M523	Three or more mononuclear heterocycles	3
OH-ALP	−15.23	(±5.06)	H481	One OH group bonded to aliphatic C	1
			H482	Two –OH groups bonded to aliphatic C	2
			H483	Three –OH groups bonded to aliphatic C	3
			H484	Four or more –OH groups bonded to aliphatic C	4
Constant	−9.50				1

[a]$R = 0.976$; $R^2 = 0.952$; $F(30,6) = 99.1$; $s = 6.67$. Descriptors, CFC, coefficients, and constants were deduced from the inhibition of ABCB11-mediated taurocholate transport by test compounds. Data taken from Hirano *et al.*[9]

0.4–0.6 μM).[13,14] Therefore, it has been suggested that troglitazone sulfate is responsible for the interaction of conjugated bile salts with hepatobiliary export in rats. Based on these animal model and *in vitro* studies, inhibition of ABCB11 by troglitazone sulfate has been implicated as a potential cause of troglitazone-induced intrahepatic cholestasis in humans.[14,15] In the year 2000, the FDA informed physicians of the removal from the market of troglitazone, which had been associated with rare but severe liver toxicity since 1997.[15]

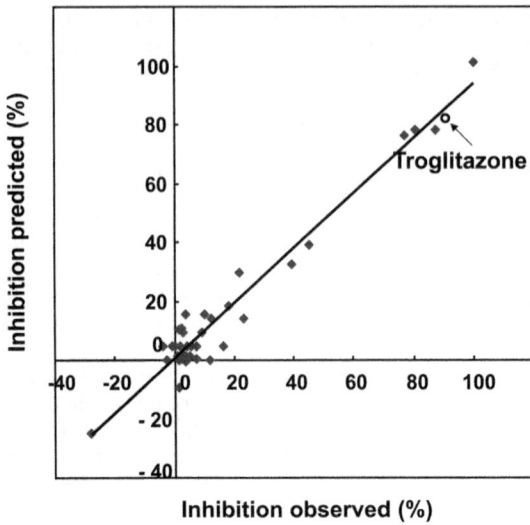

Figure 15.6 Relationship between observed and predicted values in the inhibition of taurocholate transport by the test compounds. The predicted values for the inhibition of ABCB11 by test compounds were deduced from the multiple linear regression analysis as described in the text. The inhibition by troglitazone is indicated by an open circle (o). Reprinted with permission from Hirano *et al., Mol. Pharm.*, 2006, **3**, 252–265. Copyright 2006 American Chemical Society.

15.5 Metabolism and Transport of Bile Acids

Bile is a vital secretion, essential for intestinal digestion and absorption of lipids. Moreover, bile is an important route of elimination for environmental toxins, carcinogens, xenobiotics including drugs, and their metabolites. Bile secretion is also a major route of excretion for endogenous compounds and metabolic products (endobiotics) such as cholesterol, bilirubin, and steroid hormones.[16–18] Bile is primarily secreted by hepatocytes into minute channels arranged as a network of tubules or canaliculi located between adjacent hepatocytes. Canalicular bile accounts for approximately 75% of the daily bile production in humans as it passes along the bile ductules and ducts. In humans, bile is further concentrated up to 5- to 10-fold in the gallbladder.[19] The human bile salt pool amounts to 50–60 μmol kg^{-1} of body weight and averages 3–4 g.[18]

Bile secretion is an osmotic process driven predominantly by the active excretion of organic solutes into bile canaliculi, followed by the passive inflow of water, electrolytes, and nonelectrolytes (*e.g.* glucose) from hepatocytes and across semipermeable tight junctions. The main organic solutes of bile are bile salts, phospholipids, and cholesterol, which form mixed micelles in bile. Extrusion of bile salts from the hepatocytes is also critical for liver cell viability, as the intracellular accumulation of bile salts may lead to cell death by apoptosis and/or necrosis.[20]

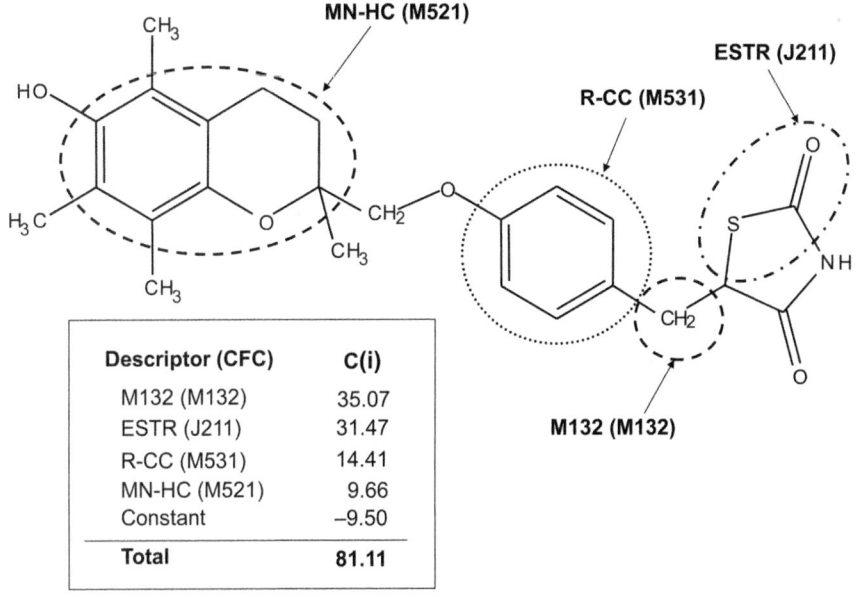

Descriptor (CFC)	C(i)
M132 (M132)	35.07
ESTR (J211)	31.47
R-CC (M531)	14.41
MN-HC (M521)	9.66
Constant	−9.50
Total	**81.11**

Figure 15.7 Chemical structure of troglitazone and its descriptors and CFCs associated with the inhibition of ABCB11-mediated taurocholate transport. Descriptors are summarized in Table 15.1, and the corresponding $C(i)$ values are presented in the inset box where the sum of $C(i)$ values is 81.11. Reprinted with permission from Hirano *et al.*, *Mol. Pharm.*, 2006, **3**, 252–265. Copyright 2006 American Chemical Society.

In humans, over 70% of the bile acid pool consists of cholic acid (~50%) and its bacterial metabolite deoxycholic acid (~20%), whereas chenodeoxycholic acid constitutes 30% of the total bile acid pool.[17] After being synthesized in hepatocytes, bile acids are conjugated with glycine or taurine (Figure 15.1). Under normal conditions, conjugated bile salts are excreted into bile by the ABCB11 protein that is expressed in the canalicular or apical domain of the hepatocyte plasma membrane. Several mutations in the *ABCB11* gene located on chromosome 2q24 have been reported to be associated with progressive familial intrahepatic cholestasis type 2 (PFIC2).[21-32] In these patients, biliary excretion of conjugated bile salts was found to be severely impaired.[22-33]

15.6 Conclusion

It has been reported that inhibition of human ABCB11 (SPGP/BSEP) after exposure to toxic xenobiotics or drug interactions has negative impacts, which include intrahepatic cholestasis and hepatotoxicity. Therefore, *in vitro* screening methods are necessary for quantifying and characterizing the inhibition of ABCB11. In line with such needs, we developed methods for *in vitro* high-speed screening and QSAR analysis to investigate the interaction of ABCB11 with a variety of compounds. The high-speed screening method and QSAR strategy are considered practical and useful approaches to identify inhibitors of ABCB11. As described herein, based on our QSAR analysis, we could identify one set of CFCs closely linked with inhibition of ABCB11. Furthermore, our high-speed screening method enabled us to analyze the kinetics of ABCB11 inhibition by test compounds, and to distinguish competitive and non-competitive inhibitors. Troglitazone was found to be a competitive inhibitor to taurocholate. Kinetics-based classification of inhibitors may further improve the accuracy of QSAR analysis and risk prediction.

Acknowledgements

Under the license agreement (License Number 2235670436990) with the American Chemical Society, Figures 15.4, 15.5, 15.6, and 15.7, as well as Table 15.1 in this chapter have been reproduced from our previous study published in *Molecular Pharmaceutics*.[9]

References

1. R. F. Service, *Science*, 2004, **303**(5665), 1796.
2. J. Mervis, *Science*, 2005, **309**(5735), 726.
3. N. Kaplowitz, Idiosyncratic drug hepatotoxicity, *Nat. Rev. Drug Discovery*, 2005, **4**(6), 489.
4. D. Schuster, C. Laggner and T. Lange, *Curr. Pharm. Des.*, 2005, **11**(27), 3545–3559.
5. International Transporter Consortium, K. M. Giacomini, S. M. Huang, D. J. Tweedie, L. Z. Benet, K. L. Brouwer, X. Chu, A. Dahlin, R. Evers, V. Fischer, K. M. Hillgren, K. A. Hoffmaster, T. Ishikawa, D. keppler, R. B. Kim, C. A. Lee, M. Niemi, J. W. Polli, Y. Sugiyama, P. W. Swaan, J. A. Ware, S. H. Wright, S. W. Yee, M. J. Zamek-Gliszczynski and L. Zhang, *Nat. Rev. Drug Discovery*, 2010, **9**, 215.
6. C. Hansch and A. Leo, *Substituent Constants for Correlation Analysis in Chemistry and Biology*. John Wiley & Sons, New York, 1979.
7. C. D. Selassie, in *Burger's Medicinal Chemistry and Drug Discovery*, ed. D. J. Abraham, John Wiley & Sons, New York, 6th edn, 2003, vol. 1, p. 1.
8. H. Saito, H. Hirano, H. Nakagawa, T. Fukami, K. Oosumi, K. Murakami, H. Kimura, T. Kouchi, M. Konomi, E. Tao, N. Tsujikawa, S. Tarui, M. Nagakura, M. Osumi and T. Ishikawa, *J. Pharmacol. Exp. Ther.*, 2006, **317**, 1114.
9. H. Hirano, A. Kurata, Y. Onishi, A. Sakurai, H. Saito, H. Nakagawa, M. Nagakura, S. Tarui, Y. Kanamori, M. Kitajima and T. Ishikawa, *Mol. Pharm.*, 2006, **3**, 252.
10. T. Ishikawa, A. Sakurai, Y. Kanamori, M. Nagakura, H. Hirano, Y. Takarada, K. Yamada, K. Fukushima and M. Kitajima, *Methods Enzymol.*, 2005, **400**, 485.

11. http://www.thomsonscientific.com/media/scpdf/chemical_index_guidelines.pdf, last accessed May 11, 2015.

12. http://scientific.thomson.com/support/patents/patinf/terms/, last accessed May 11, 2015.

13. C. Funk, C. Ponelle, G. Scheuermann and M. Pantze, *Mol. Pharmacol.*, 2001, **59**, 627.

14. C. Funk, M. Pantze, L. Jehle, C. Ponelle, G. Scheuermann, M. Lazendic and R. Grasser, *Toxicology*, 2001, **167**, 83.

15. J. E. Henney, *JAMA Oncol.*, 2000, **283**(17), 2228.

16. M. H. Nathanson and J. L. Boyer, *Hepatology*, 1991, **14**, 551.

17. M. Trauner and J. L. Boyer, *Physiol. Rev.*, 2003, **83**, 633.

18. G. A. Kullak-Ublick, B. Stieger and P. J. Meier, *Gastroenterology*, 2004, **126**, 322.

19. M. C. Carey and D. M. Small, *J. Clin. Invest.*, 1978, **61**, 998.

20. H. Higuchi and G. J. Gores, *Am. J. Physiol.: Gastrointest. Liver Physiol.*, 2003, **284**, G734.

21. S. S. Strautnieks, L. N. Bull, A. S. Knisely, S. A. Kocoshis, N. Dahl, H. Arnell, E. Sokal, K. Dahan, S. Childs, V. Ling, M. S. Tanner, A. F. Kagalwalla, A. Németh, J. Pawlowska, A. Baker, G. Mieli-Vergani, N. B. Freimer, R. M. Gardiner and R. J. Thompson, *Nat. Genet.*, 1998, **20**(3), 233.

22. L. Wang, C. J. Soroka and J. L. Boyer, *J. Clin. Invest.*, 2002, **110**(7), 965.

23. C. Pauli-Magnus, T. Lang, Y. Meier, T. Zodan-Marin, D. Jung, C. Breymann, R. Zimmermann, S. Kenngott, U. Beuers, C. Reichel, R. Kerb, A. Penger, P. J. Meier and G. A. Kullak-Ublick, *Pharmacogenetics*, 2004, **14**(2), 91.

24. C. W. Lam, K. M. Cheung, M. S. Tsui, M. S. Yan, C. Y. Lee and S. F. Tong, *J. Hepatol.*, 2006, **44**(1), 240.

25. Y. Meier, C. Pauli-Magnus, U. M. Zanger, K. Klein, E. Schaeffeler, A. K. Nussler, N. Nussler, M. Eichelbaum, P. J. Meier and B. Stieger, *Hepatology*, 2006, **44**(1), 62.

26. B. Stieger, Y. Meier and P. J. Meier, *Pflugers Arch.*, 2007, **453**(5), 611.

27. J. Noe, G. A. Kullak-Ublick, W. Jochum, B. Stieger, R. Kerb, M. Haberl, B. Müllhaupt, P. J. Meier and C. Pauli-Magnus, *J. Hepatol.*, 2005, **43**(3), 536.

28. C. Pauli-Magnus, R. Kerb, K. Fattinger, T. Lang, B. Anwald, G. A. Kullak-Ublick, U. Beuers and P. J. Meier, *Hepatology*, 2004, **39**(3), 779.

29. S. W. van Mil, W. L. van der Woerd, G. van der Brugge, E. Sturm, P. L. Jansen, L. N. Bull, I. E. van den Berg, R. Berger, R. H. Houwen and L. W. Klomp, *Gastroenterology*, 2004, **127**(2), 379.

30. K. Goto, K. Sugiyama, T. Sugiura, T. Ando, F. Mizutani, K. Terabe, K. Ban and H. Togari, *J. Pediatr. Gastroenterol. Nutr.*, 2003, **36**(5), 647.

31. P. L. Jansen, S. S. Strautnieks, E. Jacquemin, M. Hadchouel, E. M. Sokal, G. J. Hooiveld, J. H. Koning, A. De Jager-Krikken, F. Kuipers, F. Stellaard, C. M. Bijleveld, A. Gouw, H. van Goor, R. J. Thompson and M. Muller, *Gastroenterology*, 1999, **117**(6), 1370.

32. R. Kubitz, V. Keitel, S. Scheuring, K. Köhrer and D. Häussinger, *J. Clin. Gastroenterol.*, 2006, **40**(2), 171.

33. W. H. Summerskill and J. M. Walshe, *Lancet*, 1959, **2**, 686.

CHAPTER 16

Formulation for Optimizing Bioavailability

SUMA GOPINATHAN*

*E-mail: suma_gopinathan@hotmail.com

16.1 Introduction

Bioavailability describes the amount of drug that reaches systemic circulation (or the target organ) following administration. Poor bioavailability is one of the leading causes of failure in both preclinical and clinical stages of drug discovery. A drug needs to reach therapeutic levels at the target organ to be efficacious. Compounds with low bioavailability exhibit poor efficacy and greater inter-subject variability following administration.

Formulation development is the process by which a drug is modified into a form in which it can be easily administered. This is achieved by combining the active ingredient with excipients and may involve reducing the particle size of the active ingredient. Drug formulations often play a dual role in pharmaceutical development. They enable drug delivery while optimizing bioavailability. The intrinsic bioavailability of a drug depends on its physicochemical properties. Formulations can optimize the bioavailability of the drug by modulating some the physicochemical properties of the drug and also by altering the physiology of the local environment following administration. In addition to improving the bioavailability of new chemical entities (NCEs), formulation strategies are also utilized to extend

RSC Drug Discovery Series No. 49
New Horizons in Predictive Drug Metabolism and Pharmacokinetics
Edited by Alan G. E. Wilson
© The Royal Society of Chemistry 2016
Published by the Royal Society of Chemistry, www.rsc.org

patent protection by improving bioavailability and reducing the frequency of dosing.

This chapter will discuss the impact of drug formulation on some of the key parameters that have a direct impact on bioavailability.

16.2 Impact of Formulation on Key Parameters Influencing Bioavailability

A drug is considered to be 100% bioavailable following intravenous administration. For all other routes of administration, the various parameters that influence bioavailability are depicted in Figure 16.1.

16.2.1 Solubility

Solubility is one of the key challenges facing the formulation scientist. For a drug to be absorbed, it must be soluble at the site of administration. The advent of high throughput computational screening has led to a portfolio of highly lipophilic drugs. It is estimated that over 40% of all NCEs entering clinical trials today are practically insoluble in water.[1,2] It is also one of the key physicochemical parameters of the drug that can be modified by formulation development. Formulation techniques influencing solubility are depicted in Figure 16.2.

16.2.1.1 Solubilizing Excipients

In the early stages of drug discovery, the key to improving bioavailability is by the use excipients to prepare formulations in solution. The different classes of excipients employed in solubilizing NCEs have been previously described in detail.[3-5] Briefly, solubilizing excipients can be classified as:

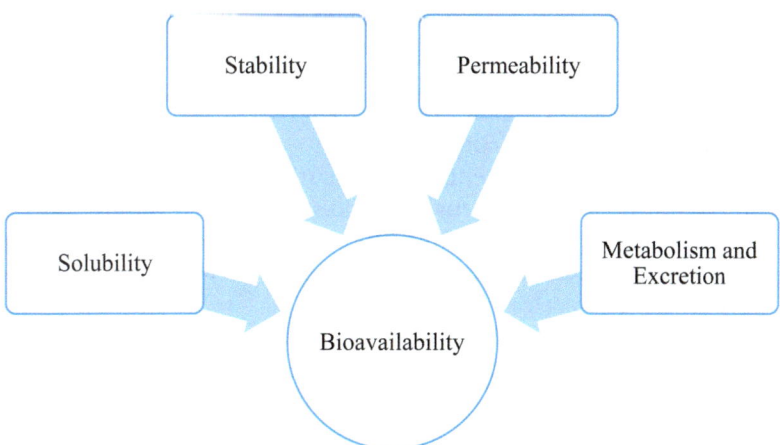

Figure 16.1 Factors impacting bioavailability.

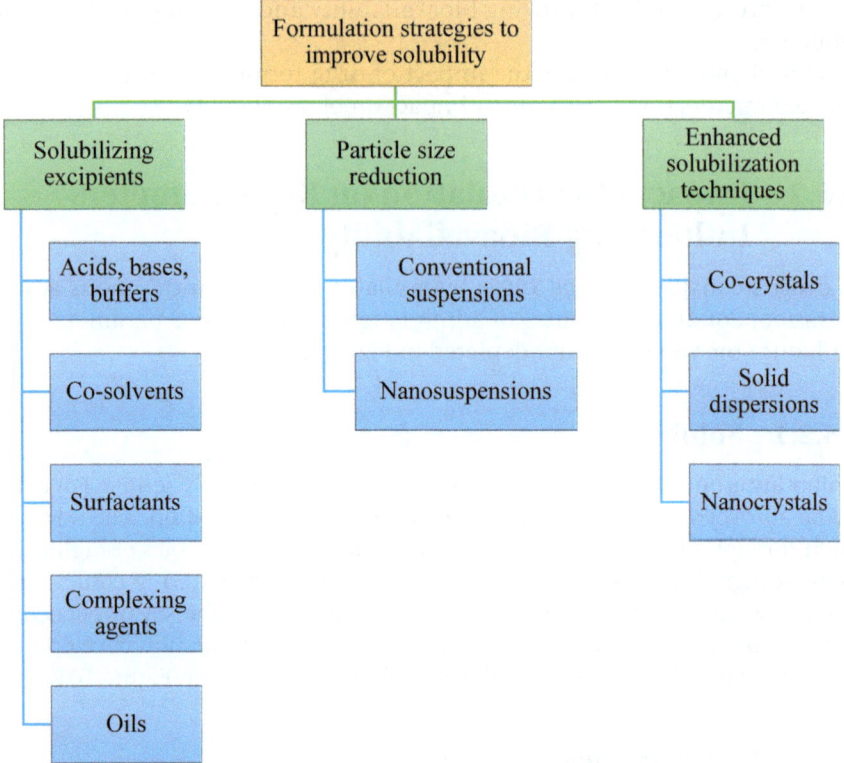

Figure 16.2   Formulation strategies to improve solubility.

1. Acids, bases and buffers: Commonly employed examples include citric acid, sodium hydroxide and phosphate buffer. For ionic compounds, the use of *in situ* salt formation and/or pH adjustment to improve solubility is a commonly employed strategy.
2. Co-solvents: These include excipients such as polyethylene glycol (PEG) and ethanol. They are water miscible organic solvents that act as powerful solubilizing agents. They are very useful in preparing aqueous solutions of lipophilic compounds.
3. Surfactants: Commonly encountered surfactants in pharmaceutical formulations include polysorbate 80 and sodium lauryl sulfate. Surfactant molecules have a hydrophilic end and a lipophilic end. They increase solubility by reducing interfacial tension between the hydrophilic–lipophilic interfaces.
4. Complexing agents: The most commonly used complexing agents are cyclodextrins. They are water-soluble molecules with a hydrophobic pocket. They solubilize lipophilic compounds by encapsulating them in the hydrophobic pocket.
5. Oils: Oils such as soybean oil and castor oils are employed to solubilize highly lipophilic compounds. They are typically employed in the preparation of emulsions or self-emulsifying drug delivery systems (SEDDS).

16.2.1.2 Particle Size Reduction

In addition to the use of excipients to enable solubilization, particle size reduction techniques are employed to improve the bioavailability of hydrophobic compounds by increasing the rate of dissolution. A decrease in particle size increases the total surface area available for dissolution thereby increasing the rate of dissolution, and leading to improved solubility at the site of absorption. Suspensions are often stabilized by the use of surfactants and viscosity enhancing agents. Conventional suspension formulations may not yield the desired improvement in bioavailability but enhanced techniques involving the formation of nanosuspensions have been shown to improve bioavailability *in vivo*.[6-12]

16.2.1.3 Enhanced Solubilization Techniques

In later stages of drug development, enhanced formulation techniques are employed. These include:

1. Co-crystals: These are formulations of crystalline materials with 2 or more molecules sharing the same crystal lattice. In pharmaceutical co-crystal formulations, the active ingredient shares a crystal lattice with one or more conformers. The interaction between the active ingredient and the conformer is by non-ionic bonds. Co-crystals are very useful in improving the solubility of non-ionizable compounds for which salt screening approaches cannot be employed to improve bioavailability. Co-crystals have been shown to modify the physicochemical properties of drugs, improving their solubility and thereby increasing their bioavailability.[13-15]
2. Solid dispersions: These formulations involve the dispersion of a hydrophobic drug within an inert hydrophilic matrix in a solid state. This enhances the wettability of the drug while reducing the particle size, allowing for an enhanced dissolution rate, and leading to improved bioavailability.[16-18] Solid dispersions are particularly attractive to the formulation scientist as they allow a high drug load.
3. Nanocrystals: These formulations involve particle size reduction of the compound to a dimension of less than 1 μm. Nanocrystals are composed entirely of the drug. They do not have any carriers. Prior to administration, they have to be dispersed in a suitable medium and are stabilized by the use of surfactants and/or polymers. They are applicable to both amorphous and crystalline material. They improve the bioavailability by increasing the saturation solubility and rate of dissolution. They have also been shown to increase cell and membrane adhesiveness, thus improving oral bioavailability.[10,19-21]

16.2.2 Stability

Drug stability has a direct impact on the bioavailability of the active ingredient. The stability of a drug determines the potency of the formulation. In early stages of pre-formulation and formulation development, it is important to have a good understanding of the stability characteristics of the drug and the possible interactions of the drug with the manufacturing process, excipients and storage containers. The stability of the drug could also be influenced by the *in vivo* environment following administration.

16.2.2.1 Common Factors Impacting Stability

The active ingredient in a pharmaceutical preparation can be labile to different stability issues. Stability can be generally categorized as physical or chemical (Figure 16.3):

1. Physical stability: Stability issues can result in a change in the physical nature of the finished product. This includes changes in color/appearance, palatability, absorption/loss of water, re-crystallization, polymorphisms and changes in suspendability. Some of these issues, such as polymorphisms and re-crystallization, directly affect the solubility of the drug, impacting bioavailability. Others, such as changes in color and smell, are often secondary changes resulting from chemical instability and can often be directly correlated to a reduction in potency. Issues such as conformational polymorphisms are difficult to address by a simple modification in the formulation. Polymorphisms

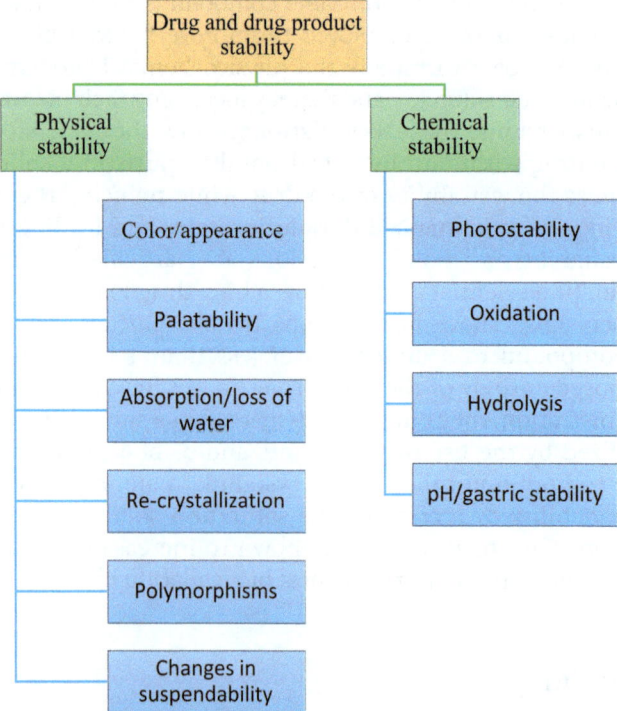

Figure 16.3   Stability issues impacting bioavailability.

are usually addressed in the drug synthesis process by rigorous control over the manufacturing process. Other issues, such as hygroscopicity, color, palatability and re-crystallization, can be improved by the use of polymers to coat the tablet or granules during the formulation process to form a protective barrier. Examples of commonly employed polymers include hydroxypropyl methylcellulose and polyvinyl alcohol.[22]

2. Chemical stability: The chemical stability of a drug can be impacted by different factors, lowering the potency of the drug and affecting its bioavailability. These include photostability, oxidation, hydrolysis and pH/gastric stability. For chemically labile drugs, chemical degradation can lead to decreased potency as well as the formation of toxic degradation products. Actively optimizing the formulation to minimize the potential for chemical degradation is critical to the success of the drug product. Formulation approaches are often very successful in addressing chemical stability issues, especially with solid dosage forms. Drugs such as furosemide, amlodipine and pantoprazole sodium are unstable when exposed to ultraviolet (UV) radiation. In addition to packaging the finished product in a light/UV resistant material such as amber colored bottles or opaque blister packaging, formulation approaches such as coating or microencapsulating the product to protect it from UV degradation have been shown to improve stability and bioavailability.[23,24] Another commonly employed formulation strategy to improve chemical stability is the use of enteric coating to protect against acidic pH and gastric stability issues. Lansoprazole is a good example of a small molecule that is unstable in the gastric environment. This compound exhibits a pH dependent stability profile and is unstable in acidic media. The stability and resulting bioavailability of the drug was improved by enteric coating of the tablet, protecting it from the acidic environment of the stomach and allowing it to be released in the alkaline intestinal environment.[25]

16.2.3 Permeability

Permeability plays a key role in the absorption and distribution of a drug. The permeability of a drug molecule is its ability to pass through biological membranes to reach systemic circulation or the site of action. While formulation development has had a significant impact on improving the solubility of a compound, its effect on permeability has remained fairly limited. This is mainly because, while solubility enhancers act by modifying the drug moiety itself, permeability enhancers operate by modifying the biological membrane. This has resulted in safety and tolerability concerns with the use of permeability enhancers. Recent studies, however, have demonstrated good tolerability profiles for permeability enhancers by different routes of administration. Commonly employed permeability enhancers include surfactants such as polysorbate 80, sodium dodecyl sulfate and polyoxyl 35 hydrogenated castor oil (KOLLIPHOR EL®);[26] bile salts such as sodium glycocholate and sodium taurodeoxycholate;[27] fatty acids such as oleic, palmitoleic and linoleic acids;[28] and chelating agents such as disodium ethylenediaminetetraacetate.[29]

16.2.3.1   Buccal Permeability

The buccal route of drug delivery offers many advantages over oral drug delivery as it bypasses first pass metabolism, theoretically enabling a faster onset of action and improved bioavailability. It is of particular interest for the non-invasive and controlled delivery of macromolecules such as proteins and peptides, as it circumvents the potential for degradation in the gastrointestinal environment.[30,31] One of the key hindrances to this route of administration is the relatively low permeability of the oral mucosa. Formulation approaches to improve permeability of the buccal mucosa includes the use of permeation enhancers such as surfactants and bile salts, and also the use of mucoadhesive agents. Studies have shown that improvements in formulation design can increase the bioavailability of different drugs when administered by the buccal route compared with the oral route.[30,32,33]

16.2.3.2   Intestinal Permeability

The intestinal ecosystem provides several barriers to the permeability of drugs. For a drug to permeate *via* the intestinal environment, it has to survive in an enzyme and microbe rich environment, pass through an outer mucus layer and finally cross the intestinal epithelial layer while avoiding efflux pumps such as P-glycoprotein (P-gp). The intestinal permeability of a drug can be improved by modulating the permeation across the intestinal epithelium with or without the use of efflux inhibitors.[34] Paracellular permeability enhancers improve the transportation of drugs (which are absorbed mainly *via* paracellular uptake) by loosening the tight junction.[35] Excipients such as disodium ethylenediaminetetraacetate and chitosan derivatives have been shown to have an effect on paracellular uptake. For drugs that are P-gp substrates, inclusion of excipients such as D-alpha-tocopheryl PEG 1000 succinate (Vitamin E-TPGS) has been shown to minimize the effect of the efflux pump and improve the oral bioavailability of drugs.[36,37]

16.2.3.3   Dermal Permeability

The use of chemical permeability enhancers to improve dermal and transdermal drug delivery has been well studied.[38–42] This is a route of drug administration where permeability enhancers have a well defined role in formulation development. In addition to their use in topical gels and ointments for improved permeability, the inclusion of permeability enhancers extends to transdermal drug delivery devices such as patches.[43] Dermal permeability enhancers function by disrupting the skin barrier, which is accomplished either by extraction or fluidization of lipid bilayers of the skin.[44] This has been associated with an increased potential for skin irritation.

16.2.3.4   Ocular Permeability

Topical ocular drug delivery is a challenging route of administration. The main challenges include the very short residence time on the corneal surface (3–5 minutes) and the relatively impermeable corneal surface. The main formulation approaches to improving ocular bioavailability are the use of bio-adhesive agents such as hydroxymethyl cellulose and gellan gum to improve corneal retention time, and the use of permeation enhancers such as benzalkonium chloride and disodium ethylenediaminetetraacetate to improve corneal permeability.[45,46] The formulation efforts to improve ocular permeability often have to be balanced with the potential for increased tolerability issues.

16.2.4   Metabolism and Excretion

The pharmacokinetic properties of a drug are intricately linked to its metabolism and excretion from the body. The impact of surfactants such as polysorbate 80 and Solutol® HS 15 on the metabolism of drugs such as midazolam has been well characterized *in vitro*, using rat hepatocytes and microsomes.[47] The effect of Solutol HS 15 on colchicine metabolism has been studied *in vivo* in rats. Solutol HS 15 was shown to increase the peak plasma concentration of colchicine and reduce the plasma clearance following intravenous administration. This has been attributed to Solutol HS 15 possibly altering the metabolism and/or the excretion of colchicine.[48]

PEGylation of drugs has been rapidly emerging as a favorable method to modify the pharmacokinetics of drug molecules.[49] It involves the linking of PEG chains to the drug molecule covalently, altering its physicochemical properties and thereby altering its absorption, distribution, metabolism and excretion (ADME) properties. PEGylation has been shown to be particularly effective in improving the pharmacokinetic profiles of proteins and peptides by increasing their molecular weight, reducing the impact of proteolytic enzymes and reducing renal clearance.[50]

16.3   Conclusion

Formulation development plays a significant role in modulating the bioavailability of a drug. The critical role of formulation in improving bioavailability by modulating the solubility of a drug has been well established. It remains one of the most widely used techniques to positively impact the bioavailability of a drug. Drug stability can be enhanced significantly by formulation development efforts. The use of coating materials and the inclusion of anti-oxidants to enable drug and drug product stability has been successfully proven, with their inclusion in many marketed products.

The use of formulation development to impact the bioavailability of a drug by modulating the permeability, metabolism and excretion of the drug has been limited. While the influence of formulation development on these parameters has been ascertained, there remain significant concerns about the safety and tolerability of excipients, and the amounts of excipient that have to be included in the drug product to have an effect. This, however, remains a viable approach to address bioavailability issues encountered in drug development.

References

1. K. T. Savjani, A. K. Gajjar and J. K. Savjani, *ISRN Pharm.*, 2012, **2012**, 195727.
2. T. Takagi, C. Ramachandran, M. Bermejo, S. Yamashita, L. X. Yu and G. L. Amidon, *Mol. Pharm.*, 2006, **3**, 631–643.
3. S. Gopinathan, A. Nouraldeen and A. G. Wilson, *Future Med. Chem.*, 2010, **2**, 1391–1398.
4. P. Li and L. Zhao, *Int. J. Pharm.*, 2007, **341**, 1–19.
5. R. G. Strickley, *Pharm. Res.*, 2004, **21**, 201–230.
6. I. Elsayed, A. A. Abdelbary and A. H. Elshafeey, *Int. J. Nanomed.*, 2014, **9**, 2943–2953.
7. I. Ghosh, S. Bose, R. Vippagunta and F. Harmon, *Int. J. Pharm.*, 2011, **409**, 260–268.
8. S. Gora, G. Mustafa, J. K. Sahni, J. Ali and S. Baboota, *Drug Delivery*, 2014, 1–11.
9. G. G. Liversidge and K. C. Cundy, *Int. J. Pharm.*, 1995, **125**, 91–97.
10. Q. Ma, H. Sun, E. Che, X. Zheng, T. Jiang, C. Sun and S. Wang, *Int. J. Pharm.*, 2013, **441**, 75–81.
11. K. Sigfridsson, A. J. Lundqvist and M. Strimfors, *Drug Dev. Ind. Pharm.*, 2009, **35**, 1479–1486.
12. K. Thadkala, P. K. Nanam, B. Rambabu, C. Sailu and J. Aukunuru, *Int. J. Pharm. Invest.*, 2014, **4**, 131–137.
13. R. Chadha, A. Saini, P. Arora and S. Bhandari, *Crit. Rev. Ther. Drug Carrier Syst.*, 2012, **29**, 183–218.
14. M. S. Jung, J. S. Kim, M. S. Kim, A. Alhalaweh, W. Cho, S. J. Hwang and S. P. Velaga, *J. Pharm. Pharmacol.*, 2010, **62**, 1560–1568.
15. A. J. Smith, P. Kavuru, L. Wojtas, M. J. Zaworotko and R. D. Shytle, *Mol. Pharm.*, 2011, **8**, 1867–1876.
16. R. Fule and P. Amin, *BioMed. Res. Int.*, 2014, **2014**, 146781.
17. T. Vasconcelos, B. Sarmento and P. Costa, *Drug Discovery Today*, 2007, **12**, 1068–1075.
18. M. Yanfei, C. Guoguang, R. Lili and O. Pingkai, *Drug Dev. Ind. Pharm.*, 2014, 1–10.
19. T. Jiang, N. Han, B. Zhao, Y. Xie and S. Wang, *Drug Dev. Ind. Pharm.*, 2012, **38**, 1230–1239.
20. V. B. Junyaprasert and B. Morakul, *Asian J. Pharm. Sci.*, 2014, **10**, 13–23.

21. V. B. Pokharkar, T. Malhi and L. Mandpe, *Pharm. Dev. Technol.*, 2013, **18**, 660–666.
22. O. Bley, J. Siepmann and R. Bodmeier, *Int. J. Pharm.*, 2009, **378**, 59–65.
23. R. Dhurke, I. Kushwaha and B. G. Desai, *PDA J. Pharm. Sci. Technol.*, 2013, **67**, 43–52.
24. A. Khames, *Expert Opin. Drug Delivery*, 2013, **10**, 1335–1343.
25. Y. Fang, G. Wang, R. Zhang, Z. Liu, Z. Liu, X. Wu and D. Cao, *AAPS PharmSciTech*, 2014, **15**, 513–521.
26. M. M. Nerurkar, P. S. Burton and R. T. Borchardt, *Pharm. Res.*, 1996, **13**, 528–534.
27. K. Morimoto, Y. Uehara, K. Iwanaga, M. Kakemi, Y. Ohashi, A. Tanaka and Y. Nakai, *Eur. J. Pharm. Sci.*, 1998, **6**, 225–230.
28. S. A. Ibrahim and S. K. Li, *Pharm. Res.*, 2010, **27**, 115–125.
29. M. Tomita, M. Hayashi and S. Awazu, *Biol. Pharm. Bull.*, 1994, **17**, 753–755.
30. J. O. Morales and J. T. McConville, *Drug Dev. Ind. Pharm.*, 2014, **40**, 579–590.
31. S. Senel and A. A. Hincal, *J. Controlled Release*, 2001, **72**, 133–144.
32. K. C. Sekhar, K. V. Naidu, Y. V. Vishnu, R. Gannu, V. Kishan and Y. M. Rao, *Drug Delivery*, 2008, **15**, 185–191.
33. M. K. Dhiman, A. Dhiman and K. K. Sawant, *AAPS PharmSciTech*, 2009, **10**, 258–265.
34. Y. Yu, Y. Lu, X. Zhao, X. Li and Z. Yin, *Die Pharm.*, 2013, **68**, 732–743.
35. H. J. Lemmer and J. H. Hamman, *Expert Opin. Drug Delivery*, 2013, **10**, 103–114.
36. K. Bogman, Y. Zysset, L. Degen, G. Hopfgartner, H. Gutmann, J. Alsenz and J. Drewe, *Clin. Pharmacol. Ther.*, 2005, **77**, 24–32.
37. M. V. Varma and R. Panchagnula, *Eur. J. Pharm. Sci.*, 2005, **25**, 445–453.
38. A. Mittal, U. V. Sara, A. Ali and M. Aqil, *Curr. Drug Delivery*, 2009, **6**, 274–279.
39. K. Hirata, F. Helal, J. Hadgraft and M. E. Lane, *Int. J. Pharm.*, 2013, **448**, 360–365.
40. A. Nawaz, S. U. Jan, N. R. Khan, A. Hussain and G. M. Khan, *Pak. J. Pharm. Sci.*, 2013, **26**, 617–622.
41. B. Dhawan, G. Aggarwal and S. Harikumar, *Int. J. Pharm. Invest.*, 2014, **4**, 65–76.
42. A. Maurya and S. N. Murthy, *J. Pharm. Sci.*, 2014, **103**, 1497–1503.
43. B. K. Rasool, U. S. Aziz, O. Sarheed and A. A. Rasool, *Acta Pharm. (Zagreb, Croatia)*, 2011, **61**, 271–282.
44. P. Karande, A. Jain, K. Ergun, V. Kispersky and S. Mitragotri, *Proc. Natl. Acad. Sci. U. S. A.*, 2005, **102**, 4688–4693.
45. I. P. Kaur and R. Smitha, *Drug Dev. Ind. Pharm.*, 2002, **28**, 353–369.
46. B. K. Nanjawade, F. V. Manvi and A. S. Manjappa, *J. controlled release*, 2007, **122**, 119–134.
47. R. C. Bravo Gonzalez, J. Huwyler, F. Boess, I. Walter and B. Bittner, *Biopharm. Drug Dispos.*, 2004, **25**, 37–49.

48. B. Bittner, R. C. Gonzalez, I. Walter, M. Kapps and J. Huwyler, *Biopharm. Drug Dispos.*, 2003, **24**, 173–181.
49. X. Zhang, H. Wang, Z. Ma and B. Wu, *Expert Opin. Drug Metab. Toxicol.*, 2014, 1–12.
50. I. Zundorf and T. Dingermann, *Die Pharm.*, 2014, **69**, 323–326.

CHAPTER 17

Systems Pharmacology Modeling

HUGH A. BARTON*[a], HARVEY J. CLEWELL, III[b],
AND MIYOUNG YOON[b]

[a]Worldwide Research and Development, Pfizer, Inc., Eastern Point Rd, MS8220-4503, Groton, CT 06340, USA; [b]The Hamner Institutes for Health Sciences, 6 Davis Drive, Research Triangle Park, NC 27709, USA
*E-mail: habarton@alum.mit.edu

17.1 Introduction

17.1.1 Systems Pharmacology Modeling

The growing interest in systems pharmacology modeling represents a movement from simpler empirical models toward more biologically realistic descriptions of determinants regulating the disposition, effectiveness, and toxicity of drugs in the body. To a large extent, the application of these models is a systems approach integrating knowledge of the biological processes regulating the concentrations of drugs at target sites and their interactions with cellular components and processes. Systems pharmacology models provide the capability to integrate information over multiple levels of biological organization, particularly for characterizing interactions between drugs and their molecular targets, including reversible binding to specific receptors, as exemplified by the binding to dihydrofolate reductase by methotrexate (MTX).[1,2] Thus, these models integrate molecular, cellular,

RSC Drug Discovery Series No. 49
New Horizons in Predictive Drug Metabolism and Pharmacokinetics
Edited by Alan G. E. Wilson

organ, and organism level processes that produce changes over time in the concentrations of the compounds, their metabolites, and bound complexes within the body, and the responses of the cells and tissues to the resulting exposure.

The main goal of systems pharmacology models is quite simple: to predict the concentration of compounds and their metabolites at target tissues and to describe their interactions with and impacts on those target tissues. While it is common for pharmaceuticals to differentiate between effects arising from interactions with the intended pharmacological target (*i.e.*, on-target effects) *versus* effects elsewhere (*i.e.*, off-target effects), in this chapter target refers more broadly to any biological molecule with which a compound interacts causing perturbations in biological processes. Once developed, the models can be used to extrapolate to various other conditions (species, routes, and dosing scenarios) because of their biological fidelity. Generally, the goal of implementing modeling for assessment of drug efficacy and safety is to understand the relationship between the administered dose and the biological sequelae of the exposure of target tissues to compounds. Pharmacokinetic (PK) modeling attempts to characterize the relationship between the administered dose and target tissue exposure. The specific steps leading from tissue exposures to the resulting tissue, organ and organism level responses are generally considered part of the pharmacodynamic (PD) modelling processes. In the past, PD models were generally empirical, utilizing relatively simple effect compartments related to plasma or tissue concentrations of an active drug. An inexorable development is the expansion of the systems approaches into the PK/PD arena.

17.1.2   Systems Pharmacology Modeling Approach

The systems pharmacology approach (Figure 17.1) involves the application of a systems biology-like approach for describing normal biological systems and their perturbations by compounds, and characterization of the exposure/dose conditions under which these perturbations become sufficiently large to pose significant health risks or achieve specific therapeutic outcomes. Perturbating biological processes can lead to either adverse outcomes (toxicity) or restoration of normal processes in a compromised tissue (efficacy). Systems pharmacology links physiologically based PK (PBPK) modeling approaches with mechanistically based models of system responses, including cellular signaling networks, which are also called computational systems biology pathway (CSBP) models. Toxicity and pharmacological efficacy arise from the interaction of the compound with the biological system, so they represent the interface of chemistry – PK (captured as the vertical component in Figure 17.1) and biology – PD (represented with the horizontal events in Figure 17.1). As systems pharmacology models become increasingly mechanistic they rely on increasingly detailed biological descriptions obtained using new experimental technologies and the expansion of computational modeling tools to characterize the system.

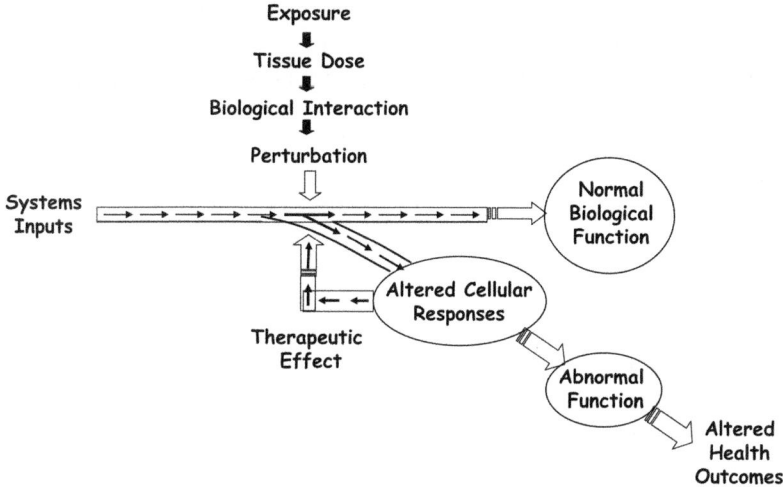

Figure 17.1 Diagram of the approach for understanding the pharmacological and toxicological effects of compounds in terms of their interaction with the biological system. The horizontal axis represents the biological component of the interaction, and the vertical axis represents the chemical component. Drugs can both restore altered biological function (efficacy) and produce altered function (toxicity). Reproduced with permission from The National Academies Press.[3]

In systems pharmacology modeling, systems of simultaneous differential equations are typically used to characterize the changes over time in the biological system. The equations are easily written and implemented in computer software that is commonly available. However, before the model can be used with confidence it has to be qualified as fit-for-purpose to address the needs for which it will be applied. This process includes evaluating the model against experimental information and, in many cases, refining it based on comparison with experimental results. The model itself can frequently be used to help design critical experiments to collect data needed for its own validation. Perhaps the most desirable feature of a systems pharmacology model is that it provides a conceptual framework for employing the scientific method in which hypotheses can be described in terms of biological processes, predictions can be made on the basis of the description, and the hypothesis can be revised on the basis of comparison with experimental data. A strength of these models is that they provide a biologically meaningful quantitative framework into which one can readily incorporate *in vitro* data or *in silico* predictions.[4] An important aspirational goal in the fields of toxicology and pharmacology is to achieve the capability to develop predictive models entirely based upon data from *in vitro* studies.

There are two competing criteria that must be balanced during model design: parsimony and plausibility. The principle of parsimony simply states that a model should be as simple as possible for the intended application (but no simpler). This "splitting" philosophy is related to that of Occam's razor: "Entities should not be multiplied unnecessarily." That is, structures and parameters should not be included in the model unless they are needed to support the application for which the model is being designed. There is no easy rule for determining the level of complexity needed in a particular modeling application. The decision as to which elements to include in the model structure for a specific application draws on all of the modeler's experience and knowledge of the biological–chemical system. The desire for parsimony in model development is driven not only by the desire to minimize the number of parameters whose values must be identified, but also by the recognition that as the number of parameters increases, the potential for unintended interactions between parameters also increases. A generally accepted rule of software engineering warns that it is relatively easy to design a computer program that is too complicated to be completely comprehended by the human mind. As a model becomes more complex, it becomes increasingly difficult to qualify its capabilities, even though concern regarding the trustworthiness of the model should increase.

Countering the desire for model parsimony is the need for biological plausibility of the model structure. The credibility of a model's predictions of behavior under conditions different from those under which the model was validated rests to a large extent on the correspondence of the model design to known biological structures and processes. Generally, a model's capability to recapitulate the observed biological system is dependent on the extent to which the model structure is biologically identifiable, meaning that specific model components represent specific biology. However, it is never possible to have complete biological identifiability, so there will always be some level of "model error", which results in systematic discrepancies between experimental observations and the model. The combination of the structural choices in the model with challenges for identification of model parameters, can result in misidentification of parameters or misspecification of the structure. This presents a challenge for model building that sometimes can be addressed by considering alternative biological hypotheses that might give rise to similar observed behavior and assessing how this impacts model fits and parameter estimates. As such, when a particular model structure improves the simulation of data, it can only be said that the model structure is "consistent" with the data, but one cannot say the model structure has been proven correct. The strongest tests of biologically based models are to make predictions for experimental results different than those used to build the model and determine the consistency with those new results. Biological model building is an art, and is best understood as an iterative process in the spirit of the scientific method.[5–7]

17.2   PBPK Modeling

17.2.1   PBPK Modeling Approach

PK is the study of the processes for absorption, distribution, metabolism, and excretion (ADME) of compounds in the body and their resulting time courses. PK models are comprised of groups of equations that simulate the time courses of compounds and their metabolites in various tissues. The value of PK modeling in pharmacology was that it provided a way to relate internal concentrations of the active form of compounds at their target sites with the doses administered to animals or human subjects. While administered doses are readily known, the disciplines of pharmacology and toxicology have long recognized that it is the internal free concentrations at the target that give rise to both adverse and beneficial effects. Relationships between tissue concentrations and administered dose are frequently complex, especially with the high doses used in toxicological studies or when biological alterations resulting from administration actually change the ADME processes, such as inducing metabolism. All PK models are fundamentally tools to characterize internal target tissues concentrations for a wide range of exposure situations.

The concept of PBPK modeling, also referred to as whole body PK modeling, was first described in the context of drug disposition, in the seminal work of Teorell.[8,9] Nevertheless, in the pharmaceutical industry noncompartmental analysis (NCA) has long been standard practice, even though NCA methods are generally only useful for summarizing the behaviors observed in a dataset (*e.g.*, volume of distribution, terminal half-life) and do not provide the advantages inherent in PBPK modeling (hypothesis testing, and prediction, *etc.*). Its principal advantages are that it is rapid and inexpensive to perform. However, in recent years there has been increasing pressure on the pharmaceutical industry to accelerate the drug development process, and PBPK modeling has repeatedly been identified as one of the technologies that could prove useful to this end.[10–12,38] Recent advances with *in silico/in vitro* based prediction tools, in particular those for absorption, distribution, and hepatic clearance, as well as the emergence of 'ready to use' PBPK software tools have enabled PBPK modeling and simulation to become a vital part of drug discovery and development.[13,14]

Unlike classical PK models, PBPK models have specific compartments for the tissues determining drug exposure, efficacy, toxicity, biotransformation, or other clearance processes. These tissues are connected by blood flow using parameters to describe them that are physiologically meaningful. This facilitates extrapolations among species by using the species-specific physiological parameters. Due to their biological structure, PBPK models can simulate a variety of conditions and extrapolate to situations that differ from those of the data used to calibrate the model.[15] PBPK models have been used effectively for interspecies extrapolation, whether among species in preclinical studies[16] or for predicting human PK based on animal data.[17,18] The biological basis of PBPK models not only facilitates interspecies extrapolations for PK, but also provides a basis for evaluating the consistency among different experimental observations and for trying to understand or explain unexpected or apparently contradictory data. For these and other reasons, particularly *in vitro* to *in vivo* extrapolation, there has been a rapid increase in recent years in pharmaceutical applications of PBPK modeling.[19–24]

Some of the early applications of PBPK modeling in drug development were for chemotherapeutic compounds[25,26] by scientists trained in chemical engineering and computational methods. Such compounds often are very toxic and achieve therapeutic efficacy only by having greater effects on rapidly dividing cancer cells compared to generally more slowly dividing normal tissues. Early successes in PBPK modeling for MTX[2] were followed by models for other chemotherapeutics, including 5-fluorouracil[27] and cisplatin.[28] These important early efforts demonstrated that realistic descriptions of physiology and metabolic pathways could be incorporated in the models effectively. This initiated activities that are now increasingly important for applying PBPK models in drug discovery and develop.[29,30] Approaches for applying PBPK modeling in pharmaceutical research have been presented[17,23] and increasingly specific software are being tailored to pharmaceutical industry needs (*e.g.*, SIMCYP, GASTROPLUS™ and PK-SIM®). As stated earlier, the availability of these PBPK modeling tools for drugs is one of the main reasons behind the recent rise of PBPK modeling in drug development.[14] Some years ago, Lüpfert and Reichel[31] predicted: "The stage is set for a wide penetration of PBPK modeling and simulations to form an intrinsic part of a project starting from lead discovery, to lead optimization and candidate selection, to preclinical profiling and clinical trials." It is now rapidly becoming a vital part of the drug discovery and development process.[32]

Historically, PK and PKPD modeling were applied later in the drug development process largely as methods to analyze data from clinical trials. A major shift has been ongoing to move modeling processes earlier in the preclinical drug discovery phase. This has been facilitated by the development of computational chemistry,[33] genomics[34] and high-throughput screening[35] methods applied in early pharmacology and "discovery toxicology".[36] PBPK modeling can complement other technologies that are increasingly used in drug discovery: quantitative structure–activity relationship (QSAR) analysis and genomics. For PBPK models, QSAR can provide estimates of compound-specific parameters, while genomics data can provide perspectives on the applicable biological processes that need to be captured by the model structure. Systems pharmacology models, representing mechanistic descriptions of pharmacokinetics and dynamics, provide a quantitative framework for integrating diverse data available early in discovery such as the physicochemical characteristics of the compound and *in vitro* data on its ADME and toxicity to predict behavior *in vivo*. This biologically constrained approach can be applied throughout drug development, building upon information for structurally or functionally related compound, as well as assessing the consistency of information obtained from studies using different *in vitro* systems or preclinical animal species. Confidence in the models can be built iteratively as additional data become available. Over time, the models can become tools for providing predictions of compound behavior in humans facilitating selection of first human dose and simulations for clinical trial design (*e.g.*, Monte Carlo simulations of population variability).

With the increased capability to characterize target concentration provided by PBPK models, investigation of the PD effects of drugs can be strengthened by comparisons with analyses focused on administered dose and even circulating blood or plasma concentrations. This can be particularly valuable when active transport processes impact free tissue concentrations, which frequently occurs in the brain, where efflux transport often limits drug exposures compared to plasma, and in the liver, where uptake transport can result in higher free concentrations. PBPK models can capture these tissue-specific processes allowing improved assessments of the likelihood for efficacy or toxicity and their potential modulation through manipulation of the dose rate and route using novel drug delivery systems. These and other attributes of PBPK models for organizing and interpreting diverse datasets, with the specific goals of understanding efficacy and toxicity, are reviving interest in applying these tools in drug development and evaluation.[37] As drug discovery has increasingly moved beyond neutral passively distributing compounds, the value of PBPK model has become more widely recognized. Similarly, with increased emphasis on early decision-making prior to expensive clinical trials, the strength of mechanistic modeling approaches to integrate diverse nonclinical data has led to the growth of preclinical modeling groups throughout the industry and academia.

The heart of a PBPK model is its mass balance equations. The equation for a compound in the liver that is metabolized *via* saturable and nonsaturable components is provided:

$$dA_L/dt = Q_L \times (C_A - C_{VL}) - k_F \times C_{Lfree} \times V_L - V_{max} \times C_{Lfree}/(K_m + C_{Lfree})$$

with A_L as the amount in the tissue (mg), Q_L as the total hepatic blood flow (combined arterial and portal), C_{Lfree} as the free concentration, C_A as the concentration in arterial blood, and C_{VL} as the venous concentration exiting the liver.

A linear (first-order) metabolic pathway described with the rate constant k_F (h^{-1}) and a saturable (Michaelis–Menten) metabolic process with maximum rate V_{max} (mg h^{-1}) and half maximal concentration K_m (mg L^{-1}) complete the equation. Non clearing tissues generally have only the initial terms describing the blood concentrations entering and exiting the tissue and the tissue blood flow. Metabolites formed through these processes may be characterized using their own whole body PBPK models or, particularly for more water soluble compounds, using simpler compartmental descriptions with a volume of distribution and clearance.

Characterizing the free concentration in the liver (C_{Lfree}) is unfortunately not entirely straight forward. For tissues that lack clearance processes (*e.g.*, metabolism, renal excretion, exhalation), it is often assumed that the free concentration in the tissue will be equal to the free or unbound concentration in the blood, *i.e.*, $C_{Tfree} = f_u \times C_B$, with C_{Tfree} as the free concentration in the tissue, f_u the free fraction in the blood and C_B the concentration of compound in the blood. However, in the liver or other tissues with substantial clearance, the free concentration will be diminished well below free blood concentrations. It should also be noted that the assumption of equal free concentrations in blood and tissue assumes a neutral compound, while charged compounds will either be excluded or concentrated due to membrane potential between

plasma and cells as well as pH differences. An alternative approach is to estimate the free liver concentration by dividing the total liver concentration by
the liver : blood partition coefficient.[2] This approximation is particularly useful for compounds whose metabolism is limited by hepatic blood flow at low
concentrations. When using *in vitro* estimates of the metabolic parameters
(V_{max}, K_m, and k_f) in the model, the definition of the *in vivo* free concentration
needs to be consistent with that applied to obtain the *in vitro* estimates of
intrinsic clearance, for example by adjusting the total incubation concentration by the fraction unbound in the presence of microsomes.

It needs to be clearly recognized that the specifics of the PBPK modeling approach can vary greatly to appropriately address the questions being
asked for different compounds in different situations. A number of excellent reviews have been written on the subject of PBPK modeling,[25,38–41] and
the literature includes examples of successful PBPK models for a wide variety of compounds that provide a wealth of insight into various aspects of
the PBPK modeling process.[25,41,42] These sources should be consulted for
further detail on the approach used to apply the PBPK methodology in
specific cases. The major areas of application include, but are not limited
to, prediction of drug–drug interactions, and the effects of age, genetics,
and disease.[42,43] The recent expansion and advances of this tool in predicting the PK of monoclonal antibodies that can then be linked to PD
modeling to eventually predict efficacy in humans,[44–46] and in predicting
the role of transporters in drug disposition and clinical drug–drug interactions[47–51] are of particular significance. Therefore, the following two
examples are meant only to illustrate the process and highlight important
considerations.

17.2.2   Examples of the Use of PBPK Modeling in Drug Development

In this section, two examples will be provided of successful PBPK models for
drugs that have been developed in the past: MTX (a cancer therapeutic) and
all-*trans*-retinoic acid (ATRA; a cancer therapeutic and skin treatment).

17.2.2.1   MTX

The MTX PBPK model is an excellent example to illustrate the iterative
nature of PBPK model development for a drug. The rationale for developing
a predictive PK model was "basing the model, as much as possible, on established, independently verifiable, physiological concepts".[2] The initial model
was developed[52] using the data from a single intravenous (iv) dose study in
CDF-1 mice conducted at a dose of 3 mg kg^{-1}, which is within the clinical
treatment ranges.

The following experimental findings were used to inform the initial model
structure for MTX. A very rapid decrease in plasma concentration and an

increase in gut lumen concentration indicated rapid uptake, tissue binding, and excretion of MTX as it is not extensively metabolized in mice; a subsequent asymptotic leveling of the concentration curves observed for all tissues suggested zero-order uptake of MTX from the gut. A rapid increase in MTX concentration in gut lumen along with a peak gut lumen to plasma concentration ratio of about 100 indicated that enterohepatic recirculation needs to be described in the model. This initial MTX model included five compartments. They are plasma, liver, muscle, kidneys, and gastrointestinal (GI) tract tissue and lumen.[52] The authors also presented simpler model structures with three compartments (liver, plasma/body, and gut lumen) or two compartments (plasma/body and gut lumen) to speed up the simulation of the associated system of equations. All versions of the model used a flow-limited transport description. However, a time delay function was incorporated to account for bile transport and holding time. Data from bile duct cannulation experiments was used to estimate biliary clearance rates. To represent GI transit time and fecal excretion delays, terms for time delay were also used in the gut lumen. Renal clearance was estimated by comparing the integrated plasma concentration with cumulative urinary excretion. The extent of plasma proteins was estimated at 25%. In general, the model predictions were in good agreement with the experimental data. However, the model overpredicted MTX concentrations in gut lumen for 60 minutes or less after exposure, which is probably due to the use of simple time delay when describing biliary transport.

To refine the initial model, Bischoff and colleagues conducted experimental studies using various dose levels of MTX in several species, including humans.[2] The additional data were consistent with the initial observations of (1) a rapid drop in plasma concentrations and a corresponding increase in gut lumen concentrations, which indicates the rapid and substantial tissue uptake and biliary secretion; (2) a peak gut lumen to plasma concentration ratio of about 100; and (3) linear binding of MTX in tissues with plasma concentrations over 0.1 μg mL^{-1}, whereas at low concentrations, mainly non-linear binding presumably to dihydrofolate reductase occurred.

The initial model was revised (Figure 17.2) to describe these more extensive data. MTX renal clearance was determined based on the comparison of the time integral of MTX plasma concentration with cumulative urine formation after intraperitoneal (ip) or iv dosing. Tissue to plasma distribution ratios were derived from constant infusion studies and/or the portion of the concentration curves from iv pulse injection experiments after initial redistribution. Constant tissue to plasma distribution ratios at high concentrations suggested linear binding, while at lower concentrations, distribution ratios represented by the sum of linear non-specific binding and strong saturable binding, which was presumed to be associated with dihydrofolate reductase.

Describing biliary secretion and GI transport of MTX using multi-compartment sub-models was an important feature of the revised model (Figure 17.2). In the original model, a mathematical time delay (step function)

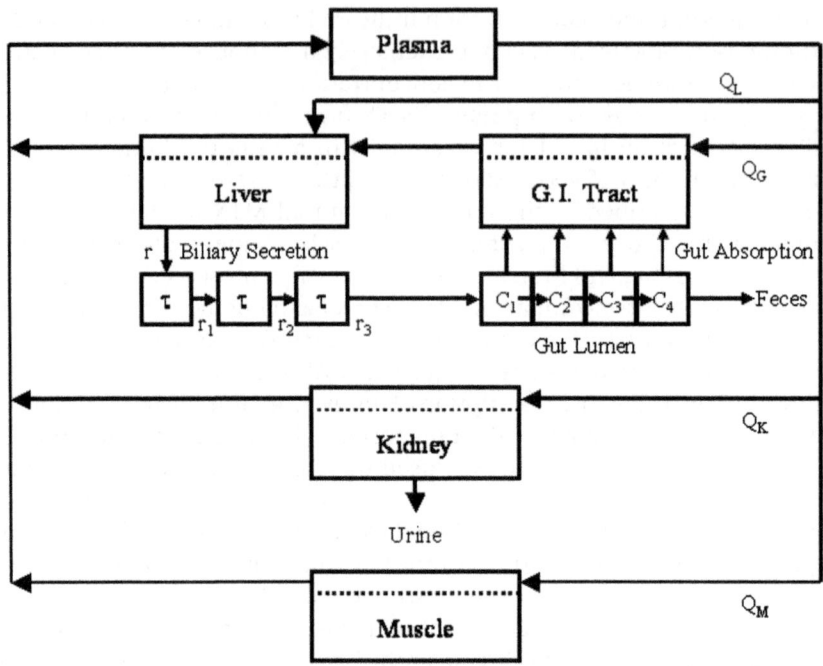

Figure 17.2   PBPK model for methotrexate. Reproduced with permission from John Wiley and Sons.[2]

was used to simulate bile formation and secretion from the liver. This caused the model to overshoot the data in this time period. The revised model used a three-compartment sub-model to represent biliary secretion, which produced a smoother "S-shaped" bile concentration efflux curve.

MTX transit through the GI tract was described using a similar approach to that used for biliary secretion. Given the tubular flow nature of the gut lumen, the time course for concentrations appearing in the feces would not be realistic if uniform mixing was assumed. Thus, the GI tract was described using four distinct regions. The feces exit from the last compartment. Although zero-order absorption from the GI tract was adequate to describe the single dose level in the initial model, more detailed description of gut absorption was required to simulate the wider range of dose levels used in the follow-up studies. Both saturable and non-saturable GI tract absorption was incorporated in the revised model. Absorption characteristics were assumed to be the same for all regions in this model. However, specific location-dependent absorption characteristics could be described with this approach if the data were available.

The consistency between experimental observations and model simulations for MTX showed that a single model structure appropriately parameterized for mouse, rat, dog, and human could reasonably describe its pharmacokinetics. The kinetics of intestinal absorption were a major uncertainty leading to the inclusion of both saturable and non-saturable absorption. Based on the observed kinetic behavior at very low doses, there was determined to be strong, saturable non-linear binding in the liver and kidney, likely arising from binding of the drug with its therapeutic target, dihydrofolate reductase.

17.2.2.2 ATRA

The ATRA PBPK model is a good example of the use of the PBPK model to provide more biologically relevant dose metrics than administered dose for assessing the human risk from a given drug, in this case, the teratogenic risk. To provide a coherent description of ATRA (tretinoin) and its metabolites' ADME across species and routes of administration, a PBPK model was developed.[18]

The PBPK model for ATRA included plasma, liver, intestinal lumen, gut, fat, skin, slowly perfused tissues, richly perfused tissues, placenta, and embryo (Figure 17.3). Saturable kinetic features were used to describe both oxidation (to the 4-oxo derivative) and glucuronidation of ATRA. Conversion to isotretinoin, the 13-*cis* isomer (13-*cis*-RA), and the subsequent metabolism of this compound were also described (not shown). For the metabolites, simpler compartmental descriptions were used, since there was no evidence indicating preferential partitioning of the metabolites into any of the body tissues. The model also included a third metabolic pathway, side chain oxidation producing CO_2. Zero-order stomach emptying and first-order uptake from the intestinal lumen were used to describe oral uptake. A two-compartment model was used to describe dermal uptake. The two compartments represented the stratum corneum and viable epidermis. Flow-limited distribution was assumed except for dermal uptake and transplacental transfer, for which diffusion limited descriptions were used. Excretion into feces and urine were described as first-order processes, with all compounds being excreted in the feces and only glucuronide conjugates being excreted in the urine. Enterohepatic recirculation of ATRA and its metabolites was also included in the model.

The physiological parameters for gestation were adopted from previously published rat gestation models,[53,54] whereas the adult animal physiological parameters were obtained from the literature.[55] Partition coefficients were obtained based on distribution studies performed with human placenta[56] and with mice.[57] The volume of distribution for ATRA was calculated to be 1.1 L kg^{-1} using these partition coefficients, which agrees with measured values. Data from rats with exteriorized bile ducts were used to estimate biliary excretion rate.[58,59] The metabolic parameters were estimated using the data from iv dosing studies in rats[58] and monkeys,[60] as well as from metabolite measurement studies.[59,61] The main species difference in the ATRA metabolism is the predominance of the oxidative metabolism in rodents,[58,59] in contrast to the predominance of the glucuronide conjugation in primates.[61]

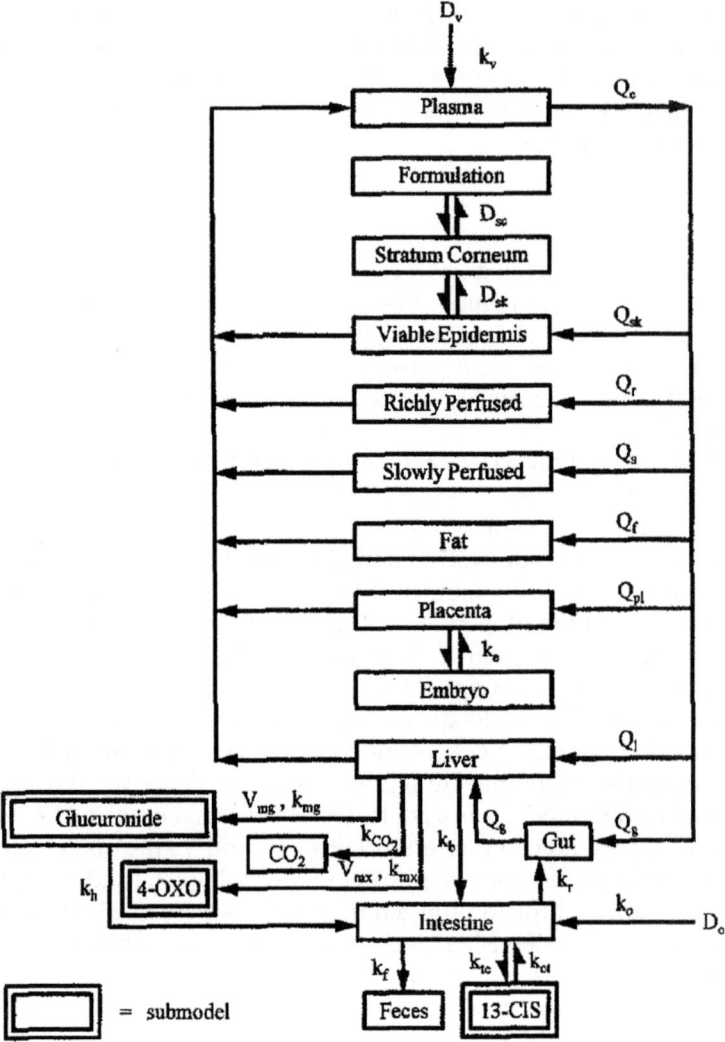

Figure 17.3   PBPK model for all-*trans* retinoic acid. Reproduced with permission from Journal of the American Academy of Dermatology.[18]

Allometric scaling was successfully used to predict plasma kinetics in human leukemia patients following oral dosing with ATRA from the monkey model for intravenous dosing.[62] For this extrapolation only the oral absorption rate was adjusted in the human simulation with all other parameters scaled from the monkey. The model also simulated the kinetics following dermal administration. While the data and classical noncompartmental analyses could only estimate combined exposure to ATRA and its metabolites, the PBPK model could separately estimate internal exposures for ATRA and its metabolites, whether active or inactive. The modeling demonstrated that the low dose rate following dermal exposure is associated with high-efficiency clearance to inactive glucuronide metabolites, whereas the greater dose rate with oral administration leads to a higher proportion of the active oxidative metabolites.

The goal of the modeling was to assess whether the human oral dose of ATRA would be expected to give rise to fetal malformations based upon the minimal teratogenic doses in primates and rodents. The appropriate dose metrics for teratogenic effects suggested by the published literature could be either C_{max} or area under the curve (AUC) for the total concentration of active retinoids. Glucuronide metabolites do not cross the placenta, so they are not included in this dose metric. Based on activity with retinoic acid receptors, the most appropriate dose measure also could be the peak concentration or AUC for ATRA alone. For either assumption, maternal plasma concentrations were considered a surrogate for fetal concentrations, based on observations of similar levels in animal studies.

For a minimal teratogenic effect, all of the dose surrogates (including administered dose) were within a factor of 2–3 across species. The most consistent dose surrogate was the C_{max} for total active retinoids, which was essentially constant across species. Based on this dose measure, the internal exposure of patients receiving oral ATRA treatment for cancer was below the threshold for teratogenic effects by about a factor of 7–10. However, this comparison assumes that the maternal plasma concentration profile is representative of fetal exposure. If one takes into consideration the longer period of organogenesis in humans (around 35 days) compared with the rodent (around 10 days), and assumes, as a worst case, fetal exposure at the maximum maternal concentration throughout the entire period, the margin of safety could be as low as 2–3. It is of interest that the kinetics of 13-*cis*-RA in the human are considerably different from those of ATRA. 13-*cis*-RA has a much longer half-life than ATRA in the human, and oxidation, rather than glucuronidation, is the dominant form of metabolism. The calculated plasma concentrations and AUCs for total active retinoids following oral treatment with 13-*cis*-RA are in the same range as those causing teratogenic effects in animals. This result is consistent with the observation of teratogenic effects associated with the human use of 13-*cis*-RA. This PBPK model was used by the US Food and Drug Administration (FDA) in their evaluation of the safety of a topical skin treatment containing ATRA.

17.3 CSBP Modeling

17.3.1 CSBP Modeling Approach

Systems pharmacology modeling requires knowledge of biology and the use of emerging *in silico*, cellular and molecular technologies to understand the mechanisms by which chemicals interact with biological systems at the cellular level to give rise to beneficial or adverse effects. Increasingly, biologists and biomedical engineers regard biological responses in terms of systems-level behaviors of dynamic networks. Molecular and cellular systems biology-based investigations have begun to map out details of the intracellular protein and gene networks mediating responses to chemical perturbations.[63,64] The availability of detailed interaction maps of protein and gene networks has provided unprecedented opportunities to explore these behaviors and provide quantitative descriptions of molecular pathways and networks that control cellular responses to various stressors.[65,66]

Cellular responses to stimulating compounds involve multiple pathways organized into networks. In large networks, there are normally huge numbers of possible interaction patterns, but biological networks consist of only a few types of circuitry patterns called network motifs. These motifs appear repeatedly throughout networks. While each motif has the same pattern of interactions, they use different genes depending on cell type and output characteristics. Ultrasensitive motifs are responsible for signal amplification and bimodal, all-or-none responses. Surprisingly, robust cell homeostasis requires the presence of ultrasensitive signaling motifs as part of negative feedback loops. In this manner, ultrasensitive motifs are likely to be at work in both adaptation (graded responses maintaining homeostasis) and adversity (quantal responses leading to new cellular phenotypes). CSBP models contain various combinations of signaling motifs that show the modulation of responses change basal, sub-threshold regions of concentration through adaptive and eventually adverse responses.

The following examples of signaling motifs[67] are intended to demonstrate that complex behaviors can be simulated using fairly simple ordinary differential equations (ODEs).

17.3.1.1   Incoherent Feed-Forward Control (Hormesis)

The following ODEs describe incoherent feed-forward control:

$$\frac{dY}{dt} = k_0 + k_1 S - k_2 GY,$$

$$\frac{dG}{dt} = k_3 + k_4 T - k_5 G,$$

$$\frac{dT}{dt} = k_6 S \left(T_{\text{tot}} - T\right) - \left(k_7 \left(T_{\text{tot}} - T\right) + k_8\right)T.$$

In this motif, T is directly regulated by the stressor S and an autocatalytic covalent modification process driven by S activates T (*i.e.*, T also catalyzes its own modification). The magnitude of the feed-forward signaling strength (referred to as gain) quantifies the induction of G by S (*via* T). When the feed-forward gain exceeds the perturbation gain, the induced stress gene activity overcompensates for the change of Y by S (Figure 17.4). As a result, there is over-adaptation, resulting in a hormetic, J-shaped dose response (Figure 17.5).[68,69]

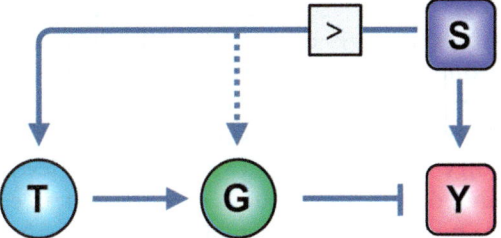

Figure 17.4 Schematic of an incoherent feedforward motif with feedforward signaling strength greater than perturbation strength. Reproduced from Environmental Health Perspectives.[67]

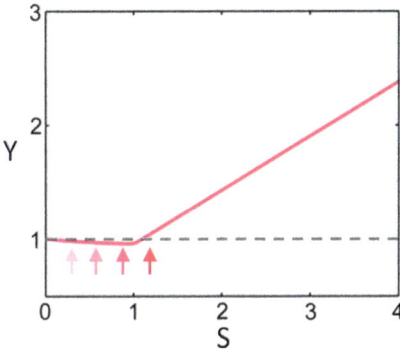

Figure 17.5 An example of greater feedforward signaling strength leads to overadaptation and hormetic steady-state response. Small arrows indicate steady-state responses of Y associated with S levels of 0.3, 0.6, 0.9, and 1.2. Reproduced from Environmental Health Perspectives.[67]

17.3.1.2 Saddle-Node Bifurcation (Switch)

The following ODEs describe positive feedback with saddle-node bifurcation:

$$\frac{dG_1}{dt} = k_1 G_2 S - k_2 G_1,$$

$$\frac{dG_2}{dt} = k_3 + k_4 \frac{G_1^n}{K^n + G_1^n} - k_5 G_2.$$

Here G_1 and G_2 are two mutually activating genes forming a positive feedback loop. S is an external signal stimulating G_1 (Figure 17.6). The Hill function in the equation for G_2 introduces ultrasensitivity, a necessary nonlinearity for generating bistability.[70,71] Depending on the level of S, both G_2 and G_1 settle into one of two discrete states. The steady-state dose response behavior between S and G_2 displays a saddle-node bifurcation (Figure 17.7).

At low levels of S, G_2 increases slightly as S increases. When a threshold value of S ("on threshold") is exceeded, the positive feedback pushes the system to the second stable steady-state with G_2 and G_1 switching abruptly to high levels. Once in the on state, the bistable system does not switch off immediately to the off state when S is reduced below the on threshold. The system switches off when S decreases to an even lower level ("off threshold"). Between the off and on threshold values of S, the system can be either on or off (thus the term bistable), with unstable saddle-node points (blue dashed line in Figure 17.7) lying in between.

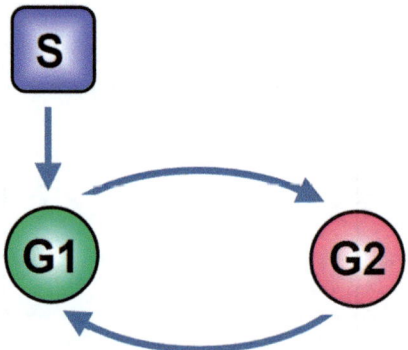

Figure 17.6   Saddle-node bifurcation motifs. Abbreviations: G_1 and G_2, gene 1 and gene 2; S, perturbing signal. The schematic of a two-gene positive feedback system in which S activates G_1 is shown. Reproduced from Environmental Health Perspectives.[67]

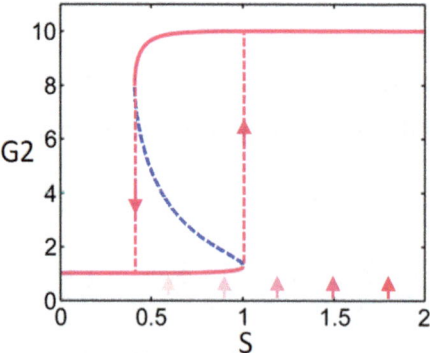

Figure 17.7   Saddle-node bifurcation motifs. Abbreviations: G_1 and G_2, gene 1 and gene 2; S, perturbing signal. The saddle-node bifurcation of G_2 shows the steady-state dose response of G_2 to S. Reproduced from Environmental Health Perspectives.[67]

17.3.1.3   Molecular Titration (Ultrasensitivity)

The following ODEs describe a molecular titration motif:

$$\frac{d[SR]}{dt} = k_1 S \cdot R - k_2 [SR],$$

$$\frac{dG}{dt} = k_3 + k_4 S - k_5 G,$$

here, the external signal S induces gene G. In addition, a high-affinity inhibitor R titrates S away into an inactive complex [SR] (Figure 17.8). In the simulation, the total amount of free R plus R bound in the [SR] complex is constant ($R_{tot} = R + [SR]$). The total amount of free S plus S bound in the complex [SR], *i.e.*, $S_{tot} = S + [SR]$, varies according to the input dose. There is a dose that causes an abrupt change in behavior with this motif, although it would not be a perfect threshold. At low levels of S_{tot}, R sequesters most S molecules due to the high-affinity binding between S and R. There is little S available for inducing G. As the level of S_{tot} approaches R_{tot}, all of R is bound by S. Any further increase in S_{tot} increases free S, which dramatically leads to the induction of G above the baseline (Figure 17.9).

Although the model described here focuses on the PD aspect of the nonlinear exposure–response relationship, this basic model for reversible binding of a compound with a receptor or target can also be important in modeling systemic or tissue PK. This was previously noted for MTX binding to its target, but it is particularly notable in modeling monoclonal antibody PK where target binding can result in substantially faster clearance at

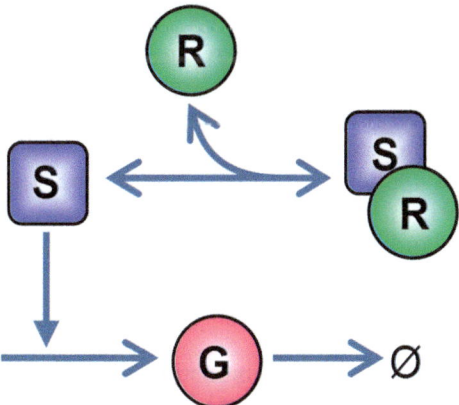

Figure 17.8   Example of an ultrasensitive motif. Abbreviations: ∅, degradation; G, gene G; R, stoichiometric inhibitor; S, stimulating signal. The schematic of a molecular titration motif where inhibitor R sequesters S, reducing the ability of free S to induce gene G is shown. Reproduced from Environmental Health Perspectives.[67]

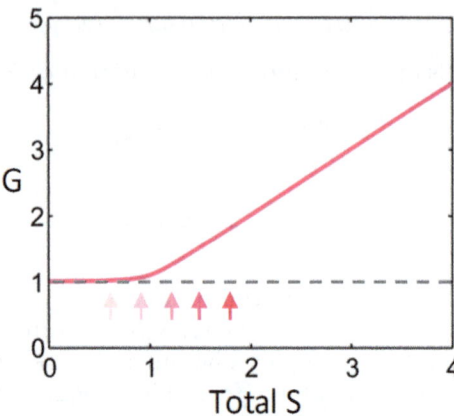

Figure 17.9   Illustration of the dynamic response of *G* to various levels of total *S*.
                    Although not a perfect threshold response, the steady-state response
                    of *G* to the total *S* level increases abruptly as total *S* increases above
                    R. Small arrows indicate steady-state responses of *G* associated with
                    S levels of 0.6, 0.9, 1.2, 1.5, and 1.8; the dashed line denotes the base-
                    line. Reproduced from Environmental Health Perspectives.[67]

lower, non-saturating concentrations. A range of target-mediated disposition models have been published.[72]

17.4   Applications of Mechanistic Modeling in Systems Pharmacology

Mechanistic or systems modeling plays an increasingly large role in drug
discovery and development efforts.[73,74] In the areas of diabetes and insulin regulation or blood pressure maintenance, mechanistic modeling has a
long history for characterizing biological feedback processes. Systems models have now been applied to a wide range of therapeutic areas including
asthma, cancer, central nervous system functions, infectious diseases and
immune function, and bone homeostasis and disease. Increasingly, efforts
are being made to model toxicity endpoints because safety findings continue
to be a major reason for compound failure during the drug discovery and
development process.

The models vary in levels of mechanistic detail and the approaches used.
Systems pharmacology (toxicology), as a term, is widely used in the literature to describe a broad range of modeling approaches, including narrowly
focused mechanistic variants of compartmental PKPD modeling, statistical
bioinformatics analyses of large scale datasets, metabolic network models,
and large multiscale mechanistic models that may include biological components and processes occurring inside cells, within tissue or organs, and at the
whole body level. Mathematically, models may use ODEs, partial differential

equations, Boolean logic, or other approaches. They may be deterministic or stochastic overall or in specific aspects. Often there is a description of the biology, *e.g.*, a deterministic model using ODEs, and then additional models are used to characterize interindividual variability and average population response (and potentially covariates that may be identified), and measurement errors. Fitting data often requires statistical models for interindividual variability and measurement errors, with the parameters estimated by appropriate methods such as nonlinear mixed effects modeling or Bayesian analyses.

While systems biology models focus on characterizing the biological system, systems pharmacology or toxicology models focus on characterizing how a drug or potential new drug would modulate the system in a healthy or diseased state. By their nature, systems pharmacology models need to include a description of the body's handling of the drug, the PK, as well as the body's response to the drug, PD. Modeling approaches for PK and PD are described in Sections 17.2 and 17.3, respectively. Models are often described as bottom-up, top-down, or middle-out, reflecting the approach to their development. Describing the fundamental mechanistic processes and biology, and building up to the overall behavior of the system is a bottom-up approach, applied for example in the development of metabolic network models. Mathematically capturing the feedback processes involved in the whole body homeostatic regulation of glucose by insulin, or blood pressure by water regulation in the kidney, represent top-down approaches that capture key aspects of the biology, but may have widely varying degrees of mechanistic detail and biological identifiability (*i.e.*, a parameter for the concentration of a specific protein or its activity). Middle-out is increasingly being used to describe models that attempt to capture critical mechanistic steps but also incorporate more empirical aspects (*e.g.*, scaling factors from *in vitro* to *in vivo*) that appear necessary to recapitulate the behavior of the intact system. The drive to use systems pharmacology models reflects the fact that drugs often specifically modulate a single target. However, the target is an element of a larger system, so that one cannot necessarily predict the response of the system based solely on what occurs at that target.

Systems pharmacology models are being applied to address a wide variety of questions. Evaluation of individual targets in pathways or the potential for modulating multiple targets with combination therapies are two major focuses. Characterization of patient populations that would benefit from a therapy, *i.e.*, personalized medicine, is another application that can impact clinical study designs in the nearer term, as well as the final applications of medical treatment. A major goal is improving the success of drug discovery and development approaches by improving the translation from a wide range of nonclinical endpoints (*i.e.*, *in vitro* assays and preclinical *in vivo* studies in various animal species) to the clinical setting. Selecting appropriate doses and dosing regimens can also be informed by systems pharmacology models.

17.4.1 Cancer

Drugs to treat cancers are a major focus of pharmaceutical discovery and development driven by the need to better treat cancers and significantly increased understanding of the biological processes underlying tumor development. Newer treatments, whether small molecules such as kinase inhibitors or biotherapeutics targeting cell surface receptors, tend to utilize specific mechanistic aspects of those biological processes to achieve efficacy. Another approach is to target agents that are broadly cytotoxic using the specificity of large molecules, such as in antibody drug conjugates (ADCs). Other efforts are ongoing to engage the immune system for tumor cell killing. Reflecting this range of contemporary drug discovery approaches, a range of modeling approaches have been applied to translate from preclinical studies to clinical settings, select targets or identify limitations of targets, identify combination treatments, and select doses and dosing regimens to maximize efficacy while limiting toxicity. These approaches characterize tumor growth and inhibition, intricacies of molecular intracellular signaling pathways, and metabolic or catabolic pathways using semi-mechanistic PKPD modeling, signaling systems modeling, and metabolic pathway analyses. These modeling approaches represent fit-for-purpose choices reflecting the different systems being modeled.

Semi-mechanistic and mechanistic PK/PD modeling has been applied to characterize tumor growth inhibition by ADCs focusing on the interactions of the ADC with its target and subsequent processing, such as internalization, and tumor growth and inhibition. Antibody drug conjugates consist of a cytotoxic small molecule payload (*e.g.*, tubulin inhibitors), an antibody to a tumor expressed target, and a small molecule to link the two. Since the PD effect is cell killing, the modeling has used several different growth equations, which were compared by Haddish-Berhane and coworkers,[75] along with proposing a hybrid model. Data for the ADC, Trastuzumab-emtansine (T-DM1) were used to demonstrate translation from preclinical studies of plasma ADC concentrations and tumor growth inhibition to clinical results. A more mechanistic description of the PK to capture tumor concentration of payload has been described for translation using ADCETRIS® (brentuximab vedotin).[76] This model explicitly captures the early PKPD effects, such as tumor target binding and internalization as well as binding to the secondary intracellular target for the payload. The rate of cell killing, k_k, is characterized as a saturable process

$$k_k = K_{k,max} \times C/(k_{C50} + C),$$

with a maximal rate ($K_{k,max}$) and a half maximal kill rate (k_{C50}). This equation, along with the sigmoid or Hill variant with exponents on the concentration and half maximal rate parameters, is widely applied for characterizing drug interactions with their targets. It has been applied to small molecule oncology drugs such as the kinase inhibitor, crizotinib,[77] as well as the ADCs.

While the focus with cytotoxic ADCs is on describing the target concentration and initial drug-target interactions with relatively simple descriptions of the subsequent cell killing processes, for therapies that target steps in cancer cell signaling processes more complex CSBP models are being applied. Several cell signaling models focus on regulation of cell growth and proliferation through the Ras/MEK/ERK pathway in responses to several external ligands (*e.g.*, VEGF, HRG, IGF-1, EGF) and apoptotic regulation *via* the PI3K/AKT pathway.[78–81] These models have between 75 and 125 state variables capturing external ligands, their binding to membrane-associated protein receptors, receptor dimerization, kinase or phosphatase activities altering phosphorylation status, recruitment of adapter proteins or enzymes, and feedback signaling processes, such as the motifs describe in Section 17.3. These models capture alternative pathways and adaptations that occur when specific steps are inhibited. Therefore, by comparison with simpler logic-based models for the same systems,[79] the systems models capture biological variation (genotypic or phenotypic), facilitate drug target selection and evaluation of the value of combinations over individual targets, and assist in translation from preclinical to clinical. Larger systems models of this kind require time and resources to build the model structure, estimate parameter values from literature or new experimental results, and test the model to demonstrate its utility. Although there are academic publications in this area, there are also publications from the pharmaceutical industry applying these models notably to novel biotherapeutic modalities such as bispecific antibodies.[80,81]

Genome-scale metabolic models represents a third variety of systems models that have been applied to cancer (reviewed in ref. 82). These models are bottom-up mechanistic representations of cellular metabolism and may utilize large scale "omics" data sets.[83] Small molecule metabolites downstream of genes and proteins may be considered to represent the integrated status of the system in the healthy state and reflect disease state alterations (reviewed in ref. 84). One could then simulate the impacts of therapies on this system, which is typically represented under steady state conditions.[85] As with the analyses using cell signaling systems models, metabolic network models can assess the value of individual targets for drugs as well as potential combination therapies modulating two or more targets.

Finally, it is worth noting that development of cancer immunotherapies is a major new direction.[86] These include those that empower the natural capabilities of the immune cells by inhibiting targets on tumor cells that evade immune surveillance as well as bispecific modalities that redirect T-cell killing using tumor specific overexpressed targets. It might be anticipated that this would lead to expanded efforts to apply modeling of immune function to cancer applications.[87] Models of immune system function have been critical for understanding diseases of that system such as human immunodeficiency virus (HIV) infection.[88] Models often have focused on specific aspects of immune function, but there have also been efforts to combine these published models into an integrated systems model,[89] and below modeling of immunogenicity of biotherapeutics is reviewed.

17.4.2   Systems Toxicology Modeling

While modeling for efficacy is complex, it is inherently as complex or more so for predicting toxicity. For evaluating safety, one is ultimately concerned about all potential impacts on targets throughout the body leading to any potentially adverse effect, in contrast with the generally more focused target interaction involved in obtaining efficacy in a specific cell, organ or system. The range of targets leading to toxicity tends to be much broader than typically engaged for efficacy, including not just specific macromolecules (*e.g.*, proteins that are receptors or enzymes), but also membranes (*e.g.*, altering fluidity and protein–protein interactions), multiple intracellular sites (*e.g.*, reactive oxygen damage to lipids, membranes, *etc.*), or physical processes (*e.g.*, crystal formation leading to nephropathy or bladder tumors). As a consequence, the term systems toxicology is used to refer to a number of quite diverse efforts attempting to predict specific toxic endpoints or organ toxicities (*e.g.*, immunogenicity, liver injury discussed below), effects of specific drugs, or global prediction of toxicity.[90]

Furthermore, many of these efforts assess whether or not toxicity might arise without consideration of drug or chemical concentration, despite the fact that exposure for pharmaceuticals, food additives, consumer products, or environmental chemicals is recognized as key to assessing their safety or associated risks.[91,92] Successful drugs generally arise from appropriately balancing concentrations adequate to modulate the target(s) to achieve efficacy while low enough to avoid toxicities that occur at higher concentrations, rather than from finding compounds that do not cause any toxicity. Predicting this balance requires accurately predicting the concentration–response relationship for efficacy and for potential toxicities. Liver injury is a particularly important endpoint occurring with small molecule drugs, while immunogenicity is a major concern for biotherapeutics, particularly proteins. Both are the subject of active efforts to develop systems models.

17.4.2.1   Liver Injury

Drug induced liver injury (DILI) is a major cause of drugs failing during clinical trials, being removed after approval, and receiving labeling language warning of potential adverse effects.[91] These findings of liver injury in humans occur despite toxicological tests in at least two animal species that are often negative and, thus, not predictive of the human experience. As a consequence, there are several ongoing efforts to develop semi-quantitative or statistical analyses[93,94] or mechanistic models[95–98] coupled with *in vitro* assays to provide input information. In addition, the fairly common observations of liver enlargement, histopathological injury, and tumors in animal toxicology studies has spawned modeling efforts to strengthen understanding of the translation of these results to humans.[99,100] Mechanistic models for DILI provide good examples of different approaches depending in part on the goals of the efforts, notably differential equation and agent-based models. Differential equation models have focused more on the mechanisms or pathways leading to adverse outcomes and the biomarkers associated with those processes, while the agent-based models have focused more on the two or three dimension structure of the liver, compound distribution throughout and dynamic changes that occur with cell death, tissue regeneration and remodeling.[100,101] An agent-based model has been used to test theories and gain insights into liver tissue regeneration following necrotic insult.[101]

One of the challenges of modeling DILI is that it represents several outcomes that can occur in livers exposed over shorter or longer periods of time. These include cytotoxicity ranging from single cells to regions of necrosis, changes in bile flow (*e.g.*, cholestasis, vanishing bile duct syndrome), and lipid accumulations (steatosis). In addition, toxic effects of drugs or environmental chemicals may be superimposed upon liver diseases arising from varied etiologies including non-alcoholic fatty liver diseases (NAFLD) due to Type 2 diabetes or cirrhosis due to chronic alcohol intake. In pharmaceutical discovery and development, effects observed in early clinical trials represent acute toxicities associated with single or short exposures while effects observed in later clinical trials or post-marketing may involve more prolonged exposures or exposure of populations with more varied genotypes and phenotypes. Thus, the goals of the modeling can play key roles in determining the modeling approach, model structure and biological content. Given the complexity of normal liver function, processing nutrients, removing waste products, and maintaining systemic concentrations of small (*e.g.*, amino acids, fatty acids, nucleosides) and large molecules (*e.g.*, plasma proteins and lipoproteins), as well as the range of diseases and toxicities that can occur in liver, it is a long term goal to have a fully comprehensive multi-scale model.

An example of a systems toxicology model in which drug concentrations in liver obtained from physiologically based PK modeling are linked with a mechanistic multi-scale toxicodynamic model is DILIsym® (http://www.DILIsym.com) (Figure 17.10). The liver in this model is described using three compartments representing the periportal, midzonal, and centrilobular regions of the liver.[97] It has submodels for biological processes important in the development of liver toxicity including glutathione depletion by reactive metabolites and synthesis, bile acid transport and homeostasis, mitochondrial function, cellular energy balances, cell death and apoptosis, and innate immune function. Building the linkages among submodels, such as between bile acid regulation and mitochondrial function, is as important as defining the contents of each submodel because they can strongly influence the overall system behavior. The model also includes a number of biomarkers measured clinically in plasma that are at least partially indicative of the form of liver injury, such as alanine aminotransferase (ALT) for necrosis, total bilirubin for altered bile acid homeostasis, fragmented keratin-18 for apoptosis, and liver specific microRNA, miR-122 for necrosis. It is an example of a "middle-out" model building approach in which critical aspects of liver biology and toxicity pathways are described and additional details at the molecular or systemic levels are added as required to capture behaviors observed with the compounds being modeled. For example, some anti-viral nucleoside analogs inhibit mitochondrial DNA synthesis leading to mitochondrial dysfunction and liver toxicity, so this mechanism could be added to the model augmenting other mechanisms leading to mitochondrial toxicity, and its absence limits the model applicability to compounds for which this mechanism is relevant.

Like several others, the model addresses reactive metabolite mediated DILI, particularly from acetaminophen exposures, for which a wide range of data are available in several species. DILIsym generally keeps the same model structure for each species, barring species specific processes, but has appropriate parameter values for mice, rats, and humans. Thus, it can capture the preferential toxicity of acetaminophen in mice and humans compared to rats, while a preferential response in rats is captured for methapyrilene, another drug associated with reactive metabolite-mediated toxicity.[104] Innate immune function has been shown to modulate even the clearly dose-dependent toxicity of acetaminophen and is an aspect of the DILIsym model.[104]

Occurrence of liver toxicity can be quite variable, so elevated serum liver enzymes may be observed in small clinical studies early in development,

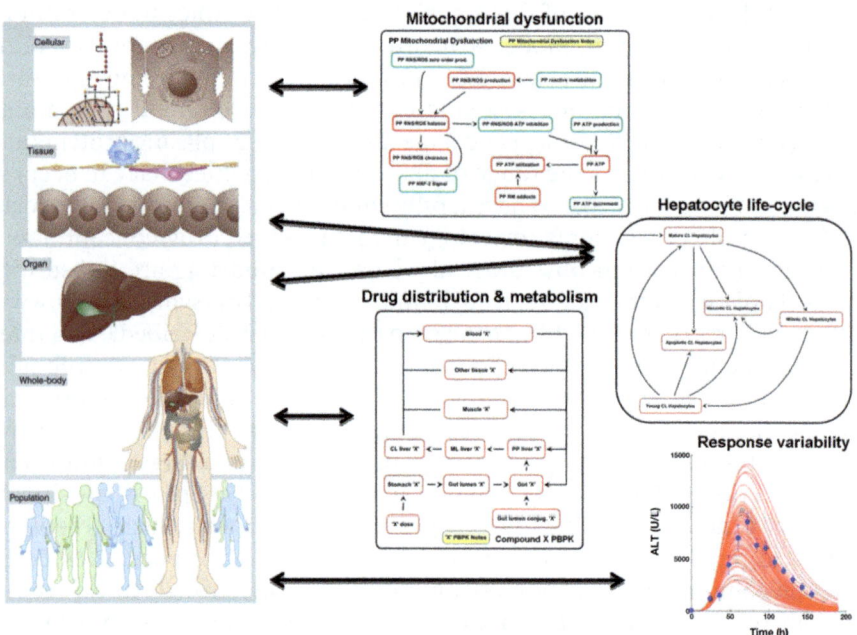

Figure 17.10   Conception of the multi-scale DILIsym™ model. The DILIsym™ model is a multi-scale representation of liver physiology, encompassing molecular and cellular interactions, variability in different zones of the liver acinus, whole-body drug distribution and metabolism, as well as variability in both drug profile and underlying physiology leading to alternate responses. Reproduced from Frontiers in Physiology and Molecular Systems Biology.[102,103]

indicating occurrence with a high frequency, while in other cases observations occur only later in large clinical trials or post-marketing, indicating low frequency, often referred to as idiosyncratic liver injury. Modeling population variability both for drug PK and for the toxicodynamic processes therefore can be quite valuable for evaluating model performance for drugs such as bosentan (8–18% incidence) or troglitazone.[105,106] Acquired immune responses have been associated with some observations of infrequent liver toxicity, but this has not been addressed yet in liver toxicity systems models.

Building systems models that describe compound PK, target tissue exposures, and multiple biological mechanisms leading to toxicity and the variability of these processes in populations offers promise for better predicting toxicity. Challenges to this approach arise from both capturing the extensive known biology as well as recognizing the frequent gaps in knowledge. Moving from the retrospective analyses involved in model building to demonstrating predictive capability is often an extended and iterative process. A key aspect is to identify the information needed as inputs for successful predictions, which ideally should be obtained from *in vitro* assays or perhaps even *in silico* predictive methods for individual model parameters (*e.g.*, tissue partition coefficient predictions in the PBPK model). *In vitro* and *in silico* sources of model inputs allows the model to be used earlier in the drug discovery process than if *in vivo* preclinical or clinical data are required.

17.4.2.2 Immunogenicity

Unwanted immune response to therapeutic proteins, particularly antidrug antibody (ADA) formation, is one of the major safety concerns for these biotherapeutic modalities. While there has been extensive mathematical modeling of the immune system, only recently have models focusing on immunogenicity been implemented. Formation of ADA can affect the PK of the therapeutic protein, often a monoclonal antibody (mAb),[107] as well the efficacy of the protein and its safety. As with other areas of systems modeling, different approaches have been applied to immune systems modeling including agent-based and differential equation models. One effort builds upon models from the literature to create a systems model explicitly directed at the primary and secondary immune responses involved in immunogenicity.[108,109] Building upon existing models facilitates development of a systems model within a shorter time frame, which is highly valued during pharmaceutical discovery and development. The model aims to integrate many known risk factors for immunogenicity, such as T- and B-epitopes on therapeutic proteins and patients' HLA genotype for predicting immune response. The model has been parameterized to the extent possible with mouse and human specific values. It describes drug (antigen) disposition and biological processes at the subcellular, cellular, and whole body levels.

The subcellular model describes antigen processing and presentation by dendritic cells, used to represent all antigen-presenting cells. Therapeutic proteins are endocytosed and digested into peptides for binding to major histocompatibility complex (MHC) class II molecules for presentation on the cell surface. Binding affinities of different T-epitopes, measured *in vitro* or predicted *in silico*, for six human subclasses play a major role in differentiating immune responses to antigens and accounting for human variability. Antigen presentation by dendritic cells activates the adaptive immune cells, causing proliferation and differentiation of T and B cells. Thus, the cellular level of this model accounts for these different cell populations (*e.g.*, naïve and memory T and B cells, short and long lived plasma cells), their interactions and growth over time. The whole body model is a simplified compartment description for the antigenic proteins and links with the cellular model by describing immune cells and antigenic proteins interacting in the plasma compartment assuming rapid movement of white blood cells between lymph organs and blood. This model recapitulates known occurrences in the immune system such as an enhanced secondary immune response, affinity maturation of antibodies, and processes of antigen presentation. Importantly, it predicts these changes in relationship to the development of ADA. The model was demonstrated to capture observations in human populations dosed with the therapeutic antibody adalimumab including a relatively high immunogenicity rate and reduced drug trough concentration in ADA positive patients.

Like all systems pharmacology or toxicology models, the immunogenicity model could be extended through incorporation of additional biology. Dendritic cell activation was described as endotoxin-driven, specifically lipopolysaccharide (LPS), which is widely used in experimental studies and exists in formulations of therapeutic proteins. The model could be expanded to account for other processes leading to dendritic cell activation, such as tissue damage. At the whole body level, the model assumes all interactions occur in plasma, but one could expand the model to include lymphoid organs where immune processes occur. Finally, as an initial model, it has undergone limited evaluation using data available for mouse immunization studies and human clinical experience. Further evaluation with clinical data will be valuable.

17.5   Conclusions

Modeling and simulation play increasingly important roles in pharmaceutical discovery and development addressing both efficacy and safety. Mathematics has long played a fundamental role in the development of basic concepts of pharmacology and PK, but the availability of vastly enhanced computing capability has influenced experimental methods and the approaches for analyzing the data. A tension now exists between well-established methods using PK/PD models for analyzing preclinical and clinical study data that restrict the model structure to only have parameters directly estimable from the specific data set and the widely perceived value of incorporating knowledge of the biological system into the analysis. Systems pharmacology models constructed by integrating PBPK with mechanistic PD models, such as

CSBP models, provide the potential to assess whether pharmacological interventions in a system will be beneficial prior to and during the costly experimental discovery and development process. Due to the resources required to develop larger systems pharmacology models, pharmaceutical modeling will continue to rely on a wide range of analyses intended to be fit-for-purpose in addressing the issues at hand. The value of bringing together the breadth of biological knowledge within a systems pharmacology modeling framework is increasingly recognized within academia, industry, and regulatory agencies worldwide.[110]

References

1. R. L. Dedrick, D. S. Zaharko, R. A. Bender, W. A. Bleyer and R. J. Lutz, *Cancer Chemother. Rep.*, 1975, **59**, 795–804.
2. K. B. Bischoff, R. L. Dedrick, D. S. Zaharko and J. A. Longstreth, *J. Pharm. Sci.*, 1971, **60**, 1128–1133.
3. National Research Council, *Toxicity Testing in the 21st Century: A Vision and a Strategy*, The National Academies Press, Washington, DC, 2007.
4. H. J. Clewell, 3rd, *Toxicol. Lett.*, 1993, **68**, 101–117.
5. A. Rescigno, J. S. Beck and A. K. Thakur, *J. Pharmacokinet. Pharmacodyn.*, 1987, **15**, 327–340.
6. F. E. Yates, *Am. J. Physiol.*, 1978, **234**, R159–R160.
7. E. R. Carson, C. Cobelli and L. Finkelstein, *The mathmatical modeling of metabolic and endocrine systems. Model formulation, identification, and validation*, John and Wiley and Sons, New York, 1983.
8. T. Teorell, *Arch. Int. Pharmacodyn. Ther.*, 1937, **57**, 205–225.
9. T. Teorell, *Arch. Int. Pharmacodyn. Ther.*, 1937, **57**, 226–240.
10. S. B. Charnick, R. Kawai, J. R. Nedelman, M. Lemaire, W. Niederberger and H. Sato, *J. Pharmacokinet. Biopharm.*, 1995, **23**, 217–229.
11. C. C. Peck, W. H. Barr, L. Z. Benet, J. Collins, R. E. Desjardins, D. E. Furst, J. G. Harter, G. Levy, T. Ludden and J. H. Rodman, *J. Pharm. Sci.*, 1992, **81**, 605–610.
12. M. Rowland, L. Balant and C. Peck, *AAPS PharmSci*, 2004, **6**, 56–67.
13. Y. Chen, J. Y. Jin, S. Mukadam, V. Malhi and J. R. Kenny, *Biopharm. Drug Dispos.*, 2012, **33**, 85–98.
14. F. Bouzom, K. Ball, N. Perdaems and B. Walther, *Biopharm. Drug Dispos.*, 2012, **33**, 55–71.
15. L. Aarons, *Br. J. Clin. Pharmacol.*, 2005, **60**, 581–583.
16. R. L. Dedrick and K. B. Bischoff, *Fed. Proc.*, 1980, **39**, 54–59.
17. H. M. Jones, N. Parrott, K. Jorga and T. Lavé, *Clin. Pharmacokinet.*, 2006, **45**, 511–542.
18. H. J. Clewell III, M. E. Andersen, R. J. Wills and L. Latriano, *J. Am. Acad. Dermatol.*, 1997, **36**, S77–S85.
19. S. A. Peters, *Physiologically-based pharmacokinetic (PBPK) modeling and simulations: principles, methods, and applications in the pharmaceutical industry*, John Wiley & Sons, 2012.

20. M. Reddy, R. Yang, M. E. Andersen and H. J. Clewell III, *Physiologically based pharmacokinetic modeling: science and applications*, John Wiley & Sons, 2005.

21. F. A. Brightman, D. E. Leahy, G. E. Searle and S. Thomas, *Drug Metab. Dispos. Biol. Fate Chem.*, 2006, **34**, 84–93.

22. D. Muzzey, C. A. Gómez-Uribe, J. T. Mettetal and A. van Oudenaarden, *Cell*, 2009, **138**, 160–171.

23. N. Parrott, H. Jones, N. Paquereau and T. Lavé, *Basic Clin. Pharmacol. Toxicol.*, 2005, **96**, 193–199.

24. A. Rostami-Hodjegan, *Clin. Pharmacol. Ther.*, 2012, **92**, 50–61.

25. M. C. Peterson and M. M. Riggs, *CPT: Pharmacometrics Syst. Pharmacol.*, 2012, **1**, e14.

26. K. Bischoff, *Fortschr. Geb. Rontgenstr Nuklearmed.*, 1966, **104**, 847–856.

27. J. M. Collins, R. L. Dedrick, M. F. Flessner and A. M. Guarino, *J. Pharm. Sci.*, 1982, **71**, 735–738.

28. F. F. Farris, R. L. Dedrick and F. G. King, *Toxicol. Lett.*, 1988, **43**, 117–137.

29. C. Lüpfert and A. Reichel, *Chem. Biodiversity*, 2005, **2**, 1462–1486.

30. I. Nestorov, *Clin. Pharmacokinet.*, 2003, **42**, 883–908.

31. C. Lüpfert and A. Reichel, *Chem. Biodiversity*, 2005, **2**, 1462–1486.

32. A. Rostami-Hodjegan, I. Tamai and K. S. Pang, *Biopharm. Drug Dispos.*, 2012, **33**, 47–50.

33. W. L. Jorgensen, *Science*, 2004, **303**, 1813–1818.

34. D. O. Ricke, S. Wang, R. Cai and D. Cohen, *Curr. Opin. Chem. Biol.*, 2006, **10**, 303–308.

35. A. Lahoz, L. Gombau, M. Donato, J. V. Castell and M. Gomez-Lechon, *Mini-Rev. Med. Chem.*, 2006, **6**, 1053–1062.

36. H. van de Waterbeemd and E. Gifford, *Nat. Rev. Drug Discovery*, 2003, **2**, 192–204.

37. K. S. Blesch, R. Gieschke, Y. Tsukamoto, B. G. Reigner, H. U. Burger and J.-L. Steimer, *Invest. New Drugs*, 2003, **21**, 195–223.

38. H. J. Clewell, M. B. Reddy, T. Lave and M. E. Andersen, *Preclin. Drug Dev. Handb.*, 2008, 1167–1227.

39. L. E. Gerlowski and R. K. Jain, *J. Pharm. Sci.*, 1983, **72**, 1103–1127.

40. K. J. Himmelstein and R. J. Lutz, *J. Pharmacokinet. Biopharm.*, 1979, **7**, 127–145.

41. M. Reddy, R. S. Yang, M. E. Andersen and H. J. Clewell III, *Physiologically based pharmacokinetic modeling: science and applications*, John Wiley & Sons, 2005.

42. M. Rowland, C. Peck and G. Tucker, *Annu. Rev. Pharmacol. Toxicol.*, 2011, **51**, 45–73.

43. P. Zhao, L. Zhang, J. Grillo, Q. Liu, J. Bullock, Y. Moon, P. Song, S. Brar, R. Madabushi and T. Wu, *Clin. Pharmacol. Ther.*, 2011, **89**, 259–267.

44. M. Chetty, L. Li, R. Rose, K. Machavaram, M. Jamei, A. Rostami-Hodjegan and I. Gardner, *Front. Immunol.*, 2014, **5**, 670.

45. Y. Cao, J. P. Balthasar and W. J. Jusko, *J. Pharmacokinet. Pharmacodyn.*, 2013, **40**, 597–607.

46. D. K. Shah and A. M. Betts, *J. Pharmacokinet. Pharmacodyn.*, 2012, **39**, 67–86.

47. R. Li, H. A. Barton, P. D. Yates, A. Ghosh, A. C. Wolford, K. A. Riccardi and T. S. Maurer, *J. Pharmacokinet. Pharmacodyn.*, 2014, **41**, 197–209.

48. A. Poirier, C. Funk, J.-M. Scherrmann and T. Lavé, *Mol. Pharmaceutics*, 2009, **6**, 1716–1733.

49. T. Watanabe, H. Kusuhara, K. Maeda, Y. Shitara and Y. Sugiyama, *J. Pharmacol. Exp. Ther.*, 2009, **328**, 652–662.

50. J. Fan, S. Chen, E. CY Chow and K. Sandy Pang, *Curr. Drug Metab.*, 2010, **11**, 743–761.

51. H. A. Barton, Y. Lai, T. C. Goosen, H. M. Jones, A. F. El-Kattan, J. R. Gosset, J. Lin and M. V. Varma, *Expert Opin. Drug Metab. Toxicol.*, 2013, **9**, 459–472.

52. K. B. Bischoff, R. L. Dedrick and D. S. Zaharko, *J. Pharm. Sci.*, 1970, **59**, 149–154.

53. E. J. O'Flaherty, W. Scott, C. Schreiner and R. P. Beliles, *Toxicol. Appl. Pharmacol.*, 1992, **112**, 245–256.

54. J. W. Fisher, T. A. Whittaker, D. H. Taylor, H. J. Clewell and M. E. Andersen, *Toxicol. Appl. Pharmacol.*, 1989, **99**, 395–414.

55. R. Brown, M. Delp, S. Lindstedt, L. Rhomberg and R. Beliles, *Toxicol. Ind. Health*, 1997, **13407**, 484.

56. M. Asai, W. Faber, L. Neth-Jessee, P. A. di Sant'Agnese, M. Nakanishi and R. K. Miller, *Placenta*, 1993, **14**, 25–33.

57. J. R. Kalin, M. E. Starling and D. L. Hill, *Drug Metab. Dispos. Biol. Fate Chem.*, 1981, **9**, 196–201.

58. B. N. Swanson, C. A. Frolik, D. W. Zaharevitz, P. P. Roller and M. B. Sporn, *Biochem. Pharmacol.*, 1981, **30**, 107–113.

59. M. H. Zile, R. C. Inhorn and H. F. DeLuca, *J. Biol. Chem.*, 1982, **257**, 3537–3543.

60. P. C. Adamson, F. M. Balis, M. A. Smith, R. F. Murphy, K. A. Godwin and D. G. Poplack, *J. Natl. Cancer Inst.*, 1992, **84**, 1332–1335.

61. J. C. Kraft, W. Slikker, Jr., J. R. Bailey, L. G. Roberts, B. Fischer, W. Wittfoht and H. Nau, *Drug Metab. Dispos. Biol. Fate Chem.*, 1991, **19**, 317–324.

62. J. R. Muindi, S. R. Frankel, C. Huselton, F. DeGrazia, W. A. Garland, C. W. Young and R. P. Warrell, Jr., *Cancer Res.*, 1992, **52**, 2138–2142.

63. E. Caron, S. Ghosh, Y. Matsuoka, D. Ashton-Beaucage, M. Therrien, S. Lemieux, C. Perreault, P. P. Roux and H. Kitano, *Mol. Syst. Biol.*, 2010, **6**, 453.

64. K. Oda and H. Kitano, *Mol. Syst. Biol.*, 2006, **2**, 0015.

65. U. Alon, *An introduction to systems biology: design principles of biological circuits*, CRC press, 2006.

66. J. J. Tyson, K. C. Chen and B. Novak, *Curr. Opin. Cell Biol.*, 2003, **15**, 221–231.

67. Q. Zhang, S. Bhattacharya, R. B. Conolly, H. J. Clewell, N. E. Kaminski and M. E. Andersen, *Environ. Health Perspect.*, 2014, **122**, 1261–1270.

68. S. Kaplan, A. Bren, E. Dekel and U. Alon, *Mol. Syst. Biol.*, 2008, **4**, 203.

69. D. Kim, Y. K. Kwon and K. H. Cho, *BioEssays*, 2008, **30**, 1204–1211.

70. D. Angeli, J. E. Ferrell, Jr. and E. D. Sontag, *Proc. Natl. Acad. Sci. U. S. A.*, 2004, **101**, 1822–1827.

71. Q. Zhang, D. E. Kline, S. Bhattacharya, R. B. Crawford, R. B. Conolly, R. S. Thomas, M. E. Andersen and N. E. Kaminski, *Toxicol. Appl. Pharmacol.*, 2013, **268**, 17–26.

72. A. P. Singh, W. Krzyzanski, S. W. Martin, G. Weber, A. Betts, A. Ahmad, A. Abraham, A. Zutshi, J. Lin and P. Singh, *AAPS J.*, 2015, **17**, 389–399.

73. B. J. Schmidt, J. A. Papin and C. J. Musante, *Drug Discovery Today*, 2013, **18**, 116–127.

74. S. A. Visser, D. R. Huntjens, P. H. van der Graaf, L. A. Peletier and M. Danhof, *J. Pharmacol. Exp. Ther.*, 2003, **307**, 765–775.

75. N. Haddish-Berhane, D. K. Shah, D. Ma, M. Leal, H. P. Gerber, P. Sapra, H. A. Barton and A. M. Betts, *J. Pharmacokinet. Pharmacodyn.*, 2013, **40**, 557–571.

76. D. K. Shah, N. Haddish-Berhane and A. Betts, *J. Pharmacokinet. Pharmacodyn.*, 2012, **39**, 643–659.

77. S. Yamazaki, L. Nguyen, S. Vekich, Z. Shen, M. J. Yin, P. P. Mehta, P. P. Kung and P. Vicini, *J. Pharmacol. Exp. Ther.*, 2011, **338**, 964–973.

78. Q. Zhang, S. Bhattacharya and M. E. Andersen, *Open Biol.*, 2013, **3**, 130031.

79. M. R. Birtwistle, D. E. Mager and J. M. Gallo, *CPT: Pharmacometrics Syst. Pharmacol.*, 2013, **2**, e72.

80. J. B. Fitzgerald, B. W. Johnson, J. Baum, S. Adams, S. Iadevaia, J. Tang, V. Rimkunas, L. Xu, N. Kohli, R. Rennard, M. Razlog, Y. Jiao, B. D. Harms, K. J. Olivier, Jr., B. Schoeberl, U. B. Nielsen and A. A. Lugovskoy, *Mol. Cancer Ther.*, 2014, **13**, 410–425.

81. D. C. Kirouac, J. Y. Du, J. Lahdenranta, R. Overland, D. Yarar, V. Paragas, E. Pace, C. F. McDonagh, U. B. Nielsen and M. D. Onsum, *Sci. Signaling*, 2013, **6**, ra68.

82. B. J. Schmidt, A. Ebrahim, T. O. Metz, J. N. Adkins, B. Ø. Palsson and D. R. Hyduke, *Bioinformatics*, 2013, **29**, 2900–2908.

83. J. Schellenberger, J. O. Park, T. M. Conrad and B. Ø. Palsson, *BMC Bioinf.*, 2010, **11**, 213.

84. L. B. Edelman, J. A. Eddy and N. D. Price, *Wiley Interdiscip. Rev.: Syst. Biol. Med.*, 2010, **2**, 438–459.

85. O. Folger, L. Jerby, C. Frezza, E. Gottlieb, E. Ruppin and T. Shlomi, *Mol. Syst. Biol.*, 2011, **7**, 501.

86. P. Kvistborg, D. Philips, S. Kelderman, L. Hageman, C. Ottensmeier, D. Joseph-Pietras, M. J. Welters, S. van der Burg, E. Kapiteijn, O. Michielin, E. Romano, C. Linnemann, D. Speiser, C. Blank, J. B. Haanen and T. N. Schumacher, *Sci. Transl. Med.*, 2014, **6**, 254ra128.

87. R. De Boer, P. Hogeweg, H. Dullens, R. A. De Weger and W. Den Otter, *J. Immunol.*, 1985, **134**, 2748–2758.

88. S. Alizon and C. Magnus, *Viruses*, 2012, **4**, 1984–2013.

89. S. Palsson, T. P. Hickling, E. L. Bradshaw-Pierce, M. Zager, K. Jooss, P. J. O'Brien, M. E. Spilker, B. O. Palsson and P. Vicini, *BMC Syst. Biol.*, 2013, **7**, 95.

90. J. P. Bai and D. R. Abernethy, *Annu. Rev. Pharmacol. Toxicol.*, 2013, **53**, 451–473.

91. S. Tujios and R. J. Fontana, *Nat. Rev. Gastroenterol. Hepatol.*, 2011, **8**, 202–211.

92. P. Morgan, P. H. Van Der Graaf, J. Arrowsmith, D. E. Feltner, K. S. Drummond, C. D. Wegner and S. D. Street, *Drug Discovery Today*, 2012, **17**, 419–424.

93. R. A. Thompson, E. M. Isin, Y. Li, L. Weidolf, K. Page, I. Wilson, S. Swallow, B. Middleton, S. Stahl, A. J. Foster, H. Dolgos, R. Weaver and J. G. Kenna, *Chem. Res. Toxicol.*, 2012, **25**, 1616–1632.

94. N. V. Morgan, J. L. Hartley, K. D. Setchell, M. A. Simpson, R. Brown, L. Tee, S. Kirkham, S. Pasha, R. C. Trembath, E. R. Maher, P. Gissen and D. A. Kelly, *Orphanet J. Rare Dis.*, 2013, **8**, 74.

95. J. G. Diaz Ochoa, J. Bucher, A. R. Pery, J. M. Zaldivar Comenges, J. Niklas and K. Mauch, *Front. Pharmacol.*, 2012, **3**, 204.

96. H. G. Holzhutter, D. Drasdo, T. Preusser, J. Lippert and A. M. Henney, *Wiley Interdiscip. Rev.: Syst. Biol. Med.*, 2012, **4**, 221–235.

97. L. K. Shoda, J. L. Woodhead, S. Q. Siler, P. B. Watkins and B. A. Howell, *Biopharm. Drug Dispos.*, 2014, **35**, 33–49.

98. K. Subramanian, S. Raghavan, A. Rajan Bhat, S. Das, J. Bajpai Dikshit, R. Kumar, M. K. Narasimha, R. Nalini, R. Radhakrishnan and S. Raghunathan, *Expert Opin. Drug Saf.*, 2008, **7**, 647–662.

99. I. Shah and J. Wambaugh, *J. Toxicol. Environ. Health, Part B*, 2010, **13**, 314–328.

100. J. Wambaugh and I. Shah, *PLoS Comput. Biol.*, 2010, **6**, e1000756.

101. S. Hoehme, M. Brulport, A. Bauer, E. Bedawy, W. Schormann, M. Hermes, V. Puppe, R. Gebhardt, S. Zellmer, M. Schwarz, E. Bockamp, T. Timmel, J. G. Hengstler and D. Drasdo, *Proc. Natl. Acad. Sci. U. S. A.*, 2010, **107**, 10371–10376.

102. S. Bhattacharya, L. K. Shoda, Q. Zhang, C. G. Woods, B. A. Howell, S. Q. Siler, J. L. Woodhead, Y. Yang, P. McMullen, P. B. Watkins and M. E. Andersen, *Front. Physiol.*, 2012, **3**, 462.

103. L. Kuepfer, *Mol. Syst. Biol.*, 2010, **6**, 409.

104. B. A. Howell, Y. Yang, R. Kumar, J. L. Woodhead, A. H. Harrill, H. J. Clewell, 3rd, M. E. Andersen, S. Q. Siler and P. B. Watkins, *J. Pharmacokinet. Pharmacodyn.*, 2012, **39**, 527–541.

105. J. L. Woodhead, K. Yang, S. Q. Siler, P. B. Watkins, K. L. Brouwer, H. A. Barton and B. A. Howell, *Front. Pharmacol.*, 2014, **5**.

106. K. Yang, J. L. Woodhead, P. B. Watkins, B. A. Howell and K. L. Brouwer, *Clin. Pharmacol. Ther.*, 2014, **96**, 589–598.

107. X. Chen, T. Hickling, E. Kraynov, B. Kuang, C. Parng and P. Vicini, *AAPS J.*, 2013, **15**, 1141–1154.

108. X. Chen, T. Hickling and P. Vicini, *CPT: Pharmacometrics Syst. Pharmacol.*, 2014, **3**, 1–10.

109. X. Chen, T. P. Hickling and P. Vicini, *CPT: Pharmacometrics Syst. Pharmacol.*, 2014, **3**, 1–9.

110. M. C. Peterson and M. M. Riggs, *CPT: Pharmacometrics Syst. Pharmacol.*, 2015, **4**, e00020.

CHAPTER 18

Pharmacokinetic–Pharmacodynamic Modeling in Drug Development with Special Reference to Oncology

MARIA LUISA SARDU[a], GIUSEPPE DE NICOLAO[a], AND ITALO POGGESI*[b]

[a]Dipartimento di Ingegneria Industriale e dell'Informazione, Universita' di Pavia, Via Ferrata 3, 27100 Pavia, Italy; [b]Quantitative Sciences/Model-Based Drug Development, Janssen-Cilag SpA, Via Michelangelo Buonarroti 23, 20093 Cologno Monzese (MI), Italy
*E-mail: ipoggesi@its.jnj.com

18.1 Introduction

18.1.1 Background

Medical knowledge, pharmaceutical and pharmacological sciences, and drug development are playing a crucial role in increasing the lifespan, improving health and quality of life. Numerous papers report statistical models that demonstrate that the use of medications is responsible for the increase in life expectancy.[1] In an econometric study, based on the launch of medications between 1982 and 2001, it was reported that the launch of new chemical entities (NCEs; *i.e.*, medications containing an active product ingredient

RSC Drug Discovery Series No. 49
New Horizons in Predictive Drug Metabolism and Pharmacokinetics
Edited by Alan G. E. Wilson
© The Royal Society of Chemistry 2016
Published by the Royal Society of Chemistry, www.rsc.org

that has not been previously approved for marketing) accounted for 0.79 years of the total increase in life expectancy (1.96 years) reported in the same period.[2] Of note, NCEs were reported to have a positive impact, while the launches of "me too" or generic drugs did not further improve longevity.[2] Naturally, these assessments are difficult and sometimes affected by methodological flaws and ideological bias.[3] However, it seems undeniable that drugs increase longevity; new drugs marketed for life-threatening medical conditions are approved if an improved survival is demonstrated compared with the current standard of care.

Over the last decades, it has become more complex and expensive for pharmaceutical industries to launch NCEs.[4] Different factors can be responsible for this. Understandably, advancements in the medical and pharmacological sciences make the approval-related regulatory requirements more stringent. Economic crises and competition pose difficulties for pharmaceutical companies, especially when the patents for their drugs expire.[5]

The quest for new targets with pharmacological relevance is becoming more difficult; while the easily accessible targets have already been researched for the development of drugs for a long time, research is now dealing with less easily "druggable" targets, *i.e.*, more difficult to target and modulate by the therapeutic intervention.[6] These difficulties are reflected in the increased rate of attrition (*i.e.*, the proportion of NCEs that fail before market approval). Kola and Landis[7] reported an average rate of success (defined as the proportion of NCEs reaching the market out of the total number of NCEs entering clinical development in a first in human study) of 11% for all therapeutic areas, *i.e.*, almost 90% of the drugs in development are stopped before approval. When the stop decisions occur at a late stage (*e.g.*, a failed Phase 3 proof of efficacy trial), this represents a huge financial loss for pharmaceutical industries, as the full amount of time, money and resources have already been spent on the development of the compound. A loss at this stage is reported to be in the range of $800 million in out of pocket costs.[5,8,9] Paul *et al.*[5] found that the most influential pharmacoeconomic aspects in the pharmaceuticals industry are the attrition rates in Phase 2 and 3 studies. Hence, even relatively minor decreases in the rate of failure during these phases (or even a shift of the attrition to an earlier development phase) may have a huge impact on the total drug development costs. For instance, for a decrease in Phase 2 attrition from 66 to 50%, a $448 million saving would be expected, on average.[5]

One of the aspects that was identified as critical to remedy this situation was a more extensive and profitable use of modeling and simulation approaches [model-based drug development (MBDD) and pharmacometrics (PMx), *etc.*].[10-13] These models involve the "development and application of pharmaco-statistical models of drug efficacy and safety from preclinical and clinical data to improve drug development knowledge management and decision-making".[10] MBDD can help to anticipate the potential failures of drugs in early stages of development, thus stopping at earlier stages the development of compounds with a low probability of technical success and diverting the resources dedicated to these projects to compounds that have a higher probability of success. Pharmacokinetic (PK)–pharmacodynamic (PD) modeling is one of the tools in this armamentarium. PK models allow the quantitative evaluation of how drugs are absorbed, distributed, metabolized and eliminated by the body of the treated species and relates an input (dose level and dosing regimen) to an output (*e.g.*, plasma or another relevant biophase concentration–time curve, or descriptive metrics for this, such as maximal, minimal or average concentration).[14] PD models, conversely, describe quantitatively the pharmacological, safety or efficacy effects of the treatment; also in this case they relate an input (concentrations or other metrics of systemic exposure to the drug) to an output (incidence, extent or duration of the considered effect).[15] PK–PD models link these different components, characterizing the interconnections between the dose (and dosing regimens), exposure to the drug (in plasma, tissue or any relevant biophase) and relevant drug effects, describing in particular their time courses. It is important to consider that a hierarchy of models can be used to interconnect the PK to the regulatory-accepted clinical endpoints *via* target interaction and activation, modulation of downstream physiological and physiopathological processes, and achievement of surrogate response rates.[16]

PK and PD models allow different scenarios to be simulated and the influence of specific variables of interest to be evaluated. Once a reasonable description and understanding of experimental data is obtained, the developed models can be adopted to investigate and/or simulate untested administration conditions (different dose levels or dosing regimens, or more specific conditions, such as the use of the drug in fasting or fed conditions), to compare different drug properties, and to test the influence of other variables on PK or PD parameters. Models can be used to evaluate risk: benefit ratios, to simulate complete clinical trials and assess the most efficient clinical trial design to allow decision making. Even after a drug enters the market, regulatory authorities may ask companies to conduct additional clinical trials for deeper investigations into relevant unclear aspects (post-marketing commitments). Whenever industries are able to provide satisfactory answers without performing an actual clinical trial, by applying modeling and simulation techniques, the cost savings can easily exceed $100 million.

18.1.2 PK–PD and PMx Analysis in Regulatory Submissions

The American regulatory authority, the US Food and Drug Administration (FDA) covers 3 important roles in protecting public health: "First, the FDA decides whether to approve a new drug for market based on the perceived benefit and risk or removes a drug from the market usually due to increased risk. Second, the FDA approves product label information. Third, the FDA provides advice to sponsors on topics such as the disease endpoint selection, development plan and trial design".[17] In 2004, the FDA itself considered boosting the contribution of PMx in drug discovery and development to be urgent.[4] Bhattaram *et al.*[18] used the term PMx to refer to "a simultaneous quantitative understanding of variables that influence pharmacokinetics

(PK) and pharmacodynamics (PD)" that can lead and support FDA decisions. In order to be able to evaluate PMx analyses conducted and submitted by the sponsors, a PMx division was formed at the FDA. PMx FDA division is the outcome of the integration of competencies from a strict collaboration between the Office of Clinical Pharmacology and the Office of New Drugs and Biostatisticians.[17] Based on the key regulatory questions discussed and established in collaborations with clinicians, statisticians and other expert consultants, the PMx FDA division examines sponsor-submitted analyses. In the case that the required answers are contained within the submission material, it reviews the work verifying its reliability. If the analyses submitted by the sponsor do not address all of the issues, the FDA PMx division itself develops models and evaluates the aspects of interest. The impact of PMx analyses on drug submissions to the FDA for obtaining approvals and/or labeling prescriptions was extensively documented by Bhattaram and colleagues.[17,18] An example reported in one of the surveys[18] was related to the approval of apomorphine (APOKYN), indicated for Parkinson's disease, based on a dose-finding (2–10 mg) study, in addition to the typical pivotal registration studies. Apomorphine was reported to have a 50% increase in exposure in subjects with renal impairment. The PMx division revised and conducted additional exposure–response analyses *via* PK–PD modeling to assess whether the maximum recommended dose proposed by the sponsor was appropriate and whether a dose adjustment was warranted in patients with renal impairment. The available data allowed it to identify a link between concentrations and both the Unified Parkinson's Disease Rating Scale (desired effect) and blood pressure (unwanted effect). The E_{max} model was used to accommodate the anti-Parkinson effect, and the plasma concentration relationship suggested that only minor benefits were expected at dose levels above 6 mg. Based on the same exposure–response analyses, the starting dose for patients with renal impairment was decreased from the proposed 2 mg to 1 mg. These recommendations were included on the label of the drug.[18]

Analyses from the PMx division helped to identify the need for additional trials and allowed the FDA to make more informed regulatory decisions.[18] Interactions between sponsors and the FDA can save time and, in some cases, clinical trials. Given the minimal costs of building models and performing PMx analyses, compared with the actual cost of a clinical trial, it is evident that PMx can play a key role in making the drug development process more efficient and less expensive.[18]

In 2009, FDA guidance for industries[19] encouraged sponsors to discuss their drug development strategies and techniques with the regulators before performing Phase IIb and III clinical studies. The poor selection of protocols and doses in these phases can jeopardize the technical and regulatory success of new drugs. Therefore, pharmaceutical industries were warmly encouraged by the FDA to integrate prior knowledge using models and use all of the available computational approaches to inform decisions during the drug development process. In this context, the potential of clinical trial simulations based on PK–PD models was actively promoted in this FDA guidance.

18.2 Typologies of PK–PD Models

Numerous PK–PD approaches, characterized by increasing complexity, can be identified and have been described in many review papers.[15,20–24] The PK–PD models can be grouped into the following categories:

(i) Static models;
(ii) Dynamic empirical models;
(iii) Dynamic semi-mechanistic models;
(iv) System-pharmacology based models.

The first type of model aims to relate time-invariant metrics of exposure with the corresponding effects by means of an empirical function (linear, log-linear or saturable). Individual plasma concentration data, area under the plasma concentration–time curve (AUC), dose, and maximal or minimal plasma concentrations can be used as static systemic exposure metrics and drivers for the PD effect. They can be obtained without the need for PK modeling, for instance *via* non-compartmental PK analysis or directly using PK measurements. Variables representing effects can be measures of clinical outcomes or causal biomarkers of drug activity, including engagement of drug targets. Typically, these models are used to describe the available data; however, they may be too crude to have predictive capabilities. An example of this kind was the sigmoid E_{max} relationship between the percentage decrease of absolute neutrophil count (ANC) and tallimustine AUC following the intravenous (IV) administration of the compound as a daily bolus injections given for 3 consecutive days in 28 day cycles.[25] Tallimustine is a minor groove DNA binder that was being evaluated as an anticancer agent. Despite the use of a simple empirical exposure–effect model, the developed model was able to accommodate the analogous ANC data obtained in a study in which the treatment was given as a single IV bolus every 28 days, suggesting that AUC (and not C_{max}) was the most relevant metric of tallimustine systemic exposure for producing the neutropenia response (Figure 18.1).

When a compartmental PK model is established, the full plasma concentration–time curve can be used as a dynamic driver for the drug effects. In particular, when the physiopathology and mechanism of action are poorly known, empirical PK–PD models attempt to describe the relationships between plasma concentration–time curves and effects without major mechanism-based assumptions. Delays in the onset of the effect can be accommodated by including effect compartments[26] or by using indirect response models.[22,27] Also in this case, models such as linear, log-linear, logistic, E_{max} or sigmoid E_{max} can be adopted to describe the relationship between the drug concentration in a biophase and the pharmacological or clinical effects.[15,21,22,28] An example of this kind is the PK–PD model used to describe estrogen suppression following the administration of exemestane, an irreversible, steroidal aromatase inactivator.[29] Plasma estrone sulfate (E1S) concentration after exemestane administration was modeled using an indirect response model (inhibition of E1S

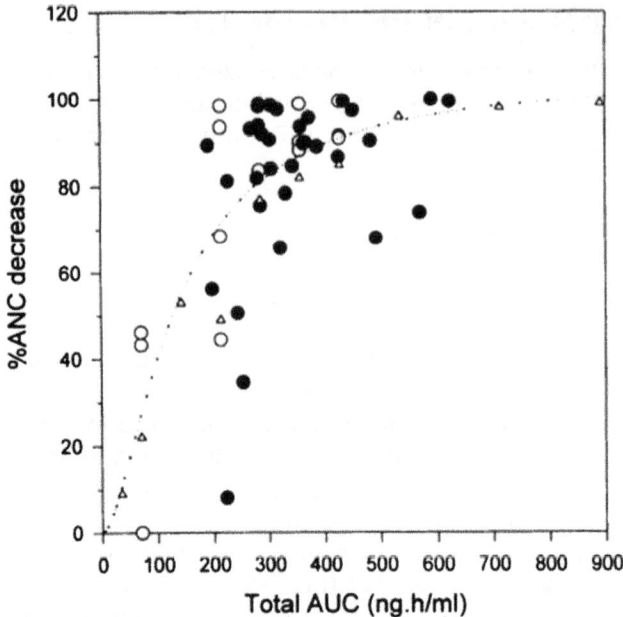

Figure 18.1 Relationship between percentage decrease in absolute neutrophil count and AUC. Dotted line: estimated model; filled circles: observations (associated with measured AUC); open circles: observations (associated with estimated AUC); dosing regimen: daily for 3 days in 28 day cycles. Open triangles: median observations obtained in a different study; dosing regimen: single dose in 28 day cycles.[25]

synthesis). The mean population estimates obtained from a food effect study were used to simulate the administration of different doses of the drug (0.5, 1, 2.5, 5 and 25 mg per day; Figure 18.2). Model predictions were in agreement with the historical data, avoiding the need for additional dose response explorations as post-marketing commitments.[29]

Mechanistic PK–PD models can be developed when a broader knowledge of the actual mechanism of action of the drug and the cascade of events governing the relationship between the target interaction and the considered endpoint (pharmacological or clinical) are known. These models try to make full use of the knowledge of the physiology and physiopathology of the system. Using these models it is generally possible to dissect system-related parameters (biology/physiology related) and drug-related parameters (*e.g.*, drug potency). As a consequence, in mechanistic or semi-mechanistic models, differences between drugs treating the same systems can be completely described simply by using a different set of drug-related parameters. These models are characterized by better predictive capabilities, and can be used to simulate different scenarios of treatment, different drug actions or systems, and can be used for extrapolations. Some examples of these will be described in more detail in the following sections.

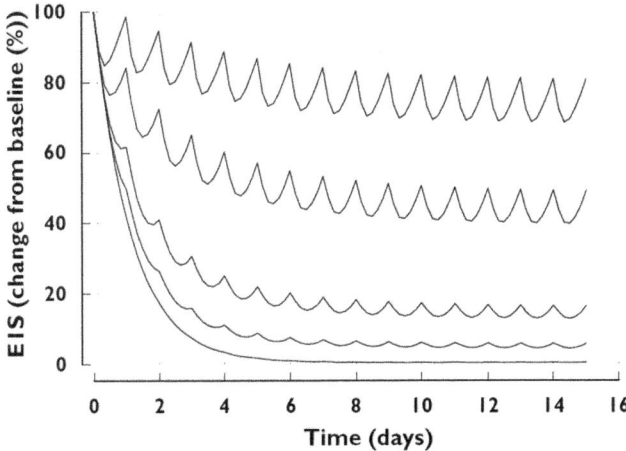

Figure 18.2 Simulated E1S concentrations (expressed as percentage of baseline) after the administration of 0.5, 1, 2.5, 5 and 25 mg per day of exemestane for a period of 15 days.[29]

When a complete mechanistic description of a particular system is available, systems pharmacology PK–PD models can be obtained. These models require a good physiological and mechanistic understanding. At present, such models are more typically used for hypothesis testing in drug research (*i.e.*, for defining paths and targets that can be used to drive a pharmacological intervention), rather than quantitatively helping the drug development process (*i.e.*, supporting the choice of the dose or dosing regimen to achieve the desired clinical effect).[23,30] On the other hand, semi-mechanistic PK–PD models, illustrated in the next section, integrate biological and mechanism-related aspects of the treated systems, maintaining a good predictive power with relatively low levels of complexity.

18.3 Examples of Semi-Mechanistic PK–PD Models

To gain a deeper insight into the role of semi-mechanistic models, in the following sections we review some examples, highlighting the models' objectives, structure and impact. All of the following applications are related to the oncology therapeutic area and cover subsequent stages of compound development, from early *in vitro* studies to the late phases of clinical development.

18.3.1 A Tumor Growth Inhibition Model for *In vitro* Data

18.3.1.1 Background

One of the first steps in the screening of anticancer drugs is the *in vitro* assessment of tumor cell growth inhibition. Tumor cells are incubated and exposed to different concentrations of the anticancer agent for different intervals of time. Cell growth inhibition is considered at different times, when the number of viable cells is measured. The inhibitory effects on cell growth are related to the initial compound concentrations. In general, the results of these experiments are summarized using IC_{50}, the concentration able to inhibit 50% of cell growth compared with controls. However, it was experimentally observed that the IC_{50} changes depending on drug concentration levels and treatment time. Hence, the effect of a drug is described as a function $E = f(c,t)$ and is often represented by a surface.[31–33] To evaluate the relative importance of drug concentration levels and treatment time on the effect, Kalns *et al.*[31] proposed a parametric model describing the effect as $E = C^n \times t$, where the parameter n indicated the relative importance of the two aspects. It was observed that, in some experimental conditions, n did not remain constant among different concentrations and times of exposure to treatment.[33] As a result, Germani and coworkers proposed a non-parametric approach, based on a neural network, to build surfaces describing the concentration–time–effect relationship.[33] Limitations of this model arise in the high computational load and the non-continuity of the surface function. Indeed, to determine effect values for non-experimental time and concentration points they resorted to interpolation, which may entail low accuracy in the predictions.

18.3.1.2   Model Description

To be able to quantitatively compare different drugs acting on the same cell lines, a smarter approach may be the identification of a drug potency parameter, independent of the experimental conditions. Del Bene *et al.*[34] developed a semi-mechanistic PK–PD model of tumor growth inhibition (TGI) *in vitro* in human cancer cells. Unperturbed and perturbed cell growth models were proposed to describe, respectively, controls and treated cells. This model aimed to mechanistically describe the dynamics of *in vitro* cell growth in different experimental conditions, to allow objective comparison of drug potencies, and to provide an analytical description of the E function.

The dynamics of untreated cell count N_u, were described by an exponential growth, in which initial conditions and rate of growth were represented by N_0 and λ_0, respectively [eqn (18.1)].

$$\frac{dN_u(t)}{dt} = \lambda_0 N_u(t)$$
$$N_u(0) = N_0$$

(18.1)

Treated cell count dynamics were described with a fourth order differential equation system [eqn (18.2)]. In this model, tumor dynamics were perturbed by the drug concentration c (assumed constant throughout the experiment). The capability of the drug to transform a cycling cell into a non-proliferating cell was described by the parameter k_2, *i.e.*, the antitumor potency. Once the drug interacts with the proliferating cells, the cells are considered to become non-proliferating and undergo a damage process (described by a 3-compartment transit model, the dynamic of which is governed by the parameter k_1) that leads to their death.

$$
\begin{cases}
\dfrac{dN_p(t)}{dt} = \lambda_0 N_p(t) - k_2 c N_p(t) \\[2mm]
\dfrac{dN_1(t)}{dt} = k_2 c N_p(t) - k_1 N_1(t) \\[2mm]
\dfrac{dN_2(t)}{dt} = k_1 N_1(t) - k_1 N_2(t) \\[2mm]
\dfrac{dN_3(t)}{dt} = k_1 N_2(t) - k_1 N_3(t)
\end{cases}
$$

$$N_t(t) = N_p(t) + N_1(t) + N_2(t) + N_3(t) \tag{18.2}$$

$$N_p(0) = N_0, \; N_1(0) = N_2(0) = N_3(0) = N_4(0) = 0$$

The model was thus characterized by two systems-related parameters, N_0 and λ_0, representing the initial number of cells and the (unperturbed) rate of proliferation of the cells, and two drug-related parameters, k_2 and k_1, related to the potency and the mode of action of the individual compounds. An important derived parameter is the threshold concentration for tumor eradication $c_T = \lambda_0/k_2$, which is the steady-state drug concentration above which regression of tumor cells can be achieved.

18.3.1.3 Model Applications and Impact

This model was adopted to describe growth inhibition of human ovarian cancer cells following treatment with ten commercial drugs and four compounds under development. The model was able to describe the experimental data well (Figure 18.3) and model parameters were identified with good accuracy. Based on parameter estimates, it was possible to perform model-based simulations to obtain continuous response surfaces against concentration and time. This allowed the prediction of effects for conditions not experimentally tested, helping in future experimental design and supporting more informed screening of compounds. In particular, a closed-form solution of the model was elaborated, which allowed an easy understanding of the minimal experimental time (*i.e.*, duration of the exposure of the cells in culture) required to assess a measurable IC_{50}. The model also allowed investigation of the most appropriate times—dependent on k_1—at which compounds with analogous modes of action could be ranked. A more thorough experiment, in which the compound concentrations are measured at different times throughout the experiment in the *in vitro* system, may provide more meaningful data.

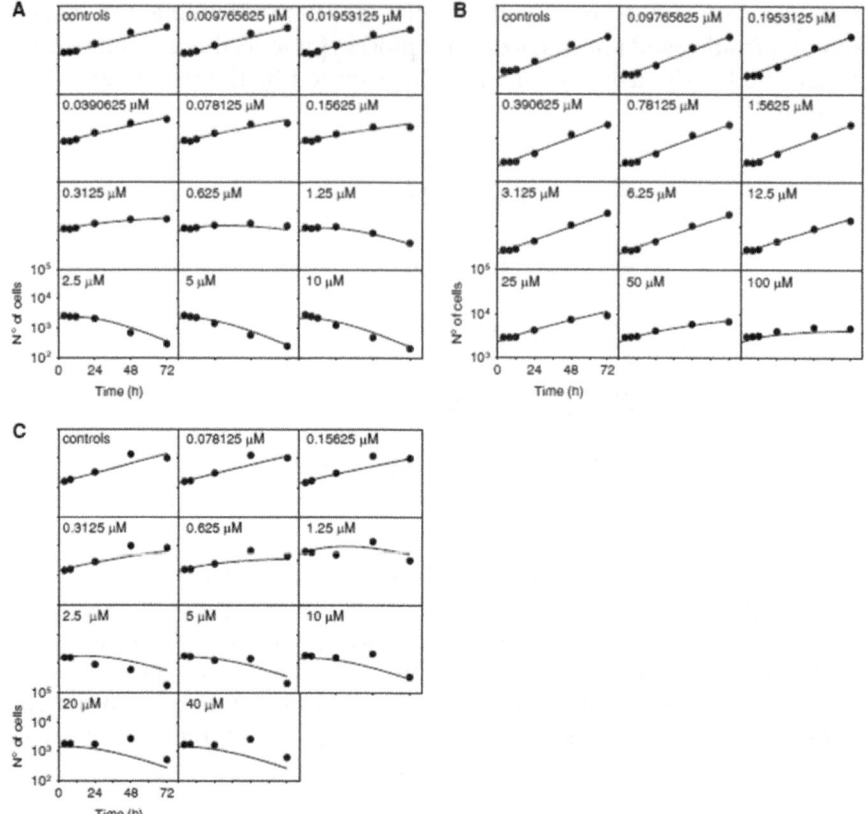

Figure 18.3   Observed (black circles) and simultaneous model-fitted tumor cell growth curves (continuous lines) for both untreated and treated A2780 human ovarian cancer cells exposed to different concentrations of doxorubicin (Panel A), fluorouracil (5-FU; Panel B) and compound C (Panel C).

18.3.2   A TGI Model for Preclinical *In vivo* Data

18.3.2.1   *Background*

After testing the *in vitro* properties, the preclinical assessment of a new anti-cancer drug is complemented with antitumor experiments *in vivo*. Indeed, the *in vivo* tests not only confirm the antitumor activity in living organisms, but deal with issues related to the PK complexities (*e.g.*, absorption, distribution to the relevant biophase and interaction with the target) and determine, *via* a pharmaco-toxicological assessment, whether the effective concentrations are actually tolerable. These studies, therefore, are of paramount importance for supporting the choice of the range of doses that should be used in the first in human studies. In the oncology context, it is typical to assess the effect of agents in xenograft experiments. In these studies, human cancer cell lines (suspension of cells or tumor fragments, grown *in vivo*) are inoculated in athymic mice. When the tumor is palpable, the animals are randomly assigned to control or treatment groups, and the treatment regimens (different compounds, dose levels and schedules) are started. To obtain tumor size measurements, main diameters are measured with a caliper and a mathematical formula is used to infer the 3D dimensions. TGI is calculated as the ratio of tumor burden in the treated *vs.* control mice. However, TGI is not a parameter, but a metric of antitumor effect, dependent on the experimental condition (duration of experiment, schedules, *etc.*). A PK–PD model defining the effect of the exposure to the drug on the trajectories of tumor volumes *vs.* time, parameterized with system and drug-related parameters could provide a more objective, experiment independent, quantitative description of the antitumor effect.

18.3.2.2 Model Description

A semi-mechanistic PK–PD model able to describe TGI dynamics in mice xenografts was developed.[35,36] This model shows some similarities with the model previously described for *in vitro* experiments. However, in the Simeoni model, the state variables do not describe cell counts but tumor masses (*e.g.*, volumes and weights).[35,36] Additionally, to drive the dynamics of the tumor, the time course of the drug concentrations, for instance obtained from a compartmental PK model, is used, instead of a constant concentration. As in the *in vitro* model,[34] the unperturbed [eqn (18.3)] and perturbed growth models [eqn (18.4)] were defined. Compared with the *in vitro* model, in which unperturbed growth was described using a single exponential phase, experimental data of control groups were considered to show two phases. Tumor masses, w, are initially described using an exponential growth with rate λ_0. This phase is followed by a linear growth with slope λ_1:

$$f_g = \begin{cases} \dfrac{\mathrm{d}w(t)}{\mathrm{d}t} = \lambda_0 w(t) & w(t) \leq w_0 \\[2mm] \dfrac{\mathrm{d}w(t)}{\mathrm{d}t} = \lambda_1 & w(t) > w_0 \end{cases} \tag{18.3}$$

$$w(0) = w_0$$

The switch between the two phases (that can be easily obtained by imposing the continuity of the model) occurs at a threshold tumor weight $w_{\mathrm{TH}} = \lambda_1/\lambda_0$.

The model for describing the perturbed growth in treated animals is analogous to the *in vitro* one, except for the unperturbed growth term of the linear phase that now depends on $x_1/w(t)$, which is the fraction of proliferating cells over the whole tumor mass, due to nutrient supply limitations.[36] For computational reasons, the growth function is approximated with a continuous function yielding the following system of differential equations:

$$
\begin{cases}
\dfrac{dx_1(t)}{dt} = \dfrac{\lambda_0 x_1(t)}{\left[1 + \left(\dfrac{\lambda_0}{\lambda_1} w(t)\right)^{\psi}\right]^{1/\psi}} - k_2 c(t) x_1(t) \\[4mm]
\dfrac{dx_2(t)}{dt} = k_2 c(t) x_1(t) - k_1 x_2(t) \\[3mm]
\dfrac{dx_3(t)}{dt} = k_1 x_2(t) - k_1 x_3(t) \\[3mm]
\dfrac{dx_4(t)}{dt} = k_1 x_3(t) - k_1 x_4(t)
\end{cases}
$$

$$
w(t) = x_1(t) + x_2(t) + x_3(t) + x_4(t) \tag{18.4}
$$

$$
x_1(0) = w_0, \; x_2(0) = x_3(0) = x_4(0) = 0
$$

Threshold concentrations for tumor eradication and properties of the models were similar to those described for the *in vitro* model. Another secondary parameter specific to the *in vivo* model is the time efficacy index (TEI), which describes the delay induced by the drug in tumor growth: $TEI = k_2 AUC/\lambda_0$. Assuming that the treatment has a finite duration, tumor mass will eventually follow a linear growth profile. The TEI indicates the time delay after which the treated tumor will achieve the same weight as the controls.

18.3.2.3 Model Application and Impact

The Simeoni model was successful in modeling tumor growth and TGI induced by the administration of numerous commercial drugs and investigational compounds in mice xenografted with different human tumor cell lines. In the original paper, human ovarian and colon xenografted mice were given three commercial and two investigational drugs.[35] Different experiments with different protocols were performed and all available data were well described by the model. The predictive power of the Simeoni model was demonstrated using internal and external validation. In the latter case, PK and tumor growth curves were simulated for an infusion experiment, starting from the model parameter estimates obtained from intermittent bolus experiments. The infusion experiment was subsequently performed and the actual data were compared with model predictions, showing outstanding agreement (Figure 18.4).

To demonstrate the relevance of the *in vivo* preclinical PK–PD model in supporting translational research between mice and humans, a further investigaton[37] based on this model aimed to predict active doses of anticancer agents in humans starting from preclinical data. Rocchetti and coworkers were able to demonstrate an outstanding correlation between the antitumor potency parameters estimated from animal data and the active doses for a panel of ten antitumor agents used in the clinic (Figure 18.5). This work

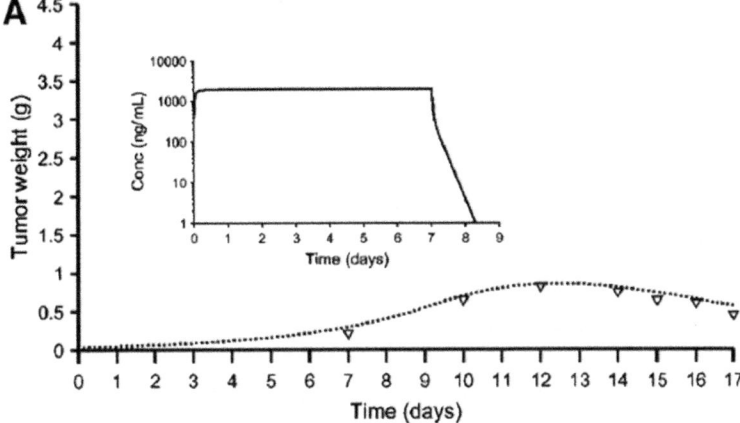

Figure 18.4 Observed and model-predicted growth curves obtained in an experiment in nude mice given an anticancer compound as a 7 day IV infusion from day 9. Inset: the concentration profile used for the predictions.

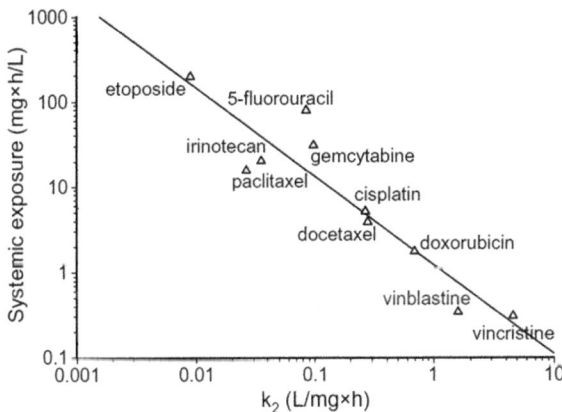

Figure 18.5 Relationship between the systemic exposures of a panel of ten drugs obtained at the midpoint of the dose range used in the clinics (cumulative doses given in 3 week cycles) and k_2 (model-based potency parameter estimated in xenografts).

opened new frontiers for anticipating the effective systemic exposure that would be needed in humans based on preclinical studies. Based on these results, it is possible to reject compounds that are characterized by active concentrations that have been demonstrated to be unsafe; for instance, new compounds for which maximum tolerated doses lead to plasma concentrations significantly lower than the threshold concentration for tumor eradication should have very little probability of having an interesting antitumor effect, and their development can be reliably be terminated or deprioritized.

18.3.3   TGI and Biomarker Modulation *In vivo* Models

18.3.3.1   *Background*

In anticancer drug development it is fundamental to investigate the relationships between TGI dynamics and biomarkers. A biomarker can be defined as "a characteristic that is objectively measured and evaluated as an indicator of normal biological processes, pathogenic processes, or pharmacologic responses to a therapeutic intervention".[38] A hierarchy of models can be used for describing the biomarker cascade, such as target engagement and activation, and physiological and physiopathological modulations.[16] This concept is also the basis of the "pharmacological audit trail" that has been used to support drug development in oncology.[39–41] Therefore, preclinical experiments collecting data on both tumor growth size dynamics and causal biomarkers can provide essential knowledge that can be more easily translated into clinical development plans than antitumor activity in experimental animal models. The mechanistic understanding of the relationships between biomarker dynamics and the corresponding TGI due to the action of an anticancer drug can provide a good basis for understanding the probability of successfully achieving a certain tumor response (and, in turn, a certain improvement in survival) based on the extent of the modulation of tumor marker dynamics. In recent years, several papers (see Table 18.1) have attempted to describe tumor growth-related biomarkers and the relationship between their modulation and antitumor effects. Here we describe the work of Bueno *et al.*[42] as an example of these semi-mechanistic PK–PD models.

Table 18.1   Summary of the models published in the literature for preclinical tumor growth inhibition and biomarker modulations.

Drug	Cell line	Biomarkers	Integration of biomarker and TGI models	References
LY2157299	Calu6, MX1	pSmad	Yes	Bueno *et al.*, 2008[42]
PF02341066	GTL16, U87MG	cMet phosphorylation	No	Yamazaki *et al.*, 2008[43]
PF04942847	MDA-MB-231	AKT	Yes	Yamazaki *et al.*, 2011[44]
PF23411066	H3122, Karpas299	ALK	No	Yamazaki *et al.*, 2012[45]
GDC-0941	MCF7.1	pAkt, pPRAS40	Yes	Salphati *et al.*, 2010[46]
Dulanermin, conatumumab	COLO205	ApopSig		Kay *et al.*, 2012[47]
LY2835219	COLO205	PHH3	Yes	Tate *et al.*, 2014[48]
PF06463922	H3122, NIH3T3	pALK	No	Yamazaki *et al.*, 2014[49]

18.3.3.2 Model Description

The work of Bueno and coworkers aimed to characterize the tumor growth inhibitory effects of a type I receptor TGF antagonist for the treatment of non-small cell lung and breast cancer in xenograft experiments.[42] They developed two integrated PK–PD models. The first biomarker dynamics (pSmad, a phosphorylated protein) were described using a type I indirect response model[27] in which the drug acted as an inhibitor of biomarker synthesis [eqn (18.5)]:

$$\frac{d\,pSmad(t)}{dt} = k_{syn}\left(1 - I_{max}\frac{c(t)^n}{c(t)^n + IC_{50}^n}\right) - k_{out}\,pSmad(t)$$

$$pSmad(0) = pSmad_{(0)} = \frac{k_{syn}}{k_{out}}$$

(18.5)

In this model, k_{syn} and k_{out} indicate the zero order synthesis and first order degradation rate constants for pSmad, respectively. The parameters I_{max} and IC_{50} describe the maximum inhibitory effect that can be induced by the drug and the concentration needed to obtain 50% of the maximum effect, respectively.

The second model describes the tumor dynamics. Analogous with the Simeoni model, tumor dynamics is driven by a delayed signal (*via* a 3 compartment transit compartment model) of biomarker inhibition, described in eqn (18.6):

$$\begin{cases} \dfrac{d\,TS}{dt} = \dfrac{k_{grw1}\left(1 - INH_2\right)TS}{\left[1 + \left(\dfrac{k_{grw1}}{k_{grw0}}TS\right)^\gamma\right]^{1/\gamma}} \\[4mm] INH_0(t) = \dfrac{pSmad_{(0)} - pSmad(t)}{pSmad_{(0)}} \\[3mm] \dfrac{d\,INH_1}{dt} = k_{tr}INH_0 - k_{tr}INH_1 \\[3mm] \dfrac{d\,INH_2}{dt} = k_{tr}INH_1 - k_{tr}INH_2 \\[2mm] TS(0) = TS_0,\ INH_0(0) = INH_1(0) = INH_2(0) = 0 \end{cases}$$

(18.6)

The unperturbed growth-related parameters k_{grw0}, k_{grw1} and γ are the same as Simeoni's λ_1, λ_0 and ψ parameters, respectively. The variable INH_0 represents the drug-induced inhibition of pSmad. INH_1 and INH_2 represent two transduced signals of biomarker inhibition.

18.3.3.3 Model Application and Impact

This semi-mechanistic PK–PD model was used to describe both pSmad and the tumor weights of breast and a non-small cell lung cancers belonging to human lines. The model was able to describe the experimental data well.

The model found different values of the mean signal propagation time (MSPT) for the non-small cell lung and breast cancer cell lines. The model was also validated using an external dataset. Based on simulations, the model was able to predict the behavior of test set experimental data and also investigate tumor size resulting from different dosing schedules not tested experimentally. In addition, it was able to build surfaces describing the percentage TGI and tumor growth delay (TGD) as a function of MSPT and steady state plasma concentration (expressed as a multiple of the IC_{50}). From the outcome of the simulations it was possible to conclude that tumor growth was inhibited less as MSPT increased.

Mechanism-based descriptions of the interactions between causal biomarkers and tumor growth dynamics can be pivotal in supporting clinical trials *via* translational approaches, as the same biomarkers can be measured in humans. Indeed, if the models are provided with a reasonable mechanistic base, and the differences between the two systems (xenografted mice and cancer patients) can be reasonably parameterized, the dynamics of tumor growth in patients can be potentially inferred by only using biomarker dynamics.

18.3.4 Tumor Growth Models for Predicting Survival in Oncology Clinical Trials

18.3.4.1 *Background*

In general, the clinical endpoint of early clinical trials in oncology is tumor response: post-treatment tumor burden, measured using imaging techniques (radiography and computer tomography scans, *etc.*), is compared to some reference measurement (for instance the pretreatment baseline), categorized, and the incidence of different responses is thus assessed at some time point during clinical treatment (or, alternatively, the best response is considered). For solid tumors, the RECIST method is used,[50] with the tumor burden quantified using the sum of the longest dimensions of pre-specified target tumor lesions. A complete response (CR) is obtained when all target lesions are below the limit of detection [and no pathological lymph nodes (>10 mm) are observed]; partial response (PR) is declared when the tumor burden is decreased by 30% compared with the baseline value; progressive disease (PD) is declared when the tumor burden is increased by at least 20% (with the smallest value observed in the study considered as the reference, with an absolute increase of at least 5 mm) or, alternatively, the appearance of new lesions; and stable disease (SD) is declared when there is neither sufficient tumor shrinkage to be qualified as PR or CR, nor sufficient tumor increase to be qualified as PD. The Phase II development of a new drug typically has the objective of achieving a target response rate, *i.e.*, a response rate that is considered sufficiently high (*vs.* the current standard of care) for treating the specified medical condition. Typically, the time courses of tumor burden are not considered and PK–PD modeling can only be examined if there is a significant correlation between the incidence of tumor response and the dose, or some metrics of systemic exposure (*e.g.*, AUC). The regulatory accepted endpoint for approval of new antitumor agents is instead survival. It is typically very difficult, if not impossible, to quantitatively translate a difference in response rate (as defined above) into a gain in survival, and to assess the drug exposures that may lead to this survival improvement. An efficient and quantitative approach to predict survival gain can be obtained only by modeling the full information contained in the time courses of tumor burden.

A very great challenge of the clinical assessments is that there is typically no information related to 'unperturbed' growth; patients can receive different lines of treatment for their conditions. To cope with the absence of unperturbed growth information, instead of having a mechanistic description of tumor progression, empirical models, such as the combination of exponentials and linear functions or sum of exponentials, are used.

18.3.4.2 Model Description

In the model proposed by Claret *et al.*,[51] tumor growth is described using an increasing exponential. Treatment effects can be described by a bimolecular decline; the tumor growth rate is thus decreased in direct proportion (using a proportionality constant that is representative of the potency of the drug) to both the tumor volume and the exposure to the drug (dose or systemic exposure), similar to what has been used for the Simeoni model.[35] In many advanced disease cases, the patients will eventually progress even if they are on treatment; this "loss of effect" of the pharmacological intervention could empirically be described using the development of a tolerance process (*i.e.*, the potency of the drug decreases with time, for instance *via* an exponential decrease). The model is given in eqn (18.7):

$$\frac{\mathrm{dTS}}{\mathrm{d}t} = K_\mathrm{L} \times \mathrm{TS} - K_\mathrm{D}(t) \times \mathrm{Exposure} \times \mathrm{TS} \tag{18.7}$$

where TS is the tumor size (in the case of solid tumors, using the RECIST method, expressed as a linear dimension), K_L is the rate of (unperturbed) tumor growth, Exposure is a metric of exposure to the drug (dose, AUC, *etc.*), and K_D is the potency of the compound, which decreases with time as described in eqn (18.8):

$$K_\mathrm{D}(t) = K'_\mathrm{D} \times e^{-\lambda \times t} \tag{18.8}$$

This relatively flexible model can accommodate a variety of trajectory shapes for the temporal evolution of the tumor dimensions. In this way, the effect of the compound on tumor growth can be quantitatively assessed. The outcome of the tumor growth model (in this case, the model-predicted tumor inhibition was estimated at week 8) is entered as a descriptor into a statistical model (*e.g.*, Cox proportional hazards model) to describe the survival of patients treated with chemotherapy agents.

18.3.4.3 Model Application and Impact

This framework was able to predict the survival expected in a Phase 3 trial of capecitabine in colorectal cancer patients based on the outcomes of a Phase 2 study; it is therefore a useful tool to support the design of Phase 3 proof of efficacy trials.

The same group extended the approach, including models of probability and duration of dose modifications (*e.g.*, due to drug toxicity) in a simulation exercise for the treatment of patients with thyroid cancer with motesanib.[52] It should be noted that, instead of using a model-predicted response at some point in time (*e.g.*, at week 8 in this case) as a descriptor of the Cox model for describing survival, the use of the TGI model parameters would provide a more integrated and quantitative basis for this approach. In this regard, a similar approach was used to model the exposure-related [*via* prostate specific antigen (PSA)] survival data obtained in Phase 3 studies of abiraterone acetate, used for the treatment of metastatic castration-resistant prostate cancer (mCRPC) patients.[53] The approach included a mixed-effects model for describing PSA trajectories (similar to the TGI model used by Claret *et al.*[51]) as a function of abiraterone exposures (described using abiraterone plasma concentrations). The model-based PSA doubling time (a summary combination of the tumor growth model parameters) was found to be a significant descriptor of the Cox proportional hazards survival model.[54]

18.3.5 Generic Hematological Toxicity Models for Describing the Nadir of Blood Counts after Treatment with Chemotherapeutic Agents

18.3.5.1 Background

Cytotoxic agents used for the treatment of cancer typically target the tissues with the highest cell turnover rate; for this reason, myelosuppression (*i.e.*, the decrease of circulating leukocytes, neutrophils or granulocytes derived from rapidly replicating bone marrow cells) is a common and important dose limiting toxicity for all of these drugs.[55] As reported previously, a simple empirical PK–PD approach is to relate a metric of drug exposure to the lowest cell count (nadir). The risk of infection in patients depends, however, on the severity and duration of myelosuppression;[30] therefore, it is of particular interest to develop PK–PD models that are able to predict the whole time course of myelosuppression. In addition, it is preferable that these models have a reasonable mechanistic basis (*i.e.*, as described in the previous sections, the models should be parameterized in terms of system-related and drug-related parameters), so that they can be translated across different systems (for instance to accommodate the decrease in specific subfamilies of leukocytes, or other blood components, such as red blood cells or platelets) and applied to different drugs.

In general, the nadir of blood counts is observed approximately between 1 and 2 weeks after the dosing of the chemotherapeutic agent; in many cases, these drugs are given once every 3 weeks, so the plasma concentrations of the drug are typically below the limit of quantification at this time. Another characteristic of this system is that after the nadir, and in absence of further treatment, the blood count typically surpasses the original baseline values. It is only after this that the counts return gradually to baseline.[56]

18.3.5.2 Model Description

In the Friberg model,[30] blood counts in the systemic circulation are modeled *via* a precursor model (with the precursor compartments representing blood counts in hematopoietic organs). This model structure explains the delayed response in the peripheral blood cells. A feedback loop is built into the model, in which the rate of progenitor cell production is modulated by the ratio of blood cells to baseline count; in this way the rebound of the system can be accommodated. According to the model, the lower the baseline value the more severe the potential toxicity. In this model, the effect of the drug is to decrease the turnover rate of the precursors. The model can be described by the following system of differential equations:

$$\frac{dProl}{dt} = k_{Prol}\left(1 - E_{drug}\right) \times \left(\frac{Circ_0}{Circ}\right)^{\gamma} - k_{tr} \times Prol$$

$$\frac{dTransit_1}{dt} = + k_{tr} \times Prol - k_{tr} \times Transit_1$$

$$\frac{dTransit_2}{dt} = + k_{tr} \times Transit_1 - k_{tr} \times Transit_2 \qquad (18.9)$$

$$\frac{dTransit_3}{dt} = + k_{tr} \times Transit_2 - k_{tr} \times Transit_3$$

$$\frac{dCirc}{dt} = + k_{tr} \times Transit_3 - k_{circ} \times Circ$$

where Prol is the amount of progenitor (proliferating) bone marrow cells, $Transit_{1-3}$ are the intermediate stages of maturation of the circulating blood cells (Circ), $Circ_0$ is the baseline circulating cell count, k_{prol} is the proliferation rate of the progenitors, E_{drug} is the inhibitory effect of the drug, γ is the parameter describing the feedback and k_{circ} represents the rate of elimination of the blood circulating cells.

It is easy to appreciate that, like typical mechanistic PK–PD models, the Friberg model dissects system-specific parameters ($Circ_0$, k_{prol}, γ and k_{circ}) and drug specific ones (E_{drug}, representing a generic inhibitory effect).

18.3.5.3   Model Application and Impact

The Friberg model was able to predict myelosuppression after the administration of numerous chemotherapeutic drugs and it is one of the most popular PK–PD models in the oncology therapeutic area. The system-related parameters were shown to be consistent in different studies, so the model can be used, with few variations,[57] for the description and prediction of myelosuppression for different chemotherapeutic drugs.[58] This has important implications as the prediction of the time courses of myelosuppression could simply be based on *in vitro* data, provided that a reasonable correlation between *in vitro* and *in vivo* cytotoxic activity can be established. Of note, models with similar structures have also been applied to other hematological processes, for instance involving red blood cell or platelet counts.[59]

18.4   Conclusions

This chapter provides a general overview of the role of the model-based approaches in drug development that have been adopted in the decision making process and requirements for market authorization and approvals, with particular reference to examples obtained in the oncology therapeutic area.

Challenges and issues related to drug development are described and discussed. In particular, the complex scenarios that pharmaceutical industries have to face to launch NCEs are described. Overall, these complexities result in a high rate of attrition.

Modeling and simulation approaches provide a fundamental contribution in optimizing drug development processes: (i) models can be used to quantitatively evaluate drug effects and establish the appropriate risk:benefit ratios for a new treatment; (ii) models can be used to simulate the outcomes of experimentally untested conditions; and (iii) models can be used to predict the outcome of individual studies or stages of the drug development process, indicating the best experimental design and the hypotheses that need to be tested to reasonably anticipate the probability of technical success. In this way, the development of compounds with a low probability of being approved can be stopped, allowing the allocation of resources to projects and programs with higher probabilities of success. The FDA itself considers it to be urgent and crucial to boost the integration of PMx expertise.

References

1. D. M. Cutler, G. Long, E. R. Berndt, J. Royer, A.-A. Fournier, A. Sasser and P. Cremieux, *Health Aff.*, 2007, **26**, 97.
2. F. R. Lichtenberg, *Int. J. Health Care Finance Econ.*, 2005, **5**, 47.
3. D. Baker and A. Fugh-Berman, *J. Gen. Intern. Med.*, 2009, **24**, 678.

4. FDA, Innovation and stagnation. Challenge and opportunity on the critical path to new medical products, FDA, March 2004, http://www.fda.gov/downloads/ScienceResearch/SpecialTopics/CriticalPathInitiative/CriticalPathOpportunitiesReports/UCM113411.pdf, accessed November 24, 2014.
5. S. M. Paul, D. S. Mytelka, C. T. Dunwiddie, C. C. Persinger, B. H. Munos, S. R. Lindborg and A. L. Schacht, *Nat. Rev. Drug Discovery*, 2010, **9**, 203.
6. A. L. Hopkins and C. R. Groom, *Nat. Rev. Drug Discovery*, 2002, **1**, 727.
7. I. Kola and J. Landis, *Nat. Rev. Drug Discovery*, 2004, **3**, 711.
8. J. A. DiMasi, R. W. Hansen and H. G. Grabowski, *J. Health Econ.*, 2003, **22**, 151.
9. C. P. Adams and V. V. Brantner, *Health Aff.*, 2006, **25**, 420.
10. R. L. Lalonde, K. G. Kowalski, M. M. Hutmacher, W. Ewy, D. J. Nichols, P. A. Milligan, B. W. Corrigan, P. A. Lockwood, S. A. Marshall, L. J. Benincosa, T. G. Tensfeldt, K. Parivar, M. Amantea, P. Glue, H. Koide and R. Miller, *Clin. Pharmacol. Ther.*, 2007, **82**, 21.
11. R. Miller, W. Ewy, B. W. Corrigan, D. Ouellet, D. Hermann, K. G. Kowalski, P. Lockwood, J. R. Koup, S. Donevan, A. El-Kattan, C. S. W. Li, J. L. Werth, D. E. Feltner and R. L. Lalonde, *J. Pharmacokinet. Pharmacodyn.*, 2005, **32**, 185.
12. L. Zhang, M. Pfister and B. Meibohm, *AAPS J.*, 2008, **10**, 552.
13. J. S. Barrett, M. J. Fossler, K. D. Cadieu and M. R. Gastonguay, *J. Clin. Pharmacol.*, 2008, **48**, 632.
14. M. S. Benedetti, R. Whomsley, I. Poggesi, W. Cawello, F.-X. Mathy, M.-L. Delporte, P. Papeleu and J.-B. Watelet, *Drug Metab. Rev.*, 2009, **41**, 344.
15. M. K. Church, M. Gillard, M. L. Sargentini-Maier, I. Poggesi, A. Campbell and M. S. Benedetti, *Drug Metab. Rev.*, 2009, **41**, 455.
16. M. Danhof, G. Alvan, S. G. Dahl, J. Kuhlmann and G. Paintaud, *Pharm. Res.*, 2005, **22**, 1432.
17. V. A. Bhattaram, *et al.*, *Clin. Pharmacol. Ther.*, 2007, **81**, 213.
18. V. A. Bhattaram, B. P. Booth, R. P. Ramchandani, B. N. Beasley, Y. Wang, V. Tandon, J. Z. Duan, R. K. Baweja, P. J. Marroum, R. S. Uppoor, N. A. Rahman, C. G. Sahajwalla, J. R. Powell, M. U. Mehta and J. V. S. Gobburu, *AAPS J.*, 2005, **7**, E503.
19. US Food and Drug Administration, Guidance for industry: End-of-phase 2A meetings, September 2009, http://www.fda.gov/downloads/Drugs/.../Guidances/ucm079690.pdf, accessed, April 10, 2015.
20. E. I. Ette and P. J. Williams, *Pharmacometrics: the science of quantitative pharmacology*, John Wiley & Sons, 2013.
21. C. Csajka and D. Verotta, *J. Pharmacokinet. Pharmacodyn.*, 2006, **33**, 227.
22. D. E. Mager, E. Wyska and W. J. Jusko, *Drug Metab. Dispos.*, 2003, **31**, 510.
23. P. H. van der Graaf and N. Benson, *Pharm. Res.*, 2011, **28**, 1460.
24. A. Bernard, H. Kimko, D. Mital and I. Poggesi, *Expert Opin. Drug Metab. Toxicol.*, 2012, **8**, 1057.

25. G. R. Weiss, I. Poggesi, M. Rocchetti, D. DeMaria, T. Mooneyham, D. Reilly, L. V. Vitek, F. Whaley, E. Patricia, D. D. Von Hoff and P. O'Dwyer, *Clin. Cancer Res.*, 1998, **4**, 53.

26. G. Segre, *Farmaco Sci.*, 1968, **23**, 907.

27. N. L. Dayneka, V. Garg and W. J. Jusko, *J. Pharmacokinet. Biopharm.*, 1993, **21**, 457.

28. J. A. Uchizono, *et al.*, *Pharmacometrics*, 2007, 529.

29. M. Valle, E. Di Salle, M. G. Jannuzzo, I. Poggesi, M. Rocchetti, R. Spinelli and D. Verotta, *Br. J. Clin. Pharmacol.*, 2005, **59**, 355.

30. L. E. Friberg, A. Henningsson, H. Maas, L. Nguyen and M. O. Karlsson, *J. Clin. Oncol.*, 2002, **20**, 4713.

31. J. E. Kalns, N. J. Millenbaugh, M. G. Wientjes and J. L.-S. Au, *Cancer Res.*, 1995, **55**, 5315.

32. N. J. Millenbaugh, M. G. Wientjes and J. L.-S. Au, *Cancer Chemother. Pharmacol.*, 2000, **45**, 265.

33. M. Germani, P. Magni, G. De Nicolao, I. Poggesi, A. Marsiglio, D. Ballinari and M. Rocchetti, *Cancer Chemother. Pharmacol.*, 2003, **52**, 507.

34. F. Del Bene, M. Germani, G. De Nicolao, P. Magni, C. E. Re, D. Ballinari and M. Rocchetti, *Cancer Chemother. Pharmacol.*, 2009, **63**, 827.

35. M. Simeoni, *Cancer Res.*, 2004, **64**, 1094.

36. P. Magni, M. Simeoni, I. Poggesi, M. Rocchetti and G. De Nicolao, *Math. Biosci.*, 2006, **200**, 127.

37. M. Rocchetti, M. Simeoni, E. Pesenti, G. De Nicolao and I. Poggesi, *Eur. J. Cancer*, 2007, **43**, 1862.

38. A. J. Atkinson, *et al.*, *Clin. Pharmacol. Ther.*, 2001, **69**, 89.

39. P. Workman, *Mol. Cancer Ther.*, 2003, **2**, 131.

40. C. H. Takimoto, *Targeted Oncol.*, 2009, **4**, 143.

41. T. A. Yap, *Nat. Rev. Cancer*, 2010, **10**, 514.

42. L. Bueno, D. P. de Alwis, C. Pitou, J. Yingling, M. Lahn, S. Glatt and I. F. Trocóniz, *Eur. J. Cancer*, 2008, **44**, 142.

43. S. Yamazaki, J. Skaptason, D. Romero, J. H. Lee, H. Y. Zou, J. G. Christensen, J. R. Koup, B. J. Smith and T. Koudriakova, *Drug Metab. Dispos.*, 2008, **36**, 1267.

44. S. Yamazaki, L. Nguyen, S. Vekich, Z. Shen, M.-J. Yin, P. P. Mehta, P.-P. Kung and P. Vicini, *J. Pharmacol. Exp. Ther.*, 2011, **338**, 964.

45. S. Yamazaki, P. Vicini, Z. Shen, H. Y. Zou, J. Lee, Q. Li, J. G. Christensen, B. J. Smith and B. Shetty, *J. Pharmacol. Exp. Ther.*, 2012, **340**, 549.

46. L. Salphati, H. Wong, M. Belvin, D. Bradford, K. A. Edgar, W. W. Prior, D. Sampath and J. J. Wallin, *Drug Metab. Dispos.*, 2010, **38**, 1436.

47. B. P. Kay, C.-P. Hsu, J.-F. Lu, Y.-N. Sun, S. Bai, Y. Xin and D. Z. D'Argenio, *J. Pharmacokinet. Pharmacodyn.*, 2012, **39**, 577.

48. S. C. Tate, S. Cai, R. T. Ajamie, T. Burke, R. P. Beckmann, E. M. Chan, A. De Dios, G. N. Wishart, L. M. Gelbert and D. M. Cronier, *Clin. Cancer Res.*, 2014, **20**, 3763.

49. S. Yamazaki, J. L. Lam, H. Y. Zou, H. Wang, T. Smeal and P. Vicini, *J. Pharmacol. Exp. Ther.*, 2014, **351**, 67.

50. E. Eisenhauer, P. Therasse, J. Bogaerts, L. H. Schwartz, D. Sargent, R. Ford, J. Dancey, S. Arbuck, S. Gwyther, M. Mooney, L. Rubinstein, L. Shankar, L. Dodd, R. Kaplan, D. Lacombe and J. Verweij, *Eur. J. Cancer*, 2009, **45**, 228.
51. L. Claret, P. Girard, P. M. Hoff, E. Van Cutsem, K. P. Zuideveld, K. Jorga, J. Fagerberg and R. Bruno, *J. Clin. Oncol.*, 2009, **27**, 4103.
52. L. Claret, J.-F. Lu, Y.-N. Sun and R. Bruno, *Cancer Chemother. Pharmacol.*, 2010, **66**, 1141.
53. S. X. Xu, *et al.*, *Genitourinary Cancers Symposium (ASCO GU)*, San Francisco, CA, January 30–February 1, 2014.
54. S. X. Xu, *et al.*, *Am. Soc. Clin. Oncol. Genitourin. Cancers Symp.*, poster presentation, 30; X. S. Xu, C. J. Ryan, K. Stuyckens, M. R. Smith, F. Saad, T. W. Griffin, Y. C. Park, M. K. Yu, A. Vermeulen, I. Poggesi and P. Nandy, *Clin. Cancer Res.*, 2015, **21**, 3170–3177.
55. E. Chatelut, J.-P. Delord and P. Canal, *Invest. New Drugs*, 2003, **21**, 141.
56. H. Takatani, H. Soda, M. Fukuda, M. Watanabe, A. Kinoshita, T. Nakamura and M. Oka, *Antimicrob. Agents Chemother.*, 1996, **40**, 988.
57. H. Hing, J. J. Perez-Ruixo, K. Stuyckens, A. Soto-Matos, L. Lopez-Lazaro and P. Zannikos, *Clin. Pharmacol. Ther.*, 2008, **83**, 130.
58. Y. M. C. Wang, W. Krzyzanski, S. Doshi, J. J. Xiao, J. J. Pérez-Ruixo and A. T. Chow, *AAPS J.*, 2010, **12**, 729.
59. W. Krzyzanski, L. Sutjandra, J. J. Perez-Ruixo, B. Sloey, A. T. Chow and Y.-M. Wang, *Pharm. Res.*, 2013, **30**, 655.

Subject Index